MANAGEMENT OF

LAPAROSCOPIC SURGICAL COMPLICATIONS

MANAGEMENT OF

LAPAROSCOPIC SURGICAL COMPLICATIONS

Edited by

KARL A. LeBLANC

Director, Minimally Invasive Surgery Institute,
Baton Rouge,
and
Clinical Associate Professor of Surgery,
Louisiana State University,
New Orleans, Louisiana, U.S.A.

MARCEL DEKKER

MARCEL DEKKER, INC.   NEW YORK • BASEL

Library of Congress Cataloging-in-Publication Data
A catalog record for this book is available from the Library of Congress.

ISBN: 0-8247-5440-9

This book is printed on acid-free paper.

Headquarters
Marcel Dekker, 270 Madison Avenue, New York, NY 10016, U.S.A.
tel: 212-696-9000; fax: 212-685-4540

Distribution and Customer Service
Marcel Dekker, Cimarron Road, Monticello, New York 12701, U.S.A.
tel: 800-228-1160; fax: 845-796-1772

World Wide Web
http://www.dekker.com

Current printing (last digit):

10 9 8 7 6 5 4 3 2 1

PRINTED IN THE UNITED STATES OF AMERICA

To my parents, Pete and Peggy.
Thank you.

Preface

> Every surgeon carries about him a little cemetery, in which from time to time he goes to pray. A cemetery of bitterness and regret, of which he seeks the reason for certain of his failures."
>
> —René Leriche, 1879–1955
> *La Philosophie de la Chirurgie.*

The growth in laparoscopic general surgical techniques has sustained since the beginnings in the late 1980's. Most of the standard open operations are now performed via a laparoscopic approach. The adoption of these methodologies has varied in the different parts of the world and even in specific centers. Surgeons realize the benefits of these technologies to the outcome of the patient. To many individuals, however, the fear of complications and the need to develop new skills has inhibited the acceptance of some of these procedures.

An understanding of the pitfalls of all operative procedures allows the surgeon the knowledge with which to avoid or prevent them. This textbook seeks to provide this understanding. The surgeon-authors of this work have tried to supply insight into the preoperative, intraoperative and postoperative expectations following the specific procedure. While I have tried to encourage each contributor to follow a standard format to the specific chapter, in many cases, the procedure described did not allow this design to be followed. This is apparent as one reviews this book.

As stated so eloquently by René LeRiche, we all endeavor to achieve success without morbidity or mortality. It is understood that the diligent surgeon will always strive to minimize complications and achieve good results. This work attempts to assist the reader in that goal. Each chapter has been written by individuals that I have selected who are the recognized leaders in their respective fields. These authors have vast knowledge of the assigned topic. Nevertheless, I implore the reader to not forget that these are opinions based upon the experience of these individuals. In many cases, there are many other opinions and sometimes quite opposite views from those that are discussed in this book. In that regard, *Management of Laparoscopic Surgical Complications* cannot be viewed as the sole authority for the prevention and treatment of these events. The reader should use this work as a basis of education and improvement in his or her technique and knowledge base. Adverse outcomes are the inevitable result of any endeavor in life. The practice of surgery in not immune to this reality. I hope this book will allow the reader some education in the identification, prevention and management of these when they occur. The undisputable facts are that despite one's best efforts, surgical complications will occur at some point in every surgeon's career.

I wish to thank all of the contributors that worked so diligently to make their own contribution as helpful and accurate as possible. Additionally, I wish to thank Marcel Dekker for the opportunity to provide a textbook for which I have seen a significant need for many years.

Karl A. LeBlanc

Contents

Contributors

Craig T. Albanese Stanford University Medical Center and Lucille Salter Packard Children's Hospital, Stanford, California, U.S.A.

Robert W. Bailey University of Miami School of Medicine, Miami, Florida, U.S.A.

Garth Ballantyne Hackensack, University Medical Center, Hackensack, New Jersey, U.S.A.

Douglas M. Bowley Department of Colorectal Surgery, John Radcliffe Hospital, Oxford, United Kingdom

Miguel Angel Carbajo Caballero Medina del Campo Hospital, Valladolid, Spain

Auxiliadora Cano University Hospital Virgen Macarena, Seville, Spain

Alfredo M. Carbonell Carolinas Medical Center, Charlotte, North Carolina, U.S.A.

J. K. Champion Videoscopic Institute of Atlanta, Atlanta, Georgia, U.S.A.

Ricardo Vitor Cohen Hospital São Camilo, São Paulo, Brazil

José Luis Lopes Correa Hospital São Camilo, São Paulo, Brazil

Federico Cuenca-Abente Mount Sinai School of Medicine, New York, New York, U.S.A.

Yves-Marie Dion Université Laval, Centre Hospitalier Universitaire de Québec, Hôpital St-François d'Assise, and Québec Biomaterials Institute, Québec, Canada

José Carlos Pinheiro Filho Hospital São Camilo, São Paulo, Brazil

Abtin Foroohar Drexel University School of Medicine, Philadelphia, Pennsylvania, U.S.A.

Fumihiko Fujita Center for Minimally Invasive Surgery, Department of Surgery, Cedars–Sinai Medical Center, Los Angeles, California, U.S.A.

Michel Gagner Mount Sinai School of Medicine, New York, New York, U.S.A.

Luca Giordano Center for Minimally Invasive Surgery, Department of Surgery, Cedars–Sinai Medical Center, Los Angeles, California, U.S.A.

Rodrigo Gonzalez Emory University School of Medicine, Atlanta, Georgia, U.S.A.

Sean P. Hedican The University of Wisconsin Medical School, Madison, Wisconsin, U.S.A.

B. Todd Heniford Carolinas Medical Center, Charlotte, North Carolina, U.S.A.

Marion C. W. Henry Stanford University Medical Center and Lucille Salter Packard Children's Hospital, Stanford, California, U.S.A.

Samuel A. Irefin The Cleveland Clinic Foundation, Cleveland, Ohio, U.S.A.

Moises Jacobs Coral Gables, Florida, U.S.A.

Michael S. Kavic St. Elizabeth Heath Center and Northeastern Ohio Universities College of Medicine, Youngstown, Ohio, U.S.A.

Stephen M. Kavic Yale University School of Medicine, New Haven, Connecticut, U.S.A.

Todd A. Kellogg The Swallowing Center, University of Washington, Seattle, Washington, U.S.A.

Kent W. Kercher Carolinas Medical Center, Charlotte, North Carolina, U.S.A.

Andrew N. Kingsnorth Department of Surgery, Postgraduate Medical School, University of Plymouth, United Kingdom

Karl A. LeBlanc Director, Minimally Invasive Surgery Institute, Boca Raton, and Department of Surgery, Louisiana State University School of Medicine, New Orleans, Louisiana, U.S.A

Juan Carlos Martín del Olmo Medina del Campo Hospital, Valladolid, Spain

Brent D. Matthews Carolinas Medical Center, Charlotte, North Carolina, U.S.A.

William C. Meyers Drexel University School of Medicine, Philadelphia, Pennsylvania, U.S.A.

Salvador Morales-Conde University Hospital Virgen Macarena, Seville, Spain

Archit Naik Drexel University School of Medicine, Philadelphia, Pennsylvania, U.S.A.

Stephen Y. Nakada The University of Wisconsin Medical School, Madison, Wisconsin, U.S.A.

Brant K. Oelschlager The Swallowing Center, University of Washington, Seattle, Washington, U.S.A.

Koji Otsuka Center for Minimally Invasive Surgery, Department of Surgery, Cedars–Sinai Medical Center, Los Angeles, California, U.S.A.

Carlos A. Pellegrini The Swallowing Center, University of Washington, Seattle, Washington, U.S.A.

Edward H. Phillips Center for Minimally Invasive Surgery, Department of Surgery, Cedars–Sinai Medical Center, Los Angeles, California, U.S.A.

Gustavo Plasencia Coral Gables, Florida, U.S.A.

Bruce J. Ramshaw Emory University School of Medicine, Atlanta, Georgia, U.S.A.

Harry Rein Longwood, Florida, U.S.A.

Vivian M. Sanchez University of Miami School of Medicine, Miami, Florida, U.S.A.

Richard M. Satava University of Washington Medical Center, Seattle, Washington, U.S.A.

Carlos Aurélio Schiavon Hospital São Camilo, São Paulo, Brazil

Levente J. Szalai Drexel University School of Medicine, Philadelphia, Pennsylvania, U.S.A.

Fabien Thaveau Centre Hospitalier Universitaire de Québec, Hôpital St-François d'Assise, Québec, Canada

Miguel Toledano Trincado Medina del Campo Hospital, Valladolid, Spain

Guy Voeller Memphis, Tennessee, U.S.A.

John M. Whitaker Minimally Invasive Surgery Institute, Baton Rouge, Louisiana, U.S.A.

Michael Williams Videoscopic Institute of Atlanta, Atlanta, Georgia, U.S.A.

1

Laparoscopic General Surgery: Overview

Karl A. LeBlanc
Minimally Invasive Surgery Institute, Baton Rouge, and Louisiana State University School of Medicine, New Orleans, Louisiana, U.S.A.

INTRODUCTION

Since the introduction of the laparoscope for the more common uses such as gynecological surgery, the field of laparoscopic general surgery has expanded gradually to more operations. As with any developing field, the laparoscopic procedures being adapted to general surgical applications have undergone many refinements over the last decade or more. We should, however, not forget the past historical accomplishments of our colleagues, who have provided us with the basis of the current clinical developments. There are many areas where minimal access surgery can still be developed and advanced. This chapter is an introduction to the realm of this surgery. Laparoscopic general surgery is no longer considered to be ''experimental''. Nearly every open procedure has been performed with the laparoscopic method with success. Now that the surgical arena has accepted this approach to many procedures, we should continue to advance its techniques while also not forgetting the past.

EARLY HISTORY

Hippocrates, in viewing the rectum, may have been the first physician to use an external device to view the interior of the human body [1]. There were many other developments subsequently but most were not of any significance until nearly 2000 years later, with the works of Ott, Kelling, and Jacobaeus, who first described thoracoscopy in the early 1900s [2–4]. Until very recently, there was essentially no further development in laparoscopic general surgery. The gynecologists, principally the Germans, mainly advanced this clinical application initially.

RECENT HISTORY

Only a relative few general surgeons developed any skills with this technology, and even those were usually limited to diagnostic laparoscopy or tubal ligation. Phillippe Mouret of Lyon, France, became the first to use the laparoscope to perform a cholecystecomy in 1987. The surgeons Eddie Joe Reddick and Leonard Schultz, who independently advanced this operation in the United States, noted its advantages. Since their pioneering work, the field of laparoscopic general surgery has expanded significantly. The limitations that initially impeded progress, such as inadequate instrumentation, have now largely been overcome. However, innovation continues to be an important hallmark of these procedures.

As surgeons became more adept with the laparoscopic technique and the new two-dimensional views obtained, the early adopters explored further possibilities. There were investigations into the treatment of inguinal hernias, appendicitis, and other organs within the abdominal cavity. At the same time, the gynecologists—the developers of this technology—adopted its use for hysterectomy.

The laparoscope was used to assist in the performance of an appendectomy in 1977, even before the advent of the cholecystecomy [5]. This procedure has been an important addition to the field, being especially useful when the diagnosis is unclear, as in the female patient or the obese individual. Some controversy does exist regarding its use in the presence of a perforation or peritonitis. Even in this situation, however, many prefer a laparoscopic technique.

French surgeons, such as Duluqc and Katkhouda, repaired inguinal hernias and treated peptic ulcer disease, respectively, via the laparoscope [6,6a]. These procedures required a higher level of technical skill and therefore they did not gain rapid acceptance by the surgical community. The treatment of peptic ulcer disease by laparoscopy is very limited because of the infrequency of the disease process and the lack of interest among most surgeons. Even today, laparoscopic repair of inguinal hernias continues to be controversial. Relatively few surgeons use this as the primary treatment option for inguinal hernia. The barriers to adoption are the increased cost, the effectiveness of open procedures, the difficulty that many have with the anatomy, and the declining reimbursement for that repair. However, a recent report of over 1.5 million cases found that the laparoscopic repair of inguinal herniation can be done at the lowest cost to society [7]. Acceptance of this procedure varies from country to country, as only about 2% of hernias are repaired in Scotland, for example, with this method, but over 30% are treated laparoscopically in Germany. In the United States, 10–15% of inguinal hernias are repaired laparoscopically, but this approach is usually limited to recurrent and bilateral hernias. Even this number is in decline because of financial disincentives to the surgeons and hospitals in the United States.

The laparoscopic repair of incisional and ventral hernias was first reported in 1993 using an expanded polytetrafluoroethylene biomaterial [8]. Since then, this procedure has continued to gain acceptance in the surgical community because of the improvement in long-term outcomes [9,10]. There are increasing numbers of reports in the literature that are quite supportive of this technique, in deference to the inguinal hernia repair. It also appears that this procedure is, in fact, less costly than that involving open prosthetic incisional hernia repair [11,12].

The successful treatment of gastroesophageal reflux disease (GERD) has been mastered by many laparoscopic surgeons [13–15]. This is quite a successful procedure that is frequently performed in an outpatient or day-case setting. With success rates that approach 90% or better, this operation would be expected to increase in frequency. However, it appears to have reached a plateau in the United States. The precise reason for this is not clear, but there does appear to be a reluctance among medical gastroenterologists to refer these patients until late in the course of their disease process. Newer technologies and effective medications may also play a role.

The treatment of achalasia has followed the success of the management of GERD [16]. This procedure is more difficult than that of the fundoplication, but it is also quite successful. The main technical discussions that are pertinent here are whether the surgeon is situated at the patient's side or between the patient's legs to perform the procedure and also the type of fundoplication to be done at the completion of myotomy.

Around the globe, bariatric surgery is expanding its role in the treatment of morbid obesity. The Roux-en-Y bypass was first reported to have been done laparoscopically by Wittgrove in 1994 [17]. Wittgrove himself has performed over 1000 of these procedures with excellent short- and long-term results. As with nearly all very technical procedures, there are a few variations in the operations, especially with regard to the method of anastomosis and the path of the small intestinal limb. One concern with this procedure is that the proliferation of this operation may be driven by market forces, so that minimally trained surgeons will come to adopt this procedure, producing many complications due to inexperience. Operations such as the adjustable gastric banding and other types of restrictive surgery may hold promise in the future, but the current ''gold standard'' is the gastric bypass. The biliopancreatic diversion and duodenal switch are complex operations that are less commonly performed but also have a substantial rate of success.

Solid organ resections were also promulgated early in the laparoscopic era. The resection of the pancreas is by far the most demanding, and only a few centers have attempted this procedure [18–20]. More common operations involve the spleen and adrenal gland [21,22,22a,22b]. Approaches to the liver and kidneys are also described [23,23a].

Laparoscopic resection of the small and large bowel are now done with some regularity. Laparoscopic adhesiolysis is sometimes performed for small bowel obstruction if the abdominal distention does not prohibit its use. Colonic resection for benign disease is a routine procedure in many areas. The use of this technique is still somewhat controversial in the setting of carcinoma. Some early reports of trocar-site recurrences stifled advances in this area. However, other studies have not found this to be a prohibitive risk, and many have found that resection is productive of more lymph tissue than the open technique [24]. The use of a larger opening for a ''hand-assisted'' procedure seems to be a beneficial contribution.

The oncologic use of laparoscopy continues to grow in other areas, as for the staging of lymphomas and, recently, the radiofrequency ablation of hepatic metastases. Certainly the latter procedure is palliative, but many patients are achieving longer survivals as these tumors are destroyed. This allows them a prolonged life expectancy that is associated with a good quality of life [24a]. The use of these ablation techniques requires a working knowledge of the intraoperative use of laparoscopic ultrasonography. The two-dimensional image must, once again, be overcome to accomplish this task. Sonography has other significant usages in identifying the common bile duct and in the staging procedures mentioned earlier.

RECENT DEVELOPMENTS

Vascular surgeons are now using the laparoscope to perform aortic bypass operations, aneurysmectomy and venous procedures [25–27]. As with the other procedures, the pioneering efforts of those willing to investigate this technology will lead others to seek the benefits that become clear with longer-term follow-up of these patients.

The most recent innovation achieving success involves the use of robotics. The initial surgical robots of this generation were merely devices designed to hold the laparoscopic camera. Today, there are devices that will perform the procedure under the active directions of the operating surgeon. In fact, many of the operations described above can now be done with the use of a robot, even in a remote situation [28,29].

THE FUTURE

Laparoscopic surgery for the general surgeon continues to develop. The current training programs are frequently inadequate to sufficiently train residents in the more complex procedures that are becoming more widespread today. The limitations in the number of residents and the work hours that they are allowed to perform have hindered the use of some of these techniques in many residency programs. Certainly most senior residents are quite capable of performing cholecystecomy and appendectomy, but operations such as bariatric surgery cannot be learned in that short experience. Consequently, fellowships are necessary to obtain the skills to perform these types of procedures.

The surgeons in practice who seek to gain this knowledge have many postgraduate courses and laboratory sessions available to them. However, the assistance of a skilled preceptor or proctor in the initial cases will be of great help in mastering the techniques of the operation being learned. In this manner, the introduction of a newly learned procedure can be advanced with the utmost safety and efficacy. Careful follow-up of the patients and close scrutiny of one's results will provide a concurrent assessment.

Innovations in optics and instrumentation, leading to the use of smaller devices, may become routine in the future. Such innovative instruments are slowly finding their way onto the market. New implantable devices and prosthetic biomaterials will probably be made that will improve the success and reach of many laparoscopic procedures.

However enthusiastically we pursue these advances, the trends in reimbursement levels may devastate future developments. The declining level of payment for laparoscopic versus open procedures coupled—with the increase in liability premiums in many areas—will undermine attempts to introduce the latest innovations to the public. Additionally, the ever-increasing cost of the newer equipment may slow the willingness of all but the larger institutions to purchase those items needed for complex laparoscopic procedures. These socioeconomic issues are rapidly becoming a drag on technological advancement and must be addressed by the government.

CONCLUSIONS

Laparoscopic general surgery has blossomed in the last decade of the twentieth century. In some measure, these changes in surgery have led many of us to follow and interpret our results carefully, with a view to improving our results. However, new and different complications have been identified along with the new and different techniques. This was not unexpected. Because of the obvious benefits of laparoscopic methods, this field will continue to evolve.

REFERENCES

1. Edmondson JM. History of the instruments for gastrointestinal endoscopy. Gastrointest Endosc 1991; 37:S27–S57.

2. Ott D. Die direkte Beleuchtung der Bauchhöhle, der Harnblase, des Dickdarms und des Uterus zu diagnostischen und operativen Zwecken. Rev Med Techn 1901; 2: 27–29.
3. Kelling G. Über Oesofagoscopie, Gastroscopie und Kölioscopie. Munch Med Wochenschr 1902; 41:259–271.
4. Jacobaeus HC. Über die Mögligkeit die Zystoscopie bei Untersuchung seröser Höhingen aus zu wenden. Munch Med Wochenschr 1910; 57:2090–2092.
5. Kok HJ. A new technique for resecting the non-inflamed non-adhesive appendix through a mini-laparotomy with the aid of the laparoscope. Arch Chir Neerl 1977; 29:195–198.
6. Katkhouda N, Moniel J. A new technique of surgical treatment of chronic duodenal ulcer without laparotomy by videocoelioscopy. Am J Surg 1991; 161:361–364.
6a. Duluqc J-L. Treatment of inguinal hernias by insertion of mesh through retroperitoneoscopy. Postgraduate General Surgery 1992; 4(2):173–174.
7. Stylopoulos N, Gazelle GS, Rattner DW. A cost-utility analysis of treatment options for inguinal hernia in 1,513,008 adult patients. Surg Endosc 2003; 17:180–189.
8. LeBlanc KA, Booth WV. Laparoscopic repair of incisional abdominal hernias using expanded polytetrafluroethylene: Preliminary findings. Surg Lap Endosc 1993; 3(1):39–41.
9. Carbajo MA, Martin del Olmo JC, Blanco JI, Toledano M, de la Cuesta C, Ferraras C, Vaquero C. Laparoscopic approach to incisional hernia. Surg Endosc 2003; 17: 118–122.
10. LeBlanc KA, Whitaker JM, Bellanger DE, Rhynes VK. Laparoscopic incisional and ventral hernioplasty: Lessons learned from 200 patients. Hernia 2003; 7:118–124.
11. Holzman MD, Purut CM, Reintgen K, et al. Laparoscopic ventral and incisional hernioplasty. Surg Endosc 1997; 11:32–35.
12. DeMaria EJ, Moss JM, Sugerman HJ. Laparoscopic intraperitoneal polytetrafluoroethylene (PTFE) prosthetic patch repair of ventral hernia. Prospective comparison to open prefascial polypropylene mesh repair. Surg Endosc 2000; 14:326–329.
13. Dallemagne B, Weerts JM, Jehaes C, Markiewicz S, Lombard R. Laparoscopic Nissen fundoplication: Preliminary report. Surg Laparosc Endosc 1991; 1:138–143.
14. Carlson MA, Frantzides CT. Complications and results of primary minimally invasive antireflux procedures: A review of 10735 reported cases. J Am Coll Surg 2001; 193(4):28–439.
15. Booth MI, Joines L, Stratford J, Dehn TCB. Results of laparoscopic Nissen fundoplication at 2–8 years after surgery. Br J Surg 2002; 89:476–481.
16. Spiess A, Kahrilas P. Treating achalasia: From whalebone to laparoscope. JAMA 1998; 280:638.
17. Wittgrove AC, Clark GW, Treblay LJ. Laparoscopic gastric bypass, Roux-en Y: Preliminary report of five cases. Obes Surg 1994; 4:353–357.
18. Klingler PJ, Tsiotos GG, Glaser KS, Hinder RA. Laparoscopic splenectomy: evolution and current status. Surg Laparosc Endosc 1999; 9:1–8.
19. Gagner M, Pomp A. Laparoscopic pylorus-preserving pancreatoduodenectomy. Surg Endosc 1994; 8(5):408–410.
20. Gagner M, Pomp A, Herrera M. Early experience with laparoscopic resections of islet cell tumors. Surgery 1996; 120(6):1051–1054.

21. Delaitre B, Maignien B, Icard P. Laparoscopic splenectomy. Br J Surg 1992; 79: 1334.
22. Carroll BJ, Phillips EH, Semel CJ, et al. Laparoscopic splenectomy. Surg Endosc 1992; 6:183–185.
22a. Gagner M, Lacroix A, Bolte E. Laparoscopic adrenalectomy in Cushing's syndrome and pheochromocytoma. N Engl J Med 1992; 323:1003.
22b. Brunt LM. The positive impact of laparoscopic adrenalectomy on complications of adrenal surgery. Surg Endosc 2002; 16:252–257.
23. Cadeddu JA, Ono Y, Clayman RV, et al. Laparoscopic nephrectomy for renal cell cancer: Evaluation of efficacy and safety: A multicenter experience. Urology 1998; 52:773–777.
23a. Fahlenkamp D, Rass Weiler J, Fornora P, et al. Complications of laparoscopic procedures in urology: experience with 2,407 procedures at 4 German centers. J Urol 1999; 162:765–771.
24. Senagore AJ, Madbouly KM, Fazio VW, Duepree HJ, et al. Advantages of laparoscopic colectomy in older patients. Arch Surg 2003; 138:252–256.
24a. Shen P, Fleming S, Westcott C, Challa V. Laparoscopic radiofrequency ablation of the liver in proximity to major vasculature: effect of the Pringle Maneuver. J Surg Oncol 2003; 83:36–41.
25. Dion YM, Gracia CR. A new technique for laparoscopic aortobifemoral graft in occlusive aortoiliac disease. J Vasc Surg 1997; 26:685–692.
26. Kolvenbach R, Cheshire N, Pinter L, Da Silva L, Deling O, Kasper AS. Laparoscopy-assisted aneurysm resection as a minimal invasive alternative in patients unsuitable for endovascular surgery. J Vasc Surg 2001 Aug; 34(2):216–221.
27. Maghraby HA. Laparoscopic varicocelectomy for painful varicoceles: Merits and outcomes. J Endourol 2002; 16:107–110.
28. Gagner M, Bein E, Hurteau R, Pomp A. Robotic interactive laparoscopic cholecystectomy (letter). Lancet 1994; 343:596–597.
29. Ballantyne GH. Robotic surgery, telerobotic surgery, telepresence & telementoring: Review of early clinical results. Surg Endosc 2002; 16:1389–402.

2

General Complications in General Surgical Procedures

Douglas M. Bowley
Department of Colorectal Surgery, John Radcliffe Hospital, OxfordUnited Kingdom

Andrew N. Kingsnorth
Department of Surgery, Postgraduate Medical School, University of Plymouth, United Kingdom

THE SURGEON/PATIENT RELATIONSHIP

Surgery creates a unique relationship between those who undergo it and those who perform it. Surgical procedures leave scars, both on the body and in the psyche. Scars, intestinal stomas, persistent discomfort, and recurrent symptoms all serve as reminders of past or present illness, risk and threat [1].

People with illness may have longed for the day when they would again feel strong and safe; they approach surgery with a mixture of hope and dread [2]. Major illness commonly causes loss of bodily functions, damage to the body image, and threat to life itself. Fear and grief are common, and the surgical treatments may be drastic and give rise to further losses. The surgical encounter itself involves pain, anesthesia, loss of autonomy, and constraints on space and time. It involves helplessness and dependence; it is something to be endured [1]. The aftermath of serious illness, particularly cancer, and its surgical treatment may impose a lifelong psychological burden [3]. The psychological consequences are not confined to the individual, as the patient's family is also likely to be affected [2].

While the cosmetic reminders of surgery—scars and intestinal stomas—can adversely affect a patient's self-image and hence quality of life [4], good functional outcomes remain critical. Where functional outcome is equivalent between surgical approaches, a lesser surgical scar confers an improved self-image and greater patient satisfaction [4]. However, in a prospective evaluation of quality of life between patients undergoing abdominoperineal excision (APE) and anterior resection (AR) for rectal cancer, patients undergoing APE consistently had a better quality of life than those undergoing sphincter-preserving surgery. Even though a stoma had been avoided, patients undergoing low AR had a worse quality-of-life score, poor function, worse body image, and more gastrointestinal and defecation-related symptoms than the other patients [5].

Information and advice given before surgery, emotional support, and the opportunity to discuss problems that are anticipated are undoubtedly valuable to patients about to undergo major surgery [6,7]. The patient needs to be prepared for both the operation and its short- and long-term consequences; the patient's need for the surgeon's support extends into the postoperative period. Other members of the patient's family, particularly his or her spouse, will also need support. Despite the prevalence of sexual dysfunction after major surgery, this is detected and treated in only a small minority of patients [6]. Establishment and maintenance of trust and a relationship of care between surgeons and patients facilitates the necessary physical and psychological transitions after major surgery. This process depends on an understanding of the extraordinary nature of the surgical experience and the pivotal role of the surgeon within it.

IMMUNE DYSFUNCTION AFTER MAJOR SURGERY

Trauma to the body from either accidental injury or controlled surgical intervention induces local changes, which are termed the inflammatory response and systemic effects; in other words, the stress response [8]. That major surgery causes disturbances to systemic immunological function has been recognized for many years [9]. Organ failure is the leading cause of death in surgical patients [10], and a causal relationship appears to exist between the extent of the surgical or traumatic injury, the postoperative metabolic and immunological changes, and the predisposition of patients to develop infectious complications and multiple organ dysfunction [11–14]. Immune dysfunction characterized by an excessive inflammatory response, together with a diminished cell-mediated immunity, appears to be responsible for the increased susceptibility to subsequent sepsis following major surgery [15].

Mechanisms of Immune Perturbation

Antigen presentation is defined as a process whereby a cell expresses antigen on its surface in a form capable of being recognized by a T cell [11]. An important contributor to the depression of cell-mediated immunity found after major trauma or surgery is explained by the depression of macrophage antigen-presentation capacity [16]. Multiple factors—including decreased metabolic activity, anti-inflammatory cytokines, prostaglandins, and nitric oxide—appear to be responsible for the depression in macrophage antigen-presenting capacity [11].

T lymphocytes also demonstrate impaired function following general surgery and trauma, which correlates with the complexity of the surgery [11]. Surgical and other trauma causes alterations in T-lymphokine release and reductions in T-lymphocyte populations; patients that develop septic complications display a predominant decrease in $CD4^+$ cells [17,18]. B-cell function is also diminished following surgical trauma [19].

The observed immunodeficiency in patients following major surgery has been found to be associated with enhanced concentrations of inflammatory cytokines [11]. There is an early release of proinflammatory cytokines, such as interleukin-1 (IL-1), IL-6 and tumor necrosis factor alpha (TNF-α), which can act to depress macrophage function. Elevated levels of anti-inflammatory cytokines, such as IL-10 and transforming growth factor beta (TGF-β), also deactivated T cells [11,15]. Numerous other mediators—such as prostaglandins and leukotrienes—also contribute to immune perturbation [11]. Although much is now known about the cellular mechanisms of immune dysfunction after major surgery and trauma, exactly how clinical manipulation of the immune response might translate into improved outcomes is still far from clear [15].

Because alterations in the immune system are proportional to the extent of injury, the physiological response to minimally invasive surgery appears to be different from that to open surgery [13]. The majority of studies have shown that although laparoscopic surgery evokes an alteration in the systemic immune response, this response is less with a minimally invasive approach [12–14,20]. The clinical consequences of these findings are obscure, but one major trial has reported superior cancer-specific survival in patients undergoing laparoscopic-assisted surgery in colonic cancer [21]. The immunological consequences of surgery, both open and minimally invasive, will demand much attention in the future.

POSTOPERATIVE PAIN

There has been a revolution in the treatment of postoperative pain over the last few years. According to a recent review analyzing pooled data on pain scores obtained from a total of nearly 20,000 patients, there has been, over the period 1973–1999, a reduction in the incidence of moderate-severe pain after surgery of 1.9% per year [22].

The traditional distinction between acute pain of recent onset and short duration and chronic pain that persists after an injury has healed, has been shown to be flawed. Processes that occur within the first day may determine an individual's response for months after injury [23]. Even brief intervals of acute pain can induce long-term neuronal remodeling and sensitization (''plasticity''), chronic pain, and lasting psychological distress [23]. Nociception elicits physiological responses even in anesthetized individuals, and minimization of pain can improve clinical outcomes [24].

Patient-controlled analgesia (PCA) is widely used and improves patient satisfaction [25]; however, meta-analysis has shown that PCA does not reduce postoperative morbidity compared to intermittent opioid therapy [25]. Nonsteroidal anti-inflammatory drugs have an opioid-sparing effect of 20–30% [26], which may be important in reducing opioid-related side effects [27]. Much attention has been paid to the contribution of epidural analgesia after surgery; continuous neuraxial blockade reduces surgical stress responses and autonomic reflexes [27]. In addition, it has been shown to be the most effective method of providing dynamic pain relief (analgesia during patient movement, such as coughing) after major procedures [28]. The risks in the placement of an epidural catheter are low; nerve damage, epidural hematoma, and infection of the central nervous system all have an incidence of less than 1 per 10,000 [29]. Permanent neurological injury is rare (0.02–0.07%); however, transient injuries do occur and are more common (0.01–0.8%). The incidence of systemic toxicity to local anesthetics has significantly lessened in the past 30 years, from 0.2–0.01%. Disturbances of micturition are a common accompaniment of epidural anesthesia, especially in elderly males. Hypotension is the most common cardiovascular disturbance associated with neuraxial blockade. Severe bradycardia and even cardiac arrest have been reported in healthy patients following neuraxial blockade, with a reported incidence of cardiac arrest of 6.4 per 10,000 associated with spinal anesthesia [30]. One meta-analysis has reported significant reductions in mortality and morbidity after major procedures with epidural anesthesia; the reduction in mortality was 30% [31]. However, the majority of patients were orthopedic, and no significant effects were found after abdominal surgery.

In major abdominal and vascular procedures, epidurals are reported to lead to a significant reduction in pulmonary complications, although when consideration is restricted to studies of thoracic epidural analgesia, statistical significance disappears [27].

A meta-analysis reported in 2001, showed that postoperative epidural analgesia, especially thoracic epidural analgesia, continued for more than 24 hr reduces the incidence of postoperative myocardial infarction [32]. In contrast to the beneficial effects of epidural analgesia in lower limb procedures on the incidence of thromboembolic complications, an analysis of six randomized controlled trials has shown that there was no significant difference in the incidence of thromboembolic complications in major abdominal and thoracic surgery with epidural or without [27]. Epidural analgesia significantly reduces the incidence of postoperative ileus [33], with a consequent reduction in respiratory morbidity and earlier introduction of enteral feeding, which may be beneficial [27].

All of these effects would be expected to have major effects on patient outcomes after major abdominal surgery, but the overall differences are surprisingly small. A recent multicenter trial [34] randomized 915 high-risk patients undergoing major abdominal surgery to intraoperative epidural anesthesia and postoperative epidural analgesia for 72 hr or to control. Mortality at 30 days was no different between the groups and only one of eight categories of morbid endpoints in individual systems (respiratory failure) occurred less frequently in patients managed with epidural techniques. Postoperative epidural analgesia was associated with lower pain scores during the first 3 postoperative days and there were no major adverse consequences of epidural catheter insertion. The authors concluded that epidurals were likely to confer substantial benefits to high-risk patients; however, those conclusions have been questioned [29], and epidural analgesia is seen by many as simply one, albeit an important, facet of a multimodal postoperative regime for the control of pain [35].

Institution of multimodal care can have dramatic results; in a study of patients undergoing colectomies, a program for accelerating recovery was evaluated that included (1) continuous thoracic epidural analgesia for 48 hr, (2) no nasogastric tubes, (3) transverse or curved abdominal incisions to reduce pain and respiratory dysfunction, (4) a liter of oral fluid on the day of operation, (5) mobilization within 8 hr of surgery, and (6) milk of magnesia. In 100 patients, defecation occurred in all but 5 patients within 72 hr and the median hospital stay was 2 days [36].

Acute pain can be viewed as the initiation phase of an extensive, persistent nociceptive and behavioral cascade triggered by tissue injury [23]; attenuation of this response will lead to clinical and economic benefits. In addition, we believe clinicians have a humanitarian mandate to provide optimal postsurgical pain relief.

Clinicians have long been aware of the influence of patient expectations on outcomes. Patients' psychological factors have been found to be crucial to the success of rehabilitation and linked to levels of postoperative pain and recovery [37]. Information given by the surgeon to patients, aside from leading to reductions in fear and anxiety about the upcoming surgery and appropriate expectations about recovery and the potential for complications, contribute toward improved health outcomes [27,37].

POSTOPERATIVE CARDIAC DYSFUNCTION

Myocardial Infarction

The rate of postoperative myocardial infarction (MI) is 0.7% after general surgery in a male population aged over 50 years [38]; however, the mortality of perioperative MI is high (17–41%) [39] and morbidity can be prolonged. Patients with perioperative MI have been found to have a 20-fold increased risk for subsequent cardiac complications in the first 6 months after surgery, and the increased risk continues for years [40].

The normal physiological response to surgery is an increase in circulating catecholamines, which leads to an increase in heart rate, myocardial contractility, and peripheral vascular resistance, all of which increase myocardial oxygen demand. Also, myocardial oxygen supply maybe decreased by hypotension, tachycardia, anemia, and hypoxia. A patient with significant coronary artery disease may not be able to cope with this and may develop myocardial ischemia [39]. In addition, perioperative activation of platelets, increased fibrinogen, and a temporary inhibition of fibrinolysis in the early postoperative period may also contribute to the increased risk of thrombotic events [39].

In a study using troponin T as a marker of myocardial injury, the peak incidence of perioperative MI was during the first 24 hr after surgery, with most MIs occurring on the first night [41]. Diagnosis of a perioperative MI can be difficult, as up to 94% of postoperative myocardial ischemic events are not associated with anginal pain [42]. When perioperative MI is present, its features include dysrhythmias, heart failure, hypotension, and impaired mental status, especially in the elderly [39].

Risk stratification of patients is based on three elements, (1) patient risk factors, (2) functional capacity of the patient, and (3) risk factors of the surgery [38]. Guidelines now exist that can guide clinicians in the evaluation of patients suffering from myocardial ischemia or at risk for it [38]. It is intuitive to suggest that revascularization of an ischemic myocardium would be protective, and pooled data from studies using historical controls suggests that coronary artery bypass grafting (CABG) prior to noncardiac surgery is significantly protective against adverse cardiac events [43]. Data from the Coronary Artery Surgery Study revealed higher perioperative mortality in patients with known coronary artery disease who underwent noncardiac surgery without a preceding CABG than in patients who did undergo a preceding coronary surgery. The protection afforded by CABG appears to last for many years; however, the operative mortality of CABG is approximately 1% [44]. Percutaneous transluminal coronary angioplasty (PTCA) has also been advocated to alleviate myocardial ischemia prior to noncardiac surgery and also as an emergency intervention in perioperative patients with evolving acute MI, in whom thrombolysis is clearly contraindicated [39]. Various interventions have been shown to reduce cardiac morbidity; a meta-analysis reported in 2001 showed that postoperative epidural analgesia, especially thoracic epidural analgesia, continued for more than 24 hr, reduces postoperative MI [32], and maintenance of perioperative normothermia, has also been shown to reduce cardiac morbidity in patients with known coronary artery disease undergoing major noncardiac surgery [45].

In a randomized, double-blind, placebo-controlled trial comparing the effect of atenolol versus placebo on overall survival and cardiovascular morbidity in patients with or at risk for coronary artery disease who were undergoing noncardiac surgery, overall mortality after discharge from the hospital was significantly lower among the atenolol-treated patients than among those who were given placebo [46]. The American College of Physicians guidelines now recommend the perioperative use of atenolol for patients with known coronary artery disease or significant coronary artery disease risk factors [47].

Treatment of a perioperative MI should be similar to treatment outside of the perioperative setting, with the exception of thrombolysis, which may be contraindicated. Treatment must include full cardiologic evaluation with attention to lipid and smoking status and cardiac rehabilitation [39].

Heart Failure

Heart failure is a syndrome where the cardiac output is insufficient for the body's need. It affects up to 10% of persons above 65 years of age in the United States [39]. The best predictor for the development of postoperative heart failure comprises symptoms and signs of its existence preoperatively [48]. However, heart failure can be precipitated by an increase in demand for cardiac output—such as anemia, hypoxia, and sepsis—or through deterioration in pump function due to MI, perioperative volume overload, pulmonary embolus, or cardiac dysrhythmia [39]. Treatment is directed at the primary cause and provision of medical therapy is directed at normalizing intravascular volume and cardiac output.

Cardiac Dysrhythmias

Cardiac dysrhythmias are common in the perioperative period; transient dysrhythmias are said to occur in approximately 80% of patients if continuous electrocardiographic (ECG) monitoring is employed, but only 5% are significant [49]. Atrial fibrillation is the commonest rhythm disturbance seen in patients undergoing noncardiac surgery, occurring in 10% of patients admitted to a surgical intensive care unit (ICU) [50]. In one study, atrial dysrythmias were associated with greater mortality and longer hospital stays, but were not the cause of death and are considered to be markers for increased mortality and morbidity [50].

The guiding principle in the treatment of perioperative cardiac dysrythmias and conduction disturbances is that the cause of the dysrythmia be identified and reversed if possible. Common causes include electrolyte disturbance, acid-base imbalance, acute volume depletion, and alterations in autonomic tone [49]. Medical therapy should be instituted according to the Advanced Cardiac Life Support (ACLS) guidelines [51].

POSTOPERATIVE PULMONARY COMPLICATIONS

Postoperative pulmonary complications (PPCs) are a major cause of morbidity, mortality, prolonged hospital stay and increased cost of health care [52]. The risk of PPCs depends on the susceptibility of the patient and the type and complexity of the surgery undertaken [53]. The incidence of PPC following abdominal surgery is approximately 20–30% [54,55], depending on the definitions used, although rates of atelectasis and pneumonia twice this great have been reported in elderly patients [56]. In a study of over 160,000 patients undergoing major noncardiac surgery, 1.5% developed pneumonia, and the 30-day postoperative mortality rate of patients with postoperative pneumonia was 21%, compared with 2% in patients without [57].

Patient-Related Factors

Significant risk factors for PPCs relate to general health and immune status, including age, functional status, weight loss, and steroid and alcohol use [57]. A prospective series of patients undergoing abdominal surgery found age > 60 years, history of cancer, impaired preoperative cognitive function, obesity (defined as body mass index > 27 kg/m^2), and positive smoking history within 8 weeks of surgery to be independent risk factors for PPCs [54]. The risk conferred by smoking is significant even for patients undergoing ambulatory surgery [58], and risk persists in the absence of demonstrable obstructive lung disease [59]. Severe obesity causes hypoxemia, and reductions in lung volume, thus increasing the work of breathing [52]. Impaired cognitive function is thought to be a risk for PPCs due to a reduced ability to cough and manage secretions [60]. Symptomatic chronic lung disease is also a risk factor for PPC [52]. Patients with abnormal chest signs have been found to be nearly six times more likely to develop PPCs than those with a normal chest examination [61].

Procedure-Related Factors

Procedure-related factors for PPCs include site of surgery, duration of anesthesia, and use of neuromuscular blockade during a procedure [52].

The presence of an upper abdominal incision or an incision across both the upper and lower abdomen has been found to be an independent predictor of PPCs [54]. Diaphragmatic dysfunction occurs after abdominal surgery, mediated by reflex inhibition and also due to splinting of the diaphragm because of pain [52]. Vital capacity may be reduced by 50–60% and impaired cough, microaspiration, and atelectasis contribute to impaired gas exchange [52].

Anesthetic drugs and techniques temporarily decrease lung volume, impair airway reflexes, limit immune function, and depress the mobilization of secretions [62]. Duration of anesthesia greater than 3 hr has been shown to increase PPCs

[63], and the presence of residual neuromuscular blockade in the postoperative period has also been shown to increase PPCs up to three times [64]. Patients receiving more than four units of blood before surgery have a significantly increased risk for developing postoperative pneumonia [57].

Risk Assessment, Prophylaxis, and Treatment

An accurate history and examination is central to the identification of patients at risk for PPCs [52]. Approximately one-third of patients with PPCs will also have cardiac complications [61], underlining the importance of comorbidity in assigning risk.

Various risk-assessment tools are available for identifying patients at risk for developing PPCs and may be useful for guiding perioperative respiratory care [57,65]. Routine preoperative spirometry does not accurately predict the risk of postoperative pulmonary complications in individual patients [52,66]; however, one simple tool to assess capacity is stair climbing. In a prospective study of patients undergoing thoracotomy or laparotomy, the incidence of postoperative cardiopulmonary complications in those unable to climb one flight of stairs was 89%. No patient able to climb seven flights of stairs developed a postoperative complication [55].

In a randomized trial assessing the value of a smoking intervention program in Denmark, the overall postoperative complication rate was 18% in the smoking intervention group and 52% in controls. Significant reductions were seen in wound-related complications, cardiovascular complications, and secondary surgery [67].

In addition to cessation of smoking, weight reduction and prophylactic treatment of at-risk patients are helpful; oral and inhaled bronchodilators, systemic steroids, and antibiotics can decrease PPCs [52]. Chest physiotherapy, lung expansion, and incentive spirometry are helpful, and chest physiotherapy is more effective if started preoperatively. Good postoperative analgesia, physiotherapy, and provision of humidification to loosen secretions are vital [52].

The importance of initial, accurate empirical therapy in improving mortality in nosocomial pneumonia has been reinforced by multiple studies [68]; protocolized treatment guidelines and antibiotic rotation policies are useful tools for reducing the frequency of antibiotic resistance and the impact of nosocomial pneumonia [68].

POSTOPERATIVE DELIRIUM AND COGNITIVE IMPAIRMENT

Delirium, or acute confusional state, is a clinical syndrome characterized by acute disruption of attention and cognition associated with increased morbidity and mortality, longer hospital stays, higher costs, poor functional recovery, and more frequent discharge to long-term-care facilities [69–71]. Despite its common occurrence, delirium is often unrecognized or misdiagnosed [72]. In a study from the Cleveland Clinic [69], patients undergoing major elective surgery were assessed using the Brigham and Women's Hospital Delirium Score [71]. Of these, approximately 11% experienced delirium in the first 4 postoperative days. Univariate factors associated with delirium included age $\geq$70 years, preexisting cognitive impairment, greater preoperative functional limitations, and a history of prior delirium. Patients' perceptions that alcohol had affected their health and the use of narcotic analgesics just prior to admission were also significantly associated with postoperative delirium [69].

Lesser degrees of postoperative cognitive dysfunction (POCD) characterized by impairment of memory and concentration are common after major surgery in the elderly, and symptoms may persist for months or years [73]. The elderly are particularly at risk, and events such as anesthesia may contribute to age-related cognitive decline even when they occurred many years previously [74]. Cognitive functions are not equally affected, with variable degrees of decline in attention, memory, visuospatial ability, and language being reported [75].

In the International Study of Postoperative Cognitive Dysfunction (ISPOCD1) comprising 1218 patients over 60 years of age, neuropsychological tests were conducted 1 week and 3 months after major surgery [74]. Oxygen saturation was measured by continuous pulse oximetry before surgery and for the first 3 nights after surgery. Blood pressure was recorded at least every 30 min for the first 24 hr after surgery. POCD was present in 25.8% of patients 1 week after surgery and in 9.9% of patients 3 months after surgery. Increasing age and duration of anesthesia, poor educational attainment, a second operation, postoperative infection, and respiratory complications were risk factors for early POCD, but only increased age was a risk for persistent POCD. Although cerebral hypoxia can lead to brain damage and monitoring of oxygen saturation has shown that hypoxemia is most severe during nights 2 and 3 after surgery, hypoxemia and hypotension were not significant risk factors at any time [74]. This finding correlates with the results of a study of 20,802 patients who were randomly assigned to monitoring with and without pulse oximetry during and after surgery. Pulse oximetry monitoring reduced the rate of hypoxemia in the operating and recovery rooms, but did not reduce the incidence of postoperative complications [76].

Early POCD complicates recovery in several ways. Delayed physical and emotional rehabilitation may postpone hospital discharge and delay return to normal activities, and there are concerns about patient safety in hazardous environments when cognitive function is impaired. Long-term POCD correlates significantly with decreased activities of daily living, suggesting that patients with POCD will necessarily become more dependent on their caregivers.

Although the risk of POCD increases with age, the ISPOCD2 study examined POCD in younger patients [77]. Using the same strict criteria for assessment of POCD as in the previous study, patients aged 40–59 years undergoing major noncardiac surgery were assessed. Cognitive dysfunction was present in 19.2% at 7 days; however, the incidence was no different from that in a control group at 3-month follow-up. Although objective evidence of POCD was absent at 3 months, subjective complaints were common, and this impression of persisting cognitive impairment was associated with depression. These results show that middle-aged patients are prone to early POCD but that the effects are temporary and may be overestimated by patients themselves. Younger patients may be helped by the recognition that the problem is genuine, but likely transient.

In the ISPOCD1 study, no relation was found between POCD and anesthetic technique; however, the ISPOCD2 study showed a clear association between postoperative epidural analgesia with local anaesthetic an early POCD [77]. The contribution that long-acting benzodiazepines make to POCD is unclear, with statistically significant correlation between reduction in memory performance and amount of benzodiazepines consumed during the first postoperative week being found by some investigators [78,79] but not by others [80].

As improvements in surgical and anesthetic techniques allow for older and sicker patients to undergo operative procedures, the incidence of acute postoperative confusion and POCD is likely to rise. Patients at risk can be identified and care pathways enhanced to minimize the morbidity attendant on these complications [69,72,74].

SURGICAL SITE INFECTION

Wound infection has undergone a change in nomenclature, and the term *surgical site infection* (SSI) is now used [81]. SSI can be classified as (1) incisional or (2) involving an organ/organ space. Incisional SSI is further classified as superficial or deep [82]. These infections are a significant predictor of mortality independent of other factors; 38% of deaths in SSI patients were attributable to infection in one study [83]. There are approximately 500,000 SSIs per year in the United States among an estimated 27 million surgical procedures [84], and SSI leads to inevitable increases in overall costs [85].

By injecting medical students with bacteria and assessing the resultant pustules, it has been shown that the number of bacteria needed to establish infection in a wound can be reduced 10,000-fold by the presence of a silk suture and that the effective dose can be reduced further if the tied suture contain tissue. The risk of wound infection is illustrated in the following equation [85]:

$$\text{Effective dose} = \frac{\text{dose of bacterial contamination x virulence}}{\text{resistance of the host}^{1}}$$

All wounds are contaminated; the key is the extent of the contamination (which can be exogenous or endogenous) and the presence of foreign material and devitalized tissue [85].

The longer a patient stays in the hospital prior to surgery, the more susceptible he or she becomes to SSI [85]. Infection increases directly with the duration of surgery, and meticulous surgical technique is critical, as hematoma formation in the wound is the leading factor in the reduction of local resistance [85].

During a 10-year infection surveillance program at the Minneapolis Veterans Administration Medical Center in the United States, there was a 2.5% overall postoperative wound infection rate, consistent with other reports [86]. In their classic paper, Cruse and Foord demonstrated the correlation between the nature of wound contamination and the incidence of infection (Table 1).

Limitations of this system of risk stratification are well recognized. One major problem is its failure to account for the intrinsic patient risk of developing an SSI. In the United States, the National Nosocomial Infections Surveillance (NNIS) collected data on 738,398 NNIS operative procedures performed during January 1992 through June 1998, including definitions of eligible patients, operations, and hospital-acquired infections [87]. In the NNIS basic SSI risk index, each operation is classified according to the traditional manner; in addition, the confounding variables of patient comorbidity [according to the American Society of Anesthesiologists (ASA) preoperative assessment score] and duration of operation are taken into consideration [87]. Standard definitions for hospital-acquired infections are used [88]. As expected, SSI rates increased significantly with increasing numbers of risk factors. Within each risk index category, SSI rates were significantly lower when laparoscopic techniques were used for cholecystectomy and colonic surgery compared to open surgery [87].

Analysis has shown significant variation in wound infection rates between different surgeons [85,89,90], and studies of nosocomial infection have found that hospitals with the lowest nosocomial infection rates had strong surveillance and prevention/control programs. Collection, calculation, and dissemination of the surgeon-specific SSI rate to surgeons lowers the SSI rate [91]. Monthly announcements of infection rates makes everyone highly aware of the hazards of infection; a reduction in the wound infection rate has been noted within 6 months

TABLE 1 Analysis of Infection Rates Related to Wound Types

	Total Number	Number Infected	%
Clean	47,054	732	15
Clean contaminated	9,370	720	77
Contaminated	442	676	152
Dirty	2,093	832	40
Overall	62,939	2,960	47

Source: From Ref. 85.

of instituting surveillance, and such improvements can be sustained for many years [85].

Several studies have suggested an association between blood transfusions and infection in surgical patients. In a survey of all patients undergoing operation for colon cancer, multivariate analysis suggested that transfusion of packed red cells after operation independently predicted wound infections. Other independent variables were the presence of a colostomy and/or drain [92].

Maintenance of perioperative normothermia and provision of supplemental perioperative oxygen are thought to reduce the risk of postoperative wound infection [93]. In a randomized trial, 421 patients having clean (breast, varicose vein, or hernia) surgery were randomly assigned to either a nonwarmed (standard) group or one of two warmed groups (local and systemic). Warming was applied for at least 30 min before surgery. Masked outcome assessments were made at 2 and 6 weeks, and significantly fewer wound infections were found in patients who underwent warming [94]. Not all studies have shown benefit from warming; no difference was found in the incidence of SSI in a study of cesarean sections [95].

Smoking is a well-recognized risk factor; one study looked at the effects of smoking on wound infection in a group of patients undergoing ambulatory surgery. In addition to a higher rate of respiratory complications, smokers developed significantly more wound infections than nonsmokers [96]. Control of remote infection prior to surgery has been shown to significantly reduce the incidence of SSI, as has appropriate control of blood sugar [97]. Obesity, malnutrition, and steroid use are all factors that increase the risk of SSI, but they may not be modifiable prior to surgery [97].

Prophylaxis is desirable and is based on a combination of preoperative preparation, surgical techniques, perioperative antibiotic prophylaxis, and postoperative wound care [98]. The first person to realize that disease could be transmitted by medical attendants was Alexander Gordon in 1795 [99]; nevertheless, attention to handwashing in the prevention of nosocomial infection is still critical today [100]. Although adhesive plastic skin drapes reduce the contamination of the wound compared to standard skin prep, no reduction has been found between the wound infection rates [85,101]. In a randomized trial, the use of an impervious wound-edge protector resulted in an 84% reduction in postoperative wound infection rates in the contaminated group when compared to those cases in which a wound protector was not used [102].

Prophylactic administration of antibiotics can decrease postoperative morbidity, shorten hospitalization, and reduce the overall costs attributable to infections [103]. However, there is considerable evidence that antibiotics are used excessively and inappropriately in the prevention and treatment of hospital-acquired infections, including SSI [104]. Timing of prophylaxis is crucial to success, yet antibiotics are often administered at the wrong time or for too long a period, with implications for the cost of patient care. Several studies have shown that the local implementation of practice guidelines can yield significant improvements in antibiotic use and the cost of surgical prophylaxis. More rational use of antibiotics is likely to benefit the treatment of future surgical patients by reducing the pressure to select for antibiotic-resistant bacterial pathogens [98].

POSTOPERATIVE NAUSEA, VOMITING, AND ILEUS

Fear of postoperative nausea and vomiting (PONV) is a leading concern for patients about to undergo surgery [105]. PONV is unpleasant and increases the risk of aspiration pneumonia; it is the leading cause of unexpected admission following planned day surgery [106]. Despite new anesthetic drugs and antiemetics, the incidence of PONV remains high; its incidence depends on numerous factors, including age, gender, obesity, anxiety, history of motion sickness, previous PONV, and the duration and type of surgery [107]. Multimodal antiemetic anesthetic regimes can reduce the incidence of PONV and improve patient satisfaction [106–108].

Postoperative ileus (POI) is defined as an impairment of gastrointestinal motility after abdominal or other surgery and is characterized by abdominal distention, lack of bowel sounds, accumulation of gas and fluids in the bowel, and delayed passage of flatus or feces [109]. POI delays enteral feeding, prolongs hospital stay, increases overall costs, and contributes to increased morbidity, especially respiratory [109].

The pathogenesis of POI mainly involves inhibitory neural reflexes and inflammatory mediators released from the site of injury. Motility of the bowel is reflexly inhibited through the sympathetic innervation of the bowel. Numerous studies demonstrate that blocking of these reflexes with epidural anesthesia can reduce the duration of POI [109]. The degree of POI also corresponds to the degree of intestinal inflammatory response [109].

POI has traditionally been accepted as a normal response to tissue injury; however, an accelerated multimodal rehabilitation program with optimal pain relief, regional anesthesia, early enteral nutrition, and early mobilization has been shown to reduce its duration. This approach also prevents reduction in lean body mass after abdominal surgery and preserves pulmonary and cardiovascular function [35,110–112]. In a randomized trial, 100 patients who were to undergo major elective surgery with an anticipated blood loss greater than 500 mL were randomly assigned to a control group that received standard intraoperative care or to a protocol group that, in addition, received intraoperative plasma volume expansion guided by an esophageal Doppler monitor to maintain maximal stroke volume. The group that achieved hemodynamic goals, guided by noninvasive monitoring, achieved an earlier return to bowel function, a lower incidence of postoperative nausea and vomiting, and decrease in length of postoperative stay [113].

Routine placement of nasogastric tubes is often undertaken in an attempt to reduce the incidence of POI. A meta-analyis of all published clinical trials comparing selective versus routine nasogastric decompression revealed that fever, atelectasis, and pneumonia were significantly less common and delay to first oral intake was significantly less in patients managed without routine nasogastric tubes. Although the study revealed significantly fewer pulmonary complications, patients managed without nasogastric tubes experienced significantly greater abdominal distention and vomiting. The authors concluded that although patients may develop abdominal distention or vomiting without nasogastric tubes, this is not associated with an increase in complications or length of stay. For every patient requiring insertion of a nasogastric tube in the postoperative period, at least 20 patients will not require nasogastric decompression [114].

The most effective method of reducing ileus is thoracic epidural blockade with local anesthetic [109]. This finding was supported by a recent Cochrane review [33]. Opioid-sparing analgesic techniques and nonsteroidal anti-inflammatory agents also reduce ileus, as does laparoscopic surgery [109]. Metoclopramide, cisapride, and erythromycin are commonly administered to reduce the duration of POI. These agents are not without potential adverse effects, and there is no evidence to support the use of metoclopramide; limited data show some benefit with cisapride. Data evaluating erythromycin are sparse, and the drug is believed to be ineffective for this indication [115].

WOUND DEHISCENCE AND INCISIONAL HERNIA

Abdominal wounds can fail early in the postoperative course, producing a burst abdomen, or, later on, leading to incisional hernia.

A feared complication, burst abdomen still occurs in approximately 0.5–2% of patients undergoing major abdominal surgery [116–118]. Introduction of the technique of mass closure—whereby a continuous mass (all layer closure with absorbable monofilament suture implemented)—has been credited with reducing the rate of burst abdomen [119], which is phenomenon is caused by mechanical failure of the suture. Predisposing factors include the suture technique, patient's age > 65 years, emergency operation, operation for cancer, hemodynamic instability, intra-abdominal sepsis, wound infection, hypoalbuminemia, ascites, obesity, steroids, pulmonary complications, and patient obesity [116–118,120]. In a modern series, mortality after burst abdomen was 16% [120].

At follow-up of 10-years, incisional hernia developed in 11% of patients who had undergone major abdominal surgery. Of these, 35% first appeared at 5 years or later [121]. The type of incision influences the incidence of wound failure. A review of 11 randomized controlled trials and 7 retrospective studies concluded that transverse abdominal incisions result in fewer wound failures than did vertical incisions [122]. Transverse incisions also lead to significantly less postoperative pain and fewer pulmonary complications [122]. The superiority of transverse incisions over vertical ones also holds true in the pediatric surgical population [123].

One important factor is the individual surgeon's technique and attention to detail; one study reported in 1999 showed no differences in the complication rate between different suture materials or between continuous and interrupted closure techniques, but there were marked individual differences in wound complication rates between surgeons [124]. This was confirmed by a further study of over 1000 patients from Sweden, which revealed that rates of incisional hernia and wound infection differed significantly between surgeons irrespective of the length of surgical experience [125].

The optimal method of abdominal closure has been studied for many years. In a meta-analysis published in 2001, mass closure was found to be the optimal technique [126]. In a further meta-analysis of 15 studies comprising a total of 6566 patients, closure by continuous rapidly absorbable suture was followed by significantly more incisional hernias than closure by continuous slowly absorbable suture or nonabsorbable suture. No difference in the incidence of incisional hernia was found between slowly absorbable and nonabsorbable sutures, but more wound pain and more suture sinuses occurred after the use of nonabsorbable suture. Similar outcomes were observed with continuous and interrupted sutures, but continuous sutures took less time to insert [127].

Following original work by Jenkins [128], suture length:wound length (SL:WL) ratio has been identified as an independent risk factor for the development of hernia. In one trial, incisional hernia occurred in significantly less patients when the SL:WL ratio was ≥4 than when it was <4 [129]. However, a SL:WL of 4 may not be adequate; in 100 consecutive patients undergoing elective or emergency laparotomy through a midline incision, suture and wound lengths were recorded. The mean SL:WL ratio: was 6.2:1. A mathematical model then found that a SL:WL ratio of 6:1 was indeed optimal [130].

Although many techniques of repair of incisional hernia have been described, the results are often disappointing. In a review of 114 patients with 135 incisional hernias, more than half the patients suffered recurrences after sutured repair during a follow-up time of 5.7 years, with a follow-up-rate of 84%. All of the patients with incisional hernias had limitations to their physical function and quality of life [131]. Repairs that include the use of mesh are considered more reliable; however, recurrence rates of up to 34% have been reported [132]. A recent retrospective review of patients undergoing elective repair of a midline incisional hernia included more than 50% of the patients with chronic lung or cardiac diseases; more than 40% had a body mass index (BMI) ≥30. A total of 62% of the patients underwent primary suture repair, whereas 38% underwent prosthetic repair. The overall recurrence rate was 45%, with a median follow-up of 45 months (range 6–73). The recurrence rate for those patients undergoing a

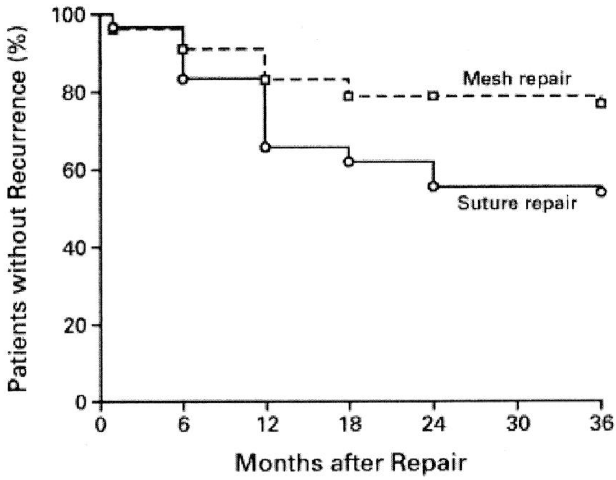

FIGURE 1 Kaplan-Meier curves for recurrence after repair of a primary or first recurrent incisional hernia. There were significantly fewer recurrences in patients who were assigned to mesh repair ($p = 0.005$) [128].

sutured repair was 54%, whereas the recurrence rate following prosthetic repair was 29%. The BMIs of patients who developed a recurrent hernia were significantly greater than those of patients whose repairs remained intact [133].

In a randomized controlled trial comparing sutured repair with mesh-based repairs among patients with primary hernias, the 3-year cumulative rates of recurrence were 43% for those who underwent sutured repair and 24% for those who underwent mesh repair (Fig. 1). The risk factors for recurrence were suture repair, infection, prostatism (in men), and previous surgery for abdominal aortic aneurysm. The size of the hernia did not affect the rate of recurrence [128].

VENOUS THROMBOEMBOLISM

The pathophysiology of venous thromboembolism (VTE) involves three factors (Virchow's triad); damage to the vessel wall, slowing down of blood flow, and an increase in coagulability [134].

Clinical risk factors include the following: increasing age, prolonged immobility, stroke or paralysis, previous thrombotic disease, cancer and its treatment, major surgery (particularly operations involving the abdomen, pelvis, and lower extremities), trauma (especially fractures of the pelvis, hip, or leg), obesity, varicose veins, cardiac dysfunction, indwelling central venous catheters, inflammatory bowel disease, nephrotic syndrome, and pregnancy or estrogen use. For surgical patients, the incidence of VTE is affected by the pre-existing factors just listed and by factors related to the procedure itself, including the site, technique, and duration of the procedure, the type of anesthetic, the presence of infection, and the degree of postoperative immobilization [134,135].

The overall incidence of deep venous thrombosis (DVT) in general surgical patients is approximately 25% in untreated patients. In surgical patients with malignant disease, the incidence of DVT approaches 30%. Clinically recognized pulmonary embolism (PE, fatal and nonfatal) is seen in approximately 1.5% of patients and fatal PE in approximately 1% [135].

The rationale for thromboprophylaxis is based on the high prevalence of VTE among hospitalized patients, the clinically silent nature of the disease in the majority of patients, and the morbidity, costs, and potential mortality associated with unprevented thrombi. Both DVT and PE produce few specific symptoms, and the clinical diagnosis is unreliable [135]. Since the first manifestation of the disease may be fatal PE, it is inappropriate to wait for symptoms and then rely on the diagnosis and treatment of established VTE. Unrecognized and untreated, DVT may also lead to long-term morbidity from the postphlebitic syndrome and may predispose patients to future episodes of recurrent VTE [136]. There is a range of interventions that may reduce the risk of thromboembolic complications after major surgery. Despite the proven benefits of prophylactic treatment, pulmonary embolism remains prevalent in general surgical patients. It is thought to account for 3% of surgical inpatient deaths [137], and in one autopsy series, it was found in 24% of 1274 surgical patients [138]. In a study reported in 1996, only 44% of surgical patients who died of PE had received prophylaxis. Patients admitted as an emergency, those managed conservatively, and those judged to be at moderate risk of thromboembolic disease were most likely not to have received thromboprophylaxis [137].

Graded compression elastic stockings (ES) reduce the incidence of leg DVT [139] and enhance the protection provided by low-dose unfractionated heparin (LDUH), but too few data are available to assess their effect on proximal DVT and PE [135]. Intermittent pneumatic compression (IPC) is an attractive method of prophylaxis because there is no risk of hemorrhagic complications. In trials comparing IPC with LDUH, both agents produced similar reductions in DVT [140]. It is not proven that IPC prevents PE (or even proximal DVT) in general surgery patients [135].

Subcutaneous injections of LDUH or low-molecular-weight heparin (LMWH) lower the risk of VTE by at least half while such treatment continues [141]. On balance, LMWH and LDUH appear to be equally efficacious in preventing DVT in general surgery patients. One distinct advantage of LMWH is that it can be administered once daily. LMWH is also less likely to cause heparin-induced thrombocytopenia and thrombosis than are standard heparin preparations [142]. Given the approximate equivalence in efficacy and safety of LDUH and LMWH in general surgery patients, cost becomes an important determinant in the choice between these drugs. In a study reported in 1999, a strategy of LMWH prophylaxis was associated with slightly fewer symptomatic cases of DVT and PE for every 1000 patients treated, with an additional cost of US $107,614 [143].

There are abundant data from meta-analyses and placebo-controlled, double-blind, randomized trials demonstrating either no increase or small increases in the absolute rates of major bleeding with the use of LDUH or LMWH [135].

A meta-analysis published in 1994 by the Antiplatelet Trialists' Collaboration, including many different types of surgical patients, concluded that perioperative antiplatelet treatment reduced the incidence of DVT in general surgery patients by 37% and PE by 71% in comparison to untreated control subjects [144]. Following on from that work, the Pulmonary Embolism Prevention (PEP) trial analyzed the use of aspirin after orthopedic surgery [145] and reported a reduction in risk of VTE by at least one-third throughout the period of increased risk. The authors extrapolated their work to conclude that aspirin could be given in a wide range of surgical groups at high risk of VTE. This conclusion has been strongly questioned by other workers [145] and is not currently recommended [135].

Whether to extend prophylaxis after discharge from hospital has been examined in a randomized study of high-risk patients undergoing major abdominal or thoracic surgery. Prolonged prophylaxis with LMWH for 3 weeks after hospital discharge did not significantly reduce the incidence of DVT as assessed by bilateral venography performed 4 weeks after surgery, compared with 1 week of in-hospital LMWH [146].

Treatment options in VTE include anticoagulation, caval filters, fibrinolytic therapy and surgical and catheter thrombectomy [134,147].

POSTOPERATIVE ADHESIONS

Adhesions after abdominal surgery are abnormal attachments between tissues or organs. Mechanical trauma to peritoneal surfaces, infection, ischemia, or the presence of bile, blood, or foreign materials in the abdominal cavity such as glove powder, gauze fluff, sutures, and prosthetic mesh are all potent causes of adhesions [148,149]. After laparotomy, almost 95% of patients are shown to have adhesions at subsequent surgery [150]; after major gynecological surgery, the incidence is 60–90% [151]. Although the majority of adhesions are asymptomatic, intestinal obstruction and strangulation, chronic pain, and infertility may result from adhesions. Approximately 1% of surgical admissions and 3% of laparotomies are estimated to be due to intestinal obstruction from adhesions [149]. In a review of 11 separate studies [152], adhesions were found to be the most common pathology in patients with chronic pelvic pain, and analysis of three studies examining the effect of adhesiolysis on chronic pelvic pain indicated significant benefits in 80% [152]. It is estimated that 15–20% of cases of infertility in women are considered to be secondary to adhesions [151]. Future surgical procedures are associated with increased morbidity, as adhesions result in more bleeding, longer laparotomies, and increased iatrogenic injury to the bowel [150].

Postoperative adhesions are the largest single cause of small bowel obstruction (SBO) and account for 65–75% of cases [153]. The type of primary abdominal operation is known to influence the development of intra-abdominal adhesions, with operations below the transverse mesocolon being particularly risky. A retrospective review of patients undergoing total or subtotal colectomy from 1985 to 1994 found that 18% of patients developed SBO caused by adhesions. The risk of adhesional SBO was 11% at 1 year, increasing to 30% at 10-years after surgery [154]. A SBO rate of 25% has been reported in long-term follow up of patients after formation of an ileal pouch [155], and this study concurs with others that have shown a cumulative probability of SBO 10 years after ileal pouch-anal anastomosis of 22% [156].

The Surgical and Clinical Adhesions Research (SCAR) study used a national linked patient data set to investigate the burden of disease caused by postoperative adhesions [153]. The initial cohort comprised over 12,000 patients undergoing lower abdominal surgery; over the following 10 years, patients were readmitted a mean of 2.2 times, and 7.3% of readmissions were directly related to adhesions. Readmissions varied according to the site of surgery, with index procedures on colon, rectum, and small intestine representing the highest number of adhesion-related readmissions. Fully 40% of all readmissions were categorized as possibly related to adhesions. The first 25% of readmissions were in the first year; however, readmissions continued to occur steadily during the 10-year follow-up with no decline over time [153].

After a single adhesive SBO, recurrence rates are high; 53% after an initial episode and 85% after second, third, or later episodes [157]. Up to one-third of cases of adhesional SBO will require operative treatment [158], and the risk of inadvertent bowel perforation during such reoperations has been recorded as 19%, thus increasing morbidity and hospital stay [159]. Independent risk factors for these bowel injuries included obesity, increasing age, and three or more previous laparotomies. The mortality in the group of patients who sustain enterotomies in this fashion is approximately 13% [159].

Cost

The economic burden of adhesions is enormous. In a recent study from the United Kingdom, mean (SD) length of stay was 16.3 days (11.0 days) for surgical treatment and 7.0 days (4.6 days) for conservative treatment of adhesive SBO. In-patient mortality was 9.8% for the surgical group and 7.2% for the conservative group. Total treatment cost per admission for adhesional SBO was almost £5000 (US$ 7950, EUR 7760) for surgically treated admissions and £1600 (US$ 2540, EUR 2480) for conservatively treated admissions [158].

Litigation

Although adhesions have been called ''an inevitable blight ··· as easily controlled as the weather'' [160], litigation not uncommonly occurs as a result of adhesions and their surgical therapy [161]. The commonest cause of litigation is delay in diagnosis (leading to gangrene and perforation of small bowel, with its consequent morbidity), visceral injury during adhesiolysis, chronic pain, and infertility [161].

Prevention Strategies

Although patients should be warned that adhesion formation is almost inevitable after laparotomy, several precautions may be taken to limit its impact. Powdered gloves should not be used. Peritoneal defects and the pelvic floor should be left open, as these rapidly reperitonealize; and the omentum may be interposed between bowel and the laparotomy wound or wrapped around anastomoses [161]. As adhesions are more likely after intraabdominal complications, meticulous surgical technique should be used [149].

Various pharmacological interventions have been tried to reduce the impact of postoperative adhesions. In a randomized trial, the severity of postoperative adhesions was reduced after placement of a bioresorbable membrane during the primary surgery [148]. Although use of such agents has not been shown to lead to any adverse outcomes, neither do they appear reduce the requirement for surgical adhesiolysis for intestinal obstruction [162]. Nevertheless, large-scale, prospective, patient-masked, controlled trials are ongoing.

TRANSMISSION OF DISEASE

Surgical gloves and drapes were originally designed to protect the patient from the surgeon; however, in recent years there has been increasing concern about transmission of blood-borne diseases from the patient to the surgeon. In 1996, the Centers for Disease Control and Prevention reported 52 health workers with documented human immunodeficiency virus (HIV) seroconversion after occupational exposure [163]. The majority of documented infections occur after contact with the blood of a patient with acquired immunodeficiency syndrome (AIDS) by means of percutaneous exposure, with a device placed in an artery or vein. Transmission may also occur through splashes, cuts, and skin contamination and, in some cases, despite postexposure, prophylaxis with zidovudine [164].

A recent survey showed that the majority of U.S. surgeons are at least moderately concerned about contracting HIV and 81% had been vaccinated against hepatitis B, although only 12% routinely used double gloves [165]. Most surgeons underestimated the risk of seroconversion after exposure to HIV and hepatitis B and C and 70% of surgeons never or rarely report needle-stick injuries [165].

The seroconversion rate after percutaneous exposure to infected blood for HIV is reported to be 1 in 300, but multiple factors influence this risk [166]. Postexposure prophylaxis is known to reduce the risk of seroconversion, and accurate knowledge concerning the risks of percutaneous exposure and the correct actions to follow after an exposure is likely to limit seroconversion [167]. The seroconversion rates for hepatitis B and C are much higher than for HIV, 6–30% for hepatitis B and 4–10% for hepatitis C [165].

Both hepatitis B and C (HBV and HCV) are associated with chronic infection ultimately leading to cirrhosis, portal hypertension, and hepatocellular carcinoma. Chronic HBV infection is seen in 1.25 million people in the United States, and 5% of acute infections are thought to result in chronic disease [168]. Chronic HCV infection is present in nearly 4 million people in the United States. It has a lower rate of transmission than HBV following needle-stick injury, but it has a 50–80% rate of chronic disease after acute infections [168]. There is no vaccine for HCV; only prevention of blood exposure will avoid the risks of this occupational infection. Risk of transmission of viral blood-borne pathogens varies around the world, with a seroprevalence rate of up to 37% being reported for HIV in sub-Saharan Africa [169].

In a large study in Italy [170], accidental exposures to blood or body fluids occurred in approximately 9% of operations. In about 2% of procedures, a parenteral-type injury, such as actual skin puncture or eye contamination, was experienced by the operating surgeon. A probabilistic model was used to predict the cumulative 30-year risk to the surgeon of contracting HBV, HCV, or HIV infection and estimate the effect of preventive strategies in reducing this risk. The current lifetime risk of acquiring HBV, HCV, and HIV infection in this study was estimated to be as high as 42.7, 34.8, and 0.54%, respectively. The adoption of preventive strategies is expected to reduce this risk to 21% for HBV, 16.6% for HCV, and 0.23% for HIV infection [170].

Education regarding the risk of exposure and seroconversion is a vital first step in changing attitudes among the surgical teams and increasing compliance with protection against blood-borne pathogens. Active immunization of surgeons against hepatitis B and prevention of blood exposure by the use of universal precautions—including face shields, impervious gowns, and double glove—is recommended to prevent occupational infection from both known and unknown blood-borne viruses carried by the surgical patient [168,170]. In addition, changes in our surgical practice, such as ''no-touch'' technique when using needles, are required to reduce the current high rate of parenteral exposures [171].

CONCLUSION

All surgeons will experience complications; the best surgeons institute strategies to reduce the risk of complications developing. The starting point in this process of risk management remains a thorough history and clinical examination.

Modern perioperative techniques, such as effective control of pain [172] using regional anesthetic techniques and balanced analgesia, cautious transfusion of blood [173], and optimal hemodynamic control during anesthesia can contribute to improved outcomes. Used in isolation, many conventional therapies have not made a dramatic impact on postoperative complications; however, interest has recently turned to a multimodal approach to reduce the incidence of postoperative problems [174].

A key factor in the success of such multimodal programs is the development of minimally invasive surgical techniques and nursing programs with emphasis on acute pain control and rehabilitation to facilitate rapid functional recovery [175]. The institution of such programs is a major task for the future; however, such efforts will undoubtedly lead to improvements in outcome for our surgical patients.

REFERENCES

1. Little JM. Ethics in surgical practice. Br J Surg 2001; 88(6):769–770.
2. Maguire P, Parkes CM. Surgery and loss of body parts. BMJ 1998; 316(7137): 1086–1088.
3. Little M, Sayers EJ, Paul K, Jordens CF. On surviving cancer. J R Soc Med 2000; 93(10):501–503.
4. Dunker MS, Bemelman WA, Slors JF, van Duijvendijk P, Gouma DJ. Functional outcome, quality of life, body image, and cosmesis in patients after laparoscopic-assisted and conventional restorative proctocolectomy: A comparative study. Dis Colon Rectum 2001; 44(12):1800–1807.
5. Grumann MM, Noack EM, Hoffmann IA, Schlag PM. Comparison of quality of life in patients undergoing abdominoperineal extirpation or anterior resection for rectal cancer. Ann Surg 2001; 233(2):149–156.
6. Maguire P, Brooke M, Tait A, Thomas C, Sellwood R. The effect of counselling on physical disability and social recovery after mastectomy. Clin Oncol 1983; 9(4): 319–324.
7. Walter PJ, Mohan R, Dahan-Mizrahl S. Quality of life after open heart surgery. 16–18 May 1991. Qual Life Res 1992; 1(1):77–83.
8. Wolf AR. Stress response in orthopaedics and trauma in paediatrics: General versus regional anaesthesia. Anaesthesia 1998; 53(suppl 2):76–78.
9. Park SK, Brody JI, Wallace HA, Blakemore WS. Immunosuppressive effect of surgery. Lancet 1971; 1(7689):53–55.
10. Carrico CJ, Meakins JL, Marshall JC, Fry D, Maier RV. Multiple-organ-failure syndrome. Arch Surg 1986; 121(2):196–208.
11. Angele MK, Faist E. Clinical review: Immunodepression in the surgical patient and increased susceptibility to infection. Crit Care 2002; 6(4):298–305.
12. Sheen-Chen SM, Chen HS, Eng HL, Chen WJ, Jawan B. Systemic immune response after laparoscopic and open cholecystectomy. World J Surg 2002; 26(12).

13. Vittimberga FJ, Foley DP, Meyers WC, Callery MP. Laparoscopic surgery and the systemic immune response. Ann Surg 1998; 227(3):326–334.
14. Karayiannakis AJ, Makri GG, Mantzioka A, Karousos D, Karatzas G. Systemic stress response after laparoscopic or open cholecystectomy: A randomized trial. Br J Surg 1997; 84(4):467–471.
15. Volk HD. Immunodepression in the surgical patient and increased susceptibility to infection. Crit Care 2002; 6(4):279–281.
16. Schinkel C, Sendtner R, Zimmer S, Faist E. Functional analysis of monocyte subsets in surgical sepsis. J Trauma 1998; 44(5):743–748.
17. Zellweger R, Ayala A, DeMaso CM, Chaudry IH. Trauma-hemorrhage causes prolonged depression in cellular immunity. Shock 1995; 4(2):149–153.
18. O'Mahony JB, Wood JJ, Rodrick ML, Mannick JA. Changes in T lymphocyte subsets following injury. Assessment by flow cytometry and relationship to sepsis. Ann Surg 1985; 202(5):580–586.
19. Abraham E, Freitas AA. Hemorrhage produces abnormalities in lymphocyte function and lymphokine generation. J Immunol 1989; 142(3):899–906.
20. Gupta A, Watson DI. Effect of laparoscopy on immune function. Br J Surg 2001; 88(10):1296–1306.
21. Lacy AM, Garcia-Valdecasas JC, Delgado S, Castells A, Taura P, Pique JM, et al. Laparoscopy-assisted colectomy versus open colectomy for treatment of non-metastatic colon cancer: a randomised trial. Lancet 2002; 359(9325):2224–2229.
22. Dolin SJ, Cashman JN, Bland JM. Effectiveness of acute postoperative pain management: I. Evidence from published data. Br J Anaesth 2002; 89(3):409–423.
23. Carr DB, Goudas LC. Acute pain. Lancet 1999; 353(9169):2051–2058.
24. Ballantyne JC, Carr DB, deFerranti S, Suarez T, Lau J, Chalmers TC, et al. The comparative effects of postoperative analgesic therapies on pulmonary outcome: cumulative meta-analyses of randomized, controlled trials. Anesth Analg 1998; 86(3):598–612.
25. Ballantyne JC, Carr DB, Chalmers TC, Dear KB, Angelillo IF, Mosteller F. Postoperative patient-controlled analgesia: Meta-analyses of initial randomized control trials. J Clin Anesth 1993; 5(3):182–193.
26. Power I, Barratt S. Analgesic agents for the postoperative period. Nonopioids. Surg Clin North Am 1999; 79(2):275–295.
27. Kehlet H, Holte K. Effect of postoperative analgesia on surgical outcome. Br J Anaesth 2001; 87(1):62–72.
28. Wheatley RG, Schug SA, Watson D. Safety and efficacy of postoperative epidural analgesia. Br J Anaesth 2001; 87(1):47–61.
29. Low J. Epidural anaesthesia and analgesia in major surgery. Lancet 2002; 360(9332):568.
30. Faccenda KA, Finucane BT. Complications of regional anaesthesia: Incidence and prevention. Drug Saf 2001; 24(6):413–442.
31. Rodgers A, Walker N, Schug S, McKee A, Kehlet H, van Zundert A, et al. Reduction of postoperative mortality and morbidity with epidural or spinal anaesthesia: Results from overview of randomised trials. BMJ 2000; 321(7275):1493.
32. Beattie WS, Badner NH, Choi P. Epidural analgesia reduces postoperative myocardial infarction: A meta-analysis. Anesth Analg 2001; 93(4):853–858.

33. Jorgensen H, Wetterslev J, Moiniche S, Dahl JB. Epidural local anaesthetics versus opioid-based analgesic regimens on postoperative gastrointestinal paralysis, PONV and pain after abdominal surgery. Cochrane Database Syst Rev 2000(4):CD001893.
34. Rigg JR, Jamrozik K, Myles PS, Silbert BS, Peyton PJ, Parsons RW, et al. Epidural anaesthesia and analgesia and outcome of major surgery: A randomised trial. Lancet 2002; 359(9314):1276–1282.
35. Basse L, Hjort JD, Billesbolle P, Werner M, Kehlet H. A clinical pathway to accelerate recovery after colonic resection. Ann Surg 2000; 232(1):51–57.
36. Basse L, Hjort JD, Billesbolle P, Werner M, Kehlet H. A clinical pathway to accelerate recovery after colonic resection. Ann Surg 2000; 232(1):51–57.
37. Mondloch MV, Cole DC, Frank JW. Does how you do depend on how you think you'll do? A systematic review of the evidence for a relation between patients' recovery expectations and health outcomes. Can Med Assoc J 2001; 165(2): 174–179.
38. Chassot PG, Delabays A, Spahn DR. Preoperative evaluation of patients with, or at risk of, coronary artery disease undergoing non-cardiac surgery. Br J Anaesth 2002; 89(5):747–759.
39. Weitz HH. Perioperative cardiac complications. Med Clin North Am 2001; 85(5): vi,1151–1169.
40. Mangano DT, Browner WS, Hollenberg M, Li J, Tateo IM. Long-term cardiac prognosis following noncardiac surgery. The Study of Perioperative Ischemia Research Group. JAMA 1992; 268(2):233–239.
41. Badner NH, Knill RL, Brown JE, Novick TV, Gelb AW. Myocardial infarction after noncardiac surgery. Anesthesiology 1998; 88(3):572–578.
42. Mangano DT, Hollenberg M, Fegert G, Meyer ML, London MJ, Tubau JF, et al. Perioperative myocardial ischemia in patients undergoing noncardiac surgery—I: Incidence and severity during the 4 day perioperative period. The Study of Perioperative Ischemia (SPI) Research Group. J Am Coll Cardiol 1991; 17(4):843–850.
43. Mangano DT. Perioperative cardiac morbidity. Anesthesiology 1990; 72(1): 153–184.
44. Eagle KA, Rihal CS, Mickel MC, Holmes DR, Foster ED, Gersh BJ. Cardiac risk of noncardiac surgery: influence of coronary disease and type of surgery in 3368 operations. CASS Investigators and University of Michigan Heart Care Program. Coronary Artery Surgery Study. Circulation 1997; 96(6):1882–1887.
45. Frank SM, Fleisher LA, Breslow MJ, Higgins MS, Olson KF, Kelly S, et al. Perioperative maintenance of normothermia reduces the incidence of morbid cardiac events. A randomized clinical trial. JAMA 1997; 277(14):1127–1134.
46. Mangano DT, Layug EL, Wallace A, Tateo I. Effect of atenolol on mortality and cardiovascular morbidity after noncardiac surgery. Multicenter Study of Perioperative Ischemia Research Group. N Engl J Med 1996; 335(23):1713–1720.
47. Palda VA, Detsky AS. Perioperative assessment and management of risk from coronary artery disease. Ann Intern Med 1997; 127(4):313–328.
48. Goldman L, Caldera DL, Nussbaum SR, Southwick FS, Krogstad D, Murray B, et al. Multifactorial index of cardiac risk in noncardiac surgical procedures. N Engl J Med 1977; 297(16):845–850.

49. Sloan SB, Weitz HH. Postoperative arrhythmias and conduction disorders. Med Clin North Am 2001; 85(5):1171–1189.
50. Brathwaite D, Weissman C. The new onset of atrial arrhythmias following major noncardiothoracic surgery is associated with increased mortality. Chest 1998; 114(2):462–468.
51. Dane FC, Russell-Lindgren KS, Parish DC, Durham MD, Brown TD. In-hospital resuscitation: association between ACLS training and survival to discharge. Resuscitation 2000; 47(1):83–87.
52. Trayner E, Celli BR. Postoperative pulmonary complications. Med Clin North Am 2001; 85(5):1129–1139.
53. Smetana GW. Preoperative pulmonary evaluation. N Engl J Med 1999; 340(12): 937–944.
54. Brooks-Brunn JA. Predictors of postoperative pulmonary complications following abdominal surgery. Chest 1997; 111(3):564–571.
55. Girish M, Trayner E, Dammann O, Pinto-Plata V, Celli B. Symptom-limited stair climbing as a predictor of postoperative cardiopulmonary complications after high-risk surgery. Chest 2001; 120(4):1147–1151.
56. Seymour DG, Pringle R. Post-operative complications in the elderly surgical patient. Gerontology 1983; 29(4):262–270.
57. Arozullah AM, Khuri SF, Henderson WG, Daley J. Development and validation of a multifactorial risk index for predicting postoperative pneumonia after major noncardiac surgery. Ann Intern Med 2001; 135(10):847–857.
58. Myles PS, Iacono GA, Hunt JO, Fletcher H, Morris J, McIlroy D, et al. Risk of respiratory complications and wound infection in patients undergoing ambulatory surgery: Smokers versus nonsmokers. Anesthesiology 2002; 97(4):842–847.
59. Wightman JA. A prospective survey of the incidence of postoperative pulmonary complications. Br J Surg 1968; 55(2):85–91.
60. Craven DE, Barber TW, Steger KA, Montecalvo MA. Nosocomial pneumonia in the 1990s: update of epidemiology and risk factors. Semin Respir Infect 1990; 5(3): 157–172.
61. Lawrence VA, Dhanda R, Hilsenbeck SG, Page CP. Risk of pulmonary complications after elective abdominal surgery. Chest 1996; 110(3):744–750.
62. Watson CB. Respiratory complications associated with anesthesia. Anesthesiol Clin North Am 2002; 20(3):275–299.
63. Celli BR, Rodriguez KS, Snider GL. A controlled trial of intermittent positive pressure breathing, incentive spirometry, and deep breathing exercises in preventing pulmonary complications after abdominal surgery. Am Rev Respir Dis 1984; 130(1):12–15.
64. Berg H, Roed J, Viby-Mogensen J, Mortensen CR, Engbaek J, Skovgaard LT, et al. Residual neuromuscular block is a risk factor for postoperative pulmonary complications. A prospective, randomised, and blinded study of postoperative pulmonary complications after atracurium, vecuronium and pancuronium. Acta Anaesthesiol Scand 1997; 41(9):1095–1103.
65. Arozullah AM, Daley J, Henderson WG, Khuri SF. Multifactorial risk index for predicting postoperative respiratory failure in men after major noncardiac surgery.

The National Veterans Administration Surgical Quality Improvement Program. Ann Surg 2000; 232(2):242–253.
66. De Nino LA, Lawrence VA, Averyt EC, Hilsenbeck SG, Dhanda R, Page CP. Preoperative spirometry and laparotomy: Blowing away dollars. Chest 1997; 111(6):1536–1541.
67. Moller AM, Villebro N, Pedersen T, Tonnesen H. Effect of preoperative smoking intervention on postoperative complications: A randomised clinical trial. Lancet 2002; 359(9301):114–117.
68. Mehta RM, Niederman MS. Nosocomial pneumonia. Curr Opin Infect Dis 2002; 15(4):387–394.
69. Litaker D, Locala J, Franco K, Bronson DL, Tannous Z. Preoperative risk factors for postoperative delirium. Gen Hosp Psychiatry 2001; 23(2):84–89.
70. Franco K, Litaker D, Locala J, Bronson D. The cost of delirium in the surgical patient. Psychosomatics 2001; 42(1):68–73.
71. Marcantonio ER, Goldman L, Mangione CM, Ludwig LE, Muraca B, Haslauer CM, et al. A clinical prediction rule for delerium after elective noncardiac surgery. JAMA 1994; 271(2):134–139.
72. Winawer N. Postoperative delirium. Med Clin North Am 2001; 85(5):1229–1239.
73. Abildstrom H, Rasmussen LS, Rentowl P, Hanning CD, Rasmussen H, Kristensen PA, et al. Cognitive dysfunction 1-2 years after non-cardiac surgery in the elderly. ISPOCD group. International Study of Post-Operative Cognitive Dysfunction. Acta Anaesthesiol Scand 2000; 44(10):1246–1251.
74. Moller JT, Cluitmans P, Rasmussen LS, Houx P, Rasmussen H, Canet J, et al. Long-term postoperative cognitive dysfunction in the elderly ISPOCD1 study. ISPOCD investigators. International Study of Post-Operative Cognitive Dysfunction. Lancet 1998; 351(9106):857–861.
75. Ancelin ML, de Roquefeuil G, Ledesert B, Bonnel F, Cheminal JC, Ritchie K. Exposure to anaesthetic agents, cognitive functioning and depressive symptomatology in the elderly. Br J Psychiatry 2001; 178:360–366.
76. Moller JT, Jensen PF, Johannesen NW, Espersen K. Hypoxaemia is reduced by pulse oximetry monitoring in the operating theatre and the recovery room. Br J Anaesth 1992; 68:146–150.
77. Johnson T, Monk T, Rasmussen LS, Abildstrom H, Houx P, Korttila K, et al. Postoperative cognitive dysfunction in middle-aged patients. Anesthesiology 2002; 96(6):1351–1357.
78. Starr JM, Whalley LJ. Drug induced dementia. Drug Safety 1994; 11:310–317.
79. Karhunen U, Jonn G. A comparison of memory function following local and general anaesthesia for extraction of senile cataract. Acta Anaesthesiol Scand 2002; 26: 291–296.
80. Rasmussen LS; Steentoft A, Rasmussen H, Kristensen PA, Moller JT. Benzodiazepines and postoperative cognitive dysfunction in the elderly. ISPOCD Group. International Study of Postoperative Cognitive Dysfunction. Br J Anaesth 1999; 83(4): 585–589.
81. Mangram AJ, Horan TC, Pearson ML, Silver LC, Jarvis WR. Guideline for Prevention of Surgical Site Infection, 1999. Centers for Disease Control and Prevention

(CDC) Hospital Infection Control Practices Advisory Committee. Am J Infect Control 1999; 27(2):97–132.
82. Nichols RL, Florman S. Clinical presentations of soft-tissue infections and surgical site infections. Clin Infect Dis 2001; 33(Suppl 2):S84–S93.
83. Astagneau P, Rioux C, Golliot F, Brucker G. Morbidity and mortality associated with surgical site infections: Results from the 1997–1999 INCISO surveillance. J Hosp Infect 2001; 48(4):267–274.
84. Nichols RL, Florman S. Clinical presentations of soft-tissue infections and surgical site infections. Clin Infect Dis 2001; 33(Suppl 2):S84–S93.
85. Cruse PJ, Foord R. The epidemiology of wound infection. A 10-year prospective study of 62,939 wounds. Surg Clin North Am 1980; 60(1):27–40.
86. Olson MM, Lee JT. Continuous, 10-year wound infection surveillance. Results, advantages, and unanswered questions. Arch Surg 1990; 125(6):794–803.
87. Gaynes RP, Culver DH, Horan TC, Edwards JR, Richards C, Tolson JS. Surgical site infection (SSI) rates in the United States, 1992–1998: The National Nosocomial Infections Surveillance System basic SSI risk index. Clin Infect Dis 2001; 33(suppl 2):S69–S77.
88. Horan TC, Gaynes RP, Martone WJ, Jarvis WR, Emori TG. CDC definitions of nosocomial surgical site infections, 1992: A modification of CDC definitions of surgical wound infections. Infect Control Hosp Epidemiol 1992; 13(10):606–608.
89. Tang R, Chen HH, Wang YL, Changchien CR, Chen JS, Hsu KC, et al. Risk factors for surgical site infection after elective resection of the colon and rectum: a single-center prospective study of 2,809 consecutive patients. Ann Surg 2001; 234(2): 181–189.
90. Wurtz R, Wittrock B, Lavin MA, Zawacki A. Do new surgeons have higher surgical-site infection rates?. Infect Control Hosp Epidemiol 2001; 22(6):375–377.
91. Haley RW, Culver DH, Morgan WM, White JW, Emori TG, Hooton TM. Identifying patients at high risk of surgical wound infection. A simple multivariate index of patient susceptibility and wound contamination. Am J Epidemiol 1985; 121(2): 206–215.
92. Ford CD, VanMoorleghem G, Menlove RL. Blood transfusions and postoperative wound infection. Surgery 1993; 113(6):603–607.
93. Sessler DI, Akca O. Nonpharmacological prevention of surgical wound infections. Clin Infect Dis 2002; 35(11):1397–1404.
94. Melling AC, Ali B, Scott EM, Leaper DJ. Effects of preoperative warming on the incidence of wound infection after clean surgery: A randomised controlled trial. Lancet 2001; 358(9285):876–880.
95. Munn MB, Rouse DJ, Owen J. Intraoperative hypothermia and post-cesarean wound infection. Obstet Gynecol 1998; 91(4):582–584.
96. Myles PS, Iacono GA, Hunt JO, Fletcher H, Morris J, McIlroy D, et al. Risk of respiratory complications and wound infection in patients undergoing ambulatory surgery: Smokers versus nonsmokers. Anesthesiology 2002; 97(4):842–847.
97. Lafreniere R, Bohnen JM, Pasieka J, Spry CC. Infection control in the operating room: current practices or sacred cows?. J Am Coll Surg 2001; 193(4):407–416.
98. Akalin HE. Surgical prophylaxis: The evolution of guidelines in an era of cost containment. J Hosp Infect 2002; 50(suppl A):S3–S7.

99. Loudon I. The cause and prevention of puerperal sepsis. J R Soc Med 2000; 93(7): 394–395.
100. Girou E, Loyeau S, Legrand P, Oppein F, Brun-Buisson C. Efficacy of handrubbing with alcohol based solution versus standard handwashing with antiseptic soap: randomised clinical trial. BMJ 2002; 325(7360):362.
101. Dewan PA, Van Rij AM, Robinson RG, Skeggs GB, Fergus M. The use of an iodophor-impregnated plastic incise drape in abdominal surgery—A controlled clinical trial. Aust NZ J Surg 1987; 57(11):859–863.
102. Sookhai S, Redmond HP, Deasy JM. Impervious wound-edge protector to reduce postoperative wound infection: a randomised, controlled trial. Lancet 1999; 353(9164):1585.
103. Page CP, Bohnen JM, Fletcher JR, McManus AT, Solomkin JS, Wittmann DH. Antimicrobial prophylaxis for surgical wounds. Guidelines for clinical care. Arch Surg 1993; 128(1):79–88.
104. Burke JP. Maximizing appropriate antibiotic prophylaxis for surgical patients: An update from LDS Hospital, Salt Lake City. Clin Infect Dis 2001; 33(suppl 2): S78–S83.
105. Eberhart LH, Morin AM, Wulf H, Geldner G. Patient preferences for immediate postoperative recovery. Br J Anaesth 2002; 89(5):760–761.
106. Akca O, Sessler DI. Supplemental oxygen reduces the incidence of postoperative nausea and vomiting. Minerva Anestesiol 2002; 68(4):166–170.
107. Gan TJ. Postoperative nausea and vomiting—Can it be eliminated?. JAMA 2002; 287(10):1233–1236.
108. Eberhart LH, Mauch M, Morin AM, Wulf H, Geldner G. Impact of a multimodal anti-emetic prophylaxis on patient satisfaction in high-risk patients for postoperative nausea and vomiting. Anaesthesia 2002; 57(10):1022–1027.
109. Kehlet H, Holte K. Review of postoperative ileus. Am J Surg 2001; 182(5A suppl): 3S–10S.
110. Kehlet H. Acute pain control and accelerated postoperative surgical recovery. Surg Clin North Am 1999; 79(2):431–443.
111. Basse L, Raskov HH, Hjort JD, Sonne E, Billesbolle P, Hendel HW, et al. Accelerated postoperative recovery programme after colonic resection improves physical performance, pulmonary function and body composition. Br J Surg 2002; 89(4): 446–453.
112. Basse L, Madsen JL, Kehlet H. Normal gastrointestinal transit after colonic resection using epidural analgesia, enforced oral nutrition and laxative. Br J Surg 2001; 88(11):1498–1500.
113. Gan TJ, Soppitt A, Maroof M, el Moalem H, Robertson KM, Moretti E, et al. Goal-directed intraoperative fluid administration reduces length of hospital stay after major surgery. Anesthesiology 2002; 97(4):820–826.
114. Cheatham ML, Chapman WC, Key SP, Sawyers JL. A meta-analysis of selective versus routine nasogastric decompression after elective laparotomy. Ann Surg 1995; 221(5):469–476.
115. Bungard TJ, Kale-Pradhan PB. Prokinetic agents for the treatment of postoperative ileus in adults: A review of the literature. Pharmacotherapy 1999; 19(4):416–423.

116. Niggebrugge AH, Hansen BE, Trimbos JB, van de Velde CJ, Zwaveling A. Mechanical factors influencing the incidence of burst abdomen. Eur J Surg 1995; 161(9): 655–661.
117. Gislason H, Gronbech JE, Soreide O. Burst abdomen and incisional hernia after major gastrointestinal operations—Comparison of three closure techniques. Eur J Surg 1995; 161(5):349–354.
118. Haddad V, Macon WL. Abdominal wound dehiscence and evisceration: contributing factors and improved mortality. Am Surg 1980; 46(9):508–513.
119. Bucknall TE, Cox PJ, Ellis H. Burst abdomen and incisional hernia: A prospective study of 1129 major laparotomies. Br Med J (Clin Res Ed) 1982; 284(6320): 931–933.
120. Pavlidis TE, Galatianos IN, Papaziogas BT, Lazaridis CN, Atmatzidis KS, Makris JG, et al. Complete dehiscence of the abdominal wound and incriminating factors. Eur J Surg 2001; 167(5):351–354.
121. Mudge M, Hughes LE. Incisional hernia: A 10 year prospective study of incidence and attitudes. Br J Surg 1985; 72(1):70–71.
122. Grantcharov TP, Rosenberg J. Vertical compared with transverse incisions in abdominal surgery. Eur J Surg 2001; 167(4):260–267.
123. Waldhausen JH, Davies L. Pediatric postoperative abdominal wound dehiscence: transverse versus vertical incisions. J Am Coll Surg 2000; 190(6):688–691.
124. Gislason H, Soreide O, Viste A. Wound complications after major gastrointestinal operations. The surgeon as a risk factor. Dig Surg 1999; 16(6):512–514.
125. Israelsson LA. The surgeon as a risk factor for complications of midline incisions. Eur J Surg 1998; 164(5):353–359.
126. Rucinski J, Margolis M, Panagopoulos G, Wise L. Closure of the abdominal midline fascia: Meta-analysis delineates the optimal technique. Am Surg 2001; 67(5): 421–426.
127. van 't RM, Steyerberg EW, Nellensteyn J, Bonjer HJ, Jeekel J. Meta-analysis of techniques for closure of midline abdominal incisions. Br J Surg 2002; 89(11): 1350–1356.
128. Luijendijk RW, Hop WC, van den Tol MP, de Lange DC, Braaksma MM, IJzermans JN, et al. A comparison of suture repair with mesh repair for incisional hernia. N Engl J Med 2000; 343(6):392–398.
129. Israelsson LA, Jonsson T. Suture length to wound length ratio and healing of midline laparotomy incisions. Br J Surg 1993; 80(10):1284–1286.
130. Varshney S, Manek P, Johnson CD. Six-fold suture:wound length ratio for abdominal closure. Ann R Coll Surg Engl 1999; 81(5):333–336.
131. Paul A, Korenkov M, Peters S, Kohler L, Fischer S, Troidl H. Unacceptable results of the Mayo procedure for repair of abdominal incisional hernias. Eur J Surg 1998; 164(5):361–367.
132. Manninen MJ, Lavonius M, Perhoniemi VJ. Results of incisional hernia repair. A retrospective study of 172 unselected hernioplasties. Eur J Surg 1991; 157(1): 29–31.
133. Anthony T, Bergen PC, Kim LT, Henderson M, Fahey T, Rege RV, et al. Factors affecting recurrence following incisional herniorrhaphy. World J Surg 2000; 24(1): 95–100.

134. Lensing AW, Prandoni P, Prins MH, Buller HR. Deep-vein thrombosis. Lancet 1999; 353(9151):479–485.
135. Geerts WH, Heit JA, Clagett GP, Pineo GF, Colwell CW, Anderson FA. Prevention of venous thromboembolism. Chest 2001; 119(1 suppl):132S–175S.
136. Prandoni P, Lensing AW, Cogo A, Cuppini S, Villalta S, Carta M, et al. The long-term clinical course of acute deep venous thrombosis. Ann Intern Med 1996; 125(1): 1–7.
137. Gillies TE, Ruckley CV, Nixon SJ. Still missing the boat with fatal pulmonary embolism. Br J Surg 1996; 83(10):1394–1395.
138. Bergqvist D, Lindblad B. A 30-year survey of pulmonary embolism verified at autopsy: an analysis of 1274 surgical patients. Br J Surg 1985; 72(2):105–108.
139. Wells PS, Lensing AW, Hirsh J. Graduated compression stockings in the prevention of postoperative venous thromboembolism. A meta-analysis. Arch Intern Med 1994; 154(1):67–72.
140. Nicolaides AN, Miles C, Hoare M, Jury P, Helmis E, Venniker R. Intermittent sequential pneumatic compression of the legs and thromboembolism-deterrent stockings in the prevention of postoperative deep venous thrombosis. Surgery 1983; 94(1):21–25.
141. Prevention of pulmonary embolism and deep vein thrombosis with low dose aspirin: Pulmonary Embolism Prevention (PEP) trial. Lancet 2000; 355(9212):1295–1302.
142. Warkentin TE, Levine MN, Hirsh J, Horsewood P, Roberts RS, Gent M, et al. Heparin-induced thrombocytopenia in patients treated with low-molecular- weight heparin or unfractionated heparin. N Engl J Med 1995; 332(20):1330–1335.
143. Etchells E, McLeod RS, Geerts W, Barton P, Detsky AS. Economic analysis of low-dose heparin vs the low-molecular-weight heparin enoxaparin for prevention of venous thromboembolism after colorectal surgery. Arch Intern Med 1999; 159(11): 1221–1228.
144. Collaborative overview of randomised trials of antiplatelet therapy—III: Reduction in venous thrombosis and pulmonary embolism by antiplatelet prophylaxis among surgical and medical patients. Antiplatelet Trialists' Collaboration. BMJ 1994; 308(6923):235–246.
145. Cohen A, Quinlan D. PEP trial. Pulmonary Embolism Prevention. Lancet 2000; 356(9225):247–1.
146. Lausen I, Jensen R, Jorgensen LN, Rasmussen MS, Lyng KM, Andersen M, et al. Incidence and prevention of deep venous thrombosis occurring late after general surgery: randomised controlled study of prolonged thromboprophylaxis. Eur J Surg 1998; 164(9):657–663.
147. Tai NR, Atwal AS, Hamilton G. Modern management of pulmonary embolism. Br J Surg 1999; 86(7):853–868.
148. Vrijland WW, Tseng LN, Eijkman HJ, Hop WC, Jakimowicz JJ, Leguit P, et al. Fewer intraperitoneal adheshions with use of hyaluronic acid-carboxymethylcellulose membrane: A randomised clinical trial. Ann Surg 2002; 235(2):193–199.
149. Luijendijk RW, de Lange DC, Wauters CC, Hop WC, Duron JJ, Pailler JL, et al. Foreign material in postoperative adhesions. Ann Surg 1996; 223(3):242–248.
150. Ellis H, Moran BJ, Thompson JN, Parker MC, Wilson MS, Menzies D, et al. Adhesion-related hospital readmissions after abdominal and pelvic surgery: A retrospective cohort study. Lancet 1999; 353(9163):1476–1480.

151. Lower AM, Hawthorn RJ, Ellis H, O'Brien F, Buchan S, Crowe AM. The impact of adhesions on hospital readmissions over ten years after 8849 open gynaecological operations: An assessment from the Surgical and Clinical Adhesions Research Study. BJOG 2000; 107(7):855–862.
152. di Zerega GS. Biochemical events in peritoneal tissue repair. Eur J Surg 1997; 163(suppl 577):10–16.
153. Parker MC, Ellis H, Moran BJ, Thompson JN, Wilson MS, Menzies D, et al. Postoperative adhesions: Ten-year follow-up of 12,584 patients undergoing lower abdominal surgery. Dis Colon Rectum 2001; 44(6):822–829.
154. Nieuwenhuijzen M, Reijnen MM, Kuijpers JH, van Goor H. Small bowel obstruction after total or subtotal colectomy: A ten year retrospective review. Dis Colon Rectum 2001; 44(6):822–830.
155. Fazio VW, Ziv Y, Church JM. Ileal pouch-anal anastomoses complications and function in 1005 patients. Ann Surg 1995; 222:120–127.
156. Meagher AP, Farouk R, Dozois RR, Kelly KA, Pemberton JH. Ileal pouch-anal anastomosis for chronic ulcerative colitis: Complications and longterm outcome in 1310 patients. Br J Surg 1998; 85:800–803.
157. Beck DE, Opelka FG, Bailey HR, Rauh SM, Pashos CL. Incidence of small-bowel obstruction and adhesiolysis after open colorectal and general surgery. Dis Colon Rectum 1999; 42(2):241–248.
158. Menzies D, Parker M, Hoare R, Knight A. Small bowel obstruction due to postoperative adhesions: Treatment patterns and associated costs in 110 hospital admissions. Ann R Coll Surg Engl 2001; 83(1):40–46.
159. van der Krabben AA, Dijkstra FR, Nieuwenhuijzen M. Morbidity and mortality of inadvertent enterotomy during adhesiotomy. Br J Surg 2000; 87:467–471.
160. Wolff BG. Invited commentary. Dis Colon Rectum 2001; 44(6):829.
161. Ellis H. Medicolegal consequences of postoperative intra-abdominal adhesions. J R Soc Med 2001; 94(7):331–332.
162. Salum MR, Lam DT, Wexner SD, Pikarsky A, Baig MK, Weiss EG, et al. Does limited placement of bioresorbable membrane of modified sodium hyaluronate and carboxymethylcellulose (Seprafilm) have possible short- term beneficial impact?. Dis Colon Rectum 2001; 44(5):706–712.
163. Centers for Disease Control and Prevention HIV/AIDS Surveillance Report. Washington, DC: US Department of Health and Human Services, 1996; 8:1–9.
164. Ippolito G, Puro V, Heptonstall J, Jagger J, De Carli G, Petrosillo N. Occupational human immunodeficiency virus infection in health care workers: Worldwide cases through September 1997. Clin Infect Dis 1999; 28(2):365–383.
165. Patterson JM, Novak CB, Mackinnon SE, Patterson GA. Surgeons' concern and practices of protection against bloodborne pathogens. Ann Surg 1998; 228(2): 266–272.
166. Cardo DM, Culver DH, Ciesielski CA. A case-control study of HIV seroconversion in health care workers after percutaneous exposure. Centers for Disease Control and Prevention Needlestick Surveillance Group. N Engl J Med 1997; 337:1485–1490.
167. Diprose P, Deakin CD, Smedley J. Ignorance of post-exposure prophylaxis guidelines following HIV needlestick injury may increase the risk of seroconversion. Br J Anaesth 2000; 84:767–770.

168. Fry DE. Hepatitis: Risks for the surgeon. Am Surg 2000; 66(2):178–183.
169. Bowley DM, Cherry R, Snyman T, Vellema J, Rein P, Moeng S, et al. Seroprevalence of the human immunodeficiency virus in major trauma patients in Johannesburg. S Afr Med J 2002; 92(10):792–793.
170. Pietrabissa A, Merigliano S, Montorsi M, Poggioli G, Stella M, Borzomati D, et al. Reducing the occupational risk of infections for the surgeon: Multicentric national survey on more than 15,000 surgical procedures. World J Surg 1997; 21(6): 573–578.
171. Corlett MP, England DW, Kidner NL, Attard AR, Fraser IA. Reduction in incidence of glove perforation during laparotomy wound closure by 'no touch' technique. Ann R Coll Surg Engl 1993; 75(5):330–332.
172. Ballantyne JC, Carr DB, Chalmers TC, Dear KB, Angelillo IF, Mosteller F. Postoperative patient-controlled analgesia: Meta-analyses of initial randomized control trials. J Clin Anesth 1993; 5(3):182–193.
173. Hill SR, Carless PA, Henry DA, Carson JL, Hebert PC, McClelland DB, et al. Transfusion thresholds and other strategies for guiding allogeneic red blood cell transfusion. Cochrane Database Syst Rev 2002(2):CD002042.
174. Kehlet H, Wilmore DW. Multimodal strategies to improve surgical outcome. Am J Surg 2002; 183(6):630–641.
175. Kehlet H, Holte K. Effect of postoperative analgesia on surgical outcome. Br J Anaesth 2001; 87(1):62–72.

3

General Laparoscopic Surgical Complications

Karl A. LeBlanc
Minimally Invasive Surgery Institute, Baton Rouge, and Louisiana State University School of Medicine, New Orleans, Louisiana, U.S.A.

INTRODUCTION

The laparoscopic application to general surgical procedures began in earnest in the latter part of the 1980s. Subsequent to that time there has been an explosion of interest and training in the various aspects of minimal-access surgery for general surgeons. At the outset of this proliferation of technology, the early innovators and early adopters identified the risks and complications associated with each procedure.

In general, these events are not significantly different from those of the open operations, but there are notable differences in the potential complications that can occur when the laparoscopic approach is undertaken. Knowledge of the clinical manifestations of these problems must be gained as one undertakes these procedures.

This textbook is designed to present the common complications seen with the various laparoscopic procedures performed today, as well as their avoidance and management. This chapter details the complications common to most laparoscopic operations. The specific events are discussed in great detail in the other parts of this book.

SURGICAL TRAINING

This is obviously not a complication but is, of course, paramount to the recognition and treatment of the patient in the operative theater. In the early years of laparoscopic surgery, the innovators developed these techniques, as only reliance on their individual skills and animal laboratory training models were available. Training centers were developed to provide rapid educational opportunities to the surgeons who were so inclined. In many instances, the surgeon attended a 2–3 day course that included didactic lectures and a hands-on animal laboratory. They then returned to the community and began their clinical experience.

Today, while this is still done in some cases, the training has changed. Many residency programs include, at least, an introduction into the field, such as the laparosocopic cholecystectomy. Several have dedicated minimally invasive surgical divisions in the department of general surgery with or without fellows. Despite the recognition that trainees are shown this technology, the majority of the laparoscopic general surgery is performed in community hospitals by ''private'' surgeons. Certainly there is a recognized lack of adequate training of some skills in residency programs—for example, inguinal hernia repair [1].

Many surgeons will continually develop their skills by attending courses and meetings. Surgeons who are performing complex procedures can easily learn the more complex operations, as the skills are transferred quickly. For example, a surgeon who can perform bowel resections and anastomoses can adopt the bariatric procedures with very little additional training. However, a surgeon who is performing only cholecystecomy cannot be expected to undertake bariatric surgery with any degree of safety. Such an individual should advance through appendectomy, fundoplication, incisional hernia repair, and other intestinal procedures. An extensive course should be attended, preferably one that includes an animal laboratory. Ideally, this would then be followed by work with a skilled and already proficient proctor who would assist the newly ''advanced'' laparoscopic surgeon in many of the procedures. This would ensure the orderly educational process while not risking an increase in any avoidable complications. However, it is recognized that this is not possible in all cases, nor is it always a requirement. Despite anyone's best efforts, however, untoward events will occur. Surgeons must be vigilant, observant, and responsive when these occur.

PREOPERATIVE EVALUATION

Generally speaking, all patients who are suitable candidates for general anesthesia can be considered for both the laparoscopic and open techniques of a given procedure. Age is not usually a factor in an otherwise healthy individual. Patients with a significant history of cigarette use, chronic obstructive pulmonary disease (especially if on steroids or supplemental oxygen), or severe cardiac disease may be a particular risk for any laparoscopic procedure. The use of CO_2 for these operations will increase minute ventilation requirements. In these individuals there may not be sufficient pulmonary capacity or cardiac reserve to respond to these physiological demands. Therefore one should consider preoperative testing that could include a chest radiograph, arterial blood gases, and/or formal pulmonary function testing. A shortened life expectancy will also influence the decision to proceed with any surgical intervention, depending on the intended operation.

The indications for the procedure will also not vary from those of the open option. In the early years of development, some surgeons tried to devise a laparoscopic procedure so that an operation could be attempted laparoscopically. This was fraught with problems. Today, we know that the minimal access technique should be equal to, if not better than, its open counterpart. In most cases, it proves to be superior.

ABDOMINAL ACCESS

The chosen method of entry into the abdominal cavity is a prime consideration. Generally, the surgeon will adopt the method that is most comfortable to him or her. As with the open method, with its many choices of abdominal incisions, the laparoscopic surgeon should be familiar with more than one method of entry so that the best technique can be used as appropriate. Each technique does require certain technical considerations to be used properly. Despite one's best efforts, complications of abdominal entry are a risk of the procedure, commonly reported at the rates shown in Table 1 [2]. The morbidity is high when this occurs and the mortality rate varies from 19–23% [3]. The study by Corson, however, reviewed litigated cases, which undoubtedly had a higher mortality rate than would occur when an injury is recognized immediately and treated promptly. It is believed that the true incidence of these complications will never be known because they are probably underreported and due to the extremely large number of patients that would have to be accumulated to achieve statistical significance.

The open, ''Hasson'' method is used extensively by many surgeons because of its known safety [4,5]. The fascia is viewed and incised. The abdomen is then entered under direct vision. Despite the fact that this technique is viewed as the

TABLE 1 Incidence of complications related to abdominal access for laparoscopy

Technique	Percentage of complications
Direct trocar	0.006–0.011
Veress needle	0.027–0.03
Open laparoscopy	0.006–0.12
First trocar	0.019–0.027
Secondary trocars	0.008–0.06

safest method, there are reports of injury to the abdominal contents during entry (Table 1). This open method is associated with fewer injuries, but visceral injury can occur in 0.048% of the patients [6]. One report noted that nearly 52% of the visceral injuries were due to open inserted trocars [7]. Vascular injuries, however, are exceedingly rare, but have been reported [8,9]. Wound infection and herniation rates range from 0.35–0.69% and 0.1–0.23% respectively [3]. If the tissue planes become indistinct during this process, one should consider relocating the point of entry or using an alternate method to obtain access to the abdomen.

Another very common choice is that of the Veress needle to insufflate the abdomen. For most procedures, this is an effective choice. The location of insertion of the needle will be dictated by the intended procedure. For example, during cholecystectomy, the needle will be placed in the umbilicus; whereas for an incisional hernia repair, the surgeon will usually opt for one of the subcostal regions, where adhesions are uncommon or not associated with intestinal involvement. Regardless of which site is chosen, it is important to utilize the saline test in the lumen of the needle to verify accuracy of placement. However, this does not always ensure that there is no inadvertent entry into bowel or a vascular structure, as the Veress needle is responsible for these types of injuries in 1.4 and 29%, respectively, of those events [6]. Others have reported that the Veress needle is the source of vascular injury in closed laparoscopy in nearly 40% of these events [10].

If the needle is placed into the bowel, the trocar and laparoscope will follow. If this occurs, the surgeon should resist the temptation to remove the trocar from the intestinal lumen. It should be left in place so that the point of injury can be found. If this trocar is removed, identification of the site of injury can be particularly difficult if one proceeds to close this defect laparoscopically. There is no absolute need to convert to the open technique if one can repair or resect the bowel (if necessary) laparoscopically. There have been scattered reports of the management of this injury without a repair because it could not be found with the use of 2-mm instruments [11].

The use of one of the ''optical'' trocars—which place the laparoscope into the device, allowing the surgeon to visualize the layers of the abdomen—is reported to be quite safe [12]. These are the nonbladed trocar (Ethicon Endosurgery, Cincinnati, OH, USA) and the Visiport (U.S. Surgical/Tyco International, Norwalk, CT, USA). The former is available in 5-, 10-, and 12-mm sizes and has a smooth, cone-shaped point with small fins on two sides to disperse the fascial fibers upon entry (Fig. 1). The latter is only available only in a 11-mm size and has a small blade that cuts as the trigger is pulled (Fig. 2). There are no known reports in the literature of significant injury resulting from the use of this type of entry, but I personally am aware of a few anecdotal reports of complications, such as vascular or bowel injury. There is indeed a learning curve associated with the use of these, because the surgeon must be aware of the appearance of

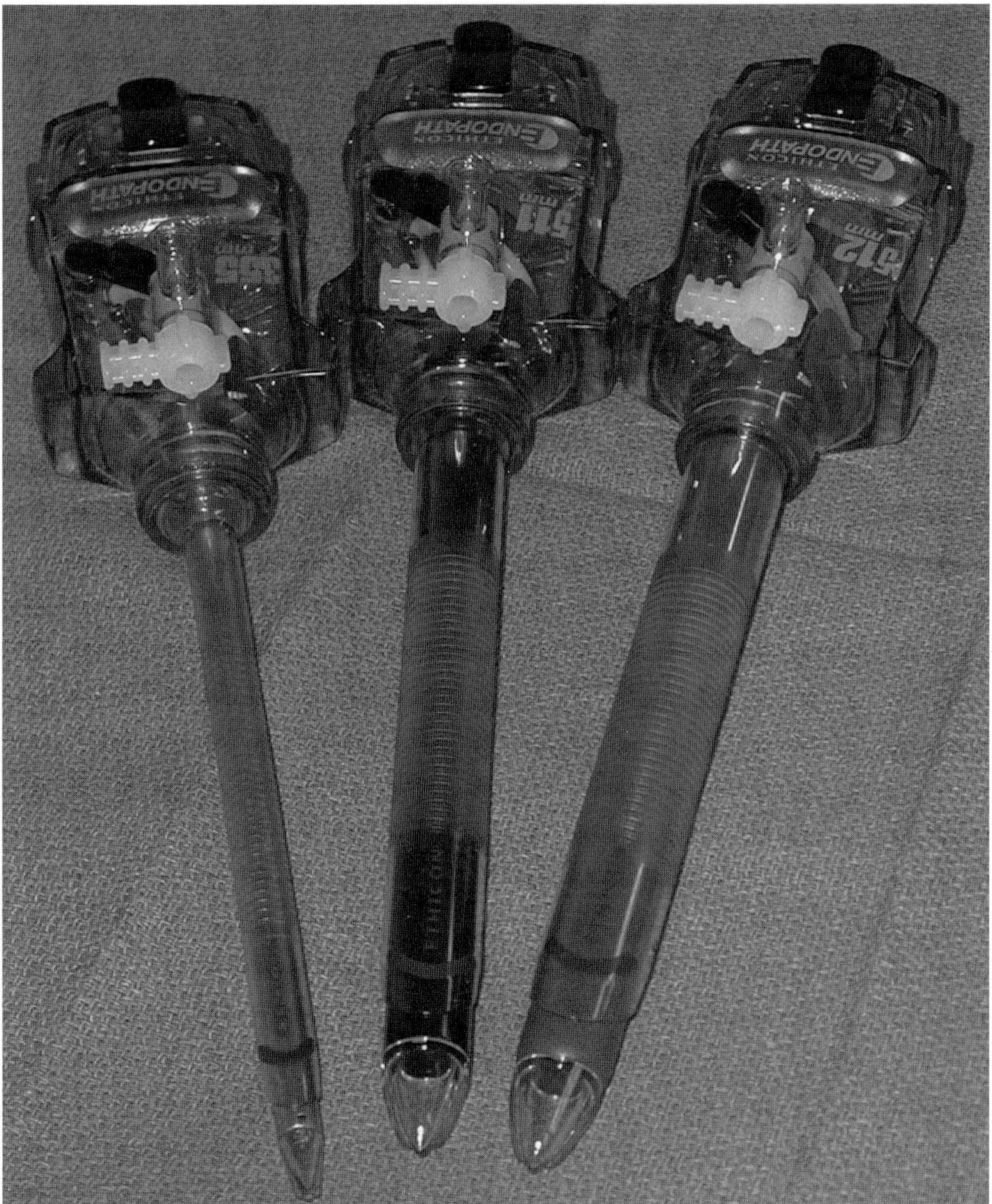

Figure 1 Ethicon Nonbladed Trocars (5 mm, 10 mm, and 12 mm).

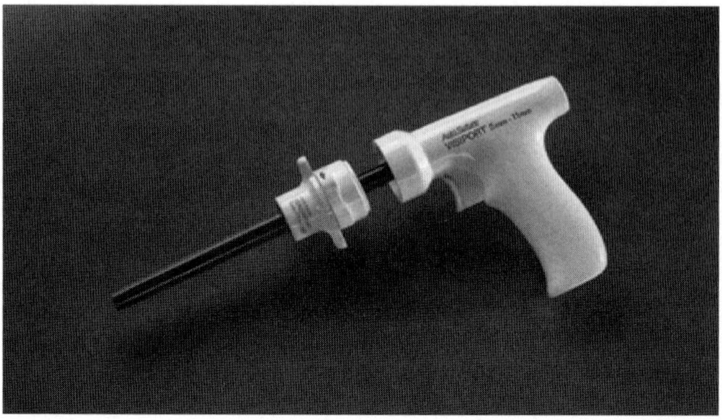

Figure 2 USSG Visiport. (Trademark of United States Surgical. Copyright 2002 United States Surgical. All rights reserved. Reprinted with the permission of United States Surgical, a division of Tyco Healthcare Group LP.)

the different layers of the abdominal wall as these devices penetrate into the abdomen.

The most common method of access to the abdomen is with the use of the closed technique, in which a sharp trocar is inserted following the creation of pneumoperitoneum. This may be done with a shielded or nonshielded trocar. These shields were formerly called ''safety,'' shields but the U.S. Food and Drug Administration did not permit this term to be used after September 1996. Their reasoning was sound, because the vast majority of the injuries that occur with closed entry are associated with the use of a shielded trocar [3,9,13,14]. The incidence of visceral injury is 0.06–0.1% and is associated with a mortality rate of 2.5% [6,15,16]. The incidence of vascular injury due to a trocar ranges from 0.003–0.25% [6,15–17]. The mortality of this type of injury is approximately 0.8%, but it can be much higher if the injury is not recognized [3,10,13].

The direct method of entry forces the trocar directly into the abdomen without the initial creation of a pneumoperitoneum. This method has been shown to have a low incidence of complications and is preferred in some centers [2,18]. Direct entry under direct visualization for the secondary trocar insertion does not eliminate the risk of injury either (Table 1). Vascular injury has been reported in 0.1% of patients caused by the introduction of these secondary trocars [19]. Therefore one should never be assured that an injury will not occur despite visualization during the insertion of any trocar. However, in the series by Usal, these injuries were eliminated by modification of the technique and careful attention to the introduction of the trocars [19].

Self-dilating trocars have recently entered the marketplace (Fig. 3). These are 2-mm instruments that are inserted in a manner similar to the Veress technique. A 2-mm laparoscope is inserted into the cannula and a pneumoperitoneum is established. This trocar site is then dilated rather than cut to accommodate the larger 10- to 12-mm instruments. While this may be a safer method, it does not eliminate injuries, as the Veress needle itself has caused several of these types of events [20]. A newer ultrasonic trocar has recently been described that requires less force than conventional trocars to achieve access [21]. It may provide a significant benefit in the future.

Perhaps the best recent investigation into these complications was that of Schäfer and colleagues [22]. Prospective data were collected on 14,243 laparoscopic procedures from 1995–1997. There were 26 injuries (an incidence of 0.182%). Thirty-five percent of these were in patients without prior abdominal surgery. Because cholecystectomy was the most common procedure, 60% of these injuries occurred during that operation. Only four of these injuries were said to be at the hands of inexperienced surgeons. The locations and types of injury are shown in Table 2. The method of entry is shown in Table 3. Obviously, this

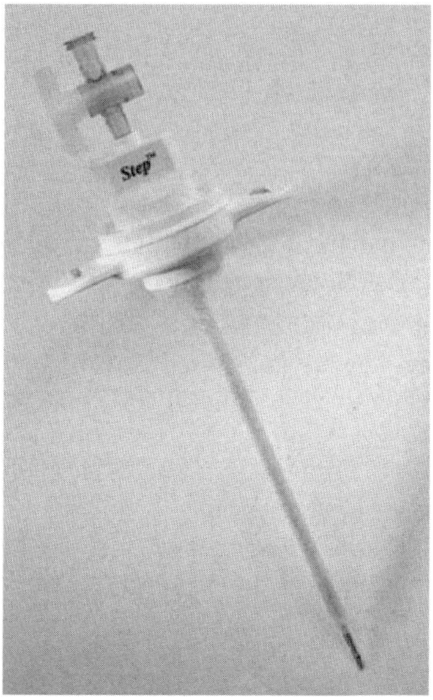

FIGURE 3 USSG One-Step Dilating Trocar. (Trademark of United States Surgical. Copyright 2003 United States Surgical. All rights reserved. Reprinted with the permission of United States Surgical, a division of Tyco Healthcare Group LP.)

TABLE 2 Location of injury based on site of abdominal entry

	Number of injuries	
Location	Trocar	Needle
Umbilical	8	3
Suprapubic	6	–
Epigastric	2	–
Left upper quadrant	2	–
Left lower quadrant	1	–
Right lower quadrant	1	–
Right upper quadrant	–	1
Unknown	1	–

confirms the conclusion of the prior discussion, that no method of entry is free from risk. Similar to other reports, there were 19 visceral and 7 vascular injuries (the Veress needle caused two of each). Repair of these injuries was performed laparoscopically in 5 (21.7%) and via laparotomy in 18 (78.2%). Three unrecognized injuries were repaired later. There was only one death, which occurred in an elderly individual with many comorbid conditions.

INSUFFLATION OF CARBON DIOXIDE

Insufflation of the abdominal cavity is a prerequisite for any laparoscopic procedure. There are a few techniques that have been performed with devices that elevate the abdominal wall during hernia repair and cholecystectomy, but these have not become commonplace. The most common problem with the use of insufflation is the placement of the CO_2 into tissues rather than into the free

TABLE 3 Method of entry and associated injury[a]

Entry method	Number	Percentage
Closed trocar	14	54
Hasson trocar	3	12
Secondary trocar	11	42
Veress needle injury	4	15

[a] These do not total to 100 because one trocar caused two injuries.

intraperitoneal cavity. Usually this is more of a nuisance than a problem, as it can make visualization difficult if the tissues adjacent to the operative field are filled with CO_2.

In procedures that are prolonged, there can be infiltration of the intraperitoneal CO_2 into tissues that are remote from the abdominal cavity. This can be more commonly seen with scrotal and penile emphysema during inguinal hernia repair or cervical emphysema during hiatal hernia repair and gastric fundoplication. These events are usually self-limited and resolve without any short- or long-term consequences. However, there have been reports of the development of tension pneumothorax related to this phenomenon [23]. Occasionally, patients may have a significant rise in the end-tidal CO_2, which can result in hypercapnia. This, however, is nearly always of little significance [24]. It is important that the anesthesia personnel be aware of this finding, because an increase in the respiratory rate can usually compensate for the rise in end-tidal CO_2 (see Chapter 5).

Occasionally, the patient with marginal cardiac reserve will not tolerate the insufflation pressures that are commonly used during laparoscopic procedures. This will be demonstrated by significant bradycardia and hypotension. It nearly always responds to atropine and/or a decrease in the amount of the insufflation.

While these problems with CO_2 are of little consequence, there is a very real risk of severe problems if insufflation into the venous system occurs. This results in an immediate gas embolism, which can occur in 0.0016–0.013% of laparoscopic patients and can frequently be a fatal event [10,25–27]. This generally occurs by direct injection of CO_2 into the venous system by the Veress needle. Patients with previous abdominal surgery may be at greater risk for this event [28]. The potential does exist for such an event by the use of the argon beam coagulator if this gas is directly injected into the venous system during its use. If such a injection occurs, the gas bubble can move centrally into the heart, where it creates an ''air lock,'' which then occludes the right ventricular outflow tract and pulmonary vasculature. The patient will then experience profound hypotension, cyanosis, and asystole. Other clinical findings include unexplained bradycardia or arrhythmia. The treatment must be rapid resuscitation, consisting of immediate cessation of the insufflation, desufflation of the abdominal cavity, the use of 100% oxygen by the anesthesiologist, and placement of the patient in a steep left lateral Trendelenburg position. A central venous line should be placed to aspirate the gas from the venous system. Fortunately, this problem is very rare, but it is fatal in 29% of the patients [28].

ELECTROSURGICAL INJURY

An integral part of practically all laparoscopic procedures is the use of tissue dissection. This usually includes the use of some type of an energy source. Even with the proper use of one of these devices, there can still be an injury to some structure that lies adjacent to the path of the current. The surgeon should have a working knowledge of the characteristics of these devices to avoid their improper usage.

The original electrosurgical device was designed to electrocoagulate the tissues. This relies on the principle that a high-frequency current can be passed through the body without consequences other than the production of heat. The amount of heat that is produced is inversely proportional to the electrode area. This can be noted with the small electrode of the monopolar cautery (less than 1 cm^2) and the larger return electrode (e.g., 100 cm^2) that is placed on the patient at a remote site. Bipolar cautery utilizes current flow only between the two electrodes of that device.

These differences can result in a burn that is not seen when monopolar cautery is used, because it can occur at a site that is not within the field of view. This current flows from the primary electrode, which is the end of the insulated cautery device, to the return electrode throughout the entire body. Therefore a thermal injury to the intestine can result if the laparoscope becomes a capacitor and touches the bowel wall. In that situation, 50–70% of the active current will be induced to the intestinal wall, resulting in at least a pinpoint burn [29]. Others have shown that this capacitance coupling can actually result in a full-thickness burn [30]. This event, however, is very unlikely if all-metal trocars are used, because the dissipation of the current in those tissues that contact that metal will avert this problem. In many areas, however, metal trocars are the exception rather than the rule. Therefore vigilance must be maintained.

Bipolar electrocautery may be safer, but it is less hemostatic. However, devices are now available (LigaSure, Valleylab, Boulder, CO) that are quite capable of coagulation of vessels up to 7 mm in diameter [31,32].

Ultrasonic devices have been available for several years. These instruments transect and coagulate tissue with high-frequency vibrations at 55,000 cps, which are generated by a series of stacked piezoelectric crystals. The scissors cut by direct cellular disruption, caused by the blades, but these also produce a cavitational effect much like that of hydrodissection ahead of the blades, which separates the tissue planes. These scissors or scalpels have been shown to produce 10 times less tissue damage than bipolar cautery with only a 1- to 3-mm spread of thermal damage rather than 2.9- to 7 mm [33–35]. This device has become popular because of this increased margin of safety. It must be remembered, however, that the improper use of this instrument can still result in a perforation if it is used in close proximity to the intestine, as contact can result in a burn that may not become manifest for a few days. This delay is the result of tissue necrosis and subsequent perforation.

Bowel injury can occur for a variety of reasons, such as traction or puncture, but the burn from electrocautery may not become manifest for several days when a perforation becomes evident [36,37]. This can take as long as 14 days and without any associated abnormal radiological or ultrasonic studies. One should be suspicious if the patient has unduly persistent abdominal pain, diffuse peritoneal signs, and fever. They may also exhibit an unexplained leukocytosis [37]. When free air is seen several days postoperatively, one must note that free air under the diaphragm will be persistent in only 38.5% of patients 24 hr after laparoscopy [38]. This finding may require the initiation of further studies if a enterotomy is suspected.

The incidence of this complication has been reported to be approximately 0.2% [37]. However, like many complications, it may be underreported. A survey at the 1993 American College of Surgeons meeting found that 18% of the respondents had had an inadvertent laparoscopic cautery injury occur in their practice but that 54% of these individuals knew of at least one other surgeon who had had such an event [39]. The true incidence of this complication may never be known.

DEEP VENOUS THROMBOSIS AND PULMONARY EMBOLISM

The etiology of deep venous thrombosis (DVT) and pulmonary embolism (PE) with laparoscopic surgery does not differ from that with open surgery. The laparoscopic surgeon was quick to adopt the use of sequential compression devices and anticoagulation during these procedures because of the need to place the patient in the reverse Trendelenburg position for many procedures. There is no standard protocol that dictates the use of either of these preventive measures, but most surgeons agree that persons at high risk should have one or both of these used during and after the operation. Such persons would include those who are obese, those with a prior history of thrombosis, or those whose operative procedure is anticipated to be a lengthy.

The incidence of DVT is approximately the same as in the open procedures, or 0.17% [40]. The risk of DVT may be procedurally related and the incidence may be skewed in smaller reported series. For example, it is rare to see a report of a PE following an incisional hernia repair, but the incidence in one report was 1% because 1 out of 100 patients experienced this complication [41]. Its occurrence is quite low, even in those patients who are at a significant risk for this problem. In one series of morbidly obese patients undergoing the gastric bypass, the incidence of PE was only 0.44% [42]. With the Silastic laparoscopic gastric band placement, there was an incidence of only 0.1% in the same risk set of individuals [43]. While very uncommon, this problem should be prevented as much as feasible with the use of sequential compression devices and/or prophylactic anticoagulation. There is a finite risk in all laparoscopic procedures (Table 4). Most authors recommend the use of some type of prophylaxis [44].

TABLE 4 Incidence of DVT/PE for selected laparoscopic procedures

Procedure	Incidence (%)
Cholecystectomy	0.139
Antireflux surgery	1.76
Colorectal surgery	0.68
Incisional hernia repair	0.2
Roux-en-Y gastric bypass	0.44
Lap Band	0.1

However, there is evidence that it may not be indicated for laparoscopic cholecystectomy [45].

POSTOPERATIVE ILEUS

A postoperative ileus is common for all intra-abdominal procedures, whether performed with a laparotomy or laparoscopically. It can generally be predicted to occur if there is a significant amount of intestinal dissection or resection or if a pronounced amount of blood remains in the abdominal cavity at the completion of the operative procedure. It is certainly a condition that is influenced by many factors. Laparoscopic techniques appear to reduce the incidence of this complication. When it does occur and is problematic, a multimodality approach should be use to treat it. This would include the limitation of the use of narcotics or other agents that are known to cause or prolong an ileus, the use of postoperative epidural anesthesia when possible, and selective application of nasogastric decompression [46].

The incidence of this event is quite variable and largely depends upon the operation that is performed. It is quite rare in inguinal hernia repair but can occur in 2.5–8% of patients that undergo an incisional hernia repair [47,48]. Antireflux surgery and colonic resection results in this problem in 6.9 and 6.2% of procedures respectively [49,50].

When this problem does occur, it may be necessary to distinguish it from acute gastric distention, as in a fundoplication or an unrecognized enterotomy following some other laparoscopic procedure [51]. Follow-up clinical examinations are important, but it may be necessary to perform a diagnostic workup, which might include a complete blood count, radiographs of the abdomen, and/or a computed tomography scan. As noted above, these can sometimes be of only minimal assistance in the determination of the diagnosis. Therefore, should the exact etiology of an ileus be in question or a more serious entity be suspected, the surgeon may have to return the patient to the operating theater for a ''second look'' to prevent an ominous result.

URINARY RETENTION

The actual incidence of this problem following laparoscopic procedures is rather difficult to quantify because of the frequent use of urinary drainage catheters for many of the operations and due to the differing definitions of this as a complication of the procedure. Despite this, it is generally recognized that the incidence of this is probably less than that in the open operations, due partly to the decrease in the use of narcotic analgesics postoperatively and the ability of these patients to mobilize more rapidly.

Retention of urine requiring a catheter is usually seen in 0.6–1.3% of patients following inguinal hernia repair. It does appear to be more common in the transabdominal preperitoneal approach than in the totally extraperitoneal approach [52,53]. This is in contrast with the 0.44% incidence following the complex Roux-en-Y gastric bypass [42]. However, with fundoplication, it can be as high as 2% of patients [49].

The precise individual etiologies are difficult to discern. However, it is obviously more common in male patients, especially those with prostatism. An initial attempt to treat this with tamulosin hydrochloride may be very beneficial in these situations. If this is not effective, insertion of a urinary catheter will be necessary, possibly resulting in a longer hospitalization for a significant number of patients. However, if the original procedure was performed on an outpatient basis, this can be managed quite successfully in an outpatient setting, if necessary with the use of home health care personnel.

TROCAR SITE HERNIATION

When laparoscopic surgery was in the purview only of the gynecologists, the incidence of herniation at the trocar site was generally considered to occur in one out of 4700 operations (0.02%). Some series have had an incidence as high as 3%, however [56]. Not surprisingly, there was (and is) an association between the size of trocar and the incidence of herniation [56,57]. Now that many general surgical procedures are commonly performed with the laparoscopic technique, more surgeons are seeing this type of complication.

This problem has been reported in several publications in the past (Table 5). While subtle, there does appear to be a trend toward an increasing incidence of this problem. The early use of laparoscopic cholecystectomy provides the majority of the operations in most series that resulted in trocar site herniation, usually at the umbilical site [63]. This is rather obvious, as this is the most commonly used site for the larger trocar used to place the laparoscope and

TABLE 5 Incidence of trocar site herniation

Author	Year	Number of procedures	Incidence (%)
Delaitre	1992	6,091	0.016
Saviano	1993	1,712	0.06
Go	1993	6,076	0.08
Bernard	1993	19,696	0.03
Buccianti	1995	981	0.5
Corcione	1997	19,320	0.21
Coda	1998	1,287	1.0
Bowrey	2001	320	3.0

to extract the gallbladder. The overall incidence of trocar site herniation appears to be approximately 0.13%. As noted earlier, the majority of these reports follow cholecystectomy, but this complication can follow other procedures as well.

The incidence of these hernias will be increased in patients who experience significant weight gain postoperatively. The increase in the intra-abdominal pressure will amplify the risk of herniation. This occurs with any abdominal operation. Other etiologies include malnutrition, steroid usage, and advanced age. The extraction of any specimen from the abdominal cavity that requires an enlargement of the trocar site or the repeated manipulation of instruments during the procedure can increase the likelihood of hernia development.

To avoid these difficulties, all port sites larger than 5 mm should be closed with either an absorbable or nonabsorbable fascial suture. This can be done with either a direct approach or with one of the percutaneous suture closure devices available for that purpose. This does not always eliminate the risk of hernias, as these have been reported at a 5-mm port site [64]. However, this is quite rare. The use of noncutting or self-dilating trocars may diminish the risk of this problem, as the defects created are approximately 3 mm in diameter [65,66] (Figs. 1 and 3). The increasing use of 2- to 3-mm instruments and trocars will also reduce the likelihood of these hernias, but it will not eliminate them [67].

Another infrequently discussed method to reduce the incidence of these hernias and resultant intestinal incarceration, such as a Richter's hernia, is the manner in which the CO_2 is released from the abdominal cavity. One should remove all trocars under direct vision when possible. Those trocars that cannot be visualized should not have their valves open at the time of removal. This can cause the bowel to be drawn into the trocar and pulled into the fascial defect, resulting in an acute hernial incarceration within the trocar that can appear as either a small bowel obstruction and/or a Richter's hernia [64,68]. Treatment can be either laparoscopically or by means of a laparotomy.

Trocar hernias that develop in the nonacute setting should be approached as would any other hernia of the abdominal wall. That is, a direct approach by either an open or a laparoscopic technique can be used. The use of suture closure alone may suffice, but the use of a prosthetic biomaterial should be considered if the defect is large or the patient is at high risk for recurrence.

MORTALITY

The mortality associated with laparoscopic operations is not significantly different from that of the open counterparts. As expected, the incidence of this adverse outcome varies with the procedure that is performed (Table 6). Not unexpectedly, the older population with more comorbid conditions represents the greatest risk of mortality. This is increased with those individuals who require emergent surgery to treat the presenting illness.

The most common procedure, cholecystectomy, has a low mortality that is generally associated with severe illness, associated cardiac problems, and an elderly population. In one series, the only mortalities (2.8%) were seen in those patients that were in the 80- to 95-year of age group [69]. Laparoscopic antireflux surgery carries a 0–1% mortality risk, which is usually associated with perforation of either the esophagus or the stomach, especially with larger paraesophageal hernias [54,55,70].

Incisional and inguinal hernias are rarely associated with mortality. However, they are known to occur and usually remain unreported. Only one series

TABLE 6 Mortality associated with selected laparoscopic procedures[a]

Procedure	Percentage
Adrenalectomy	0.5
Antireflux procedures	1
Roux-en-Y gastric bypass	0.9
Lap Band	0.53
Cholecystectomy	0.18
Genitourinary procedures	0.08
Hernia, incisional	0.02
Hernia, inguinal	0.1

[a] These percentages are representative incidences of these complications. In most reported series, there are no deaths. Therefore it should be assumed that all of these numbers range from zero to the number shown.

of incisional hernia repair recorded a death, and it is difficult to find a report of such an event following inguinal hernia repair [72,73]. Even in these series, the deaths were not related to operative complications but rather to cardiac or hepatic disease. However, intestinal injury can predispose the patient to significant risk of death in these and other procedures, such as complications associated with genitourinary procedures [74].

Operations on the morbidly obese patient carry an especial risk due to the complex nature of most such operations, such as the Roux-en-Y gastric bypass. This procedure carries a risk of death on the order of 0.4–0.9%, despite the many risk factors associated with these patients. The usual cause of death is a gastrointestinal complication such as torsion of the Roux limb, anastomotic leakage, sepsis, or pulmonary embolism [42,71]. This appears to be common in the early experiences of the procedure [42]. Somewhat surprisingly, a recent publication on the Lap Band procedure reported that it was associated with a mortality rate of 0.53%, due to myocardial infarction and pulmonary embolism [43]. This re-emphasizes the fact that good preoperative evaluation and excellent postoperative care can still be associated with death as a consequence of the patient's preexisting condition.

CONCLUSION

Laparoscopic surgery is a safe approach to the abdominal operations performed today. Preoperative preparation of the patient should be performed, as with any open procedure. While there may be certain additional considerations with the laparoscopic patient, usually this does not involve any significant change. Complications that are somewhat unique to the minimally invasive approach exist; they are recognized by most and generally avoided. However, despite the best care and skill, there is a finite risk that one of a myriad of adverse events will eventuate. We must prevent those that are preventable and treat those that are not.

REFERENCES

1. DeTurris SV, Cacchione RN, Mungara A, Pecoraro A, Ferzli GS. Laparoscopic herniorrhaphy: beyond the learning curve. J Am Coll Surg 2002; 194(1S):65–73.
2. Jacobson MT, Osias J, Bizhang R, Tsang M, et al. The direct trocar technique: An alternative approach to abdominal entry for laparoscopy. JSLS 2002; 6:169–174.
3. Corson SL, Chandker JG, Way LW. Survey of laparoscopic entry injuries provoking litigation. J Am Assoc Gynecol Laparosc 2001; 8(3):341–347.
4. Nuzzo G, Giuliante F, Tebala GD, Vellone M, Cavicchioni C. Routine use of open technique in laparoscopic operations. J Am Coll Surg 1997; 184:58–62.
5. Zaraca F, Catarci M, Gossetti F, Mulieri G, Carboni M. Routine use of open laparoscopy: 1006 consecutive cases. J Laparoendosc Adv Surg Tech 1999; 9(1):75–80.

6. Bonjer HJ, Hazebroek EJ, Kazemier G, Giuffrida MC, Meijer WS, Lange JF. Open versus closed establishment of pneumoperitoneum in laparoscopic surgery. Br J Surg 1997; 84:599–602.
7. Wherry DC, Marohn MR, Malanoski MP, Hetz SP, Rich NM. An external audit of laparoscopic cholecystectomy in the steady state performed in medical treatment facilities of the Department of Defense. Ann Surg 1996; 224:145–154.
8. Hanney R, Alle K, Cregan P. Major vascular injury and laparoscopy. Aust NZ J Surg 1995; 65:533–535.
9. Soderstrom RM. Injuries to major blood vessels during endoscopy. J Am Soc Gynecol Laparosc 1997; 4(3):395–398.
10. Sigman HH, Fried GM, Garzon et al. GM. Risk of blind versus open approach to celiotomy for laparoscopic surgery. Surg Laparosc Endosc 1993; 3:296–299.
11. Berry MA, Rangraj M. Conservative treatment of recognized laparoscopic colonic injury. JSLS 1998; 2:195–196.
12. Melzer A, Kipfmuller K, Groenemeyer DH, Seibel R, Buess G. Ports, trocars/cannulae, and access techniques. Semin Laparosc Surg 1995; 2:179–204.
13. Apelgren KN, Scheeres DE. Aortic injury. A catastrophic complication of laparoscopic cholecystecomy. Surg Endosc 1994; 8:689–690.
14. Saville LE, Woods MS. Laparoscopy and major retroperitoneal vascular injuries (MRVI). Surg Endosc 1995; 9:1096–1100.
15. Hashizume M, Sugimachi K. Needle and trocar injury during laparoscopic surgery in Japan. Surg Endosc 1997; 11:1198–1201.
16. Deziel DJ, Millikan KW, Economou SG, et al. Complications of laparoscopic cholecystectomy: A national survery of 4,292 hospitals and an analysis of 77,604 cases. Am J Surg 1993; 165:9–14.
17. Chandler JG, Corson SL, Way LW. Three spectra of laparoscopic entry access injuries. J Am Coll Surg 2001; 192:478–491.
18. Byron JW, Markenson G, Miyazawa K. A randomized comparison of Veress needle and trocar insertion for laparoscopy. Surg Gynecol Obstet 1993; 177:259–262.
19. Usal H, Sayad P, Hayek N, Hallak A, et al. Major vascular injuries during laparoscopic cholecystecomy. Surg Endosc 1998; 12:960–962.
20. Feste JR, Bojahr B, Turner DJ. Randomized trial comparing a radially expandable needle system with cutting trocars. JSLS 2000; 4:11–15.
21. Matsumoto S, Kawabe N, Mizuno Y, Shirasugi N, et al. The ultrasonic trocar provides an easy, sharp, bloodless, and repeatable approach to the abdominal cavity. JSLS 2002; 6:401–405.
22. Shäfer M, Lauper M, Krähenbähl L. Trocar and Veress needle injuries during laparoscopy. Surg Endosc 2001; 15:275–280.
23. Whiston RJ, Eggers KA, et al. Tension pneumothorax during laparoscopic cholecystectomy. Br J Surg 1991; 78:1325.
24. Kent RB. Subcutaneous emphysema and hypercarbia following laparoscopic cholecystectomy. Arch Surg 1991; 126:1154–1156.
25. Corwin CL. Pneumoperitoneum. In: Scott-Connor CEH, ed. The SAGES Manual: Fundamentals of Laparoscopy and GI Endoscopy. New York: Springer-Verlag, 1999, 37–42.

26. Mintz M. Risks and prophylaxis in laparoscopic surgery: A survey of 100,000 cases. Reprod Med 1977; 18:269–272.
27. Schulman D, Aronson HB. Capnography in the early diagnosis of carbon dioxide embolism during laparoscopy. Can Anaesth Soc J 1984; 31:455.
28. Cottin V, Delafosse B, Viale J-P. Gas embolism during laparoscopy. Surg Endosc 1996; 10:166–169.
29. Soderstrom RM. Electrical safety in laparoscopy. In: Phillips JM, ed. Endoscopy in Gynecology. Downey, Calif.: American Association of Gynecology and Laparoscopy, 1978, 306–311.
30. Voyles CR, Tucker RD. Education and engineering solutions for potential problems with laparoscopic monopolar electrosurgery. Am J Surg 1992; 164:57–62.
31. Kennedy JS, Stanahan PL, Taylor KD, Chandler JG. High-burst strength, feedback-controlled bipolar vessel sealing. Surg Endosc 1998; 12:876–878.
32. Heniford BT, Matthews BD, Sing RF, Backus C, et al. Initial results with an electrothermal bipolar vessel sealer. Surg Endosc 2001; 5:799–801.
33. Reidel HH, Corts-Kleinwort G, Semm K. Various coagulation techniques tested in a rabbit model. Endoscopy 1984; 16:47–52.
34. Amaral JC. Depth of thermal injury: Ultrasonically activated scalpel versus electrosurgery. Surg Endosc 1995; 9:226.
35. Hoenig DM, Chrostek CA, Amaral JF. Laparosonic Coagulating shears: Alternative method of hemostatic control of unsupported tissue. J Endourol 1996; 10(5): 431–433.
36. Deziel DJ, Millikan KW, Economou SG, Doolas A, et al. Complications of laparoscopic cholecystectomy: A national survey of 4,292 hospitals and an analysis of 77,602 cases. Am J Surg 1993; 165:9–14.
37. Schrenk P, Woisetschläger R, Rieger R, Wayand W. Mechanism, management, and prevention of laparoscopic bowel injuries. Gastrointest Endosc 1996; 43(6):572–574.
38. Farooqui MO, Bazzoli JM. Significance of radiologic evidence of free air following laparoscopy. J Reprod Med 1976; 16(3):119–125.
39. Tucker RD. Laparoscopic electrosurgical injuries: Survey results and their implications. Surg Laparosc Endosc 1995; 5:311–317.
40. Carlson MA, Frantzides CT. Complications and results of primary minimally invasive antireflux procedures: A review of 10735 cases. J Am Coll Surg 2001; 193(4): 428–439.
41. Rosen M, Brody F, Ponsky J, Walsh RM, et al. Recurrence after laparoscopic ventral hernia repair. Surg Endosc 2003; 17:123–128.
42. Oliak D, Ballantyne GH, Weber P, Wasielewski A, et al. Laparoscopic Roux-en-Y gastric bypass. Surg Endosc 2003; 17:405–408.
43. Angrisani L, Furbetta F, Doldi SB, Basso N, et al. Lap Band adjustable gastric banding system. Surg Endosc 2003; 17:409–412.
44. Nguyen NT, Luketich JD, Friedman DM, et al. Pulmonary emobolism following laparoscopic antireflux surgery: A case report and review of the literature. JSLS 1999; 3:149–153.
45. Blake AM, Toker SI, Dunn E. Deep venous thrombosis prophylaxis is not indicated for laparoscopic cholecystecomy. JSLS 2001; 5:215–219.

46. Luckey A, Livingston E, Tache Y. Mechanisms and treatment of postoperative ileus. Arch Surg 2003; 138:206–214.
47. Morena-Egea A, Castillo Bustos JA, Aguayo JI. Day surgery for laparoscopic repair of abdominal wall hernias. Hernia 2002; 6:21–25.
48. LeBlanc KA, Whitaker JM, Bellanger DE, Rhynes VK. Laparoscopic incisional and ventral hernioplasty: Lessons learned from 200 patients. Hernia 2003; 7:118–124.
49. Pohl D, Eubanks TR, Omelanczuk PE, Pellegrini CA. Management and outcome of complications after laparoscopic antireflux operations. Arch Surg 2001; 136: 399–403.
50. Hamel CT, Hildebrandt U, Weiss EG, Feifelz G, Wexner SD. Laparoscopic surgery for inflammatory bowel disease. Surg Endosc 2001; 15:642–645.
51. Ben-Haim M, Kuriansky J, Ral R, Zmora O, et al. Pitfalls and complications with laparoscopic intraperitoneal expanded polytetrafluoroethylene patch repair of postoperative ventral hernia. Surg Endosc 2002; 16:785–788.
52. Ramshaw B, Abiad F, Voeller G, Wilson R, Mason E. Polyester (Parietex) mesh for total extraperitoneal laparoscopic inguinal hernia repair. Surg Endosc 2003; 17: 498–501.
53. McCloud JM, Evans DS. Day-case laparoscopic hernia repair in a single unit. Surg Endosc 2003; 17:491–493.
54. Carlson MA, Frantzides CT. Complications and results of primary minimally invasive antireflux procedures: a review of 10735 reported cases. J Am Coll Surg 2001; 193(4):428–439.
55. Flum DR, Koepsell T, Heagerty P, Pellegrini CA. The nationwide frequency of major adverse outcomes in antireflux surgery and the role of surgeon experience, 1992–1997. J Am Coll Surg 2002; 195:611–618.
56. Bowrey DJ, Blom D, Crookes PF, Bremner CG, Johansson JL, Lord RV, Hagen JA, DeMeester SR, DeMeester TR, Peters JH. Risk factors and the prevelance of trocar site herniation after laparoscopic fundoplication. Surg Endosc 2001; 15:663–666.
57. Montz FJ, Holschneider CH, Munro MG. Incisional hernia following laparoscopy: A survey of the American Association of Gynaecologic Laparoscopists. Obstet Gynecol 1994; 84:881–884.
58. Delaitre B, Testas P, Dubois F, et al. Complications des cholécystectomies par voi coelioscopique. A propos de 6,091 observations. Lyon Chir 1992; 88:170–175.
59. Saviano MS. Analisi di uno studio multicentrico su 1712 casi di colecistectomia-video laparoscopica. Atti Giornate Chirurgia Endo-Laparoscopica e Mini-Invasiva. L'antologia, 1993.
60. Go PM, Scholand F, Gouma DJ. Laparoscopic cholecystectomy in the Netherlands. Br J Surg 1993; 80:1180–1184.
61. Buccianti P, Decanini L, Chiarugi M. Analisi delle complicanze in quasi 1000 colecistectomie laparoscopiche. Archivo e Atti della Societa Italiana di Chirurgia, 97 Congresso, Trieste, 8–11 Ottobre, 1995, Vol Comunicazione. Roma: Edizioni Luigi Pozzi, 1995:157–158.
62. Corcione F, Titilo O, Damiano I, Cascone U. Post-laparoscopy incisional hernias: An epidemiologic investigation in Italy. Hernia 1997; 1(suppl1):55.
63. Coda A, Bossotti M, Ferri F, Mattio R, et al. Incisional hernia and fascial defect following laparoscopic surgery. Surg Laparosc Endosc Percut Tech 2000; 10(1): 34–38.

64. Reardon PR, Preciado A, Scarborough T, Matthews B, et al. Hernia at 5-mm laparoscopic port site presenting as early postoperative small bowel obstruction. J Laparoendosc Adv Surg Tech 1999; 9:532–525.
65. Bhoyrul S, Mori T, Way LW. Radially expanding dilation: A superior method of laparoscopic trocar access. Surg Endosc 1996; 10:775–778.
66. Romagnolo C, Minelli L. Small bowel occlusion after operative laparoscopy: Our experience and review of the literature. Endoscopy 2001; 33:88–90.
67. Bergemann JL, Hibbert ML, Harkins G, et al. Omental herniation through a 3-mm umbilical trocar site: Unmasking a hidden umbilical hernia. J Laparoendosc Adv Surg Tech A 2001; 11:171–173.
68. Wegener ME, Chung D, Crans C, Chung D. Small bowel obstruction secondary to incarerated Richter's hernia from laparoscopic hernia repair. J Laparoendosc Surg 1993; 3(3):173–176.
69. Brunt LM, Quasebarth MA, Dunnegan DL, Soper NJ. Outcomes anaylsis of laparoscopic cholecystectomy in the extremely elderly. Surg Endosc 2001; 15:700–705.
70. Terry M, Smith CD, Branum GD, Galloway K, et al. Outcomes of laparoscopic fundoplication of gastroesophageal reflux disease and paraesophageal hernia. Surg Endosc 2001; 15:691–699.
71. Schauer PR, Ikramuddin S, Gourash W, et al. Outcomes after laparoscopic Roux-en-Y gastric bypass for morbid obesity. Ann Surg 2000; 232:515–529.
72. Koehler RH, Voeller G. Recurrences in laparoscopic incisional hernia repairs: A personal series and review of the literature. JSLS 1999:293–304.
73. Phillips EH, Arregui M, Carroll BJ, et al. Incidence of complications following laparoscopic hernioplasty. Surg Endosc 1995; 9:16–21.
74. Fahlenkamp D, Rassweiler J, Fornara P, et al:. Complications of laparoscopic procedures in urology: Experience with 2,407 procedures at 4 German centers. J Urol 1999; 162:765–771.

4

Adrenalectomy

Vivian M. Sanchez and Robert W. Bailey
University of Miami School of Medicine, Miami, Florida, U.S.A.

INTRODUCTION

Bartolomeo Eustachius first described the anatomy of the adrenal gland in 1563 [1]. In 1886, Fraenkel was the first to describe a patient with an adrenal tumor [2]. The first description of laparoscopic adrenal surgery in the literature was by Higashihara in 1992 using an abdominal lift technique combined with CO_2 insufflation [3]. Gagner went on to popularize the currently used technique later in 1992 [4]. In the last 10 years, the laparoscopic approach has evolved to become the standard of care for removal of the adrenal gland in most situations. Laparoscopic adrenalectomy is a safe and effective procedure with morbidity rates of less than 11% and mortality rates less than 1% [5].

Anatomy

A thorough understanding of the anatomy is essential to the safe performance of laparoscopic adrenal surgery. Although the left and right glands are symmetrically imbedded in Gerota's fascia and are in close proximity to the diaphragmatic crura, they have different anatomical relationships to the surrounding viscera. The right adrenal gland is bordered by the inferior vena cava on its medial side, the liver on its superior and anterior aspect, and the kidney posteriorly and laterally. At times, the second portion of the duodenum may drape the inferior aspect of the gland. Complete exposure of the organ therefore may sometimes require a Kocher maneuver. The left adrenal gland is bordered by the spleen and pancreas superiorly, the aorta medially, the renal hilum inferiorly, and the kidney posteriorly. In laparoscopic surgery, these anatomical relationships are important during the initial approach and exposure of the adrenal gland. On the right, the right lobe of the liver must first be retracted superiorly before dissection of the gland can begin. On the left, the splenic flexure of the colon and the inferior attachments of the spleen must also be mobilized in order to expose the adrenal gland.

The arterial supply to the adrenal gland is symmetrical bilaterally. Each gland is supplied by the superior, middle, and inferior adrenal arteries, which arise from the inferior phrenic artery, abdominal aorta, and renal artery, respectively (Fig. 1). These arteries usually branch frequently and early, making it appear as if there were many small vessels supplying the gland rather than a true hilum. The venous drainage of the glands is mostly through one main or central adrenal vein. In addition, the right adrenal gland typically has several small accessory veins that empty along its medial aspect directly into the vena cava. These small branches can easily be injured leading to some troublesome bleeding during the operative procedure (Fig. 2). The main right adrenal vein typically drains from the superior border of the gland directly into the posterolateral aspect of the inferior vena cava. The right adrenal vein is usually quite short, only 0.5–1.0

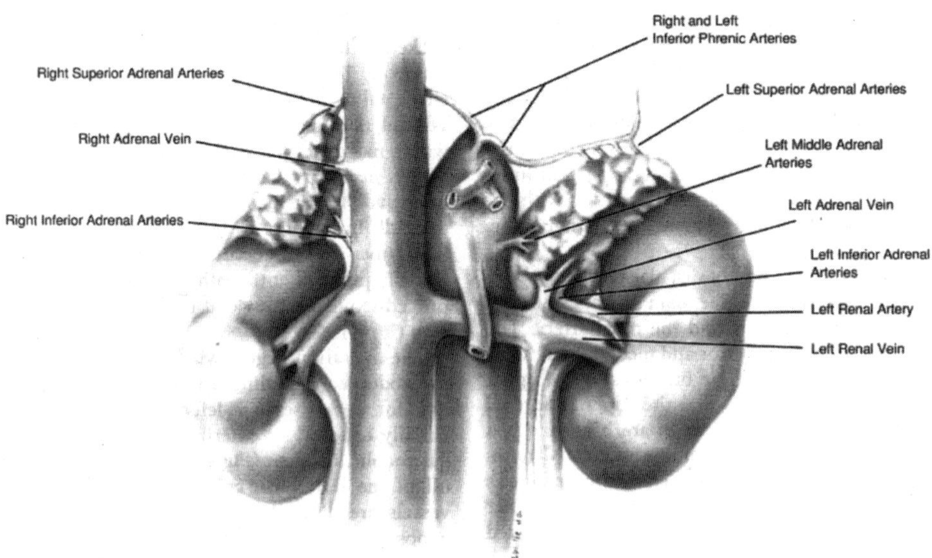

FIGURE 1 Anatomy of adrenal gland. (From Ref. 33.)

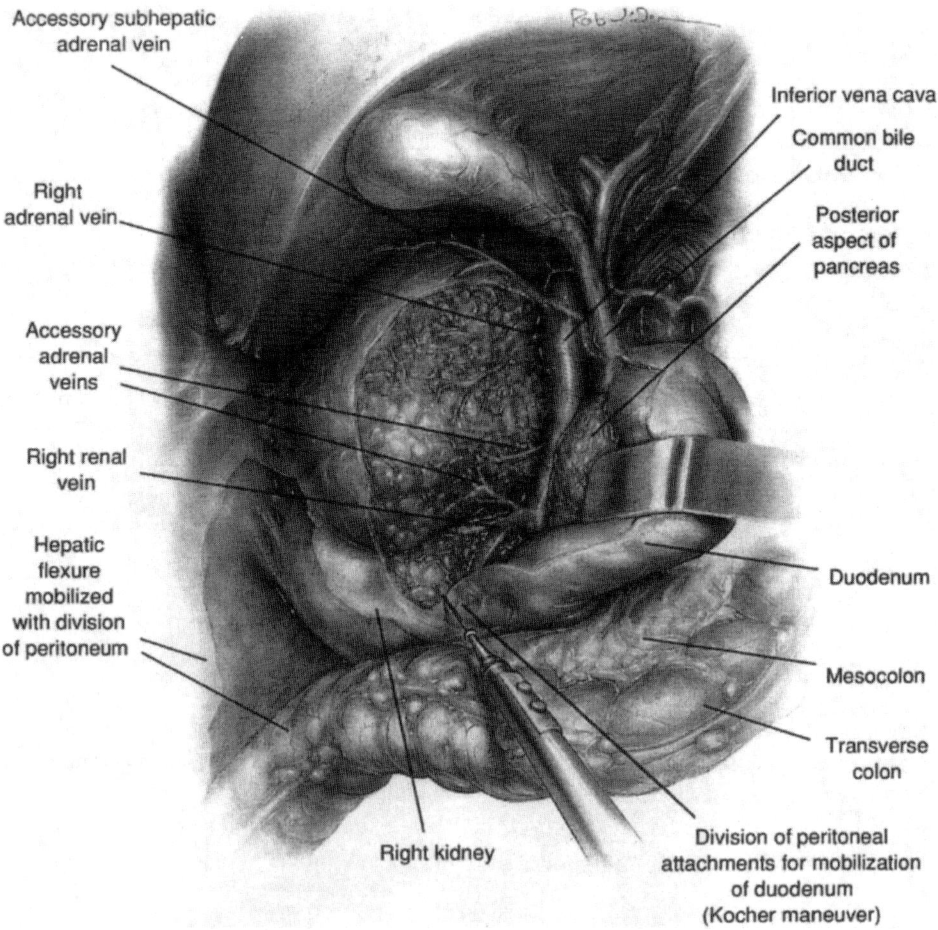

Figure 2 Accessory adrenal veins and their anatomic location. (From Ref. 33.)

cm in length, making its dissection and ligation difficult, with little room for error. The left adrenal vein most commonly empties into the left renal vein and is longer than the right adrenal vein; it is 2–3 cm in length. Furthermore, variations of these venous drainage patterns occur in 5–6% of cases and can predispose to intraoperative bleeding [6]. Some examples include a right adrenal vein that empties into the hepatic veins and an anomalous or aberrant left adrenal vein that is seen in association with variations of the left renal vein. A detailed knowledge of these vascular relationships is critical to avoiding many of the complications encountered during laparoscopic adrenalectomy. It is also important for the surgeon to be knowledgeable about the endocrine function of the adrenal gland, since the majority of adrenalectomies are performed for overproduction of one the adrenal hormones. Although small in size, weighing only 4–6 g each, the adrenal gland has two distinct anatomical and functional regions. The outer region, the adrenal cortex, is characteristically yellow in color and has three discrete zones. The zona glomerulosa secretes aldosterone, the zona fasciculata secretes cortisol, and the zona reticularis secretes androgens and estrogens. The inner region, the adrenal medulla, is of neural crest origin and is responsible for the secretion of catecholamines such as epinephrine and norepinephrine. This region is highly vascular and rich preganglionic sympathetic innervation.

Indications

The current indications for laparoscopic adrenalectomy include both functional, hormone-producing lesions and nonfunctional lesions. Either type may be benign or malignant. The most common indications for laparoscopic adrenalectomy are Conn's syndrome (primary hyperaldosteronism, 38%), Cushing's syndrome (21%), nonfunctioning adrenal masses (21%), pheochromocytoma (17%), and malignancy (3%) [5,7] (Fig. 3).

Incidentalomas are typically nonfunctioning adrenal lesions discovered unexpectedly during abdominal computed tomography (CT) or magnetic resonance imaging (MRI) that is being performed for other diagnostic purposes. The incidence of such masses as detected by CT is between 0.4–4.4% [8]. While any functional adrenal adenoma regardless of size should be resected, the management of incidentalomas is a little more complex and controversial. It is generally agreed that lesions larger than 5 cm or those with evidence of rapid growth on a repeat CT scan should be removed. Lesions smaller than 3 cm can simply be observed,

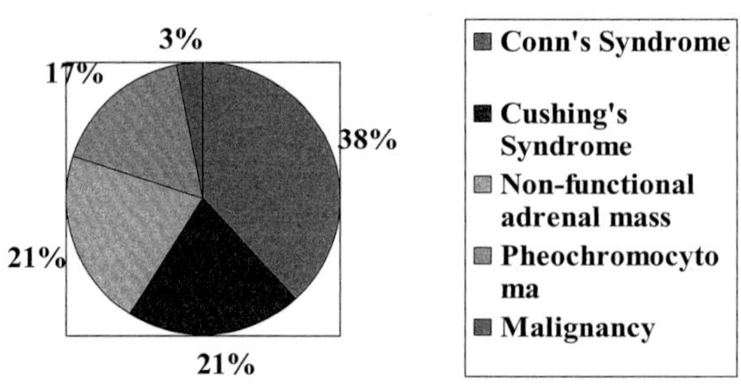

FIGURE 3 Common indications for laparoscopic adrenalectomy. (Adapted from Ref. 5.)

while those between 3 and 5 cm may need closer evaluation and often come to surgery [7,9]. Given the low morbidity and quick recovery following laparoscopic adrenalectomy, some centers even advocate the routine removal of all lesions greater than 4 cm.

Other less common indications for adrenalectomy include adrenocortical hyperplasia, virilizing/feminizing tumors, benign adrenal lesions, and metastatic disease. Adrenocortical hyperplasia, otherwise known as Cushing's disease, is a condition that may require bilateral adrenalectomy if medical therapy has been unsuccessful. Virilizing or feminizing tumors, usually seen in childhood, are rare but well-established indications for adrenalectomy. Additional indications for surgery include benign lesions, such as angiomyolipoma, adrenal cysts and pseudocysts, and isolated metastatic lesions (usually originating from melanoma or from lung, breast, or colon cancer), which are also indications for laparoscopic adrenalectomy. Metastatic disease was formerly considered a relative contraindication to surgery. However, as more experience has been gained, recent studies suggest that it can be done safely with recurrence rates similar to those of an open approach [10,11]. Even primary adrenal cancers without evidence of direct invasion can be safely removed laparoscopically; however, concern remains over the risk of local tumor recurrence [11].

Tumor size has also been used to determine whether or not a particular lesion is amenable to laparoscopic removal. Tumor size is of concern for two reasons. The first relates to the risk of harboring occult malignancy within the mass itself. Adrenal masses greater than 4 cm have a 22% probability of harboring a malignant tumor [12]. Tumor size is also important due to the obvious limitations it imposes on the surgeon's ability to gain adequate exposure and vascular control. For these reasons, previous studies have advocated the removal of large tumors (> 6 cm) via an open approach. However, a recent study by MacGillivray and colleagues [13] did not demonstrate any significant difference in operative time, blood loss, hospital stay, or locoregional recurrence between a laparoscopic and an open approach for tumors between 6 and 12 cm.

Absolute contraindications to laparoscopic adrenalectomy are few. Adrenocortical cancer with direct invasion of contiguous structures or renal vein involvement usually mandates an open approach so that an en bloc resection may be performed. Uncontrolled coagulopathy, portal hypertension, and enlargement of the right hepatic lobe (preventing exposure of the right adrenal gland) are other examples. In addition, the general contraindications associated with all types of laparoscopic procedures, such as severe cardiac or pulmonary dysfunction, will always need to be considered prior to embarking on a laparoscopic adrenalectomy.

IDENTIFICATION OF COMPLICATIONS

The overall mortality rate associated with laparoscopic adrenalectomy is quite low, with a cited incidence of 0.5% [14]. The overall morbidity rate following laparoscopic adrenalectomy is also acceptable, usually being in the range of 8–12% [14,15]. Unfortunately, complications following adrenal surgery are often iatrogenic in nature and occur as a result of perioperative bleeding or overwhelming sepsis from a missed intraoperative bowel injury.

One of the largest published reviews [5] of laparoscopic adrenalectomy, which summarizes the experience with 1522 patients, found an overall complication rate of 10.9% (range 4–15%) and a mortality rate of 0.3% (Table 1). The most common complication following laparoscopic adrenalectomy is bleeding, which and can be expected in 5% of cases [5,16]. It is usually due to injury or avulsion of an adrenal vein at or near its junction to the vena cava or renal vein [17]. Some 2–5% of all patients undergoing adrenalectomy will require blood transfusion [5,18]. Conversion to an open procedure is usually required in these cases in order to gain adequate control of the bleeding source. Published conversion rates are in the range of only 1.6–4%, with 30% of these conversions being performed solely for the control of bleeding [5,14,18].

Other major complications include infectious problems (1.6%), wound complications (1.4%), pulmonary complications such as pneumonia, effusions, atelectasis and pleural tears leading to pneumothorax (0.9%), and visceral injury (0.7%). Deep venous thrombosis as well as urinary and cardiac complications are less likely to occur and are reported in less than 0.5% of cases [5,19]. Other rarely reported complications include pulmonary embolus, incisional hernia, and rare instances of injury to the kidney, ureters, spleen, pancreas, and liver.

Complications of laparoscopic adrenalectomy specific for adrenal malignancy include port site recurrence, local recurrence, and diffuse peritoneal dissemination of disease. There is still debate as to whether or not a laparoscopic approach should be used in dealing with adrenal malignancies, especially primary adrenal cancers. Unfortunately, information regarding adrenalectomy for cancer is scarce, and it is difficult to draw any strong conclusions. The major indication for surgery in most series is for isolated adrenal metastases. Among the two largest series [10,11] reporting on this topic, only one [11] included patients who presented with primary adrenal cancer. The incidence of local recurrences in this study was 13%, all occurring in those patients who had a primary adrenal malignancy. The incidence of local recurrences was 0% in the other study, where no patients had primary adrenal cancer. This experience is to be contrasted to that from open surgery, where the locoregional recurrence rate is as high as 60% [11]. Fortunately, regardless of the type of malignancy, the incidence of port site recurrence and diffuse peritoneal dissemination appears to be 0% [10,11]. Overall, the existing data, although limited in scope, suggest that laparoscopic adrenalectomy for isolated metastatic disease to the adrenal gland and for primary adrenal cancer confined to the adrenal gland is safe and does not compromise the oncological outcome.

TABLE 1 Complications and Mortality During Laparoscopic Adrenalectomy

Author, Year	Number of Patients	Total Complications	Deaths	Bleeding	Transfusions	Conversions	Organ Injury	Wound	GI	DVT	Infectious	Pulmonary
Kebebew, 2002 [11]	176	9 (5.1%)	1(0.5%)	1(0.5%)	ND[a]	0	0	1(0.5%)	0	0	1(0.5%)	1(0.5%)
Pilinger, 2002 [34]	59	4 (6.7%)	0	1(1.7%)	1(1.7%)	3(5.1%)	0	1(1.7%)	0	0	0	0
Brunt, 2001 [5]	1522	166 (10.9%)	5(0.3%)	71(4.7%)	27(1.8%)	ND	11(0.7%)	22(1.4%)	6(0.7%)	7(0.5%)	24(1.6%)	14(0.9%)
Gagner, 1997 [14]	100	12(12%)	0	4(4%)	2(2%)	3(3%)	0	0	1(1%)	3(3%)	1(1%)	3(3%) two pulmonary emboli
Total	1,857	191(10.2%)	6(0.3%)	77(4.1%)	30(1.7%)	6(1.8%)	11(0.6%)	24(1.3%)	7(0.4%)	10(0.5%)	26(1.4%)	18(1.0%)

Abbreviations: GI = gastrointestinal; DVT = deep venous thrombosis; ND = no data.

Complications of laparoscopic adrenalectomy may also occur as a result of the hormonal imbalances created by functional adenomas. One of the most common medical conditions seen with these tumors is hypertension. This may occur as a result of all three of the common functional conditions (primary hyperaldosteronsim, pheochromocytoma, and Cushing's syndrome). In addition to hypertension, patients with functional tumors are at risk for other metabolic problems, such as hypokalemia (Conn's syndrome), malignant hypertension, stroke, flushing and arrhythymias (pheochromocytoma), and diabetes (Cushing's syndrome). In addition, the mere treatment of these tumors, especially their surgical removal, may lead to sudden decreases in high levels of circulating hormones. These changes may lead to hypotension, acute adrenal insufficiency (Addisonian crisis), and hypoglycemia. By contrast, adrenal manipulation during surgery for pheochromocytoma may lead to the sudden release of catecholamines. This may lead to severe, uncontrolled hypertension, stroke, myocardial infarction, and even intraoperative mortality. Interestingly, it appears that patients with pheochromocytomas are more likely to be selected for an open procedure than for a laparoscopic approach [5].

PREOPERATIVE EVALUATION

A thorough and well-directed preoperative evaluation of patients with adrenal pathology is paramount to a successful outcome. The surgeon must have an excellent working knowledge of the specific disease process requiring surgical intervention. Since many adrenal lesions are found incidentally, workup of these lesions mandates a detailed history and physical examination directed toward the underlying etiology of the adrenal disease. The patient's history is carefully evaluated for the presence of hypertension, diabetes, muscular weakness, paresthesias, polyuria and polydipsia, diaphoresis, palpitations, flushing, headaches, easy bruising, prior cancer, weight loss or weight gain, changes in body habitus, or a family history of multiple endocrine neoplasia (MEN) type II. The patient should be examined for the presence of prior abdominal or flank incisions, skin fragility, poor wound healing, central obesity, facial hirsutism, moon facies, buffalo hump appearance, depressive psychosis, and virilization/feminization characteristics.

Finally but perhaps most important, the functionality of any adrenal lesion must be thoroughly evaluated, usually by extensive preoperative testing. The initial laboratory screening tests used to determine the functionality of an incidental adrenal mass include a serum potassium level; glucose tolerance test; 24-hr urinary metanephrine, vanillylmandelic acid, and catecholamine levels; plasma catecholamine levels; and 24-hr urinary free cortisol levels (Table 2).

TABLE 2 Initial Screening for the Functionality of an Adrenal Mass

• Serum	• Urine (24-hr)
– Potassium	– Metanephrines
– Glucose tolerance	– Catecholamines
– Catecholamines	– Vanillylmandelic acid (VMA)
	– Free cortisol

All patients found to have an adrenal mass should have a chest radiograph to evaluate the potential for metastatic disease, as the most common primary malignancy to metastasize to the adrenal gland is lung cancer. If there is a known history of cancer, the cancer should be thoroughly staged and any extra-adrenal lesion biopsied. Extra-adrenal metastasis would indicate disseminated disease; thus these patients would be better served by a course of chemotherapy rather than by surgery.

Specific Preoperative Hormonal Evaluation

Conn's Syndrome (Primary Hyperaldosteronism)

Conn's syndrome presents with signs and symptoms related to overproduction of aldosterone. This entity is due to an autonomous solitary adreno cortical adenoma in 80% of cases [8]. The remaining 20% are due to bilateral cortical hyperplasia (idiopathic hyperaldosteronism) resulting in excess hormone production. Most aldosterone-producing adenomas are less than 2 cm in diameter; they are unilateral in 95% of cases [8]. The syndrome is characterized by hypertension (as a result of intravascular volume expansion from sodium retention), hypokalemia (<3.5 mmol/L), headaches, muscular weakness, paresthesias, polyuria, and polydipsia. Often, unexplained hypokalemia is the first sign to suggest the presence of an aldosteronoma.

The workup for aldosteronoma includes measurements of morning (8 a.m.) plasma aldosterone and renin levels. The patient with an aldosterone-secreting adenoma has an elevated plasma aldosterone level associated with a decreased plasma renin level. If the ratio of plasma aldosterone to plasma renin is greater than or equal to 20, a diagnosis of primary hyperaldosteronism is almost guaranteed. It is impossible to interpret data when a patient is on medications that might affect aldosterone or renin levels, such as spironolactone. Such medications should be stopped for at least 6 weeks prior to measuring the appropriate hormone levels [8]. If there is any question as to the diagnosis, a 24-hr urine aldosterone may be obtained, with levels greater than 20 μ/day suggesting primary hyperaldosteronism. On rare occasions, renal vein sampling for aldosterone is necessary, usually in cases where the tumor cannot be localized by preoperative imaging studies. Localization of aldosteronomas with renal vein sampling may be required in cases of unilateral adrenal hyperplasia—an extremely rare circumstance. In such cases, it may be impossible to determine from the CT or MRI alone which is the affected gland. The other indication for venous sampling is bilateral adrenal hyperplasia. It this case, both adrenal glands would have to be removed in order to provide a complete surgical cure. Therefore one might prefer to document that both glands are actively producing abnormally high levels of aldosterone before recommending such aggressive surgical treatment. Due to the serious side effects resulting from bilateral adrenalectomy, however, this disease is usually treated with aggressive medical therapy, not surgery [20]. Unfortunately, venous sampling is difficult to perform and the success rate is dependent on the experience of the interventional radiologist. Success rates may vary from 74–93% [21].

Cushing's Syndrome

Cushing's syndrome results from an excess production of glucocorticoids. It can be caused by a number of conditions, including a pituitary adenoma secreting excess ACTH (Cushing's disease), ectopic production of adrenocorticotropic hormone (ACTH)—usually due to an underlying malignancy such as lung or pancreatic cancer or a thymoma—or finally, excess cortisol secretion due to an adrenal adenoma, adrenal hyperplasia, or an adrenal carcinoma. Adrenal adenomas account for only 10–20% of all causes of Cushing's syndrome [8]. Cushing's disease caused by a pituitary adenoma is the most common etiology of excess cortisol production. Physical features include skin friability, easy bruising, central obesity, purple striae, poor wound healing, facial hirsutism, hypertension, glucose intolerance, hypokalemia, moon facies, buffalo hump appearance, and depressive psychosis. The pattern of onset of symptoms is important. Rapidly progressing signs of cortisol excess are more common with ectopic ACTH production, seen with rapidly growing primary tumors. Cushing's syndrome caused by an adrenal adenoma or hyperplasia typically has a more gradual onset of symptoms. Adrenal carcinomas often produce additional androgens, making hirsutism and virilization a more common phenomenon, which is not usually seen with adenomas or ectopic ACTH production [22].

If Cushing's syndrome is suspected, several tests may be used to help establish the diagnosis. The most useful screening test is a 24-hr urinary free cortisol level. Normally, very little free cortisol is excreted in the urine. If the levels are elevated, a diagnosis of hypercortisolism is likely. Also, patients with Cushing's syndrome do not exhibit the normal diurnal variation in plasma cortisol levels. Therefore comparison of morning and evening cortisol levels may offer insight. The next step is to confirm a diagnosis of hypercortisolism and determine the source of the excess cortisol production. Baseline cortisol levels will be elevated in cases of adrenal adenomas or cortical carcinomas. However, the levels are usually much higher in patients with cancer than in those with a benign adenoma. If the cortisol secretion level is greater than 150 μg/24 hr, the workup should proceed to a low-dose (1 mg) dexamethasone suppression test. In this test, 1 mg of dexamethasone is given between 11 p.m. and 12 a.m. and a fasting cortisol level is then obtained at 8 a.m. the following morning. Normally, low-dose dexamethasone will suppress normal amounts of pituitary-derived ACTH, thus decreasing cortisol. However, in patients with Cushing's syndrome, the cortisol remains elevated despite the low-dose suppression ($>$ 10 μg/dL). The cortisol levels in patients with adrenal neoplasms or ectopic ACTH-producing tumors will not usually be suppressed by either low- or high-dose dexamethasone. Other tests—such as plasma ACTH levels and metyrapone stimulation—may help to differentiate between pituitary, adrenal cortex or ectopic cortisol production sites. Plasma ACTH levels are usually low when the cortisol is excreted from an adrenal source, elevated or normal with a pituitary adenoma, and markedly high in patients with ectopic ACTH production [23].

Pheochromocytoma

Pheochromocytomas are tumors that secrete excess quantities of catecholamines, primarily epinephrine and norepinephrine. The characteristic signs and symptoms of this condition are uncontrolled and labile hypertension (occasionally paroxysmal in nature), headaches, diaphoresis, and feelings of apprehension or anxiety. These symptoms tend to wax and wane and typically occur in identifiable episodes or attacks. The attacks are characterized by diaphoresis, apprehension, and tachycardia and usually last from 15–60 min.

Pheochromocytomas are associated with distinct patterns of presentation. They are familial in 10–20% of cases, extra-adrenal in 10%, bilateral in 10%, and malignant in 10%. They are seen in the pediatric age group in 10%. This unique pattern gives rise to the so-called rule of tens for this disease entity.

The three familial syndromes associated with pheochromocytoma are MEN II, neurofibromatosis (von Recklinghausen's syndrome), von Hippel–Lindau disease, and hereditary paraganglioma syndrome [24]. If seen in association with a familial condition, pheochromocytomas are more likely to be multiple or bilateral. Therefore CT scans performed in this subgroup of patients should be assessed for the presence of an extra-adrenal pheochromocytoma. If there is any difficulty in accurately localizing the tumor, an iodine-125 (^{125}I) metaiodobenzylguanidine (MIBG) scan should be performed to help detect the presence of an extra-adrenal disease.

Patients suspected of having a pheochromocytoma should have 24-hr urinary measurements of metanephrine, catecholamines, and vanillylmandelic acid (VMA). Plasma levels of catecholamines should also be obtained. A diagnosis of pheochromocytoma can be confirmed with elevations in these hormonal levels. False-positive tests can result when patients are taking drugs such as phenothiazines, methyldopa, or monoamine oxidase inhibitors; therefore the patient's history should be carefully screened for this.

Preoperative Evaluation of a Suspected Adrenal Cancer

Malignant tumors of the adrenal cortex are typically functional in 50% of cases and can lead to hirsutism and virilization. High cortisol levels (>5000 nmol) in a 24-hr urine collection associated with a low plasma ACTH level can be diagnostic. A 24-hr urine collection for 17-ketosteroid should also show elevated levels. Plasma dehydroepiandrosterone (DHEA) levels may also be elevated in these patients. Less than 10% of adrenal cancers are smaller than 8 x 6 cm at the time of presentation, with the median size ranging from 10–12 cm [8]. These lesion can show radiographic evidence of local invasion, with possible extension into the inferior vena cava. Lymphadenopathy may also be apparent. Adrenal cancers have a lower lipid content on CT and MRI than adenomas and can have areas of central low attenuation due to tumor necrosis and calcifications [9,22]. Only 8% of adrenal cancers are smaller than 6 cm at the time of presentation [9]. However, lesions larger than 6 cm have a higher likelihood of malignancy. If adrenal cancer is suspected preoperatively, consideration should be given to using an open approach, especially if there are signs of local invasion.

Virilizing Tumors

Virilizing tumors are rare, but unfortunately they are often malignant. They should be suspected in cases of precocious puberty and facial hirsutism. If such a tumor is clinically suspected, a 24-hr urine collection for 17-ketosteroid, plasma testosterone, and DHEA should be obtained.

Diagnostic Imaging

CT scanning with fine 3-mm cuts through the adrenal glands is the diagnostic imaging test of choice for the evaluation of adrenal lesions. Intravenous contrast should be used except in cases of pheochromocytoma, where it can precipitate a hypertensive crisis. An adenoma characteristically appears as a homogenous lesion with smooth, encapsulated margins. MRI is also useful in the evaluation of adrenal pathology, especially in evaluating T2-weighted images of pheochromocytomas. Evidence of portal hypertension should be carefully noted, as this is a relative contraindication for laparoscopic adrenalectomy.

Tissue Sampling

The performance of a biopsy or fine-needle aspiration of adrenal lesions is controversial. Some authors speculate that preoperative biopsy will break the tumor's capsule and make tumor seeding and skin implantation more likely. Perhaps the greatest role of tissue sampling is in assessing for metastatic disease in situations where the finding of metastatic disease will change the management strategy. Studies demonstrate that fine-needle aspirates are less than 60% sensitive in correctly identifying adrenal pathology. Biopsy of pheochromocytomas can precipitate a hypertensive crisis and should be avoided. In general, fine-needle aspiration of adrenal lesions is not recommended.

PREOPERATIVE MEASURES TO PREVENT AVOIDABLE COMPLICATIONS

Most of the complications associated with laparoscopic adrenalectomy are directly related to intraoperative techniques. The few avoidable complications include deep venous thrombosis (DVT), brachial nerve and skin injuries related to patient positioning, hypertension, hypokalemia, and cardiac complications. Preoperative imaging should also be carefully reviewed to assess for aberrant renal veins or any other abnormal vascular anatomy that could lead to intraoperative complications.

Preoperative Measures in Specific Functional Adenomas

Patients with Conn's syndrome have potential complications related to hypertension and hypokalemia. Blood pressure control should be optimized preoperatively, and this will often require multiple agents. Spironolactone should be administered to decrease both intravascular volume and hypertension. Prazosin can also be used with good results for blood pressure control. Patients should consume no more than 150 mEq/day of sodium. Potassium should be corrected to keep levels $>$3.5 mEq. Ultimately, only the removal of the aldosteronoma will correct the severe hypertension. A substantial improvement in the blood pressure can be expected in 90% of patients [25].

Patients with Cushing's syndrome have problems directly related to their disease entity that require specific attention. These patients have friable skin that, as a result of exposure to excess glucocorticoids, is palpably thin and susceptible to easy bruising. Osteoporosis is also a major component. Therefore, in positioning these patients for laparoscopic adrenalectomy, they must be padded, and their skin protected; gentle care must be taken to prevent iatrogenic fractures and skin breakdown in placing these patients in the lateral decubitus position. Most importantly, patients with functional cortisol-producing adenomas have pituitary-adrenal axis suppression and atrophy of the contralateral gland. This makes them susceptible to Addisonian crisis, also known as acute adrenal insufficiency. As a result, all patients undergoing unilateral or bilateral adrenalectomy for hypercortisolism should receive perioperative steroids. The current recommendation for steroid administration is 50–60 mg of hydrocortisone on the day of surgery and for the first 24 hr thereafter [26]. Some advocate using a cortisol-lowering medication such as ketoconazole or RU-486, an antiglucocorticoid agent.

Patients with pheochromocytoma have specific potential complications related to excess catecholamines, such as hypertensive crisis, arrhythmias, and stroke. Induction of anesthesia and surgical resection without perioperative blockade is associated with an unacceptably high mortality rate of up to 50% [24]. Alpha-antagonists should be started at least two weeks before surgery for preoperative blood pressure control. The most commonly used agent is phenoxybenzamine at a dose of 10 mg every 12 hr. This dosage can be titrated based on blood pressure; some use nasal congestion as an endpoint for the titration of alpha blockade. A preoperative dose of phenoxybenzamine of 1 mg/kg given at the midnight before surgery is also recommended by Walther [24]. Beta blockade can be initiated *after* initial treatment with phenoxybenzamine for persistent tachycardia greater than 100. There is some controversy; however, most will agree that beta blockade should not be used as first-line therapy to prevent unopposed alpha effects and exacerbation of hypertension. The medications should be titrated slowly so as to prevent episodic bursts of tachycardia and hypertension. In difficult cases of blood pressure control, metyrosine, a tyrosine hydroxylase inhibitor, can be used. Walther advocates its use as combination therapy even if blood pressure is well controlled with phenoxybenzamine, since it decreases tumor catecholamine content by 50–80% if used for 2 weeks preoperatively. Finally, patients should be volume loaded with intravenous fluids the day prior to the procedure.

INTRAOPERATIVE MEASURES TO PREVENT COMPLICATIONS

Patient Positioning and Operating Room Setup

Proper setup of equipment and personnel in the operating room is essential to a laparoscopic adrenalectomy. The surgeon and assistant/camera holder will usually stand on the same side of the patient (Fig. 4A). Patient positioning is critical to preventing complications, since laparoscopic adrenalectomy relies on gravity to aid with proper exposure. Proper exposure is the key to adequately visualizing the anatomy. First, a roll is placed underneath the axilla and the flanks are lined up with the break in the table. The table is then flexed and the kidney elevated to maximize exposure. The hips are secured to the table to prevent the patient from slipping. The superior arm is suspended and gently padded to prevent brachial plexus injuries (Fig. 4B).

In general, patients should have pneumatic compression stockings placed prior to the induction of anesthesia. The use of prophylactic thromboembolic

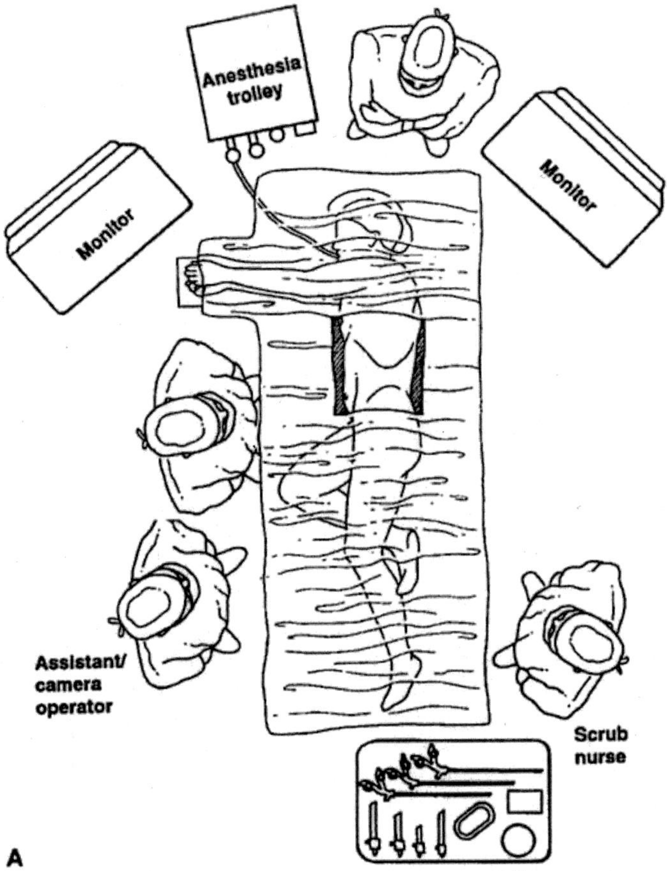

A

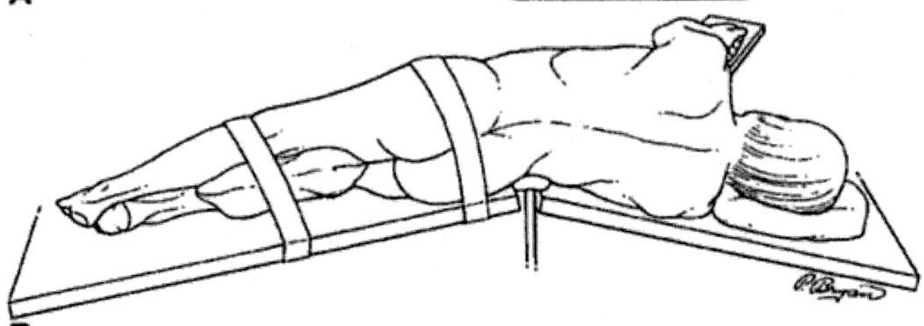

B

FIGURE 4 A. Operating room setup for a laparoscopic left adrenalectomy. The patient and room are reversed for a laparoscopic right adrenalectomy. B. Proper patient positioning during a lateral transabdominal approach to laparoscopic adrenalectomy. Note that the patient is supported, often using a beanbag, with the table break at the iliac crest. The knees are slightly flexed. The arm is gently positioned on an armrest. (From Ref. 15.)

medication is controversial, as the rate of DVT is low, at only 0.5%, in laparoscopic adrenalectomy. Since laparoscopic adrenalectomies are considered clean cases, preoperative antibiotics are not indicated. Bowel preparation is usually not indicated.

Operative Technique

There are three laparoscopic techniques used to perform laparoscopic adrenalectomy. The first and most favored technique in over 90% of cases is the *lateral transabdominal approach* [7,14]. It involves placing the patient in a lateral decubitus position with the affected adrenal on the up side (Fig. 4). This approach utilizes gravity to assist with traction and exposure. Its main disadvantage is that patients must be repositioned if the opposite adrenal must be excised. It can also be difficult if dense adhesions are encountered from previous abdominal surgery. It is the most popular technique because of the familiar anatomy, easy exposure, and large working area. The second approach is the *anterior transperitoneal approach*. This can be a useful technique if a bilateral adrenalectomy is indicated. Unfortunately, the surgeon loses natural retraction and more ports are then needed to retract adjacent structures. This approach can also be difficult if dense intra-abdominal adhesions are found. Another option is the *posterior retroperitoneal approach*, which requires that the patient be placed in a prone jackknife position. All dissection is performed in the retroperitoneal space, never entering the peritoneum. This technique is useful for patients with prior abdominal operations. Its main disadvantage is that vascular control can de difficult to obtain if bleeding occurs. In addition to the small working space, the area can become even smaller if the peritoneum is entered inadvertently during dissection, making visualization even worse.

There does not appear to be any significant difference in outcomes among these three approaches, so surgeon preference will determine the operative technique [27].

Lateral Transperitoneal Approach

With this technique, the surgeon stands facing the patient with the table rotated slightly away from him or her. Patients should be prepped from beyond the midline anteriorly to the midline posteriorly and from the costal margin superiorly down to the iliac crests inferiorly. If the patient has had prior abdominal operations, an open Hassan technique should be used to enter the abdomen.

The patient should be placed in reverse Trendelenburg to allow intra-abdominal structures like the colon and small bowel to fall caudally and thus maximize exposure. Three to four 10-mm trocars are placed 2–3 cm underneath the costal margin (Figs. 5 and 6). The trocars should be at least 5 cm apart so as to prevent inadvertent conflict between the instruments. A 30-degree camera

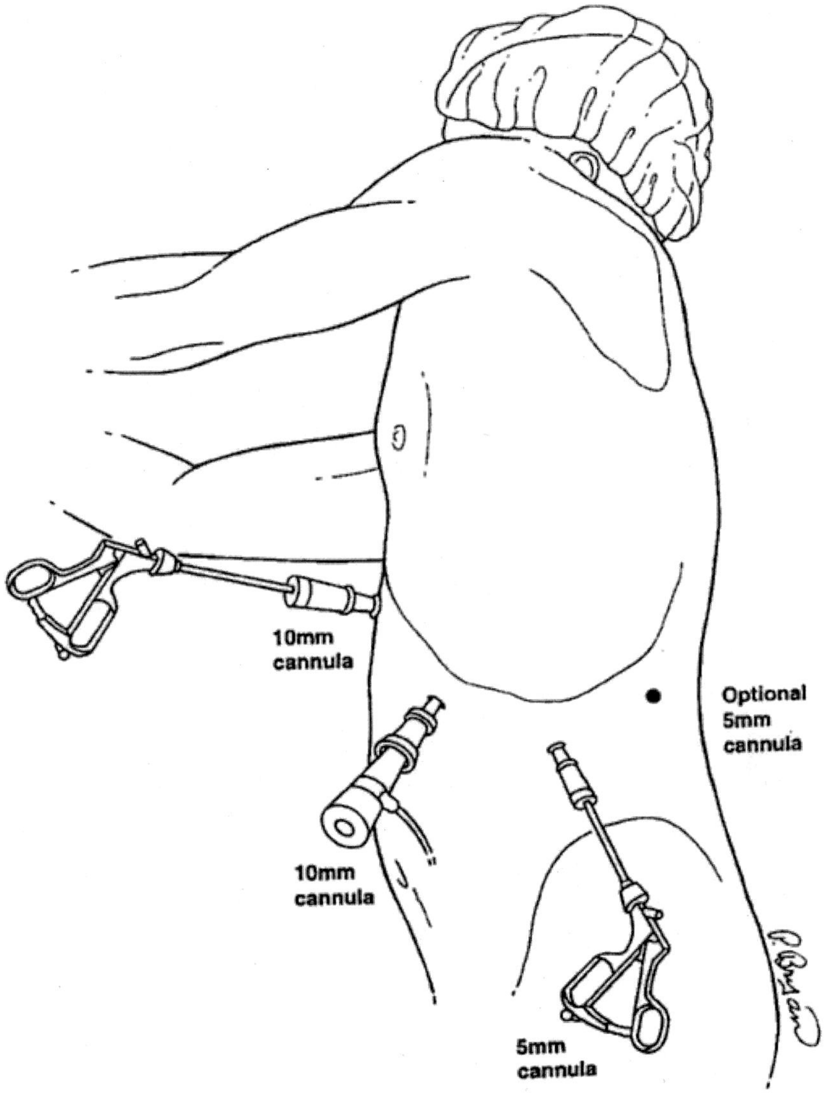

Figure 5 Port placement for a lateral transabdominal laparoscopic approach to the Left adrenal gland. Note that usually only three ports are used and an optional fourth port can be placed laterally if more exposure is needed. (From Ref. 15.)

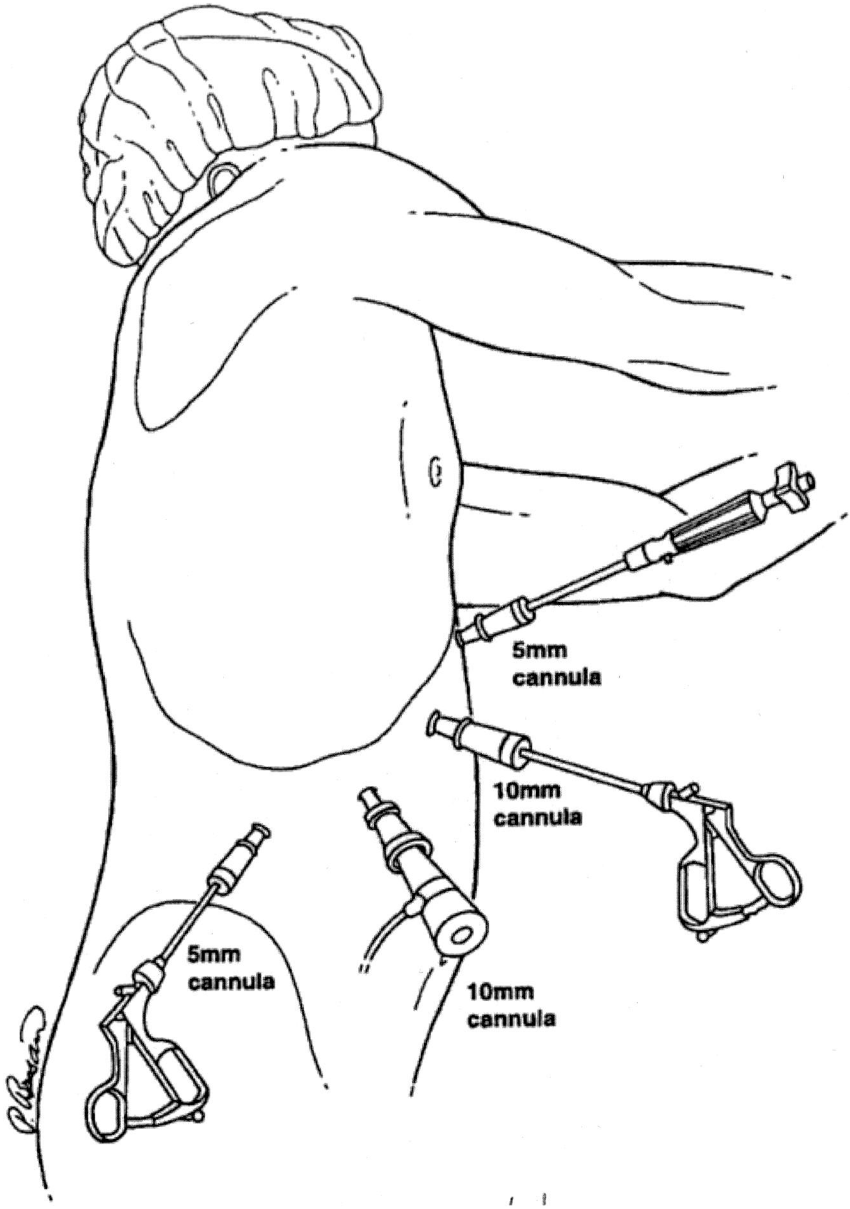

Figure 6 Port placement for lateral transabdominal approach to the right adrenal gland. Note that four ports are used and that the medial most port is used to secure the liver retractor. (From Ref. 15.)

should be used to maximize exposure. Some surgeons use only 5-mm ports with a 5-mm 30-degree scope. The entire abdomen is assessed, looking for evidence of metastatic disease or other pathology.

For a laparoscopic left adrenalectomy, the spleen and colon are mobilized medially as a unit to expose the lienorenal ligament. The dissection should be carried all the way up to the diaphragm. This allows the spleen to fall medially, exposing the retroperitoneal space. The adrenal gland, the adrenal mass, and the adrenal vein are identified. Gerota's fascia should not be entered until adequate identification of all structures is performed, since it is such a highly vascular area and bleeding can be encountered. Laparoscopic ultrasound may be useful in this identification. Grasping the perinephric fat, dissect the medial and inferior pole. Be sure to avoid grasping the adrenal gland or tumor directly, as the tissue may tear and bleed. One pitfall involves dissecting out the lateral attachments too early. This allows the adrenal to flip forward, so that the surgeon loses exposure of the hilum. After the medial and inferior portions of the adrenal are dissected, the adrenal vein should be visible. Control of the vessel can be obtained with a right-angle dissector. As dissection is continued upward, adrenal branches of the inferior phrenic vessels are ligated. Clip and divide the adrenal vein last except in cases of pheochromocytoma, where it should be clipped first. The vein should be clipped with at least two clips on each side to prevent inadvertent slips. The adrenal is then placed in an impermeable nylon bag and withdrawn through the original trocar site. The trocar site may have to be extended slightly. Finally, all 10-mm ports are closed to prevent postoperative hernias.

For a laparoscopic right adrenalectomy, the positioning is, of course, reversed from that used for the left adrenalectomy. The surgeon works through the two most lateral ports with a dissector and scissors. The fan retractor should be placed several centimeters below the costal margin in the most anterior, epigastric region to allow the angle of retraction to be parallel to the undersurface of the right lobe of the liver. The lateral right hepatic attachments are divided along with the right triangular ligament. The right hepatic lobe is mobilized cephalad and medially. The adrenal gland is identified after the peritoneum is entered and the liver retracted. The fan retractor is placed through the lateral most post. Care should be taken to stabilize the fan retractor so as to prevent inadvertent liver injury. A Kocher maneuver may be needed to fully expose the adrenal gland. The inferolateral edge of the right adrenal gland is identified and dissected inferiorly. The adrenal branches of the inferior phrenic vein are clipped and divided as the dissection is completed upward. Dissection is then carried caudally to identify the adrenal vein, which is clipped and divided.

Technical Considerations to Prevent Intraoperative Complications

- Use local anesthesia pre-emptively at port sites to minimize postoperative pain.

- Always inspect the abdomen thoroughly for extra-adrenal disease.
- Use of specialized equipment and instrumentation:
  - Ultrasonic tissue dissector
  - 30-degree laparoscope
  - Right-angle clip applier
  - Laparoscopic ultrasound to help identify small adrenal lesions
  - Use of a hand-assist device for large tumors
  - Impermeable and durable specimen retrieval bag
- Mobilize the spleen and colon as a single unit to prevent damage to the spleen.
- Preserve the adrenal capsule in cases of malignancy. The capsule must be preserved carefully and contact with the skin through the ports avoided.
- Do not morcellate adrenal lesions, so as to preserve architecture.
- Maintain close communication with the anesthesiologist in cases of pheochromocytoma.
- Use of sponges, placed laparoscopically, to control bleeding.

Intraoperative Management of Pheochromocytoma

The intraoperative management of pheochromocytoma deserves special mention. Its successful operative management depends on invasive monitoring and central access to anticipate and attend to rapid blood pressure shifts, volume management, minimal grasping of the tumor, and early ligation of the vein. The anesthesiology team must work closely with the surgeons. Agents such as halothane, which sensitize the myocardium to catecholeamines, should be avoided [24]. Surgeons must notify anesthesia when the tumor is being manipulated so that changes can be anticipated. Sodium nitroprusside is the drip of choice for the control of hypertension, since it can be rapidly titrated. Despite all efforts, however, systolic blood pressure changes as high as 200 mmHg can be expected in 67% of cases [28,29]. Tachycardia should be controlled with intravenous administration of beta blockers [24]. Hypoglycemia may also occur secondary to the sudden withdrawal of catecholamines. This can result in uncontrolled hypotension if the condition is not anticpated. Frequent blood sugar checks should be performed intraoperatively after the adrenal vein is ligated. The treatment is volume replacement with dextrose.

POSTOPERATIVE MEASURES TO PREVENT COMPLICATIONS

Postoperative complications following laparoscopic adrenalectomy may present in many forms. Potential problems include bleeding, ileus, hematomas, atelectasis, deep venous thrombosis (DVT), hypotension, hypoglycemia, and adrenal insufficiency (addisonian crisis). Several general measures should be routinely employed to prevent postoperative complications. Early ambulation may help to prevent DVT and incentive spirometry may prevent atelectasis. Antihypertensive medications should be carefully managed to prevent hypo- or hypertension and serum hematocrit levels should be checked regularly during the immediate postoperative period to assess for bleeding. Serial glucose monitoring may help to prevent hypo- or hyperglycemia and potassium levels should be checked. Perioperative steroids should be routinely administered to patients with Cushing's syndrome.

Patients undergoing unilateral adrenalectomy for hypercortisolism should be maintained on 50–60 mg of hydrocortisone per day on the day of surgery and for the first 24 hr thereafter. Once a patient is tolerating oral intake, 25 mg/day of hydrocortisone (or equivalent, such as prednisone) should be started. Oral steroids should be continued until an ACTH-stimulation test has demonstrated a normal pituitary-adrenal axis. The recovery of this axis can take up to 2 years. Bilateral adrenalectomy will require the replacement of mineralocorticoids or the administration of fluodrocortisone acetate (Florinef) for life.

CLINICAL SIGNS AND WORKUP FOR SUSPECTED POSTOPERATIVE COMPLICATIONS

Bleeding

Intraoperative bleeding is usually recognized immediately. Treatment consists of suction to maximize visualization; therefore the suction device should be open and available for all cases of laparoscopic adrenalectomy. The introduction of a sponge into the peritoneal cavity can also help hold pressure and improve visualization. Postoperative bleeding should be suspected if the patient has unexplained tachycardia, hypotension, or shoulder pain. A hematocrit should be obtained postoperatively if there is any suspicion of bleeding.

Organ Injury

Intraoperatively, careful inspection of the abdomen prior to closure, with meticulous attention to evaluation of the colon, is key. Postoperatively, unexplained tachycardia, mental status changes, hypotension, and abdominal pain are signs of potential injury to other organs and should be worked up aggressively. Early exploration, laparoscopically or otherwise, is indicated.

Wound Complications

Early wound complications are usually infectious. Careful tissue handling and sterility is the key to prevention of these. If cellulitis is suspected, oral antibiotics should be started in a timely manner. Late wound complications include hernias, chronic pain, and numbness. These can be avoided by the closure of port sites larger than 5 mm and maintaining a distance from the costal margin while placing ports, so as to avoid injury to the intercostal bundle.

Pulmonary Complications

If respiratory insufficiency develops early postoperatively, the diagnosis of a pneumothorax from diaphragmatic injury should be considered. A chest x-ray should be obtained. If a pneumothorax is visualized and is small, it can be observed with serial films. If the pneumothorax is large, enlarges on serial imaging, or is a tension pneumothorax, rapid decompression with a chest tube is indicated.

Although DVT is rare, usually being documented in less than 1% of cases, pulmonary emboli should be considered in any patient with unexplained tachycardia or a new onset of respiratory distress. An arterial blood gas should be obtained to check for hypoxemia and respiratory alkalosis; a duplex scan of the lower extremities may detect the presence of lower extremity thrombus. Although these studies may be highly suggestive of a pulmonary embolus, a definite diagnosis can be made only by a spiral CT scan with intravenous contrast or a pulmonary angiogram. Treatment consists of careful anticoagulation or placement of an anti-embolus filter.

Respiratory insufficiency can also occur in patients with Cushing's syndrome because of their abnormal body habitus as well as the possibility of an addisonian crisis.

Addisonian Crisis

Any patient undergoing surgery for Cushing's syndrome is at risk for the development of acute adrenal insufficiency (Addisonian crisis). Hypotension, hypoglycemia, hyponatremia, fever, mental status changes, confusion, and weakness are all signs of the condition. Often the early signs are subtle and can manifest as lethargy. If addisonian crisis is suspected, hydrocortisone 100 mg IV should be administered and then continued for 24 hr at a dosage of 100 mg IV every 8 hr. To prevent Addisonian crisis from developing, surgeons should have a high awareness of it, carefully write for tapering of the steroid dosage and check a metabolic profile the morning after surgery to check for hyponatremia and hypoglycemia.

If a patient who has undergone a unilateral adrenalectomy for hypercortisolism shows signs of persistent hypercortisolism, incomplete resection or bilateral disease should be considered.

Nelson's Syndrome

Nelson's syndrome is a late condition that occurs in less than 10% of patients having bilateral adrenalectomies [30]. It is a result of a locally invasive and enlarging pituitary macroadenoma that produces elevated levels of ACTH. The tumor is believed to develop as a feedback mechanism due to the lack of hormonal secretion after bilateral adrenalectomy. The enlarging pituitary macroadenoma leads to visual symptoms, headaches, increased skin pigmentation, and gynecomastia due to hyperprolactinemia. The treatment is usually transphenoidal pituitary resection.

Conn's syndrome

Patients should be monitored for postoperative hypotension and their medications adjusted accordingly. Success rates for a unilateral aldosteronoma resection are between 60 and 80%. Prognostic factors associated with a higher success rate are age less than 44, preoperative response to spironolactone, hypertension for less than 5 years, and, on pathology, absence of multinodular disease.

Mineralocorticoid deficiency after aldosteronoma excision is a known entity and is characterized by salt wasting, hyponatremia, and hyperkalemia. The treatment is fluodrocortisone acetate (Florinef).

Pheochromocytoma

Catecholamine levels should be evaluated approximately 6 weeks after surgery to confirm complete excision of the pheochromocytoma [24]. Residual hypertension is reported in 27–38% of cases and is attributed to essential hypertension [24,31]. If hypertension persists in the setting of elevated catecholamines, a MIBG scan should be performed to rule out recurrent disease.

In summary, laparoscopic adrenalectomy is now the standard of care for the removal of adrenal masses [15] except perhaps in cases of suspected malignant disease with invasion of surrounding structures. The technique is safe and has few complications, many of which can be prevented preoperatively, intraoperatively and postoperatively [32].

REFERENCES

1. Eustachius B. Tabulae anatomicae clarissimi viri bartholomaei Eustachii quas, 1563 (Republished in Rome in 1714 by Lancisius JM, Gonzagae F.).
2. Frankel F. Ein Fall von doppelseitigem vdllig latent verlaufenen Nebenneirentumor und gleichzeitiger Nephritis mit Vergnderungen am Circulationapparat und Retinitis. Virchows Arch Pathol Anat Physiol 1886; 103:244–263.
3. Higashihara E, Tanaka Y, Horie S, Aruga S, Nutahara K, Homma Y, Minowada S, Aso Y. A case report of laparoscopic adrenalectomy. Nippon Hinyokika Gakkai Zasshi 1992; 83:1130–1133.
4. Gagner M, Lacroix A, Bolte E. Laparoscopic adrenalectomy in Cushing's syndrome and pheochromocytoma. N Engl J Med 1992; 323:1033.

5. Brunt LM. The Positive impact of laparoscopic adrenalectomy on complications of adrenal surgery. Surg Endosc 2002; 16:252–257.
6. Sebe P, Peyroumaure M, Raynaud A, Delmas V. Anatomic variation in the drainage of the principal adrenal veins: The results of 88 venograms [abstr]. Surg Radiol Anat 2002; 24:222–224.
7. Quinn TM, Rubino F, Gagner M. Laparoscopic adrenalectomy. In: Souba WW. ACS Surgery: Principles and Practice. Danbury, Con.: Web MD Professional Publications, 2002; 1–18.
8. Brunt LM, Moley JF. Adrenal incidentaloma. World J Surg 2001; 25:905–913.
9. Thompson GB, Young WF. Adrenal incidentaloma. Curr Opin Oncol 2003; 15: 84–90.
10. Heniford BT, Arca MJ, Walsh RM, Gill IS. Laparoscopic adrenalectomy for cancer. Semin Surg Oncol 1999; 16:293–306.
11. Kebebew E, Siperstein AE, Clark OH, Duh QY. Results of laparoscopic adrenalectomy for suspected and unsuspected malignant adrenal neoplasms. Arch Surg 2002; 137:948–953.
12. Bernini GP, Miccoli P, Moretti A, Vivaldi MS, Iacconi P, Salvetti A. Sixty adrenal masses of large dimensions: hormonal and morphologic evaluation. Urology 1998; 51:920–925.
13. MacGillivray DC, Whalen GF, Malchoff CD, Oppenheim DS, Schichman SJ. Laparoscopic resection of large adrenal tumors. Ann Surg Oncol 2002; 9:480–485.
14. Gagner M, Pomp A, Henford BT, Pharand D, Lacroix A. Laparoscopic adrenalectomy: Lessons learned from 100 consecutive procedures. Ann Surg 1997; 222: 238–247.
15. Smith CD, Weber CJ, Amerson JR. Laparoscopic adrenalectomy: New gold standard. World J Surg 1999; 23:389–396.
16. Hallfeldt KK, Mussack T, Trupka A, Hohenbeicher F, Schmidbauer S. Laparoscopic lateral adrenalectomy versus open posterior adrenalectomy for the treatment of benign adrenal tumors. Surg Endosc 2003; 17:264–267.
17. Meraney AM, Samee AA, Gill IS. Vascular and bowel complications during retroperitoneal laparoscopic surgery. J Urol 2002; 168:1941–1944.
18. Guazzoni G, Cestari A, Montorsi F, Lanzi R, Rigatti P, Kaouk J, Gill IS. Current role of laparoscopic adrenalectomy. Eur Urol 2000; 40:8–16.
19. Rutherford JC, Stowasser M, Tunny SM, Klemm SA, Gordon RD. Laparoscopic adrenelectomy. World J Surg 1996; 20:758–761.
20. Welbourn RB. Survival and causes of death after adrenalectomy for Cushing's disease. Surgery 1985; 97:16–20.
21. Young WF. Primary Aldosteronism, Management issues. Ann NY Acad Sci 2002; 970:61–76.
22. Ng L, Libertino JM. Adrenocortical carcinoma: Diagnosis, evaluation and treatment. J Urol 2003; 169:5–11.
23. Goldfarb DA. Contemporary evaluation and management of Cushing's syndrome. World J Urol 1999; 17:22–25.
24. Walther MM. New therapeutic and surgical approaches for sporadic and hereditary pheochromocytoma. Ann NY Acad Sci 2002; 970:41–53.

25. Shen WT, Lim RC, Siperstein AE, Clark OH, Schecter WP, Hunt TK, Horn JK, Duh QY. Laparoscopic vs open adrenalectomy for the treatment of primary hyperaldosteronism. Arch Surg 1999; 134:628–631.
26. Salem M, Tainsh RE, Bromberg J, Loriaux DL, Chernow B. Perioperative glucocorticoid coverage: A reassessment 42 years after emergence of a problem. Ann Surg 1994; 219:416–425.
27. Naya Y, Nagata M, Ichikawa T, Amakasu M, Omura M, Nishikawa T, Yamaguchi K, Ito H. Laparoscopic adrenalectomy: Comparison of transperitoneal and retroperitoneal approaches. BJU Int 2002; 90:199–204.
28. Walz MK, Peitgen K, Neumann HPH, Janssen OE, Philipp T, Mann K. Endoscopic treatment of solitary, bilateral, multiple, and recurrent pheochromocytomas and paragangliomas. World J Surg 2002; 26:1005–1012.
29. Gotoh M, Ono Y, Hattori R, Kinukawa T, Ohshima S. Laparoscopic adrenalectomy for pheochromocytoma: Morbidity compared with adrenalectomy for tumors of other pathology. J Endourol 2002; 16:245–249.
30. Grabner P, Hayer-Jensen M, Jervell J, Flatmark A. Long-term results of treatment of Cushing's disease by adrenalectomy. Eur J Surg 1991; 157:461–464.
31. Favia G, Lumachi F, Polistina F, D'Amico DF. Pheochromocytoma, a rare cause of hypertension: Long-term follow-up of 55 surgically treated patients. World J Surg 1998; 22:689–693.
32. Fernandez-Cruz L, Taura P, Saenz A. Laparoscopic approach to pheochromocytoma: Hemodynamic changes and catecholamine secretion. World J Surg 1996; 20:762–768.
33. McHenry CR, Wolfe MS. Open anterior left adrenalectomy. In: Operative Technique in General Surgery. Duh QY, ed. Philadelphia: WB Saunders, 2002; 4:289.
34. Pillinger SH, Bambach CP, Sidhu S. Laparoscopic adrenalectomy: a 6 year experience of 59 cases. Anz J Surg 2002; 72:467–470.

5

Anesthesia

Samuel A. Irefin
The Cleveland Clinic Foundation, Cleveland, Ohio, U.S.A.

INTRODUCTION

The aim of laparoscopic surgery is to minimize trauma and achieve a satisfactory therapeutic result. The laparoscope has evolved from a diagnostic tool to an instrument that can be used to perform an ever-increasing range of surgical procedures. Compared with traditional open procedures, the laparoscopic approach for surgical procedures is associated with less postoperative pain, shorter hospital stays, more rapid return to normal activities, reduced overall adverse events, and significant cost savings [1]. With improvements in anesthetic techniques and the introduction of new fast-acting drugs, it is now possible to perform many laparoscopic procedures in an outpatient setting safely and comfortably for both patient and surgeon.

In the case of any new surgical procedure, there must be a critical analysis of related complications. This is very necessary in the case of minimally invasive surgery, because more extensive procedures are being performed in older and sicker patients with significant coexistent cardiopulmonary disease. Therefore, it is important that the benefits of laparoscopic procedures be weighed against potential complications. The incidence of anesthesia-related adverse events is remarkably low. In addition to a high incidence of minor morbidities such as pain and nausea/vomiting, the most common anesthesia-related complications are attributed to hypoventilation and cardiopulmonary arrest [2]. Most of the intraoperative anesthesia-related complications of laparoscopic surgery are due to traumatic injuries sustained during blind trocar insertion and physiological changes associated with patient positioning and the creation of pneumoperitoneum. The creation of pneumoperitoneum and assumption of the Trendelenburg position have several potential hemodynamic and respiratory consequences. These complications can be detected earlier if the anesthesiologist is aware of the expected physiological changes during laparoscopy, as well as the consequences of the potentially life-threatening complications.

CARDIOVASCULAR COMPLICATIONS

The initiation of pneumoperitoneum imposes both mechanical and physiological changes on the cardiovascular system. The extent of these changes will depend on the intra-abdominal pressure attained, the patient's intravascular volume, the volume of carbon dioxide absorbed, surgical conditions, ventilatory technique, and the anesthetic agent employed [3]. The response to laparoscopy by the cardiovascular system can be subdivided into three components: preload, cardiac, and afterload. At intra-abdominal pressures of 10–20 mmHg, venous pressure is decreased [4]. The decrease in venous return is counteracted by the overall stimulatory effect of absorbed CO_2 [5]. Venous return is also moderately augmented in the head-down position in normotensive and normovolemic patients [6]. During laparoscopy with intra-abdominal pressures of less than 20 mmHg, systemic and central venous pressures, as well as venous resistance, usually increase [7]. Mean arterial blood pressure and myocardial filling pressure are also increased during laparoscopy. These changes are accompanied by a fall in cardiac index with little change in heart rate [8]. Creation of pneumoperitoneum and laparoscopy can influence the cardiovascular responses based on the patients intravascular volume, pre-existing cardiopulmonary status, neurohormonal factors, and perhaps, patient medication and the anesthetic agents used. Preload, as shown by a minimally changed venous return, is not changed significantly by laparoscopy. As far as cardiac performance is concerned, there is a slight decrease in stroke volume, but the heart rate is increased during laparoscopy [9]. As a result, there is a minimal change in cardiac output. Afterload is augmented during laparoscopy as a result of increases in arterial pressures and arterial resistance. The overall effect of laparoscopy on the cardiovascular system is a hyperdynamic state in which the work of circulating the blood is increased. Although laparoscopic surgery is tolerated well by most patients, cardiovascular changes can have adverse consequences for those with limited cardiac reserve [10]. Cardiomyopathy, untreated congestive heart failure, and moderate to severe ischemic heart disease should be considered relative contraindications to laparoscopic surgery.

Major cardiovascular complications associated with laparoscopic surgery include hypotension, hypertension, dysrhythmias, and cardiac arrest [11]. Most of the cardiac arrests were noted to occur during induction of pneumoperitoneum

[12]. As a result of alterations in hemodynamic variables during laparoscopy, the patient may have a limited capacity to compensate for minimal additional insults, and this can lead to sudden deterioration.

Significant bradycardia, nodal rhythm, atrioventricular dissociation, and asystole have been reported during laparoscopy [13]. These have been noted to occur during insertion of the Veress needle or trocar and the induction of pneumoperitoneum, and are due to a vagal reflex that occurs with the insufflation of gases. Treatment of these dysrhythmias consist of prompt interruption of surgical stimulation or, if necessary, administration of an anticholinergic drug. Tachyarrhythmias that occur during laparoscopy are due to increased concentrations of carbon dioxide and catecholamines. Ventricular extrasystoles, bigeminy, and fusion beats may be the earliest manifestations of hypoxemia and must be carefully interpreted and treated. On the electrocardiographic tracings, deviation of the electrical axis to the left, increased R-wave amplitude, and T-wave inversion can be produced by excessive distention due to pneumoperitoneum. Treatment in this situation is deflation of the pneumoperitoneum.

There have been case reports of acute cardiovascular collapse during Nissen fundoplication due to cardiac tamponade [14]. Surgical disruption of esophageal hiatus during Nissen fundoplication can result in CO_2 insufflation into the mediastinum, resulting in cardiac tamponade. The anesthesiologist must maintain a high index of suspicion for this lethal complication. Immediate treatment includes decompression of the mediastinum. Cardiovascular function is minimally affected if the intra-abdominal pressure is maintained at or below 15 mmHg.

PULMONARY COMPLICATIONS

Creation of pneumoperitoneum involves frequent intraperitoneal insufflation of CO_2 through a Veress needle while the patient is in a 15- to 20-degree Trendelenburg position. With the creation of pneumoperitoneum during laparoscopy, there is a reduction in lung volumes, increase in peak airway pressures, and decrease in pulmonary compliance secondary to increased intra-abdominal pressure and patient positioning. These changes may be more marked in obese, elderly, or debilitated patients and may be worsened by placement of surgical packs and retractors in the upper abdomen.

CO_2 is the gas most commonly used for surgical laparoscopy. The peritoneal cavity is a well-vascularized surface that generally allows for rapid absorption [15]. Although CO_2 absorption during laparoscopy is well tolerated by most patients, severe hypercapnia can occur in those with severe pulmonary disease and a limited capacity to eliminate CO_2. Moderate hypercapnia is stimulatory to the cardiovascular system overall, via the interplay of central stimulation and peripheral depression. In severe hypercapnia has direct cardiodepressive predominate [16]. Moderate hypercapnia has a stimulatory effect on the cardiovascular system due to a proportionate rise of endogenous epinephrine and norepinephrine. By contrast, severe hypercapnia has a direct cardiodepressive effect on the cardiovascular system. Although there is an abrupt rise of endogenous epinephrine associated with severe hypercapnia, this effect is, to a certain extent, offset by a decreased sensitivity of target organs when pH is reduced. Hence, significant depression of the cardiovascular system by severe hypercapnia occurs despite an increase in circulating catecholamines.Severe hypercapnia can result in pulmonary vasoconstriction, resulting in pulmonary hypertension, right ventricular ischemia, or infarction. Hypercapnia can also increase the systemic vascular resistance and reduce cardiac index in patients with pre-existing cardiovascular disease. Cardiovascular collapse, severe acidosis, and fatal dysrhythmias may occur. The respiratory acidosis associated with hypercapnia is responsible for many of the ill effects of hypercapnia, although CO_2 has some direct effects as well. Hypercapnia may also accompany acute respiratory insufficiency. Acute respiratory insufficiency during laparoscopy may result from altered pulmonary mechanics, pneumothorax, pneumomediastinum, cardiogenic pulmonary edema secondary to increased intrathoracic pressure, or gas embolism.

Measures to prevent hypercapnia include avoidance of subcutaneous emphysema, lower insufflation pressure, intermittent desufflation during prolonged procedures, increased minute ventilation, and appropriate patient selection. Since most laparoscopic procedures are performed under general anesthesia with mechanical ventilation, hypercapnia can be easily controlled with an increase in minute ventilation.

There is restriction of diaphragmatic motion due to increased abdominal pressure and lung volume with initiation of pneumoperitoneum [17]. Pulmonary dead space is not altered by laparoscopy, but functional residual capacity is decreased. Total respiratory compliance is decreased and the work of breathing is increased due to an increase in airway pressures [18]. Hypoxemia may result from decreased functional residual capacity. Excess effort is usually not clinically significant when laparoscopy is performed under general anesthesia and mechanical ventilation is employed. However, in patients with pulmonary disease, the application of positive end-expiratory pressure (PEEP) may be required to compensate adequately [19].

Extraperitoneal gas may localize to several tissue planes or spaces. Subcutaneous emplysema is the most common manifestation of this condition and usually occurs secondary to incorrect placement of the insufflation needle or leakage around the laparoscopic port. Subcutaneous emphysema is generally harmless, but it may predispose to hypercapnia (acute or delayed) if it is extensive. Since properitoneal or retroperitoneal gas is not limited by the subdiaphragmatic peritoneum, it can move along the great vessels cephalad through the diaphragmatic hiatus and into the chest to cause pneumomediastinum. A congenital defect of the diaphragm (patent pleuroperitoneal canal), through which insufflated gas can pass into thoracic cavity, can result in pneumothorax and pneumomediastinum. Tension pneumothorax has been reported during laparoscopy and has the potential to result in severe cardiopulmonary insufficiency [20]. Undetected pneumothorax and pneumomediastinum can be life-threatening. Subcutaneous emphysema of the neck, chest wall, and face should alert the anesthesiologist to the possibility of associated complications. If there is clinical evidence of tension pneumothorax, immediate chest tube decompression is indicated.

Venous gas embolism is a rare but potentially lethal complication of laparoscopy. This complication results from the direct injection of gas into the venous system and usually occurs during the initial insufflation through a Veress needle. The gas bubble can move centrally, where it blocks the right ventricular outflow tract and pulmonary vasculature. This can result in profound hypotension, cyanosis, and asystole [21]. An important characteristic suggesting gas embolism is cardiopulmonary collapse that occurs during insufflation. The end-tidal CO_2 tracing, capnometry, can be a sensitive indicator of venous gas embolism. A sudden decrease in CO_2 tracings on capnography suggests gas embolism [22]. Treatment of gas embolism must be swift. This includes immediate desufflation of the pneumoperitoneum, application of 100% oxygen, initiation of a steep left lateral Trendelenburg position, and general resuscitation maneuvers. Aspiration of gas from the right ventricle may be attempted if a central venous catheter is in place. To avoid gas embolism, intravascular placement of the insufflation needle should be ruled out by aspirating the needle for the presence of blood before gas is instilled into the abdomen.

TRENDELENBURG POSITION

In the 1860s, Friedrich Trendelenburg, the renowned Leipzig urologist, confronted with the need to improve operative access to the viscera of the lower abdomen and pelvis, popularized the high pelvic posture that still bears his name. During World War I, this position was advocated for treatment of shock. Over the past century, the Trendelenburg position has been modified from the original posture advocated by Trendelenburg. It is now used in diverse situations, with application found in low, high, and reverse Trendelenburg positions. Presently, variations of the Trendelenburg position are also used in pelvic surgery to improve cerebral blood flow, treat venous air embolism, engorge cervical vessels for central venous catheter placement, prevent pulmonary aspiration at the onset of vomiting, correct pulmonary ventilation/perfusion mismatch, and achieve a high level of spinal or epidural anesthesia. Many of these applications are controversial because all present risks as well as benefits.

The Trendelenburg position causes physiological changes in the respiratory and circulatory systems during laparoscopy. Pulmonary function changes associated with a Trendelenburg position will depend on the patient's age and weight, the anesthetic agents used, and the intraoperative ventilatory techniques. The work of breathing is increased and the vital capacity is reduced in the Trendelenburg position [23]. These changes may be worsened by the placement of surgical packs and retractors in the upper abdomen. Obese patients especially do not tolerate the steep Trendelenburg position. The increased weight of the abdominal viscera on the diaphragm and the weight of the chest wall further decrease compliance and increase the risks of atelectasis and hypoxemia.

In Trendelenburg position, there is a potential for right mainstem endobrochial intubation and hypoxemia. This is because the endotracheal tube, firmly secured at its proximal end to the mandible, does not always move along with the trachea as the diaphragm displaces the lung and carina cephalad [24]. The anesthesiologist must pay special attention to the position of the endotracheal tube after each change in the patient's posture.

In Trendelenburg position, the patient's age, intravascular volume status, associated cardiac disease, anesthetic drugs, and ventilation mode may influence cardiovascular changes. The circulatory mechanics of the patient with heart disease are different from those of the normal person, so that such a patient might not tolerate the added blood volume in the central circulation that may result from Trendelenburg position. It is widely believed that Trendelenburg position improves cardiovascular function by increasing venous return and, hence, cardiac output. However, the physiological effects of the head-down position in normotensive, normovolemic patients have been shown to be associated with minimal changes in arterial pressure and cardiac output despite an increase in indices of cardiac filling [25]. Increases in central venous pressures may worsen acute glaucoma; with generous intraoperative fluid administration, edema of the periorbital tissues and tissues of the head and neck may occur. Edema may compromise the airway in the period immediately after the extubation of the trachea.

POSTOPERATIVE COMPLICATION OF LAPAROSCOPY

Laparoscopic surgery is associated with a high incidence of minor postoperative morbidity. Over 95% of patients had some symptoms 24 hr after laparoscopy [26]. Neck, shoulder, and abdominal pain is most common. Majority of patients also complain of sore throat due to irritation from the endotracheal tube, backache, headaches, nausea, and weakness. Although some of these complications are outside the control of the anesthesiologist, pain, nausea, and vomiting are extremely common and can be influenced by the anesthetic technique.

One of the advantages of laparoscopy is that it causes substantially less severe and prolonged discomfort compared to the corresponding open procedure. However, postoperative pain can still be considerable. Prevention and treatment of postoperative pain can be accomplished with local anesthesia infiltration, nonsteroidal anti-inflammatory drugs (NSAIDs), and opioid analgesics. Combinations of these modalities may also be employed. Simple infiltration of laparoscopic portals with local anesthetic should reduce pain arising from the small skin incisions. The pain that follows tubal ligation can be reduced by the application of local anesthetic directly to the fallopian tube or injection into the mesosalpinx [27]. This will allow reduced postoperative use of opioids and fewer hospital admissions. NSAIDs as sole agents are not as effective for immediate postoperative pain control. Their effect in the majority of patients is to reduce the need for opioids. Given sufficiently early in the postoperative period, NSAIDs may be effective in many patients to render discomfort tolerable after the opioids have worn off. Opioids, which are the mainstay of postoperative pain therapy, are utilized in the perioperative period in laparoscopic surgery. The use of opioids perioperatively constitutes a risk factor for postoperative nausea and vomiting. Balanced analgesia has been demonstrated to be highly efficacious in patients undergoing laparoscopic surgery [28]. This entails pain-management concept combining analgesia with fewer side effects of the drugs combined, which is achieved by administering the combination of opioids, NSAID, and local infiltration of the skin and subcutaneous tissue with local anesthetic. Using this modality, pain scores have been demonstrated to be consistently lower 48 hr after laparoscopy.

The laparoscopic approach to any intra-abdominal operation is associated with a high risk of nausea and vomiting in the perioperative period. The incidence of emetic sequelae after laparoscopy, under general anesthesia, exceeds 50% [29]. These unpleasant side effects are common after laparoscopic surgery, irrespective of anesthetic technique, and may contribute to delayed discharge [30]. The symptoms of nausea and vomiting are multifactorial in origin, and causative factors can be identified and predicted [31]. The use of postoperative opioids, female gender, history of motion sickness, history of migraine, duration of operation, and previous history of nausea and vomiting have been demonstrated, in a predictive model for risk assessment, as significant independent variables with a marked association with postoperative nausea and vomiting [32]. The most important patient characteristic influencing the incidence of postoperative nausea and vomiting seems to be a previous history of postoperative nausea and vomiting. Although routine antiemetic prophylaxis for postoperative nausea and vomiting is not widely accepted clinical practice, it can be justified in high-risk patients in order to reduce the incidence and severity of undesirable morbidity after laparoscopic surgery. Currently available pharmacological agents with antiemetic properties involve at least four receptor sites of action at which the emetic response can be blocked [31]. None of these agents is effective as a single therapy for the prevention of nausea and vomiting. Four receptor sites appear to play major roles in mediating the emetic response. These are the dopamine, histamine (H_1), cholinergic muscarinic, and 5-hydroxytryptamine type 3 (5-HT_3). Pharmacological agents can block these receptors, and this appears to be the mechanism of action of currently used antiemetic drugs. In the perioperative period, agents that act as antagonists at dopaminergic and serotonin receptors are used to control emesis. The anticholinergic and antihistaminic agents have been associated with a variety of unacceptable side effects, including dysphoria, sedation, lethargy, and dry mouth, when used in doses administered as antiemetic agents. As a result of the multifactorial etiology of postoperative nausea and vomiting, combination therapy of two pharmacological agents that act at different receptor sites may be more efficacious than the use of a single agent alone after laparoscopic surgery. The combination of a serotonin receptor antagonist and doperminergic receptor antagonist has been demonstrated in recent studies to be clinically and statistically superior to either agent alone in complete response, time to first emetic episodes, number of emetic episodes, and incidence and severity of nausea. These agents can also be combined in recommended dosages with dexamethasone for the prophylactic treatment of nausea and vomiting. In addition to pharmacologic agents, various other measures can be taken to prevent nausea and vomiting after laparoscopic surgery. Adequate hydration with about 20 mL/kg, suction of the stomach with an orogastric tube before the end of surgery, and avoidance of opiates, unless necessary, will help to prevent nausea and vomiting after laparoscopic surgery.

CONCLUSION

Laparoscopy has evolved from a diagnostic tool into a powerful therapeutic modality applicable to virtually every surgical subspecialty. Anesthetic techniques have also evolved with all forms of laparoscopy. Laparoscopic surgery has reduced postoperative morbidity, shortened hospital stays, and moved many procedures into the outpatient arena. Laparoscopy is remarkably safe; yet potentially life-threatening complications may occur. As with all surgical procedures, prevention and proper patient selection is the key to avoiding complications. High-risk patients should be clearly identified from the outset. Cooperation and consultations between the surgeon and the anesthesiologist are vital during laparoscopic surgery. The anesthesiologist must maintain a high index of suspicion for sudden cardiopulmonary complications during laparoscopy. These may include profound vasovagal reaction, cardiac dysryhthmia, excessive intra-abdominal pressure, acute blood loss, myocardial dysfunction, tension pneumothorax, severe respiratory acidosis, venous gas embolism, cardiac tamponade, and anesthetic drug–related complications. Vigilant monitoring and resuscitation equipment are essential to avoid serious complications should a surgical misadventure occur. The likelihood of a surgical misadventure increases as more complex procedures are attempted. The availability of rapid, short-acting anesthetics, analgesics, and muscle relaxants can provide for prompt recovery even after prolonged laparoscopic procedures. Laparoscopic surgery is safe, but there is no substitute for cooperation between the surgeon and the anesthesiologist in avoiding lethal complications.

REFERENCES

1. Cunningham AJ, Brill SJ. Laparoscopic cholecystectomy: Anesthetic implications. Anesth Analg 1993; 76:1120–1133.
2. Peterson HB, De Stefano F, et al. Deaths attributable to tubal sterilization in the United States, 1977 to 1981. Am J Obstet Gynecol 1983; 146:131.
3. Liu SY, Leighton T, Davis I, et al. Prospective analysis of cardiopulmonary responses to laparoscopic cholecystectomy. J Laparoendosc Surg 1991; 1:241–246.
4. Lenz RJ, Thomas TA, Wilins DG. Cardiovascular changes during laparoscopy. Studies of stroke volume and cardiac output using impedance cardiography. Anaesthesia 1976; 31:4.
5. Price HL. Effects of carbon dioxide on the vascular system. Anesthesiology 1960; 21:652.
6. Gentili DR, Benjamin E, Berger SR, Iberti TJ. Cardiopulmonary effects of the head-down tilt position in elderly post-operative patients: A prospective study. South Med J 1988; 81:1258.
7. Kashtan J, Green JF, Parsons EQ, Holcroft JW. Hemodynamic effects of increased abdominal pressure. J Surg Res 1981; 30:249.
8. McLaughlin JG, Scheeres DE, Dean RJ, et al. The adverse hemodynamic effects of laparoscopic cholecystectomy. Surg Endosc 1995; 9:121.
9. Ho HS, Gunther RA, Wolfe BM. Intraperitoneal carbon dioxide insufflation and cardiopulmonary functions. Arch Surg 1992; 127:928.
10. Cunningham AJ, Brill SJ. Laparoscopic Cholecystectomy: Anesthetic implications. Anesth Analg 1993; 76:1120.
11. Shifran JL, Adelstein L, Finkler NL. Asystolic cardiac arrest: A rare complication of laparoscopy. Obstet Gynecol 1992; 79:840.
12. Brantley JC, Riley PM. Cardiovascular collapse during laparoscopy: A report of two cases. Am J Obstet Gynecol 1988; 159:735.
13. Myles PS. Bradyarrhythmias and laparoscopy: A prospective study of heart rate changes and laparoscopy. Aus NZ J Obstet Gynaecol 1991; 31:171.
14. Farlo J, Thawgathuria D, Mikhail M, et al. Cardiac tamponade during laparoscopic Nissen fundoplication. Eur J Anaesthesiol 1998; 15:246.
15. Collins JM. Inert gas exchange of subcutaneous and intraperitoneal gas pockets in piglets. Respir Physiol 1981; 46:391.
16. Cullen D, Eger E. Cardiovascular effects of carbon dioxide in man. Anesthesiology 1974; 41:345.
17. Alexander GD, Brown EM. Physiologic alterations during pelvic laparoscopy. Am J Obst Gynecol 1969; 105:1078.
18. Drummond GB, Martin LV. Pressure-volume relationships in the lung during laparascopy. Br J Anaesth 1978; 50:261.
19. Ekman LGet al. Hemodynamic changes during laparoscopy with positive end-expiratory pressure ventilation. Acta Anaesth Scand 1988; 32:447.
20. Whiston RJ, Eggers KA, et al. Tension pneumothorax during laparoscopic cholecystectomy. Br J surg 1991; 78:1325.
21. Root B, Levy MN, et al. Gas embolism death after laparoscopy delayed by ''trapping'' in portal circulation. Anesth Analg 1978; 57:232.

22. Schulman D, Aronson HB. Capnography in the early diagnosis of carbondioxide embolism during laparoscopy. Can Anaesth Soc J 1984; 31:455.
23. Schiller WR. The Trendelenburg position. Surgical aspects. In: Martin JT, ed. Positioning in Anesthesia and Surgery. 2nd ed.. Philadelphia: Saunders, 1987, 117.
24. Heinonen J, Takki S, Tammisto T. Effect of the Trendelenburg on tilt and other procedures on the position of endotracheal tubes. Lancet 1969; 1:850.
25. Wilcox S, Vandam LD. Alas poor Trendelenburg and his position! A critique of its uses and effectiveness. Anesth Analg 1988; 67:574.
26. Collins KM, Docherty PW, Plantevin OM. Post-operative morbidity following gynaecological outpatient laparoscopy: A reappraisal of the service:. Anaesthesia 1984; 39:819.
27. Smith BE, MacPherson GH, deJonge M, et al. Rectus sheath block and mesosalphinx for diagnostic laparoscopic sterilization. Anaesthesia 1991; 46:875.
28. Michalolakou C, Chung F, Sharma S. Pre-operative multimodal analgesia facilitates recovery after ambulatory laparoscopic cholecystectomy. Anesth Analg 1996; 82: 44.
29. Thune A, Applegren L, Haglind E. Prevention of post operative nausea and vomiting after laparoscopic cholecystectomy. A prospective randomized study of metoclopramide and transdermal hyoscine. Eur J Surg 1995; 161:265.
30. Kapur PA. The big ''little'' problem. Anesth Analg 1991; 73:243.
31. Watcha MF, White PF. Post operative nausea and vomiting. Its etiology, treatment and prevention. Anesthesiology 1992; 77:162.
32. Palazzo M, Evans R. Logistic regression analysis of fixed patient factors for postoperative sickness: A model for risk assessment.. Br J Anaesth 1993; 70:135.

6

Appendectomy

Michael S. Kavic
St. Elizabeth Heath Center and Northeastern Ohio Universities College of Medicine, Youngstown, OhioU.S.A.

Stephen M. Kavic
Yale University School of Medicine, New Haven, ConnecticutU.S.A.

INTRODUCTION

The appendix had been recognized as an independent organ for millennia. More than 4000 years ago, ancient Egyptians noted the presence of the appendix during their funeral preparations and referred to it as the ''worm'' of the bowel [1]. Its function and role in disease, however, remained obscure.

From the late Middle Ages to the preindustrial period, many physicians noted during postmortem studies that the appendix was involved with foreign bodies and abscesses. They did not, however, believe that the appendix was the cause of right-lower-quadrant abdominal inflammation. Rather, they thought that the observed abscess or infectious process originated in the cecum. Inflammation of the cecum was referred to as *typhlitis* and *perityphlitis*—terms used to describe infectious processes of the iliac fossa.

Reginald H. Fitz, a pathologist at Harvard University in the late nineteenth century, was the first to describe the signs and symptoms of acute appendicitis [2]. He coined the term *appendicitis* in 1886 and advocated surgical intervention as a management option for this disease. Although the concept was novel at the time, the revolutionary aspect of Fitz's insight was not so much that he recommended surgical intervention for appendicitis but that he recognized the existence of a disease process originating at the appendix; if left untreated, the disease could proceed to perforation and abscess.

Charles McBurney, a general surgeon and Fitz's contemporary, described the point of maximal tenderness in the right lower quadrant associated with acute appendicitis [3]. This point, which now bears his name, is located one-third of the distance between the right anterosuperior iliac spine and the umbilicus; it corresponds to the anatomic base of the appendix. McBurney helped popularize the ''gridiron'' incision for appendectomy and, along with Fitz, was a strong advocate of early surgical intervention for acute appendicitis [4].

McBurney's technique for operative removal of a diseased appendix remained relatively unchanged for almost a century. His procedure was and is a good operation. The open approach to appendectomy has remained the ''gold standard'' because it is a safe and efficacious procedure that results in minimal morbidity and near zero mortality.

Kurt Semm, a German gynecologist, was the first to radically change McBurney's procedure when he performed the first laparoscopic appendectomy on May 30, 1980 [5,6]. Semm's technique employed a laparoscope to visualize the appendix. Endosutures were used to secure the mesoappendix prior to division, and pretied Roeders loops were used to ligate the skeletonized appendix, which was then amputated between the fixed Roeders loops. The technique was efficient, effective, and frugal.

Appendicitis is a common surgical emergency. In excess of 270,000 appendectomies are performed each year in the United States [7]. Persons between 10 and 19 years of age have the highest incidence of appendicitis, with males having a higher rate than females for all age groups. The lifetime risk for appendicitis has been estimated at 8.6% for males and 6.7% for females [8].

In cases of presumed appendicitis, two adverse outcomes must be considered in the management of the disease: (1) perforation of the appendix with the possibility of contamination, peritonitis, abscess, and sepsis and (2) misdiagnosis, which can result in the removal of a normal appendix. To reduce the potential of a perforated appendix, surgeons have traditionally accepted that approximately 10–20% of procedures for possible acute appendicitis will reveal noninflamed, histologically normal appendices [9,10].

APPENDICITIS

The underlying cause of acute appendicitis is that of obstruction of the appendiceal lumen [11]. Typical causes of obstruction are fecalith, hypertrophy of submucosal lymphoid tissue, or kinking of the appendiceal wall. Less common causes of appendiceal obstruction include obstruction secondary to foreign bodies, intestinal worms, or vegetable seeds.

Proximal occlusion of the appendix causes a closed-loop obstruction and consequent distention of the distal appendix. Mucosal inflammation in the distal segment is followed by ulceration and ultimately inflammation of the entire appendiceal wall. Stagnation distal to the obstruction allows for overgrowth of both anaerobic and aerobic organisms. Progressive distension eventually leads to vascular occlusion and infarction of the antimesenteric border. Perforation with frank peritonitis and abscess formation can occur.

Patients with acute appendicitis usually present with right-lower-quadrant pain, which may have begun in the periumbilical region, along with fever and emesis [12]. A leukocytosis of 11,000 to 18,000 white blood cells (WBCs) per cubic milliliter is common in acute appendicitis, with a ''left shift'' (increase in the percentage of neutrophils and immature band forms). Although plain abdominal radiographs may demonstrate a fecalith, for the most part these studies are nonspecific. Computed tomography (CT) studies are more accurate than plain films [13]. Typically, CT is utilized for patients with acute abdominal pain and uncertain history, physical, and/or laboratory findings. Ultrasound, which is very operator-dependent, can be useful and may demonstrate a ''bulls-eye'' in the right lower quadrant, signifying a distended appendix [14].

TECHNIQUE OF LAPAROSCOPIC APPENDECTOMY

Once a diagnosis of acute appendicitis is made, the patient is prepared for surgical intervention and the operating room. Larson et al. enumerated several factors that make the laparoscopic approach to appendectomy inherently appealing: superior visualization, identification of lesions in structures other than the appendix, reduced tissue trauma, the potential for more rapid return to normal activity, good exposure in obese patients, and decreased wound surface area to serve as a focus for infection [15]. The capability of establishing a diagnosis through superior visualization is particularly important in female patients of childbearing years, in whom the diagnosis may be less certain [16].

Since Kurt Semm initially described laparoscopic appendectomy in 1980 [17], dramatic changes in technology and instrumentation have occurred; undoubtedly these designs will continue to evolve. As a result, Semm's technique has undergone numerous revisions and adaptations. However, what follows is one common approach to laparoscopic appendectomy.

A preoperative antibiotic, usually a broad-spectrum cephalosporin, is given intravenously. After induction of general anesthesia, the patient remains in the supine position on the operating table. The abdomen is prepped with antiseptic (povidone-iodine) and the umbilicus is carefully cleansed. Pneumoperitoneum is then established, either through the closed technique (use of the Veress needle) or the ''open'' technique (Hasson blunt port insertion).

In the closed technique, a Veress needle is passed transumbilically. During needle insertion, upward traction is maintained on the skin with towel clips. Traction on the skin should be applied whenever trocars or needles are inserted into the abdomen in order to give the operator better control of the thrusting hand and insertion device. Typically, a 10-mm cannula is preferred at the umbilical site so that a 10-mm laparoscope, with its superior visual field and light intensity capabilities, may be used.

An open laparoscopy technique may also be used to initiate laparoscopic access. A 2-cm incision is made in the skin about the umbilicus. Dissection is carried down through all layers of the abdomen to the peritoneum, which is opened under direct vision. A Hasson-type cannula is inserted and secured to the abdominal wall or the underlying fascia [18].

The camera is then introduced via the umbilical cannula. Laparoscopic examination of the entire abdomen is first performed to rule out other pathology, such as a Meckel's diverticulum, Crohn's disease, mesenteric adenitis, or, in the female patient, pelvic genital tract disease. This important step helps confirm the region of pathology and serves as a guide for placement of additional working ports.

Additional 5-mm trocars and cannulas are brought in under direct laparoscopic vision. Operating ports are sited so that the surgeon can appropriately

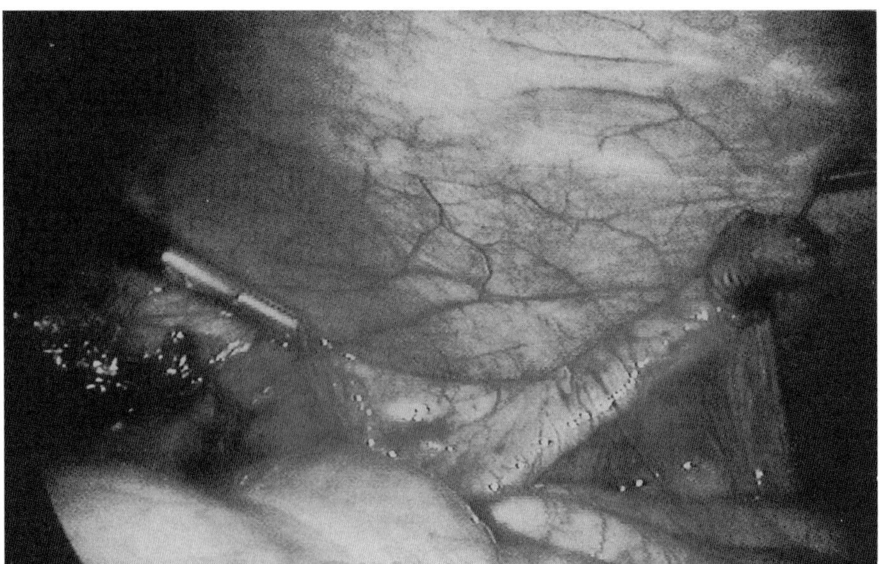

Figure 1 Roeders loop affixed to tip of appendix.

triangulate the diseased organ. Generally, cannulas should be placed at least four fingerbreadths distant from one another to prevent them from interfering with one another (''dueling''). A three-port technique may be used, with ports in the mid–left lower quadrant and the suprapubic or right lower quadrant positions.

Next, the appendix is mobilized. It may be necessary to divide the lateral peritoneal attachments of the cecum and right colon to expose the appendix completely. The tip of the appendix is usually friable in acute appendicitis and easily torn with laparoscopic graspers. To minimize this possibility, a pretied Roeders endoloop may be affixed to the tip of the appendix. The loop is tightened and the end of the suture cut long. Traction to the tail of the suture is then applied to elevate and maneuver the appendix (Fig. 1). In this way, multiple applications of the grasper to the appendix are eliminated and the risk of tearing is lessened.

An opening is made into the mesoappendix at the base of the appendix and the mesoappendix is divided with an EndoGIA stapling unit (U.S. Surgical Corporation, Norwalk, CT), harmonic scalpel, ultrasonic dissector, or serial clamping, division, and ties with pretied suture loops (Figs. 2 and 3). After the mesoappendix has been divided, the base of the appendix is secured and divided (Fig. 4). If the appendix is tenaciously bound down, it may be necessary to remove it in a retrograde fashion. In this instance, the base of the appendix is first divided

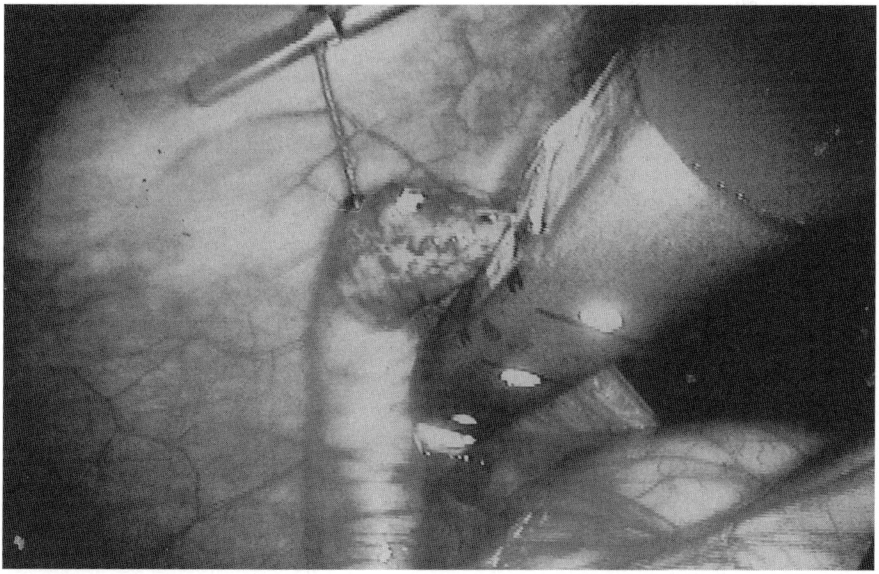

FIGURE 2 Stapling of mesoappendix.

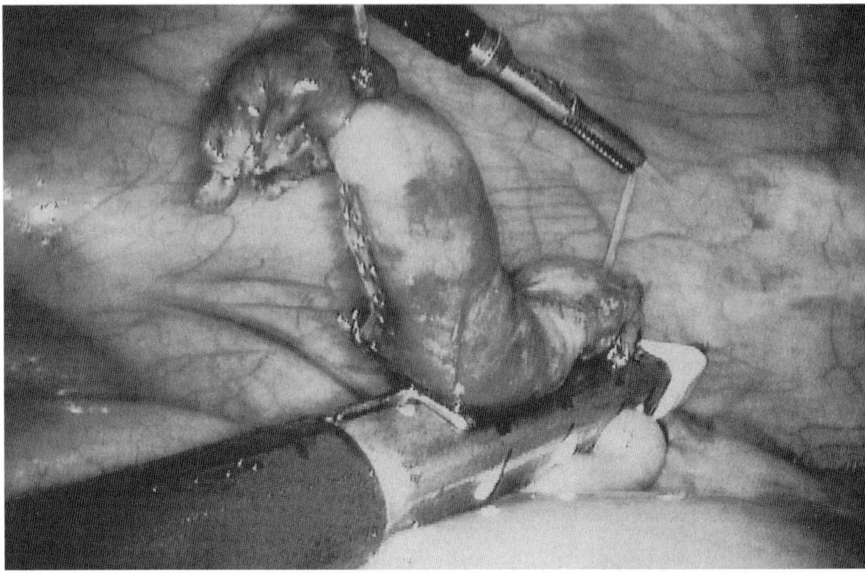

Figure 3 Stapling of mesoappendix.

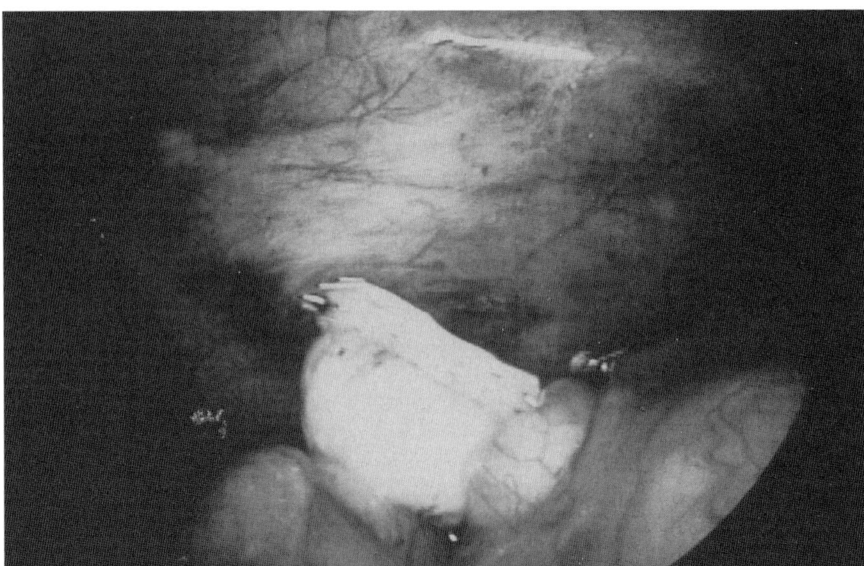

Figure 4 Stapled appendiceal stump.

between endoloops or with an EndoGIA stapler. The mesoappendix is then secured.

Staple leg length should be considered in using the EndoGIA. Standard intestinal staple cartridges have a leg length of 3.5 mm and are suitable for congested or edematous tissues. Vascular staples, which have a shorter leg length of 2.5 mm, should be employed on isolated vascular structures or tissue without significant edema or swelling.

To protect a friable appendix and limit contamination, the amputated appendix should be placed in an endoscopic retrieval bag and removed through the 10-mm cannula site (Fig. 5). If there has been any contamination (Fig. 6), the operative site must be irrigated with a copious amount of saline, typically several liters in volume, and antibiotics continued throughout the postoperative period (Fig. 7). There is some evidence that the addition of a local anesthetic to irrigation fluid may decrease postoperative shoulder pain, providing an added benefit [19].

To minimize the possibility of port-site herniation, all cannula defects 10 mm in diameter and greater are closed with fascial suture. All cannulas are withdrawn and CO_2 is allowed to evacuate. The fascial sutures are tied with the knots placed in a subcutaneous position. It is important to maintain upward traction on the fascial sutures while CO_2 is being evacuated to prevent omentum or intestine

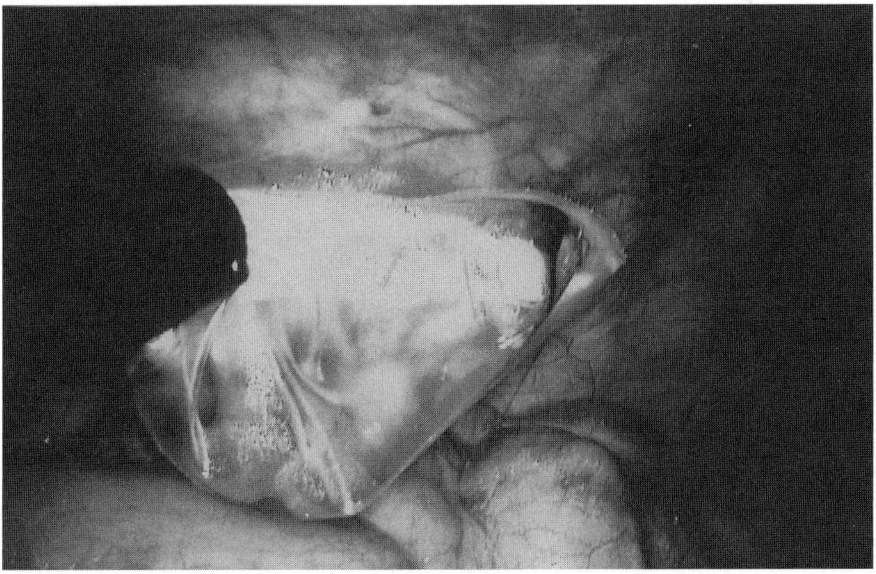

FIGURE 5 Amputated appendix within retrieval bag.

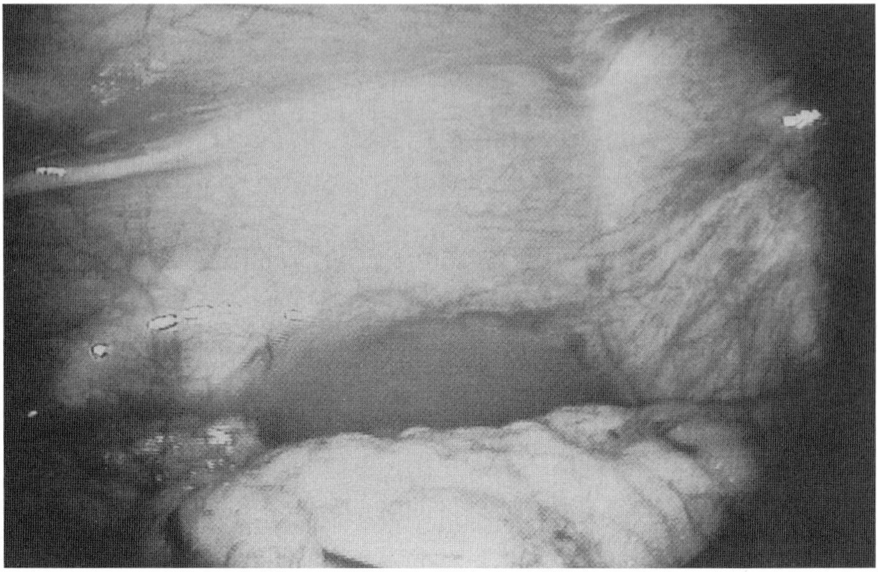

Figure 6 Pus in right lower quadrant secondary to perforated appendix.

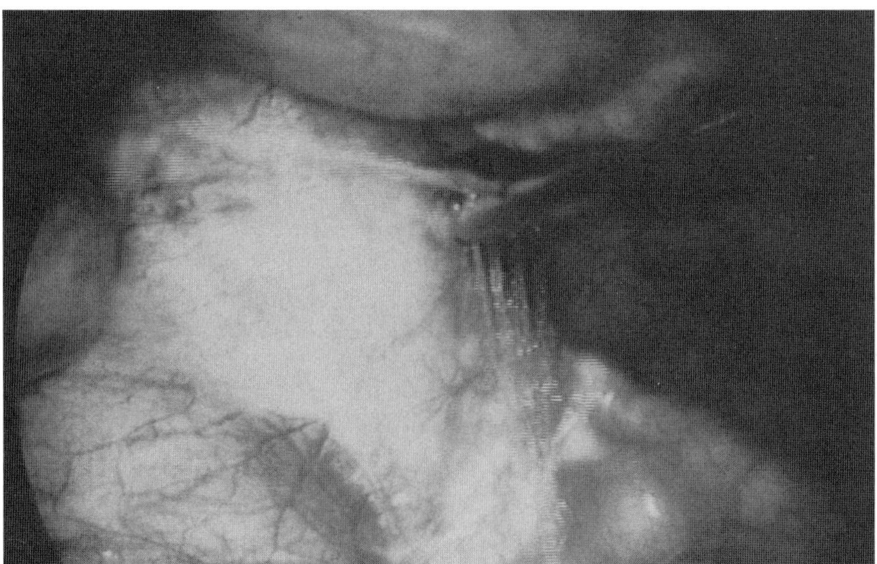

Figure 7 Irrigation of the appendiceal fossa.

from being drawn into the cannula sites. Subcutaneous and subcuticular suture complete the wound closure. Steri-strips help maintain the skin edges in apposition.

Many variations of this basic technique have been developed. Some surgeons have aimed to determine the optimal number of ports required for appendectomy, including, in the extreme, only a single port site [20]. Others have performed the procedure during transvaginal hysterectomy [21]. Laparoscopic appendectomy has also been performed using 2-mm minilaparoscopy instruments [22]. The appendix itself has been removed using a wire snare [23] or ultrasonically activated scalpel [24]. An additional maneuver has been the introduction of a finger through a port site in cases of complicated appendicitis [25].

COMPLICATIONS OF APPENDECTOMY

The complications of appendicitis include those associated with the disease itself and those of its operative treatment. These operative complications fall into three broad categories: those related to any operation requiring general anesthesia, those related to access to the right lower quadrant, and those related specifically to removal of the appendix. Each of these potential complications is examined in turn below.

COMPLICATIONS OF GENERAL ANESTHESIA

A full review of anesthetic complications in laparoscopic appendectomy is beyond the scope of this chapter (see Chapter 5). However, laparoscopic appendectomy requires general anesthesia and is associated with all the potential complications that such a condition entails. For instance, hypothermia may result from exposure, and neuropathies may be related to patient positioning. Any general surgical procedure also predisposes the patient to a variety of postoperative complications that are not specific to the procedure itself. Nonspecific but significant complications such as pulmonary embolism [26], ileus [27], urinary tract infection [28], and myocardial infarction [29] have all been described following laparoscopic appendectomy.

COMPLICATIONS OF OPEN APPENDECTOMY

Complications that have been historically associated with open appendectomy are listed in Table 1.

TABLE 1 Complications of Appendectomy

Wound infection
Intra-abdominal abscess
Fecal fistula
Intestinal obstruction
Liver abscess
Tubal infertility
Right inguinal hernia

Appendiceal perforation has been reported to occur in 19–32% of patients undergoing appendectomy and is primarily related to a delay in seeking medical attention. The very young and very old have been particularly susceptible to perforation. Up to 40% of patients less than 10 years of age, present with a perforated appendix; as many as 90% of those over 60 years of age, may also present with a perforation [30]. In the elderly, a delay in presentation may be related to difficulty in accessing medical care, fear of hospitalization or difficulties in communicating, or an altered pain response [31]. Others have suggested that the disease pathology of appendicitis is different in the elderly and that progression is more rapid in this subgroup because of decreased lymphoid tissue or blood supply in the elderly appendix [32].

Perforation is followed by infection, which is usually polymicrobial in character. Organisms commonly isolated include *Escherichia coli*, *Streptococcus*, *Pseudomonas aeruginosa*, and *Bacteroides* [33,34]. Interestingly, even with the addition of newer diagnostic modalities—including ultrasound, CT, and laparoscopy—no significant reduction of perforated appendix has been noted in the modern era [31].

Appendiceal abscess occurs in about 2–3% of patients with acute appendicitis and perforation. Abscess is less common than diffuse peritonitis. Complications related to an appendiceal abscess following perforation include wound infection, fecal fistula, small bowel obstruction, and recurrent abscess [17].

Wound infection is the most common reported complication to follow open appendectomy and can occur in upwards of 30% of cases [35]. Wound infection is more frequent in patients who have a perforated appendix than in those with an intact appendix.

Pelvic abscess has been reported in 1.4–18% of patients undergoing appendectomy. Evidence of an abscess is delayed and is usually not manifest for 5–10 days after the procedure [36]. The symptoms of pelvic abscess may be vague and include abdominal discomfort, loose bowel movements, and fever. CT-guided drainage has proven to be an effective tool in managing these abscesses.

Abscess secondary to appendiceal stump leakage after open appendectomy has been reported to occur in 0.5% of cases [37]. It is thought that the previously common practice of stump inversion with purse-string suture may compromise vascular supply and lead to cecal wall necrosis, perforation, and abscess [30]. For this reason, many authors have recommended ligation and amputation of the appendix without stump inversion. There has been no reported difference in postoperative infection when the appendiceal stump has not been inverted, and this method does not result in the development of a cecal mass, as occasionally seen after stump inversion [38].

Right inguinal hernias are three times more common in patients who have undergone open appendectomy than in the general population [39]. Although an exact cause for this phenomenon has not been identified, possible factors may include ilioinguinal and iliohypogastric nerve injury secondary to the abdominal incision [40]. Surgical trauma related to the abdominal incision may also incite direct damage to the transversus abdominis, internal oblique muscle and shutter mechanism of the groin, predisposing to hernia formation.

COMPLICATIONS OF LAPAROSCOPIC APPENDECTOMY

It is important to bear in mind that a laparoscopic approach to abdominal disease frequently results in reduced morbidity and decreased postoperative pain. However, regardless of the procedure performed, the primary disease process and its effect on the patient must never be forgotten. Infection is the main antagonist of the surgeon treating appendicitis. If the infection is confined to the appendix, the surgeon's task is easier and the patient's chance for full recovery is more promising once the diseased organ has been removed. If the appendix is perforated and infection has spread, management is more involved. But in both instances, infection and all of its possible ramifications must be brought into the equation and the patient treated appropriately. Minimal access does not change disease pathophysiology, and the surgeon must not be seduced into thinking a patient is doing well just because he or she is without postoperative pain. The whole patient and the whole disease must be treated.

A laparoscopic approach incurs potential complications inherent in performing an intracavitary procedure remote from that body cavity. These complications have been recently reviewed elsewhere [41]. Complications associated with laparoscopic access to the abdominal cavity may be broadly classified into three groups: abdominal wall injuries, vascular injuries, and visceral injuries [42]; they are outlined in Table 2. A more complete listing of complications specifically reported after laparoscopic appendectomy is presented in Table 3.

The rate of wound infection, which can be as high as 30% following open appendectomy, is reported to be about 0.1% following laparoscopic procedures [35,43]. Strict attention to cleansing the umbilicus of all debris and proper sterili-

TABLE 2 Complications of Laparoscopic Access

Skin infection
Subcutaneous emphysema
Hemorrhage
Visceral perforation
Gas embolism
Vascular injuries

zation of laparoscopic instruments may reduce this incidence even further. The majority of studies suggest that wound infections occur infrequently, at rates similar to those of open surgery [70], with most randomized studies demonstrating fewer infections in laparoscopic appendectomy than in the open cohort [44,45,49].

A systematic review of studies comparing laparoscopic and open appendectomies was performed by Sauerland et al. and published in 2002 [46]. The meta-analysis of 39 separate investigations concluded that wound infections were significantly reduced in laparoscopic appendectomy (odds ratio 0.5), but abscess formation was significantly increased (odds ratio 2.8). Intra-abdominal abscess remains one of the more feared complications of appendectomy, be it performed by laparoscopic or open techniques. The responsible organisms include those typically associated with the gastrointestinal tract. In one of the largest published series, the overall rate of abscess formation was 0.4% in laparoscopic procedures, including perforated and gangrenous appendicitis [47]. The rate of abscess formation in this and in many centers is comparable to abscess formation following open procedures [48,49].

However, other research highlights our incomplete understanding of the effects of laparoscopy on the infectious process that accompanies clinical appendicitis. Nordentoft et al. conducted a randomized study in 23 adult patients with bacteremia at the time of appendectomy [50]. Interestingly, half of the patients who underwent laparoscopic appendectomy had culture-documented bacteremia, whereas none of the patients who underwent open appendectomy had bacteremia. The significance of this finding may be debated because of the obvious size limitations of the study and because there was no increase in rates of abscess formation in the laparoscopic group. However, in a separate report, one patient developed a left-sided scrotal abscess following laparoscopic appendectomy [76]. This does implicate pneumoperitoneum as a possible etiological factor in facilitating transit through a processus vaginalis and subsequent abscess development.

Appendiceal rupture may also occur during aggressive laparoscopic manipulation due to decreased tactile sensation [51]. Perhaps the most important concept in the assessment of laparoscopic appendectomy is that the principles of good

TABLE 3 Complications of Laparoscopic Appendectomy

Vascular injury[59]
Bowel perforation[68]
Gas embolism[60]
Ileus[61,62]
Small bowel obstruction
Foreign body[63]
Cecal volvulus[64]
Midgut volvulus[65]
Adhesions
Hemorrhage
Intra-abdominal[66]
Hematoma
Abdominal wall[68]
Parietal wall[67]
Scrotal[68]
Infection
Wound infection[69,70]
Abscess
Intra-abdominal[71]
Appendiceal stump[72,73]
Pelvid[74]
Hydrocele[75]
Scrotal[76,77]
Sepsis[78]
Local (stump) complications
Retained fecalith[79]
Stump appendicitis[80–82]
Leak[83]
Fistula[84]
Hernia
Inguinal
Port site[66]
Pregnancy loss (pneumoamnion)[85]

open surgical technique must be honored in the laparoscopic environment. Specifically, careful dissection, appropriate tissue handling, adequate hemostasis, secure stump closure, and proper fascial approximation must occur to minimize the risks of complications.

Stump complications may occur more often during laparoscopic appendectomy if care is not taken to ensure proper closure. Multiple reports have been published detailing the hazards of inadequate closure, including stump appendicitis [73] as well as intestinal perforation [83]. To minimize the risks of these complications, it remains essential to adhere to the fundamentals of proper surgical conduct. For example, appropriate antibiotics must be given for simple, gangrenous, and perforated appendicitis. Adequate supervision of surgical residents is also necessary.

Most importantly, the appendiceal stump must be secured completely, without ischemia. There is no need for invagination of the stump, making the laparoscopic operation significantly less challenging. Insufficient evidence exists to recommend a definitive surgical approach to the treatment of the stump. However, one multicenter trial including 253 patients compared stump closure with ligature to stump closure with a linear stapling device [52]. Although both modalities resulted in fewer complications than open appendectomy, closure with a stapling device was the superior technique. Surgeons experienced with these staplers recognize some of their limitations: the potential for stapler misfire, the inevitable spillage of excess staples into the abdominal cavity, and increased cost. For these reasons, the optimal technique of stump closure remains somewhat controversial.

Should a stump complication occur, a number of treatment options exist. In the stable patient, relaparoscopy may be performed for definitive management. Percutaneous drainage is also available for abscess drainage or to temporize a developing fistula. Last, laparotomy remains the ultimate means of controlling intra-abdominal pathology. The surgeon must always retain a high level of suspicion for complication and utilize adjunct studies, such as CT scanning, to hasten their diagnoses.

Subcutaneous emphysema may arise from initial superficial placement of the insufflation needle or dislodgement of the cannula used for intraoperative insufflation into the subcutaneous tissues. CO_2 is injected under pressure into subcutaneous spaces, which may ascend into the neck and face. The body usually rapidly reabsorbs CO_2, and tissue emphysema is usually well tolerated. Hypercarbia, however, can occur with a rise in end-tidal CO_2 and a fall in pH. These changes are often easily managed with controlled ventilation by the anesthesiologist [53]. It may be necessary to discontinue CO_2 insufflation during this time and evacuate the pneumoperitoneum while the anesthesiologist manages the patient's ventilation needs.

Hemorrhage from the abdominal wall secondary to port placement is usually due to transection of the inferior epigastric vessels or their branches in the lower abdomen [17]. Inferior epigastric vessels (recall that that inferior epigastric artery is accompanied by two epigastric veins) may be avoided by inserting trocars *lateral* to the rectus sheath under direct laparoscopic vision. Epigastric vessels as well as unnamed vascular channels of the abdominal wall may also be transilluminated with the laparoscope and thereby avoided during trocar insertion.

The risk of hemorrhage from laceration of the aorta or external iliac vessels can be lessened by strict and constant attention to technique. No trocar or cannula should be inserted without countertraction on the abdominal wall. A tense pneumoperitoneum may provide sufficient countertraction; however, the procedure is safer if the surgeon applies countertraction with the aid of a towel clip and uses the nondominant hand to support the abdominal wall. Additionally, if the surgeon extends the third digit of the thrusting hand, this finger will help limit incursion of the trocar and provide an additional measure of safety.

Mild to moderate bleeding from abdominal wall trocar sites can be controlled with bipolar or monopolar desiccation. Larger transected vessels should be secured with suture ligature. There are special needles for passage of suture via port sites, including the Semm emergency needle [54], Gore needle, and Carter-Thomason closure system. In general, the cannula at the bleeding port site should be left in place. Using any of the above needles, suture is passed through the fascia into the abdomen, where it is caught and held with a laparoscopic grasping instrument. The needle is repositioned and passed through the fascia 180 degrees opposite to the initial suture placement. Under direct laparoscopic visualization, the intra-abdominal suture is passed to the needle now in an intra-abdominal position, secured to that needle, and withdrawn. Several sutures can be passed in this fashion, allowing the bleeding vessel to be secured and fascia of the port site closed. The long ends of the suture are held with hemostats and the needle is transferred to other cannula sites for fascial closure.

Gas embolism can result from insufflation of CO_2 or other gases into a major vessel or venous channel [55]. Devices such as the argon beam coagulator utilize a low-flow stream of inert gas to maintain the beam of electrical energy in position. This gas, if directed at a venous channel, may gain entrance, leading to a gas embolism. Obstruction of right heart outflow can occur with gas embolism and subsequent cardiovascular collapse. Emergency treatment of gas embolism is outlined in Table 4.

Visceral trauma can occur at any time during a laparoscopic procedure from the initial introduction of trocar and cannulas to the completion of the

TABLE 4 Emergency Treatment for Gas Embolism

Discontinue CO_2 insufflation
Evacuate pneumoperitoneum
Place the patient in the head-down, left lateral decubitus position
Insert CVP[a] line for aspiration of gas embolism (right internal jugular position preferred)
Maintain vigorous ventilatory support

[a] Central venous pressure.

procedure. Visceral injuries may be life-threatening but indolent, as they may occur away from the region of interest. Distended hollow organs such as the stomach and urinary bladder can be protected from injury by preoperative decompression—i.e., orogastric tube and Foley catheter [56]. Patients who have undergone previous open operative procedures are at increased risk for visceral injury because of the presence of adhesions. Careful dissection of the bowel and closure of all iatrogenic serosal tears are necessary when dense adhesions are encountered.

Visceral trauma secondary to puncture with the Veress needle can usually be managed expectantly. If there is little lateral damage from passage of the Veress needle, the intestine will usually seal spontaneously without untoward sequelae. Of course, larger tears must be repaired primarily. The repair can be performed laparoscopically or via open laparotomy. Lacerations to solid organs such as the liver and spleen must be managed according to the degree of injury. As important as managing an injury is, it is perhaps more important to recognize that an injury has occurred. For this reason, a diagnostic abdominal survey visualizing all of the abdomen and its content before and after the operative procedure should be routine during any laparoscopic operation.

Children and persons of small body habitus should be carefully assessed prior to a laparoscopic procedure. Their small frames and thin abdominal walls dictate that the appropriate laparoscopic instrumentation be available and used. There is a decreased intra-abdominal working space in patients of small build, and incursions of trocars and laparoscopic instruments must be carefully managed lest intra-abdominal vascular and visceral injury occur. The principles of countertraction and extension of the third digit must be followed. In many instances, open exploration utilizing a small McBurney incision may be the safest and most expeditious way to perform appendectomy in children [17].

Port-site hernias have been an ongoing problem since the advent of laparoscopic surgery. They remain a potentially serious problem yet one that is readily preventable. Any port site 10 mm in diameter or greater should be closed with fascial suture reliably placed under laparoscopic visualization [57,58]. Port sites smaller than 10 mm in diameter, if vigorously manipulated and stretched, should also be closed with fascial suture.

CONCLUSION

In experienced hands, laparoscopic appendectomy is a safe, viable alternative to open appendectomy for the treatment of acute appendicitis. Whether the procedure is performed via open laparotomy or minimally invasive laparoscopy, the potential of infection must always be borne in mind by the operating surgeon. Patients with perforation, peritonitis, or abscess must be treated for their infection. The fact that minimally invasive surgery is accompanied by lessened immediate postoperative pain does not diminish the importance of treating the patient for infection and its sequelae. Intravenous antibiotics, adequate hydration, and support of nutrition are all important. The surgeon must not be lulled into a false sense of security by a patient who has little discomfort after laparoscopic appendectomy. In treating the whole patient and anticipating the possibility of infectious sequelae, the likelihood of complications will be minimized.

REFERENCES

1. Herrington JL. The vermiform appendix: Its surgical history. Contemp Surg 1991; 39:36–43.
2. Fitz RH. Perforating inflammation of the vermiform appendix with special reference to its early diagnosis and treatment. Trans Assoc Am Phys 1886; 1:107–144.
3. McBurney C. The incision made in the abdominal wall in cases of appendicitis with a description of a new method of operating. Ann Surg 1894; 20:38.
4. McBurney C. Experience with early operative interference in cases of disease of the vermiform appendix. NY State Med J 1889; 50:676–687.
5. Semm K. Endoscopic appendectomy. Endoscopy 1983; 15:59–64.
6. Litynski GS. Highlights in the History of Laparoscopy. Frankfurt: Barbara Bernert Verlag, 1996:136.
7. Hall MJ, Owings MF. 2000 National Hospital Discharge Survey. Advance data from vital and health statistics, no 329. Hyattsville. MD: National Center for Health Statistics, 2002.
8. Addis DG, Shaffer N, Fowler B, Tauxe RV. The epidemiology of appendicitis and appendectomy in the United States. Am J Epidemiol 1990; 132:910–925.
9. Detmer DE, Nevers LE, Sikes ED. Regional results of acute appendicitis care. JAMA 1981; 246:1318–1320.
10. Flum DR, Morris A, Koepsell T, Dellinger EP. Has misdiagnosis of appendicitis decreased over time. JAMA 2001; 286:1784–1753.
11. Lally KP, Cox CS, Andrassy RJ. Appendix. In Townsend CM, ed. Sabiston Textbook of Surgery. 16th ed.. Philadelphia: Saunders, 2001, 917–928.
12. Silen W. Cope's Early Diagnosis of the Acute Abdomen. 18th ed.. New York: Oxford University Press, 1991:67–84.
13. Birnbaum BA, Balthazar EJ. Computed tomography of appendicitis and diverticulitis. Radiol Clin North Am 1994; 32:885–898.
14. Rossi P, Covarelii P, Mosci F, Bisacci R, Sensi B, Moggi L. Ultrasonography in management of acute appendicitis. Surg Endosc 1996; 149:619–621.
15. Larson GM, Cheadle WG, Polk HC. Appendectomy for acute appendicitis. In Ballantyne GH , Leahy PF , Modlin IM, eds. Laparoscopic Surgery. Philadelphia: Saunders, 1994, 220.
16. Kavic MS. Laparoscopic appendectomy. In Grochmal S, ed. Minimal Access Gynecology. Oxford. UK: Radcliff Medical Press, 1995, 149–16.
17. Kavic MS, Semm K. Laparoscopic appendectomy. In Kavic MS , Levinson CJ , Wetter PA, eds. Prevention and Management of Laparoendoscopic Complications. Miami. FL: Society of Laparoendoscopic Surgeons, 1999, 35.

18. Hasson HM. Modified instrument and method for laparoscopy. Am J Obstet Gynecol 1971; 110:886–887.
19. Cunniffe MG, McAnena OJ, Dar MA, Calleary J, Flynn N. A prospective randomized trial of intraoperative bupivacaine irrigation for management of shoulder-tip pain following laparoscopy. Am J Surg 1998; 176:258–261.
20. Rispoli G, Armellino MF, Esposito C. One-trocar appendectomy. Surg Endosc 2002; 16:833–835.
21. Pelosi MA, Pelosi MA. Vaginal appendectomy at laparoscopic-assisted vaginal hysterectomy: A surgical option. J Laparoendosc Surg 1996; 6:399–403.
22. Schier F. Laparoscopic appendectomy with 1.7-mm instruments. Pediatr Surg Int 1998; 14:142–143.
23. Chikamori F, Kuniyoshi N, Shibuya S, Takase Y. Laparoscopic appendectomy with the help of a wire snare. Surg Today 2001; 31:560–563.
24. Martin del Olmo JC, Blanco Alvarez JI, Carbajo Caballero MA, de la Cuesta de la Llave C, Vaquero Peurta C, Arenal J. Laparoscopic appendectomy by ultrasonically activated scalpel in acute appendicitis: Preliminary report. J Laparoendosc Adv Surg Tech A 2002; 12:111–113.
25. Katkhouda N, Mason RJ, Mavor E, Campos GM, Rivera RT, Hurwitz MB, Waldrep D. Laparoscopic finger-assisted techniques (fingeroscopy) for treatment of complicated appendicitis. J Am Coll Surg 1999; 189:131–133.
26. Cox MR, McCall JL, Toouli J, Padbury RTA, Wilson TG, Wattchow DA, Langcake M. Prospective randomized comparison of open versus laparoscopic appendectomy in men. World J Surg 1996; 20:263–266.
27. Klinger A, Henle KP, Beller S, Rechner J, Zerz A, Wetscher GJ, Szincz G. Laparoscopic appendectomy does not change the incidence of postoperative infectious complications. Am J Surg 1998; 175:232–235.
28. Tucker O, Rashid Al-Faqih S, El-Amin O, Zaki A. Laparoscopic appendicectomy: Review of 331 cases over 7 years, in a Saudi Arabian hospital. Endoscopy 2002; 34:639–642.
29. Pedersen AG, Petersen OB, Wara P, Ronning H, Qvist N, Laurberg S. Randomized clinical trial of laparoscopic versus open appendicectomy. Br J Surg 2001; 88: 200–205.
30. Cooperman M. Complications of appendectomy. Surg Clin North Am 1983; 63: 1233–1247.
31. Hui TT, Major KM, Avital I, Hiatt JR, Margulies DR. Outcome of elderly patients with appendicitis. Effect of computed tomography and laparoscopy. Arch Surg 2002; 137:995–1000.
32. Fruend HR, Rubinstein E. Appendicitis in the aged: Is it really different. Am Surg 1984; 50:573–576.
33. Lau WY, Teoh-Chan CH, Fan ST, Yam LOC, Lau KF, Wong SH. The bacteriology and septic complications of patients with appendicitis. Ann Surg 1994; 200:576–581.
34. Christou NV, Turgeon P, Wassaf R, Rotstein O, Bohnen J, Potvin M. Management of intra-abdominal infections. Arch Surg 1996; 131:1193–1201.
35. Gilmore OJA, Martin TDM. Aetiology and prevention of wound infection in appendectomy. Br J Surg 1974; 61:281–287.

36. Finne CO. Transrectal drainage of pelvic abscess. Dis Colon Rectum 1978; 23: 293–297.
37. Sihha AP. Appendectomy: An assessment of the advisability of stump invagination. Br J Surg 1977; 64:499–500.
38. Engstrom L, Fenyo G. Appendectomy: assessment of stump invagination versus simple ligation: A prospective randomized trial. Br J Surg 1985; 72:971–972.
39. Arnbjornsson E. Development of right inguinal hernia after appendectomy. Am J Surg 1983; 143:174–175.
40. Avsar FM, Sahin M, Arikan BU, Avsar AF, Demirci S, Elhan A. The possibility of nervus ilioinguinalis and nervus hypogastricus injury in lower abdominal incisions and effects on hernia formation. J Surg Res 2002; 107:179–185.
41. Schafer M, Lauper M, Krahenbuhl L. Trocar and Veress needle injury during laparoscopy. Surg Endosc 2001; 15:275–280.
42. Miranda CS, Carvajal AR, Escobar P. Complications of operative laparoscopy. Gynaecologic Endosc 2000; 9:161–165.
43. Phillips JM. Complications in laparoscopy. Int J Gynaecol Obstet 1977; 15:157–162.
44. Merhoff AM, Merhoff GC, Franklin ME. Laparoscopic versus open appendectomy. Am J Surg 2000; 179:375–378.
45. Ozmen MM, Zulfikaroglu B, Tanik A, Kale IT. Laparoscopic versus open appendectomy: Prospective, randomized trial. Surg Laparosc Endosc 1999; 9:187–189.
46. Sauerland S, Lefering R, Neugebauer EA. Laparoscopic versus open surgery for suspected appendicitis. Cochrane Database of Systematic Reviews 2002; 1: CD001546.
47. Katkhouda N, Friedlander MH, Grant SW, Achanta KK, Essani R, Paik P, Velmahos G, Campos G, Mason R, Mavor E. Intraabdominal abscess rate after laparoscopic appendectomy. Am J Surg 2000; 180:456–461.
48. Golub R, Siddiqui F, Pohl D. Laparoscopic versus open appendectomy: A metaanalysis. J Am Coll Surg 1998; 186:545–553.
49. Chung RS, Rowland DY, Li P, Diaz J. A meta-analysis of randomized controlled trials of laparoscopic versus conventional appendectomy. Am J Surg 1999; 177: 250–256.
50. Nordentoft T, Bringstrup FA, Bremmelgaard A, Stage JG. Effect of laparoscopy on bacteremia in acute appendicitis: A randomized controlled study. Surg Laparosc Endosc Percut Tech 2000; 10:302–304.
51. Flowers JL. Appendectomy. In Bailey RW , Flowers JL, eds. Complications of Laparoscopic Surgery. St. Louis: Quality Medical Publishing, 1995, 165.
52. Ortega AE, Hunter JG, Peters JH, Swanstrom LL, Schirmer B. the Laparoscopic Appendectomy Study Group. A prospective, randomized comparison of laparoscopic appendectomy with open appendectomy. Am J Surg 1995; 169:208–213.
53. Kent RB. Subcutaneous emphysema and hypercarbia following laparoscopic cholecystectomy. Arch Surg 1991; 126:1154–1156.
54. Semm K. Pelviscopy—Operative guidelines. Technical section. Table 4–9.1. Instruments for emergencies. WISAP, 1992.
55. Mintz M. Risks and prophylaxis in laparoscopic surgery: A survey of 100,000 cases. Reprod Med 1977; 18:269–272.

56. Soderstrom RM, Levy BS. Bowel injury during laparoscopy: Causes and medicolegal questions. Contemp Obstet Gynecol 1986; 27:41–45.
57. Hogdall C, Rodsen JU. Incarcerated hernia following laparoscopy. Acta Obstet Gynecol Scand 1987; 66:735–736.
58. Williams MD, Flowers SS, Fenoglio ME, Brown TR. Richter hernia: A rare complication of laparoscopy. Surg Laparosc Endosc 1995; 5:419–421.
59. Juricic M, Bossavy JP, Izard P, Cuq P, Vaysse P, Juskiewenski S. Laparoscopic appendicectomy: Case reports of vascular injury in two children. Eur J Pediatr Surg 1994; 4:327–328.
60. Cottin V, Delafosse B, Viale JP. Gas embolism during laparoscopy: A report of seven cases in patients with previous abdominal surgical history. Surg Endosc 1996; 10:166–169.
61. Piskun G, Kozik D, Rajpal S, Shaftan G, Fogler R. Comparison of laparoscopic, open, and converted appendectomy for perforated appendicitis. Surg Endosc 2001; 15:660–662.
62. Huang M-T, Wei P-L, Wu C-C, Lai I-R, Chen RJ, Lee W-J. Needlescopic, laparoscopic, and open appendectomy: A comparitive study. Surg Laparosc Endosc Percut Tech 2001; 11:306–312.
63. Nottingham JM. Mechanical small bowel obstruction from a loose linear cutter staple after laparoscopic appendectomy. Surg Laparosc Endosc Percutan Tech 2002; 12: 289–290.
64. McIntosh SA, Ravichandran D, Wilmink AB, Baker A, Purushotham AD. Cecal volvulus occurring after laparoscopic appendectomy. J Soc Laparoendosc Surg 2001; 5:317–318.
65. Cuadra SA, Khalife ME, Char DJ, Wax MR, Halpern D. Intestinal obstruction from midgut volvulus after laparoscopic appendectomy. Surg Endosc 2002; 16:215.
66. Wullstein C, Barkhausen S, Gross E. Results of laparoscopic versus conventional appendectomy in complicated appendicitis. Dis Colon Rectum 2001; 44:1700–1705.
67. Bakshi GK, Agrawal S, Shetty SV. A giant parietal wall hematoma: Unusual complication of laparoscopic appendectomy. J Soc Laparoendosc Surg 2000; 4:255–257.
68. Peiser JG, Greenberg D. Laparoscopic versus open appendectomy: Results of a retrospective comparison in an Israeli hospital. Israeli Med Assoc J 2002; 4:91–94.
69. Bhadnarkar DS, Bhagwat S, Punjani R. Port-site infection with Mycobacterium chelonei following laparoscopic appendicectomy. Indian J Gastroenterol 2001; 20: 247–248.
70. Klingler A, Henle KP, Beller S, Rechner J, Zerz A, Wetscher GJ, Szinicz G. Laparoscopic appendectomy does not change the incidence of postoperative infectious complications. Am J Surg 1998; 175:232–235.
71. Paik PS, Towson JA, Anthone GJ, Ortega AE, Simons AJ, Beart WR. Intra-abdominal abscesses following laparoscopic and open appendectomies. J Gastrointest Surg 1997; 1:188–193.
72. Filippi de la Palavesa MM, Vaxmann D, Campos M, Tuchmann C, Guth S, Dietemann JL. Appendiceal stump abscess. Abdom Imaging 1996; 21:65–66.
73. Chikamori F, Kuniyoshi N, Shibuya S, Takase Y. Appendiceal stump abscess as an early complication of laparoscopic appendectomy: Report of a case. Surg Today 2002; 32:919–921.

74. Frizelle FA, Hanna G. Pelvic abscess following laparoscopic appendicectomy. Ann R Coll Surg Engl 1995; 77:467–468.
75. Lantsberg L, Mor I, Levy I, Khoda J. Infected hydrocele following laparoscopic appendectomy: case report. Surg Laparosc Endosc 1997; 7:262.
76. Kollis J, Gallery RM. Left scrotal abscess complicating laparoscopic appendicectomy. Aust NZ J Surg 1996; 66:568–569.
77. Thakur A, Buchmiller T, Hiyama D, Shaw A, Atkinson J. Scrotal abscess following appendectomy. Pediatr Surg Int 2001; 17:569–571.
78. Frazee RC, Bohannon WT. Laparoscopic appendectomy for complicated appendicitis. Arch Surg 1996; 131:509–511.
79. Strathern DW, Jones BT. Retained fecalith after laparoscopic appendectomy. Surg Endosc 1999; 13:287–289.
80. Courouclis M, Blackberg M. A case report. Stump appendicitis two months after laparoscopic appendectomy (Swedish). Lakartidningen 1999; 96:3062.
81. Marcoen S, Onghena T, van Loon C, Vereecken L. Residual appendicitis following incomplete laparoscopic appendectomy. Acta Chir Belg 1999; 177:39–40.
82. Milne AA, Bradbury AW. ''Residual'' appendicitis following incomplete laparoscopic appendectomy. Br J Surg 1996; 83:217.
83. Pier A, Gotz F. Laparoscopic appendectomy in 625 cases: from innovation to routine. Surg Laparosc Endosc 1991; 1:8–13.
84. Schreiber JH. Early experience with laparoscopic appendectomy in women. Surg Endosc 1987; 1:211–216.
85. Friedman JD, Ramsey PS, Ramin KD, Berry C. Pneumoamnion and pregnancy loss after second-trimester laparoscopic surgery. Obstet Gynecol 2002; 99:511–513.

7

Bariatric Surgery

Michael Williams and J. K. Champion
Videoscopic Institute of Atlanta, Atlanta, Georgia, U.S.A.

INTRODUCTION

Morbid obesity remains a significant public health issue associated with a tremendous expenditure of resources. The increasing prevalence of morbid obesity and its complications, along with the success of present bariatric procedures, has resulted in an exponential increase in the number of bariatric procedures performed by general surgeons today. The decision to embark on a bariatric surgical practice should be made only after careful and comprehensive planning with a multidisciplinary approach. Bariatric surgery is now considered one the most litiginous of all surgical specialties. The purpose of this chapter is to increase the reader's awareness of potential complications and to discuss the management and perioperative care involved in these cases, which can help to limit the potential complications of laparoscopic bariatric surgery.

The identification of complications related to bariatric surgery requires intraoperative and perioperative vigilance. The management of complications begins with avoidance by appropriate surgical training and patient selection. Ideally, surgeons should undergo a preceptorship, such as the program offered by the American Society of Bariatric Surgeons, to ensure acquisition of the basic qualifications. The ability to suture laparoscopically, tie intracorporeal knots, and perform a hand-sewn two-layer anastamosis, if necessary, are the minimal skills that a competent laparoscopic bariatric surgeon must have mastered prior to embarking on direct patient care.

Appropriate patient selection during the surgeon's learning curve is paramount in limiting potential complications. We recommend that surgeons initiating laparoscopic bariatric procedures begin by selecting patients with a body mass index of less than 50 or weight less than 350 lb, a gynecoid body habitus, and no history of open abdominal surgical procedures so as to avoid a conversion to an open operation.

LAPAROSCOPIC ROUX-EN-Y GASTRIC BYPASS

The laparoscopic Roux-en-Y gastric bypass (LRYGB) has combined the traditional benefits of minimally invasive surgery with the proven efficacy of weight control via gastric bypass and is one of the most popular bariatric procedures performed in the United States today. The Roux-en-Y gastric bypass has resulted in 90% of patients losing 50–75% of their excess weight and maintaining this weight loss for up to 15 years [1]. Wittgrove et al. first reported the laparoscopic Roux-en-Y gastric bypass in 1994 [2]. LRYGB has all the conventional complications of open gastric bypass and the general complications of a laparoscopic approach. Here our discussion focuses on the unique complications associated with LRYGB, such as internal herniations, postoperative stenosis, and complications of calibration and construction.

Internal Hernias

There is an inherently increased risk of internal hernias associated with LRYGB as compared to open Roux-en-Y gastric bypass. It has been postulated that the increased incidence of internal herniation is related to the lack of tactile sensation in closing the potential hernia sites during LRYGB and reduced adhesions associated with a laparoscopic approach. Closure of the defect should be tight enough to prevent internal herniation, yet an excessively tight closure would promote scar formation and possible kinking of the adjacent bowel. Potential hernia sites that should be closed include the transverse mesocolon defect in the retrocolic approach, the jejunojejunostomy mesenteric defect, and the space between the mesentery of the Roux limb and transverse colon (Petersen hernia). The reported incidence of internal hernia formation through the mesocolic window range from 0.7–3.25% [3–6]. The antecolic technique of Roux limb passage eliminates the defect in the transverse mesocolon; however, herniation through an omental window or mesenteric defect may also result in bowel obstruction.

A high index of suspicion is paramount in the diagnosis of internal hernia after LRYGB. Internal hernia with intermittent closed-loop obstruction may progress to gangrenous bowel with subtle clinical signs or symptoms. Patients may present with an acute onset of severe epigastric or periumbilical pain associated with nausea and vomiting, hematemesis, or fever. In a series of patients with an internal hernia after LRYGB followed by Filip et al., all patients were tachycardic at presentation [7]. Plain abdominal x-rays are usually inconclusive, but contrast abdominal films may reveal a point of obstruction (Fig. 1). Computed tomography (CT) scanning may provide a diagnosis but may not be attainable due to the weight limitation of the scanner. In patients with persistent abdominal pain and inconclusive imaging studies, we proceed with laparoscopic exploration.

Morbidly obese patients presenting with typical signs, symptoms, and radiological studies consistent with obstruction or patients with atypical symptoms but a high index of suspicion should receive definitive therapy with laparoscopic or open exploration without undue delay. The surgeon's decision to proceed with laparoscopic versus open exploration is based on his or her individual skills and comfort level. We use a laparoscopic approach utilizing the previous incisions. Once a transition site or internal hernia has been identified, the bowel is reduced and the defect approximated with nonabsorbable sutures. If the viability of the bowel is unequivocally compromised, a resection with primary reconstruction

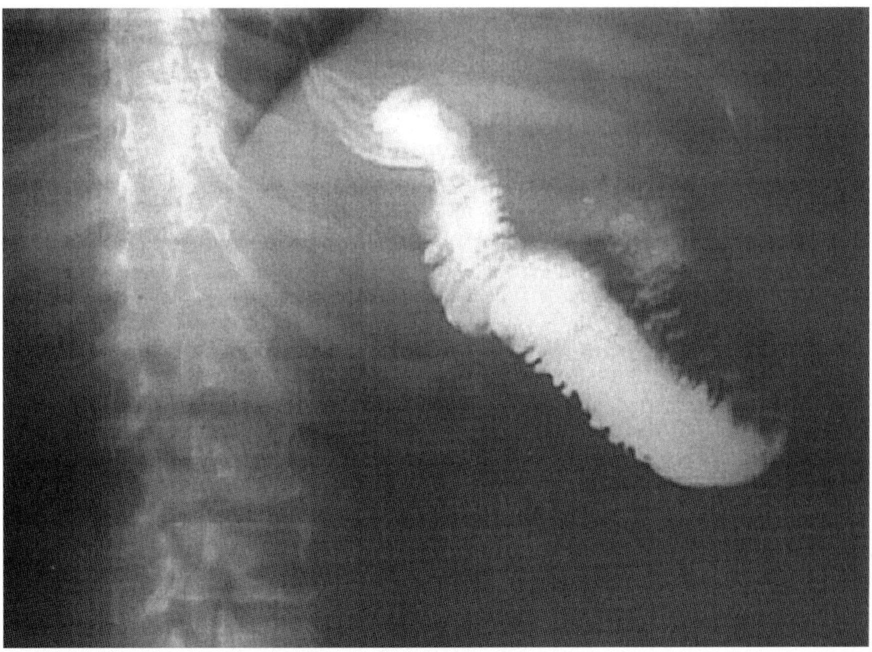

Figure 1 Barium swallow demonstrating obstruction 20 cm below gastrojejunostomy secondary to internal hernia at mesocolon window defect.

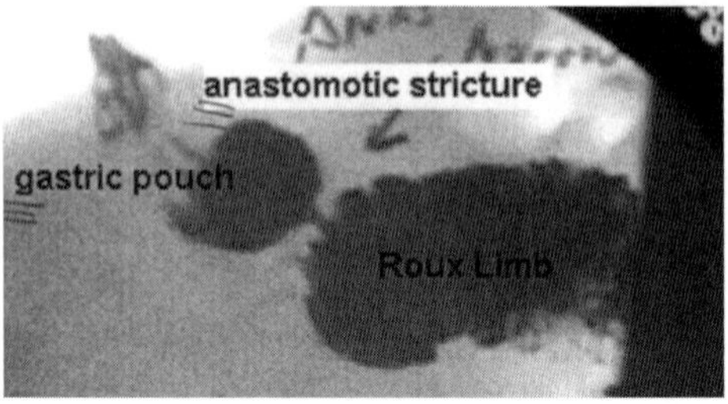

FIGURE 2 Barium swallow with a stricture at the gastrojejunostomy.

should be performed. In cases of equivocal bowel viability a second look operation should be considered.

Stoma Stenosis

Stricture of the gastrojejunostomy, also known as stoma stenosis, may also complicate the postoperative recovery following a LRYGB. The rate of stoma stenosis has been reported as 0–10%, with an average of 5–8% in our experience [8]. Ischemia has been proposed as the mechanism of stenosis. Patients with stenosis usually present with a history of progressive food intolerance (as the diet is advanced from liquids to solids). Patients may experience nausea and vomiting of undigested food shortly after meals. We investigate any patient who cannot advance to solids by 6 weeks after extensive diet counseling. A barium swallow may identify a stomal stricture but has a high false-negative rate (Fig. 2). Gastroscopy, however, is a definitive test and provides the examiner with the opportunity to perform a balloon dilatation of the gastrojejunostomy. We perform our own endoscopies and define a stenosis as any outlet through which we cannot pass our 10-mm gastroscope. We have successfully dilated each stenosis without requiring surgical revision due to stricture; however, we had two perforations requiring surgical repair after dilatation associated with the 18-mm balloon. We have not experienced any perforations from pneumatic dilation with a 15-mm balloon to date and, based on our outcomes, we no longer advocate dilation with the 18-mm balloon. Patients in our practice have required one to four dilations over time, but over 90% require one episode of dilation to treat their stoma stenosis. To decrease the incidence of stoma stenosis, intraoperative vigilance to prevent pouch devascuarization and excessive tension should be maintained.

POUCH CONSTRUCTION AND CALIBRATION

The challenge with adoption of a minimally invasive approach of an established procedure is to perform the same operation without compromising technique for laparoscopic access. The long-term success of open gastric bypass depends on a measured and calibrated pouch of less than 30 mL, a stoma outlet of 12-mm, and a Roux limb of 100 cm. Many laparoscopic bariatric surgeons unnecessarily ''eyeball'' pouch construction, outlet diameter, and Roux limb length without a method of calibration [5,6]. The pouch should be calibrated with a balloon or bougie; the outlet with a bougie, gastroscope, or circular stapler anvil; and the Roux limb accurately measured with an endoscopic ruler. The distortion of lens magnification, lack of depth perception, and absence of tactile sensation associated with laparoscopic surgery creates a potential failure in technique, mandating subsequent revisions unless the problem is addressed at the initial procedure.

The technique of the laparoscopic formation of the gastrojejunostomy has spawned a new set of complications. The three common techniques currently used are the circular stapler, linear stapler, and hand-sewn anastamosis. When the circular stapler is passed transorally, it has been reported to lodge in the esophagus or to cause esophageal lacerations. Passing the anvil per os and withdrawing the stapler through the abdominal wall has resulted in a 10% incidence of wound infection despite antibiotic bowel preparation [5]. A modification to avoid the infection risk associated with the transoral route was to insert the anvil via a gastrostomy, which we employed in 1995 and which was later popularized by Scott and Dela Torre [11]. Our solution was to develop the linear stapler technique, so that the stapler could be inserted via a standard 12-mm trocar [12]. In patients with significant hiatal hernias, we mobilize the distal esophagus to ensure an adequate intra-abdominal length, and the crura is approximated with nonabsorbable sutures.

A leak from an anastomotic line is a dreaded complication of a LRYGB. Higa and Boone employ a hand-sewn anastomosis to avoid the technical issues of laparoscopic stapling; this was initially thought to reduce leak rates [13]. However, leaks still occur with the hand-sewn approach, and the challenge of a running suture line is beyond all but a handful of laparoscopic bariatric surgeons; its utilization has therefore been limited. In our opinion there is no significant difference in leak rates between the three principal techniques, and the outcome is probably most dependent on surgeon skill and training. The learning curve for laparoscopic gastric bypass is generally accepted as comprising 100 cases [5,13]. Leaks may be more common with a laparoscopic gastric bypass, particularly early in the learning process; therefore we strongly urge laparoscopic surgeons to assess for leaks at the end of the case, prior to closing. Leaks may be tested by flooding the field with saline to cover the staple and suture lines and instilling air via a gastroscope or by instilling methylene blue via a nasogastric tube with a bowel clamp occluding the Roux limb. We identified 31 intraoperative leaks in our first 823 laparoscopic gastric bypasses (4%) but had only 1 (0.12%) leak postoperatively from the gastrojejunostomy. It is a good policy to utilize a drain in your first 100 cases until you establish a known leak rate. A postoperative swallow

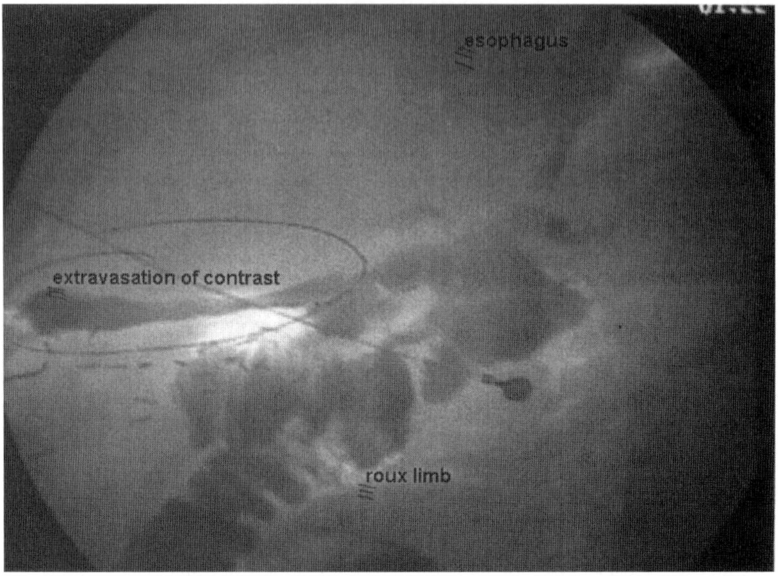

FIGURE 3 Gastrografin swallow after Roux-en-Y gastric bypass revealing leakage of contrast.

of meglumine distrizoate (Gastrografin) is also recommended to assess possible missed leaks during the learning process (Fig. 3). It is important to know that a negative Gastrografin swallow does not rule out a leak at the gastrojejunostomy or at the other sites where leaks can occur (enteroenterostomy, distal stomach staple lines, or iatrogenic injury at remote sites).

Excluded Stomach

Complications such as hemorrhage, distention, or perforation may occur at the gastric remnant. The diagnosis of complications of the gastric remnant and duodenum is often delayed due to the relative isolation of this gastrointestinal segment from conventional radiological and endoscopic evaluation.

In patients presenting with gastrointestinal bleeding following gastric bypass, the excluded stomach should be considered in the diagnostic workup. In a retrospective review of 3000 gastric bypasses, Printen et al. identified an incidence of 0.3% of symptomatic bleeding from the bypassed pouch; resection of the distal pouch was curative in all cases [14]. Melena and hematemesis were the most common presenting symptoms. Sinar and colleagues [15] described the use of a pediatric colonoscope to evaluate the gastric remnant via a retrograde technique.

Fobi and colleagues [16] advocate placement of a radio-opaque marker to identify the site of the gastrostomy in the excluded stomach during the primary Roux-en-Y gastric bypass. If preoperative assessment of the gastric remnant is not performed or appears equivocal, we advocate intraoperative endoscopy of the excluded stomach prior to subtotal gastrectomy.

Acute distention or perforation of the excluded stomach may occur due to an obstruction at the jejunojejunostomy, creating a closed-loop obstruction. Patients with severe gastric distention may present with nausea and abdominal pain. Persistent gastric distention leads to staple-line disruption unless the gastric remnant is vented with a gastrostomy or the obstruction at the jejunojejunostomy is repaired. We advocate placement of a gastrostomy during the primary LRYGB if compromise of the jejunojejunostomy is suspected. A leak from the gastric remnant staple line is relatively obscure from standard radiographic evaluation; in patients presenting with classic signs of sepsis—such as, tachycardia, tachypnea, fever, malaise, and leukocytosis—we advocate a laparoscopic exploration despite a negative radiological assessment.

LAPAROSCOPIC VERTICAL BANDED GASTROPLASTY

The vertical banded gastroplasty evolved from the shortcomings of horizontal gastroplasty and was developed in 1980 by Mason [17]. The benefits of minimally invasive surgery have led to the development and popularization of laparoscopic vertical banded gastroplasty (LVBG). This procedure also involves the unique complications associated with a minimally invasive technique and shares all the traditional morbidity of the open gastroplasty [17,18]. Like the LRYGB, the LVBG requires advanced skills in stapling and laparoscopic suturing. Complications such as leaks and stoma stenosis may also occur with LVBG and usually present with the typical signs and symptoms, as discussed with LRYGB (Fig. 4). The intraoperative complications unique to the laparoscopic approach include staple-line bleeding and misfiring of staples, uncontrolled intra-abdominal bleeding, and pouch misconstruction.

Endoscopic staplers are mechanical devices associated with a definite incidence of malformed staples, misfires, or malfunctions as previously reported [19]. Laparoscopic surgeons must be prepared to repair and protect staple misfires with an intracorporeal oversewing of staple lines. Locking of an endoscopic stapler in place is a rare complication that may occur during LVBG or LRYGB. If a surgeon encounters this rare complication, he or she may attempt to pry the jaws of the stapler open with graspers. If anatomical conditions permit, placement of an additional endoscopic stapler via an alternate trocar site may allow a wedge resection of the tissue locked within the jaws of the stapler thus allowing removal of the stapler with the encompassed segment of tissue. Failure of these maneuvers should be followed by an open conversion to dislodge the device.

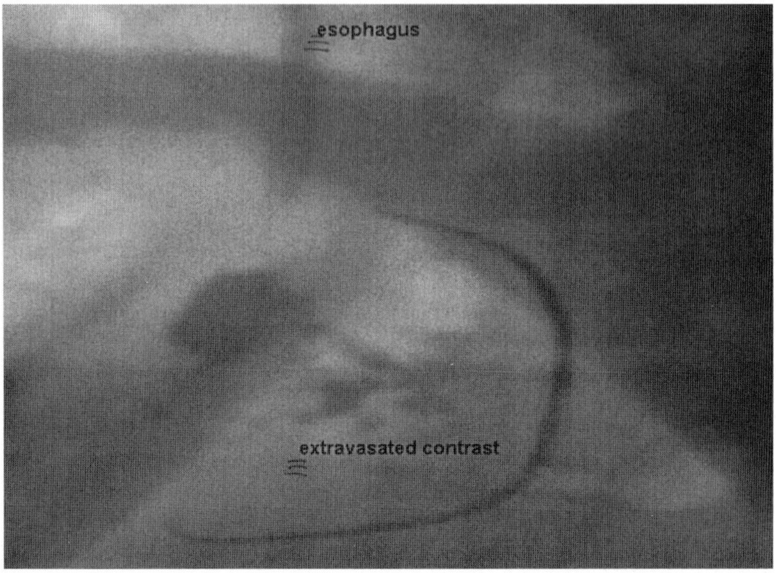

FIGURE 4 Gastrografin swallow after laparoscopic vertical banded gastroplasty with staple-line extravasation.

Uncontrolled intra-abdominal hemorrhage is a serious potential complication of LVGB. Significant bleeding may occur during perigastric dissection for band placement, division of the short gastric vessels, splenic injury, or lesser sac dissection from branches of the splenic vessels, a procedure that can perforate the posterior gastric wall. Control of massive unexpected bleeding can be achieved by laparoscopic compression and waiting 4–5 min if temporary control is achieved. Invariably the bleeding point will slow at that point and permanent ligation can be achieved. It is imperative that the surgeon and assistants remain calm. We maintain a second suction setup with a 10-mm suction probe and a second insufflator in the operating room suite, which can be activated immediately if massive bleeding occurs. Persistent bleeding of more than 500-mL or intraoperative hypotension is managed by conversion to an open procedure. It is well to remember the caveat that a conversion to open is not a complication; rather, it reflects good surgical judgment in the face of a problem. Hemorrhage from the staple line is a commonly observed event and is easily controlled with hemaclips or interrupted sutures. We are very meticulous with hemostasis, since the use of perioperative anticoagulants for prophylaxis of venous deep thrombosis may cause delayed postoperative bleeding.

Pouch misconstruction can occur with the laparoscopic technique if calibration of the pouch and stoma is not employed. The LVBG relies on the accurate construction of a vertically oriented pouch of less than 30 mL with a controlled outlet, which is calibrated and measured. We calibrate the pouch by measuring 5 cm with a laparoscopic ruler from the angle of His along the lesser curve to create a window into the lesser sac for ultimate placement of the mesh band. A 50F blunt-tip bougie is then positioned along the lesser curve to be used as a stent as the stomach is staple-transected to create the pouch. This technique ensures a 5 by 3 cm pouch, which we have measured to hold 20 mL. The mesh band (1.5 by 7 cm) is overlapped 1 cm on either end to create a 5-cm-diameter band stabilizing the outlet at 12 mm around a 30F bougie. The final quality control of pouch construction is verification on endoscopy during surgery. We confirm that the pouch has the appropriate volume, there is no staple line hemorrhage or leak, and the stoma is patent, allowing a 10-mm gastroscope to pass into the distal stomach. As an alternative to the bougie technique, balloon devices are also available to assist the surgeon with accurate pouch calibration.

LAPAROSCOPIC ADJUSTABLE GASTRIC BAND

Placement of a laparoscopic adjustable gastric band (LAGB) is a restrictive bariatric procedure that is relatively safe and effective. Kuzmark first introduced the adjustable gastric band in 1986 [20]. The first surgeon to implant the adjustable band laparoscopically was Belachew in 1993 [21]. The U.S. Food and Drug Administration approved the Lap-Band System (Inamed Health, Santa Barbara, CA) in June 2001. Complications specifically associated with the LAGB include perforation, erosion, slippage, infection, mechanical port problems, and malposition with pouch enlargement or esophageal enlargement.

Perforation

Perforation of the gastric wall during band placement is a potentially lethal complication. Patients with gastric perforation may present with fever, tachycardia, leukocytosis, abdominal pain, or peritonitis. Perforation usually occurs during blunt retrogastric dissection. The principal cause of mortality after perforation is a delay in diagnosis. We routinely test for gastric wall perforations by performing an intraoperative gastroscopy with insufflation of air while the stomach is immersed in irrigation fluid. A routine gastrografin swallow is also obtained on the first postoperative day to rule out leakage.

Erosion

Erosion of the LAGB usually presents as loss of satiety or weight gain. Patients may complain of epigastric discomfort or hematemesis. In patients presenting with reservoir infection, erosion with subsequent bacterial migration along the tubing should be ruled out as an inciting cause. Band erosion may occur in 1–4% of patients. Radiological examination is usually nondiagnostic; diagnostic confirmation is obtained by visualization of the band during endoscopy. We prefer to manage band erosion via a laparoscopic approach. The site of the band can be located by following the connection tubing from the abdominal wall. Adhesions, which often cover the site of the band, are sharply divided and the buckle of the band should also be cut with laparoscopic shears. The band, tubing, and access port should be removed and the damaged gastric wall repaired with interrupted sutures. Gastroscopy or methylene blue can be used to test the integrity of the repair. These patients may be considered for future bariatric procedures to continue loss of excess weight, including replacement of the LAGB on an individual basis. There is speculation that band erosion may be reduced by avoiding excessive anterior fixation with compression of the gastric wall against the buckle.

Slippage

Slippage of the LAGB has been reported as the most common late complication and the most common cause of reoperation. O'Brien, at the Minimally Invasive Surgery for Morbid Obesity and GERD Related Topics Course in 2002, reported an incidence of 15% in his group's experience. Slippage may occur anteriorly or posteriorly, with posterior slippage occurring most commonly if anterior fixation sutures are utilized. Band slippage may be caused by inappropriate placement, inadequate fixation, or maladaptive eating behavior (binge eating and recurrent vomiting). Slippage occurs because the stomach wall distal to the band usually slides proximally through the band and creates an enlarged proximal pouch. Patients with band slippage may present with vomiting, heartburn, reflux, food intolerance, sleep disturbance, or persistent cough. The diagnosis of slippage is confirmed by a barium swallow demonstrating pouch dilation and posterior slippage. An abdominal radiograph demonstrating a horizontal or tilted band may suggest slippage (Fig. 5).

The initial management of band slippage should be conservative. All fluid should be removed from the band and the patient observed for symptoms. If the symptoms resolve and the patient maintains weight control, observation may be continued without intervention. If the patient starts to regain weight, however, then band fills are resumed in increments of 1 mL over 4–6 weeks until the patient starts to achieve weight control. Patients with recurrent or persistent symptoms are treated with revisional surgery. Belachew et al. have cited the risk of recurrent prolapse due to posterior slippage as almost 100% [22]. Revisional surgery may be performed laparoscopically or open, and we replace the band with a new pathway via the pars flaccida. Slippage may be prevented intraoperatively by

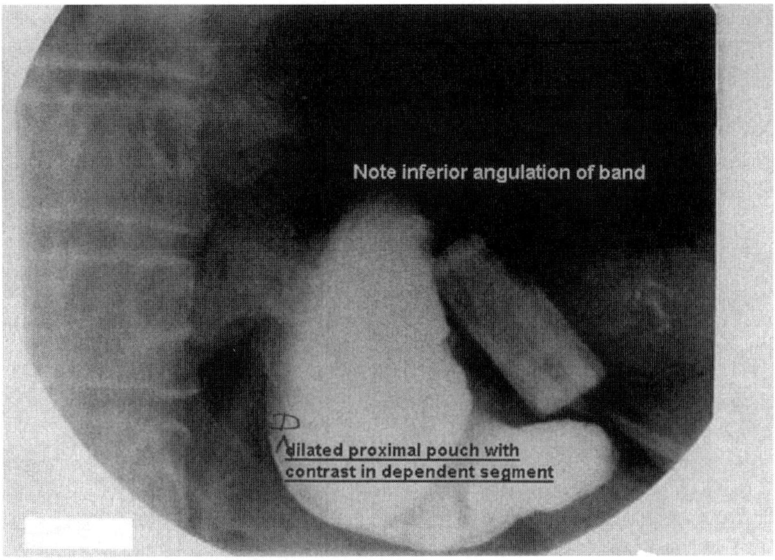

FIGURE 5 Posterior slippage of laparoscopic adjustable gastric band presenting with obstructive symptoms 1 year after surgery.

opening the lesser sac to identify inadvertent malpositioning of the band within the lesser sac space. If the band is identified within the lesser sac, additional posterior fixation stitches around the band should be placed.

Infection

Infection of the LAGB is another potential complication, which may require reoperation for definitive therapy. LAGB infections are usually associated with the access port and are caused by a breach in sterile technique during implantation or band adjustments. Mild infections without purulent discharge or tissue reaction may be treated with a trial of oral antibiotics. Moderate infections may require local drainage or debridement as well as antibiotic coverage. Infections associated with purulent drainage should be treated with explantation of the access port, placing the tubing completely within the abdominal cavity. The patient should receive a course antibiotics tailored to the bacterial species isolated. A new reservoir is then placed at an alternate site 6 weeks later. It is prudent to perform endoscopy and rule out erosion as a cause of bacterial migration along the tubing prior to replacement of the access port.

Esophageal/Pouch Enlargement

Enlargement of the esophagus or pouch may occur as a result of binge eating or malposition of the band. Patients who develop pouch enlargement due to maladaptive eating behavior should be treated with behavior modification. Pouch/esophageal enlargement may also occur due to a severely restrictive stoma. These patients usually experience recurrent bouts of emesis and excessive weight loss, exceeding the average weight loss of gastric-band patients in our practice. Treatment is initiated by removal of fluid from the band and obtaining a barium swallow. If the symptoms persist or the barium swallow reveals a persistent enlargement of the pouch, the band should be replaced using either the pars flaccida or perigastric technique.

Tubing and Access Port Problems

Potential complications of the LAGB include mechanical problems with the tubing, such as tubing breaks or leaks, and loss of fixation, leading to difficult port access. Szold et al. reported port complications in 18 out of 715 patients who received a LAGB [23]. Most tubing breaks occurred prior to mid-1999, when a revised connection of the tubing was introduced and a tie to secure the tubing to the port was no longer required. Inadvertent needle sticks of the tubing may lead to leaks. Leaks or tubing breaks cause loss of fluid, which is manifest by a loss in the sense of restriction. We test for leaks by simply measuring the volume of fluid with needle aspiration. If a discrepancy exists between fluid placed into the port and the amount aspirated, the port site can be mobilized and tested under local or general anesthesia. A localized tubing leak may be repaired or a break managed by replacing the access port. The access port may rotate if inadequate fixation sutures are placed, which can lead to difficulty in port access. Localizing the port with fluoroscopy and identifying the appropriate angle at which to insert the needle under fluoroscopic visualization may allow successful port access. To minimize potential mechanical problems with the access port and tubing, it is important to make sure that the tubing passes in a smooth line into the abdominal cavity without kinking or looping of the tubing and to ensure adequate fixation of the port.

CONCLUSION

Meticulous surgical technique, vigilance, and knowledge of potential complications are essential components of avoiding complications of laparoscopic bariatric surgery. Major complications such as leaks, bleeding, bowel obstructions, and pulmonary embolus may occur with each of the aforementioned procedures. Leaks or perforation may occur at any anastamosis or staple line or secondary to inadvertent thermal injury. Classic signs and symptoms of leaks may occur with leakage of enteric contents anywhere along the gastrointestinal tract; a negative radiological examination should be followed by an operative exploration to rule out leaks at relatively obscure sites such as the enteroenterostomy or the gastric remnant. Early identification and treatment is paramount to limiting the clinical sequelae of potential complications of bariatric procedures.

REFERENCES

1. Pories WJ, Swanson MS, MacDonald KG, et al. Who would have thought it? An operation proves to be the most effective therapy for adult-onset diabetes mellitus. Ann Surg 1995; 222:339–352.
2. Wittgrove AC, Clark GW, Treblay LJ. Laparoscopic gastric bypass, Roux-en Y: Preliminary report of five cases. Obes Surg 1994; 4:353–357.
3. Higa KD, Booone KB, Ho T, Davies OG. Laparoscopic Roux-en-Y gastric bypass for morbid obesity: Technique and preliminary results of our first 400 patients. Arch Surg 2000; 135:1029–1034.
4. Higa KD, Boone KB, Ho T. Complications of the laparoscopic Roux-en-Y gastric bypass: 1,040 patients—What have we learned. Obes Surg 2000; 10:509–513.
5. Schauer PR, Ikramuddin S, Gourash W, et al. Outcomes after laparoscopic Roux-en-Y gastric bypass for morbid obesity. Ann Surg 2000; 232:515–529.
6. Wittgrove AC, Clark GW. Laparoscopic gastric bypass, Roux-en-Y: 500 patients: Technique and results, with 3–60 month follow-up. Obes Surg 2000; 10:233–239.
7. Filip JE, Mattar SG, Bowers SP, Smith CD. Internal hernia formation after laparoscopic Roux-en-Y gastric bypass for morbid obesity. Am Surg 2002; 68(7):640–643.
8. Champion JK. The route of the roux in laparoscopic gastric bypass-does it matter. Obes Surg 2001; 11:159.
9. Wittgrove AC, Clark GW. Laparoscopic gastric bypass, Roux-en-Y—500 patients: Technique and results, with 3–60 month follow-up. Obes Surg 2000; 10(3):233–239.
10. Champion JK, Hunt T, DeLisle N. Laparoscopic vertical banded gastroplasty and Roux-en-Y gastric bypass. Obes Surg 2000; 10:378–379.
11. Dela Torre RA, Scott JS. Laparoscopic Roux-en-Y gastric bypass: A totally intra-abdominal approach—Technique and preliminary report. Obes Surg 1999; 9: 492–497.
12. Champion JK, Hunt T, DeLisle N. Laparoscopic vertical banded gastroplasty and Roux-en-Y gastric bypass. Obes Surg 1999; 9:123.
13. Higa KD, Boone KB, Ho T. Complications of the laparoscopic Roux-en-Y gastric bypass: 1,040 patients—What have we learned. Obes Surg 2000; 10(6):509–513.
14. Printen KJ, LeFavre J, Alden J. Bleeding from the bypassed stomach following gastric bypass. Surg Gynecol Obstet 1983; 156(1):65–66.
15. Sinar DR, Flickinger EG, Park HK, Sloss RR. Retrograde endoscopy of the bypassed stomach segment after gastric bypass surgery: Unexpected lesions. South Med J 1985; 78(3):255–258.
16. Fobi M, Lee H, Holness R, et al. Gastric bypass operation for obesity. World J Surg 1998; 22:925–935.

17. Mason EE, Doherty C, Cullen JJ, Scott D, Rodriguez EM, Maher JW. Vertical gastroplasty: Evolution of vertical banded gastroplasty. World J Surg 1998; 22(9): 919–924.
18. Balsinger BM, Poggio JL, Mai J, Kelley KA, Sarr MG. Ten and more years after vertical banded gastroplasty as primary operation for morbid obesity. J Gastrointest Surg 2000; 4:598–605.
19. Champion JK. Incidence of endostapler malfunction during laparoscopic bariatric surgery. Obes Surg 2000; 10:131.
20. Kuzmak L. A review of 7-yeas experience with silicone gastric banding. Obes Surg 1991; 1:403–408.
21. Belachew M, Legrand M, Jacquet N. Laparoscopic placement of adjustable silicone gastric banding in the treatment of morbid obesity: An animal model experimental study; A video film, a preliminary report. Obes Surg 1993; 3:140.
22. Belachew M, Legrand MJ, Defechereaux TH, et al. Laparoscopic adjustable silicone gastric banding in the treatment of morbid obesity. A preliminary report. Surg Endosc 1994; 8:1354–1356.
23. Szold A, Abu-Abeid S. Laparoscopic adjustable silicone gastric banding for morbid obesity. Results and complications in 715 patients. Surg Endosc 2002; 16:230–233.

8

Cholecystectomy

Fumihiko Fujita, Koji Otsuka, Luca Giordano, and Edward H. Phillips
Ceders-Sinai Medical Center, Los Angeles, California, U.S.A.

INTRODUCTION

The laparoscopic technique of cholecystectomy (LC) has almost completely replaced the open one for the treatment of symptomatic gallstones. The advantages of LC include reduced postoperative recovery time, shorter hospitalization, reduced pain, improved cosmesis, and rapid return to normal activities [1–3]. Though there was much less surgical trauma for the majority of patients undergoing LC, there was an increased incidence of certain complications, such as bile duct injuries and strictures [4–6].

The laparoscopic technique is not for every situation. While there are no absolute contraindications to LC, there are relative ones; these are multiple prior abdominal surgeries, diffuse peritonitis, cirrhosis of the liver, or known gallbladder carcinoma. In these situations, the decision whether or not to proceed with the laparoscopic technique is based on judgment and the skill level of the operating surgeon. The decreasing number of contraindications to LC and the decreasing conversion rate parallel the increased experience of surgeons and the significant advances of laparoscopic surgical instrumentation [7].

The common complications specific to laparoscopic cholecystectomy, as well as their prevention and treatment, are discussed in this chapter.

BILE DUCT INJURY

Bile duct injury is a serious complication that can be life-altering and even fatal. Prior to laparoscopic cholecystectomy, the incidence of bile duct injuries was 0.1–0.3% [8,9]. During the LC era, the estimated incidence of major bile duct injuries has risen to an estimated 0.4–0.6% [4,10–12].

The most common injury occurs when the common bile duct is misidentified and thought to be the cystic duct. If the misidentification is not recognized, an excisional injury follows. The common hepatic duct is usually divided just beneath the bifurcation. Occasionally, the excision involves the bifurcation, and the right and left bile ducts require separate repairs. Excisional injuries usually result in significant early and long-term morbidity as they are difficult to repair and often stricture. Careful identification of the cystic duct and its junction with the gallbladder is always required to avoid this injury. The underside of the gallbladder must be dissected and followed to its adhesion to the liver bed to ensure that the common hepatic or right hepatic duct is not adherent to it.

Another injury that occurs during the initial dissection of the cystic duct is due to the injudicious use of cautery. This leads to a remote thermal injury of the common duct and may result in a delayed leak or stricture. These injuries may present days, weeks, or months after the initial surgery and often require reconstruction. This can be avoided by the sparing use of cautery until the anatomy is identified. Dissection should be performed bluntly. Suction and patience should be used until the dissection is completed.

The most likely causative factors of bile duct stricture include thermal or laser injury, excessive manipulation, and mechanical trauma to the common bile duct and bile duct vessels during the operative dissection [13]. The most common site of a bile duct stricture associated with LC is in the common hepatic duct or at the bifurcation of the right and left ducts (Bismuth types 3, 4, and 5) (Table 1) [5]. Patients with these injuries tend to present later in their postoperative course, sometimes 4–6 weeks to several months after the initial procedure.

TABLE 1 Bismuth Classification of Bile Duct Strictures

Type 1:	Low common hepatic duct stricture (>2 cm of hepatic duct stump)
Type 2:	Mid common hepatic duct stricture (<2 cm of hepatic duct stump)
Type 3:	Hilar stricture with no residual common hepatic duct but hilar confluence intact
Type 4:	Destruction of hilar confluence (right and left hepatic ducts separated)
Type 5:	Combined common hepatic duct and aberrant right hepatic duct injury

Table 2 Bile Duct Injury: Mechanism and Pattern

Mechanism	Pattern
Misidentification	Incision in CBD, Excision of CHD
Clipped CBD when clipping cystic duct	Partial or complete obstruction of CBD
Electrocautery	Stricture of CBD or CHD, delayed bile leak
Misidentification of right hepatic duct	Excision, bile leak, obstruction

Abbreviations: CBD-common bile duct, CHD-common hepatic duct.

Repair of bile duct injuries usually requires hepaticojejunostomy Roux-en-Y reconstruction. The best treatment is prevention. The main patterns and the etiology of bile duct injuries are summarized in Tables 2 and 3.

Preoperative Evaluation

The surgeon must always perform a thorough preoperative evaluation of all patients. Comorbid illnesses should be identified. Similarly, elderly patients can be expected to have a higher incidence of comorbidities and more complications following LC. Evidence of prior surgery should suggest the presence of adhesions or abdominal wall hernias, which can complicate the laparoscopic technique.

While many bile duct injuries occur during an ''easy'' case from misidentification of the ducts, acute cholecystitis carries the most significant risk for bile duct injury. A history of prior severe cholecystitis and present acute exacerbation is probably the worst combination, as acute inflammation (edema, bleeding) is superimposed on chronic scar tissue. Acute cholecystitis not only makes the surgical dissection more difficult, but also makes these patients have nearly twice the incidence of common bile duct (CBD) stones (18%) compared to uncomplicated cases [14]. Cirrhosis of the liver or morbid obesity is also a risk factor because of the difficulty in exposing the hilum.

Table 3 Bile Duct Injury: Etiologies

Poor visualization	Obesity, bleeding due to cirrhosis, prior surgery, inexperience, obscured operative field
Difficult anatomy	Acute cholecystitis, variant anatomy
Technique	Improper use of cautery, traumatic dissection, improper retraction

Patients with acute cholecystitis usually complain of right-upper-quadrant pain, nausea, or vomiting. Murphy's sign is frequently present. Schafer et al. [15] demonstrated that it was possible to predict the severity of inflammation by using laboratory (white blood cell count, C-reactive protein) demographic (age, gender), and individual (American Society of Anesthesiologists classification, duration of symptoms) findings. Physical examination may reveal an abdominal mass or palpable gallbladder.

Laboratory assessments should include an ultrasound, serum bilirubin, glutamyl transferases, alkaline phosphatase, and amylase (if acute), and albumin and prothrombin if cirrhosis is suspected.

Abdominal ultrasound (US) is the most useful test for the detection of possible gallbladder calculi, evaluation of the thickness of the gallbladder wall, and measurement of the common duct diameter. Computed tomography (CT) may succeed where US fails because of intestinal gas and/or obesity, and it provides excellent definition of the anatomy, especially when a tumor is suspected. Endoscopic retrograde cholangiopancreatography (ERCP) can provide precise definition of biliary and pancreatic anatomy. ERCP should be considered preoperatively for patients with severe cholangitis or those with unremitting severe pancreatitis or for patients suspected of having pancreatic or biliary tumors. Magnetic resonance cholangiopancreatography (MRCP) is noninvasive and can replace ERCP in selected patients, especially to diagnose common bile duct calculi. Percutaneous transhepatic cholangiography (PTC) is useful for patients with a history of a Billroth II gastrojejunostomy when MRCP is nondiagnostic. In our opinion, MRCP should not be used instead of an intraoperative cholangiogram in patients suspected of harboring common duct stones. Even in the most suspicious circumstances, preoperative ERCP fails to show stones in 50% of patients [62]. Consequently, even if laparoscopic duct exploration is not available, open duct exploration or postoperative ERCP is preferable to subjecting half of the patients to a negative invasive test. Other than the previously mentioned preoperative indications, endoscopic sphincterotomy should be reserved for those cases with CBD stones that are not surgical candidates or those who have retained CBD stones after attempted surgical removal.

Preoperative Measures for Prevention of the Avoidable Complications

Bleeding and inflammation are risk factors for bile duct injury. In acute cholecystitis, severe inflammation of the porta hepatis can make dissection and identification of the cystic duct and artery difficult. The back wall of the gallbladder may also be fused to the liver from inflammation, resulting in bleeding when dissected

[16]. In these patients with severe inflammation, the use of antibiotics before the operation is recommended. However, there is really nothing that can be done acutely to significantly decrease the inflammation except to postpone the procedure to a later date—at least 6 weeks later. If a patient has a first attack, the edema and inflammation usually dissect easily. But if the patient has had multiple previous attacks of cholecystitis, it may be worth trying to "cool the patient off" with antibiotics. If the patient does not improve during a 48-hr trial, surgery will have to be performed urgently. However, if the gallbladder is palpable or an empyema is suspected, surgery should be undertaken after stabilization and antibiotic administration.

Cholangitis is a risk factor for systemic septic complications and hepatic abscess. Stones in the bile ducts are the most common cause of extrahepatic obstructive jaundice and cholangitis. An obstructed biliary tree becomes colonized rather quickly, usually with gram-negative bacteria. The resulting cholangitis becomes an important potential source of bacteremia and systemic infection. Early surgical or endoscopic decompression is indicated. ERCP with endoscopic sphincterotomy and even stent placement is indicated preoperatively.

Intraoperative Measures to Prevent Complications

Good visualization is one of the most important factors in preventing complications intraoperatively. Visualization is improved by using a 30-degree endoscope and good laparoscopic equipment. If visualization is not adequate, the procedure should be converted to an open one. The other consideration of visualization is exposure. The infundibulum of the gallbladder and the region of the porta hepatis must be clearly in view on the operating monitor prior to beginning any dissection. Additionally, the operative field must not be obscured by the stomach, duodenum, colon, omentum, or liver [17]. An additional 5-mm working port can be placed to add a retractor to improve exposure. If exposure is suboptimal, the procedure should be converted to an open one.

The gallbladder fundus should be elevated over the liver by an atraumatic grasper and fixed to the patient so the exposure is fixed and no assistant is required to maintain it. This allows the assistant to work with two hands via an additional working port for an extra retractor or grasper (Fig. 1).

The dissection should start high up on the gallbladder where the fat begins to hide the infundibulum. In cases of acute and chronic cholecystitis, the anatomy may be obscured and the porta hepatis may not be distinguishable from the body of the gallbladder. By bluntly stripping the fat off, where the wall of the gallbladder becomes obscure by itself, inadvertent injury to a common duct that has scarred to a contracted body of the gallbladder or Hartman's pouch can be avoided.

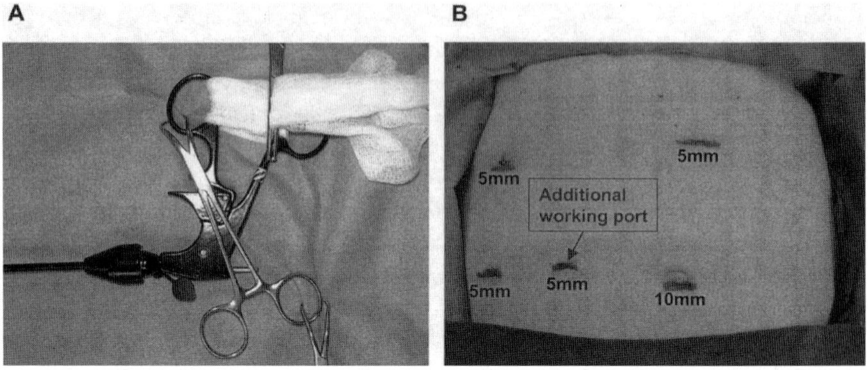

Figure 1 A. The grasper is secured to the patient's drapes. B. Additional trocar to control bleeding or improve exposure in difficult cholecystectomy.

Dissection of the lateral Hartman's pouch can identify the common duct laterally where there is no cystic artery (except in the 10% of cases of a replaced right hepatic artery). Sometimes, the infundibulum and Hartman's pouch wrap around the porta hepatis laterally and the inflammation obscures the duct and hilar anatomy. By bluntly stripping away the fat, the surgeon can sweep the duct away from the body of the gallbladder and can feel the structures as firm bands, alerting him or her to the possibility of the bile duct being ''higher'' than usual. Again, lateral blunt dissection can unwrap the body and infundibulum from the porta hepatis and allow for identification of the posterolateral common duct.

If the body of the gallbladder cannot be fully dissected (360 degrees), it is safer to transect the gallbladder transversely high up on the body, empty the stones, and dissect the lower half of the gallbladder from the top down (Fig. 2). The origin of the cystic duct can also be identified from within the gallbladder. A cholangiogram through the open gallbladder can verify the anatomy. If at this point the anatomy is not clear (note that there has been no division of any tubular structure), the procedure should be converted to an open one. Some authors have demonstrated that laparoscopic subtotal cholecystectomy is a safe, feasible, and effective procedure, allowing removal of a difficult gallbladder and reducing the need for open conversion [16,18,19]. On the other hand, Raj et al. [20] recommend a routine fundus-down approach, which might lower the rate of injury to the common bile duct to that of open cholecystectomy. Whichever approach is used, no clips should be placed and no incisions made into a tubular structure until the cystic duct's infundibular junction and the junction of the body of the gallbladder with the liver have been identified with certainty.

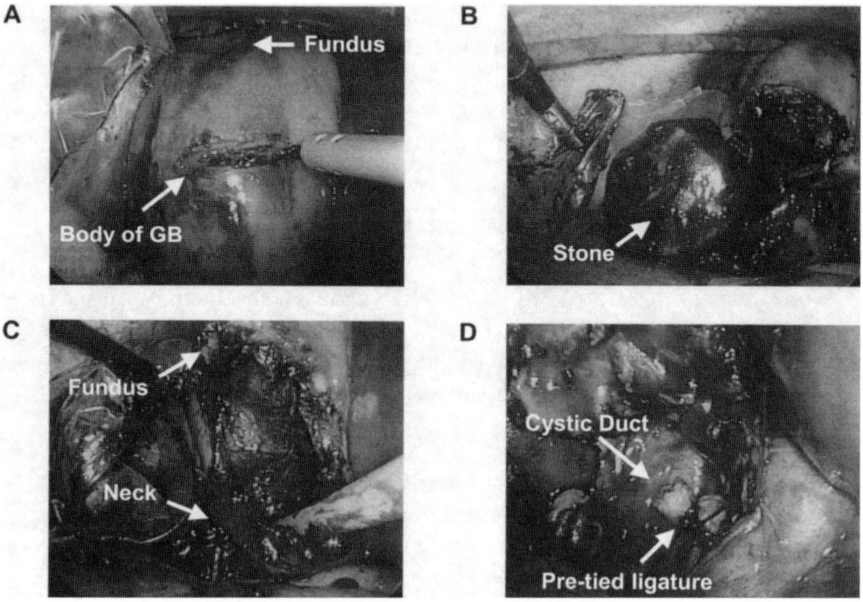

FIGURE 2 The technique for transections the gallbladder. A. The gallbladder (GB) is transected. B. The stone is removed. C. The gallbladder is dissected off the liver bed using the top-down technique; the cystic duct is cannulated through the opening into the gallbladder to obtain an intraoperative cholangiogram. D. A pretied ligature on cystic duct.

Intraoperative cholangiography (IOC) is an important adjunct to the prevention of excisional bile duct injuries [21]. IOC can confirm the anatomy and exclude other abnormalities. In some cases, the operative plan will be altered on the basis of cholangiography. While cholangiography does not appear to decrease the absolute incidence of biliary injuries, the injury level—and thus the severity, morbidity, late sequelae, and costs—are reduced by IOC [22]. If the common duct is misidentified as the cystic duct, a small lateral incision is the end result if a cholangiogram is performed instead of an excision of the common hepatic duct.

Some argue that IOC can be the cause of morbidity and complications itself. One possible pattern of cystic duct injury has been ascribed to unrecognized mechanical injuries to the posterior wall of the cystic duct during introduction of a cholangiocatheter [23]. Avoidance of the use of rigid catheters can easily prevent these injuries. Additionally, excessive force during manipulation of the catheter into the cystic duct should be avoided.

Bile leak from the cystic duct can be reduced by not using electrocautery to divide the duct. Additionally, if the cystic duct is large or edematous, a pretied loop, rather than a clip, should be used to provide a more secure closure. Again, electrocautery should not be used to dissect the cystic duct. Electrocautery can cause a thermal injury that is not recognized at the time of surgery, leading to necrosis of the cystic duct and subsequent bile leak.

Postoperative Clinical Signs and Management of Bile Duct Injury

Acute bile duct injuries are usually associated with bile leaks; therefore, a patient's complaint of abdominal pain is unexpected following LC [13,21]. Sometimes patients will present with pulmonary symptoms similar to pulmonary embolus, as the bile irritation of the diaphragm causes chest and shoulder pain with tachypnea and tachycardia. The physical examination will usually reveal peritonitis, guarding, rigidity, icterus, or jaundice. Rarely will a bile leak not produce physical findings. Bile in the peritoneal cavity usually results in chemical and subsequent bacterial peritonitis. This is manifest clinically by shortness of breath, nausea, vomiting fever, tachypnea, and tachycardia. Jaundice is caused by complete or partial obstruction—a sign of bile duct injury and not merely a cystic duct leak. The bilirubin level is usually under 3.0 when bile is absorbed from the peritoneal cavity without an element of sepsis or obstruction. A proposed algorithm for the management of suspected bile duct injury is shown in Fig. 3.

US and CT examinations are very helpful to identify complications after surgery. An ultrasound examination should be performed for evaluation of patients who are suspected of having an abnormal fluid accumulation in the subhepatic space. Dilated extrahepatic and intrahepatic biliary ducts can also be found if obstruction is present.

If an obstruction is suspected, ERCP should follow. This procedure can be both diagnostic and therapeutic, as a stent can be inserted if needed. Percutaneous transhepatic cholangiography (PTC) is needed in some cases and will show the level of damage in cases of complete bile duct obstruction or transection and allows for placement of a drainage catheter. Furthermore, a percutaneous drain in the bile collection should be placed under CT or US guidance as it decreases morbidity, sepsis, and pain.

Chronic or delayed bile duct injuries, such as strictures, present more insidiously. Anorexia, ileus, or abdominal pain that does not resolve as quickly as would be expected should alert the surgeon to the possibility of a bile duct injury [21]. Delayed injuries can be evaluated with MRCP, but these usually require an ERCP for dilation or stenting.

Treatment

Most bile duct injuries should be treated with Roux-en-Y hepaticojejunostomy. The exceptions are when the injury is a lateral incision or a clip injury that can

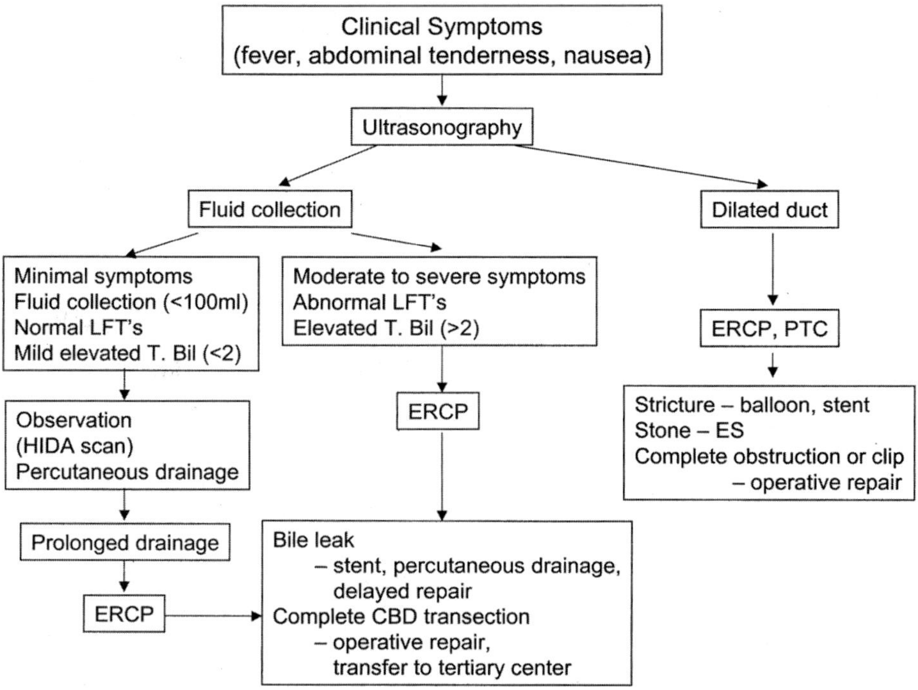

FIGURE 3 The algorithm for management of suspected bile duct injury. HIDA scan-99m-technetium hepatobiliary iminodiacetic acid scan; ERCP = endoscopic retrograde cholangiography; PTC = percutaneous transhepatic cholangiography; ES = endoscopic sphincterotomy; CBD = common bile duct; LFT = liver function test; T. Bil = total bilirubin

be repaired primarily or with a T tube or stent. This is true whether the injury is discovered at the time of the initial operation or days to weeks after the initial procedure. All excisional or thermal injuries need to be treated with a Roux-en-Y hepaticojejunostomy.

If the surgeon is not able, by circumstance or skill, to perform a Roux-en-Y hepaticojejunostomy, a drainage catheter should be placed into the severed bile ducts and the area drained with closed suction catheters. Later, after having been stabilized, the patient can be transferred to a facility with experience in treating these injuries. Some surgeons have argued that it is best to leave the severed bile duct ligated so that it will dilate and make subsequent repair easier. This is not necessary. Modern surgical experience and techniques of anastomosis have obviated the need for that type of treatment. It is considered best to maintain hepatic function by drainage rather than ligation of the duct, which interferes with the normal processes of the liver.

If the injury is chronic, a nonsurgical approach should be investigated. If a stricture is short, hydrostatic balloon dilatation and placement of biliary stents can be performed endoscopically or percutaneously. There are some data suggesting that endoscopic and radiological approaches have higher success rates in the management of anastomotic strictures than repeated surgical attempts [24].

BILE LEAK

Bile leak following LC is a major problem because it usually results in biliary peritonitis. Bile may escape from the liver bed, unrecognized accessory ducts, the cystic duct stump, or a bile duct injury. Cystic duct leaks are more likely to occur in the setting of acute cholecystitis, when the cystic duct stump is broad, there is scissoring of the cystic duct clip, or the surgeon cannot adequately visualize and confirm accurate clip placement at the time of operation [25,26]. Alternatively, a leak may be caused by the injudicious use of cautery that results in devascularization of the cystic duct [26–28].

Postoperative Management of Bile Leak

An ultrasonic examination is usually the first study performed and, in this scenario, will confirm a subhepatic or subphrenic fluid collection. If the hemoglobin is stable and the bilirubin is elevated, a bile leak should be considered. Radionuclide hepatobiliary scans with ^{99m}Tc-IDA (technetium 99m–labeled iminodiacetic acid) can also help to detect the accumulation of isotopes outside the biliary tree, which documents an ongoing bile leak [21]. When a leak is identified or suspected, ERCP can not only demonstrate the leak but also allow for transampullary stent placement [17].

Treatment

Cystic duct bile leak, leak from accessory bile ducts or leaks from the liver bed should be managed nonoperatively. Endoscopic nasobiliary or transampullary stent placement, combined with percutaneous drainage, has been found to be excellent therapy [7,29,30]. Though minor bed leaks can be treated with percutaneous drainage alone, a bile duct stent decreases the time needed to heal the leak.

However, asymptomatic or minimally symptomatic subhepatic collections are unlikely to be caused by significant or persistent bile leakage; these very small subhepatic bile accumulations can be managed with observation alone or percutaneous drainage. On the other hand, a patient who is significantly symptomatic and has a documented bile collection or active bile duct leak with peritoneal signs should have endoscopic stenting and percutaneous drainage. Only those patients who continue to deteriorate with uncontrolled leakage should undergo surgery, laparoscopic or open [31,32].

BLEEDING

Intraoperative bleeding during LC can occur from several sites. Minor bleeding may occur at trocar insertion sites in the abdominal wall. Bleeding from liver laceration may occur due to excessive retraction on the gallbladder, or it may be secondary to injury from an instrument or trocar. Bleeding from inflamed tissue due to acute cholecystitis is common, and bleeding from the cystic artery is not unusual. Injury to the hepatic artery or portal vein is rare.

Preoperative Evaluations to Prevent Complications

Close attention should be paid to patients to diagnose comorbidities that predispose to bleeding, such as hepatic or hematological diseases. In all of these cases, preoperative evaluations of hemoglobin, platelet count, and liver function are required. Any abnormalities should be corrected preoperatively if possible.

Intraoperative Management of Bleeding

Bleeding from trocar insertion sites in the abdominal wall is usually self-limited but may occasionally prove to be troublesome. It is best dealt with by passing an absorbable suture through the abdominal wall into the peritoneal cavity and then back out above and below the working port site. Bleeding from a liver laceration is best treated by benign neglect. Temporary insertion of a gauze sponge into the peritoneal cavity can serve to apply pressure to the injury. Most liver bleeding that can be stopped with cautery would have stopped with pressure. Rarely, a major vein is near the surface of the liver and suturing is required. Bleeding from the portal vein is usually associated with bile duct injury and should be considered a criterion for converting to the open technique. If an errant grasper punctures the porta hepatis and bleeding occurs, it is safer to apply pressure with a gauze sponge rather than making indiscriminate use of clips or cautery.

Injury to the cystic artery (or if a clip comes off) results in significant bleeding that can obscure visualization. The bleeding vessel should be grasped, if visible, or pressure applied to slow the bleeding. The field should be thoroughly suctioned before clips or a pretied ligature is applied. Of course, no further dissection should be initiated until the bleeding is under control and the patient hemodynamically stable. Blind clipping or the application of electrocoagulation current is dangerous in such a situation and should not be done lest an injury to the bile duct occur. If the bleeding is exigent or uncontrollable, the patient should be opened immediately. Bleeding from the gallbladder bed may be controlled easily by using coagulation current or argon beam coagulation. The key to preventing this is to maintain a dissection plane as close to the gallbladder as possible. Otherwise, gauze packing is effective in stopping this bleeding as well.

In dealing with bleeding (just as when anatomy is obscure), adding an additional working port provides access for an additional instrument to improve exposure or for suctioning that is needed to efficiently and safely identify the bleeding site and control it.

CONVERSION TO OPEN

Conversion rates for both acute and chronic cholecystitis have been reported to range from 2–20% (average 5%) [33–37]. Inability to delineate the anatomy secondary to adhesions or inflammation, unexpected operative findings, and iatrogenic injuries are the most common reasons for conversion [3,33]. If, after a predetermined period of time, the anatomy is still not clear, conversion should be considered.

There are some predictive factors for conversion of laparoscopic to open cholecystectomy. These include morbid obesity, thickened gallbladder wall [38], advanced age, presence of cardiovascular disease, male gender, acute cholecystitis, and severe inflammation [3,37].

Conversion to an open operation should not be viewed as a complication or as the result of inexperience, but as an exercise in good judgment. Various reasons associated with conversion are summarized in Table 4.

LAPAROSCOPIC CHOLECYSTECTOMY AND CIRRHOSIS

Until recently, cirrhosis has been considered to be an absolute or relative contraindication to LC [39,40]. But Morino et al. reported that Child-Pugh A and Child-Pugh B patients could undergo LC safely [41]. Careful attention should be paid to diagnosing cirrhosis preoperatively. A high index of suspicion is needed, as some cases are unsuspected and difficult to diagnose.

If hypertrophic collateral venous circulation above the abdominal wall (''caput medusae'') is present, an umbilical port should be avoided to prevent

TABLE 4 Reasons for Conversion to Open Surgery

Unclear anatomy
Bleeding or vascular injury
Bile duct injury or suspected injury
Bowel injury (duodenum, colon)
Gall bladder carcinoma

injury to an umbilical vein. A left-lower-quadrant site is best for the initial puncture. Once the cystic duct is identified, blunt dissection should be avoided to minimize bleeding and all tissues should be clipped and cut. Sometimes, subtotal cholecystectomy should be performed to prevent massive blood loss from the varicosities in the gallbladder bed. The anterior wall of the gallbladder may be excised with electrocoagulation, leaving a rim of the posterior wall attached to the liver. In these cases, the mucosa of the remaining posterior wall should be dessicated with electrocoagulation or argon beam coagulation [42]. All access ports should be checked internally for bleeding just before completion of the procedure.

Postoperative Management of Bleeding

Bleeding is an important postoperative complication and tends to occur within the first 24 hr of surgery. Surgeons should check the vital signs carefully, as tachycardia can be the first sign of bleeding. If a drain was placed during the initial operation, it may be clotted, and lack of output should not dissuade one from considering hemorrhage as a cause of cardiovascular collapse.

When bleeding is suspected by changes in vital signs and a fall in hemoglobin, the patient should initially be resuscitated with crystalloid simultaneously with analysis of prothrombin time, platelet count, and, if indicated, clotting factors. Blood should be typed and cross-matched if the patient's status allows. If the patient is unstable and the use of blood that has not been cross-matched is necessary, immediate surgical exploration is required. If they are bleeding more slowly, as evidenced by easily stabilized vital signs, patients should undergo ultrasound to diagnose intraperitoneal fluid. Sometimes significant hemorrhage can occur in the abdominal wall. A CT scan can diagnose these hematomas. In the acute setting, abdominal wall bleeding can be occult clinically. But as a rule, unstable patients suspected of postoperative bleeding should be immediately returned to the operating room.

INTRAPERITONEAL SPILLAGE OF STONES AND BILE

Iatrogenic gallbladder perforation during LC is common and occurs in as many a 40% of cases [43,44], often leading to spillage of bile and gallstones into the peritoneal cavity. It has been reported that spilled stones can lead to intra-abdominal abscesses [45–50], wound infections [50–53], small bowel obstruction [54,55], empyema [50,56,57], and even colocutaneous fistula [49].

Intraoperative Measures to Prevent this Complication

Retrieval of gallstones spilled during LC can be challenging because of difficulty in exposing the perihepatic or subhepatic space [58]. The authors recommend that every effort should be made to remove all the stones once spillage has occurred. First, insert a specimen bag into the peritoneal cavity and place it above the liver. Use a closed grasper to elevate the right lobe of the liver while using another grasper to push down on the right colon and duodenum to expose the subhepatic space and then the suprarenal space. Stones are always in these two areas. Judicious irrigation can sometimes help, as some stones float. A large-bore suction device (Probe-plus II with stone retrieval attachment; Ethicon) can remove small stones and bile [58]; otherwise a chest tube that fits through a 10-mm trocar with the side holes cut off can be used to capture larger stones. Larger stones must be grasped and placed in the specimen bag.

If the gallbladder is inflamed and distended and perforation is likely, it is helpful to place a gauze sponge into the subhepatic space to catch stones should a perforation occur. If the gallbladder becomes perforated, the site of perforation can be temporarily closed using an Endoloop (Ethicon EndoSurgery, Cincinnati, OH, USA), thus limiting further stone spillage. The perforated gallbladder should be removed from the abdomen, using a specimen bag, via the umbilical trocar site (or the site of the largest trocar) to avoid contamination of the wound. Any bile in the abdomen should be irrigated with normal saline and suctioned until the return is clear.

Rupture of the gallbladder during extraction from the umbilical port site is extremely frustrating and time-consuming. It is difficult to remove stones from the omentum. Replacing the port and visualizing the area with the laparoscope can facilitate retrieval of the stones, but if there are many it is usually easier to widen the umbilical incision and remove them under direct vision. Of course, this can be avoided by exercising patience and using a specimen bag during gallbladder extraction.

Postoperative Management

Spillage of bile and stones can lead to an intra-abdominal abscess or a wound infection. Symptoms such as fever, abdominal pain, or wound erythema should alert one to these possibilities. If stone spillage occurred during LC and not all were removed, prophylactic antibiotic use is recommended, especially in imunosuppressed patients; in this instance, a second-generation cephalosporin could be adequate. Bacterial culture of the removed stones may be helpful for selecting the antibiotics to be used. If an abscess is diagnosed and stones are present, percutaneous drainage and prolonged antibiotic administration will usually be successful. Percutaneous intubation of the abscess cavity and stone retrieval has even been performed in some cases. Repeat drainage and antibiotics can treat a single recurrence, but a third recurrence should lead to surgical intervention [48,59].

COMMON BILE DUCT STONES

Since common bile duct (CBD) stones occur in at least 10% of patients undergoing LC, any discussion of complications must take these patients into account. The incidence of CBD stones is 18% in patients with acute cholecystitis, and unsuspected CBD stones occur in 4% of patients undergoing laparoscopic cholecystectomy. Intraoperative cholangiography will diagnose these stones and appropriate treatment will prevent postoperative complications of cholangitis, hepatic abscess, pancreatitis, and chronic abdominal pain. The pre-, intra-, and postoperative treatment of these patients is discussed in a separate chapter.

POSTOPERATIVE PANCREATITIS

Pancreatitis can occur from hypotension or drug reaction or be idiopathic, but when it occurs after LC, gallstone pancreatitis must be considered [60]. Gallstone migration with transient blockage of the ampulla of Vater can cause this complication [61]. Initially, all patients should be managed with intravenous fluids, bowel rest, and pain control [60]. In the vast majority, the stone will pass spontaneously, the amylase will decrease over the next few days, and the patient will recover. However, an MRCP should be done to prove that there are no other stones present. But the fact remains that MRCP can miss an impacted stone in the ampulla. If the pancreatitis does not improve in 24–48 hr, ERCP should be performed. Of course, an intraoperative cholangiogram can diagnose the presence of CBD stones, and laparoscopic duct exploration can remove them in 90% of instances.

CONCLUSION

Despite careful preparation, unexpected scenarios can sometimes be encountered during laparoscopic cholecystectomy. These situations can lead to unfortunate sequelae, but their prompt and adequate management will surely reduce morbidity and mortality. In addition, constant attention to any comorbidity that may exist will significantly aid in the minimization of the occurrence of some of these most feared complications.

REFERENCES

1. Wongworawat MDet al. The impact of prior intra-abdominal surgery on laparoscopic cholecystectomy. Am Surg 1994; 60(10):763–766.
2. Lujan JAet al. Laparoscopic cholecystectomy vs open cholecystectomy in the treatment of acute cholecystitis: A prospective study. Arch Surg 1998; 133(2):173–175.
3. Kanaan SAet al. Risk factors for conversion of laparoscopic to open cholecystectomy. J Surg Res 2002; 106(1):20–24.

4. Adamsen Set al. Bile duct injury during laparoscopic cholecystectomy: A prospective nationwide series. J Am Coll Surg 1997; 184(6):571–578.
5. Lillemoe KDet al. Postoperative bile duct strictures: Management and outcome in the 1990s. Ann Surg 2000; 232(3):430–441.
6. Melton GBet al. Major bile duct injuries associated with laparoscopic cholecystectomy: Effect of surgical repair on quality of life. Ann Surg 2002; 235(6):888–895.
7. Bailey R, Gluck E. Cholecystectomy. In . Bailey R , Flowers J, eds. Complications of Laparoscopic Surgery. St Louis: Quality Medical Publishing, 1995:77–127.
8. Roslyn JJet al. Open cholecystectomy. A contemporary analysis of 42,474 patients. Ann Surg 1993; 218(2):129–137.
9. Strasberg SM, Hertl M, Soper NJ. An analysis of the problem of biliary injury during laparoscopic cholecystectomy. J Am Coll Surg 1995; 180(1):101–125.
10. Wherry DCet al. An external audit of laparoscopic cholecystectomy in the steady state performed in medical treatment facilities of the Department of Defense. Ann Surg 1996; 224(2):145–154.
11. Windsor JA, Pong J. Laparoscopic biliary injury: More than a learning curve problem. Aust NZ J Surg 1998; 68(3):186–189.
12. Fletcher DRet al. Complications of cholecystectomy: Risks of the laparoscopic approach and protective effects of operative cholangiography: A population-based study. Ann Surg 1999; 229(4):449–457.
13. Davidoff AMet al. Mechanisms of major biliary injury during laparoscopic cholecystectomy. Ann Surg 1992; 215(3):196–202.
14. Phillips EHet al. Laparoscopic cholecystectomy in acute cholecystitis. Am Surg 1992; 58(5):273–276.
15. Schafer M, Krahenbuhl L, Buchler MW. Predictive factors for the type of surgery in acute cholecystitis. Am J Surg 2001; 182(3):291–297.
16. Ransom KJ. Laparoscopic management of acute cholecystitis with subtotal cholecystectomy. Am Surg 1998; 64(10):955–957.
17. Onaitis M, Cbekan E. Complications of laparoscopic cholecystectomy. In Pappas T , Chekan Eubanks S, eds. Atlas of Laparoscopic Surgery. Norwalk. CT: Appleton & Lange, 1999, 14.1–14.12.
18. Michalowski Ket al. Laparoscopic subtotal cholecystectomy in patients with complicated acute cholecystitis or fibrosis. Br J Surg 1998; 85(7):904–906.
19. Chowbey PKet al. Laparoscopic subtotal cholecystectomy: A review of 56 procedures. J Laparoendosc Adv Surg Tech A 2000; 10(1):31–34.
20. Raj PK, Castillo G, Urban L. Laparoscopic cholecystectomy: Fundus-down approach. J Laparoendosc Adv Surg Tech A 2001; 11(2):95–100.
21. Rossi RLet al. Laparoscopic bile duct injuries. Risk factors, recognition, and repair. Arch Surg 1992; 127(5):596–601; discussion 601–602.
22. Carroll BJet al. Routine cholangiography reduces sequelae of common bile duct injuries. Surg Endosc 1996; 10(12):1194–1197.
23. Deyo GA. Complications of laparoscopic cholecystectomy. Surg Laparosc Endosc 1992; 2(1):41–48.
24. Millis JMet al. Management of bile duct strictures. An evolving strategy. Arch Surg 1992; 127(9):1077–1082; discussion 1082–1084.

25. Hanazaki Ket al. Bile leakage resulting from clip displacement of the cystic duct stump: A potential pitfall of laparoscopic cholecystectomy. Surg Endosc 1999; 13(2): 168–171.
26. Christoforidis Eet al. The endoscopic management of persistent bile leakage after laparoscopic cholecystectomy. Surg Endosc 2002; 16(5):843–846.
27. Benson EA. Is ischaemia a possible factor in the aetiology of bile duct stricture. Br J Clin Pract 1981; 35(3):97–104.
28. vanSonnenberg Eet al. Complications of laparoscopic cholecystectomy: Coordinated radiologic and surgical management in 21 patients. Radiology 1993; 188(2): 399–404.
29. Liguory Cet al. Endoscopic treatment of postoperative biliary fistulae. Surgery 1991; 110(4):779–83; discussion 783–784.
30. Woods MSet al. Cystic duct leaks in laparoscopic cholecystectomy. Am J Surg 1994; 168(6):560–3; discussion 563–565.
31. Ress AMet al. Spectrum and management of major complications of laparoscopic cholecystectomy. Am J Surg 1993; 165(6):655–662.
32. Soper NJet al. Diagnosis and management of biliary complications of laparoscopic cholecystectomy. Am J Surg 1993; 165(6):663–669.
33. Sanabria JRet al. Risk factors in elective laparoscopic cholecystectomy for conversion to open cholecystectomy. J Am Coll Surg 1994; 179(6):696–704.
34. Alponat Aet al. Predictive factors for conversion of laparoscopic cholecystectomy. World J Surg 1997; 21(6):629–633.
35. Schrenk P, Woisetschlager R, Wayand WU. Laparoscopic cholecystectomy. Cause of conversions in 1,300 patients and analysis of risk factors. Surg Endosc 1995; 9(1): 25–28.
36. Wiebke EAet al. Conversion of laparoscopic to open cholecystectomy. An analysis of risk factors. Surg Endosc 1996; 10(7):742–745.
37. Bingener-Casey Fet al. Reasons for conversion from laparoscopic to open cholecystectomy: A 10-year review. J Gastrointest Surg 2002; 6(6):800–805.
38. Rosen M, Brody F, Ponsky J. Predictive factors for conversion of laparoscopic cholecystectomy. Am J Surg 2002; 184(3):254–258.
39. Cuschieri Aet al. The European experience with laparoscopic cholecystectomy. Am J Surg 1991; 161(3):385–387.
40. Gadacz TR, Talamini MA. Traditional versus laparoscopic cholecystectomy. Am J Surg 1991; 161(3):336–338.
41. Morino Met al. Laparoscopic cholecystectomy in cirrhosis: Contraindication or privileged indication. Surg Laparosc Endosc Percutan Tech 2000; 10(6):360–363.
42. Tuech JJet al. Laparoscopic cholecystectomy in cirrhotic patients. Surg Laparosc Endosc Percutan Tech 2002; 12(4):227–231.
43. Peters JHet al. Complications of laparoscopic cholecystectomy. Surgery 1991; 110(4):769–777; discussion 777–778.
44. Soper NJ, Dunnegan DL. Does intraoperative gallbladder perforation influence the early outcome of laparoscopic cholecystectomy. Surg Laparosc Endosc 1991; 1(3): 156–161.
45. Catarci Met al. Lost intraperitoneal stones after laparoscopic cholecystectomy: Harmless sequela or reason for reoperation. Surg Laparosc Endosc 1993; 3(4):318–322.

46. Mellinger JDet al. Delayed gallstone abscess following laparoscopic cholecystectomy. Surg Endosc 1994; 8(11):1332–1334.
47. Carlin CB, Kent RB, Laws HL. Spilled gallstones—complications of abdominal-wall abscesses. Case report and review of the literature. Surg Endosc 1995; 9(3): 341–343.
48. Maldjian C, Stancato-Pasik A, Shapiro RS. Abscess formation as a late complication of dropped gallstones. Abdom Imaging 1995; 20(3):217–218.
49. Patterson EJ, Nagy AG. Don't cry over spilled stones? Complications of gallstones spilled during laparoscopic cholecystectomy: Case report and literature review. Can J Surg 1997; 40(4):300–304.
50. Horton M, Florence MG. Unusual abscess patterns following dropped gallstones during laparoscopic cholecystectomy. Am J Surg 1998; 175(5):375–379.
51. Wetscher Get al. Subcutaneous abscess due to gallstones lost during laparoscopic cholecystectomy. Endoscopy 1994; 26(3):324–325.
52. Bour ES, Gifford RR. Gallstone umbilical sinus tract formation following laparoscopic cholecystectomy. Arch Surg 1995; 130(9):1007–1008.
53. Rioux Met al. Delayed peritoneal and retroperitoneal abscesses caused by spilled gallstones: A complication following laparoscopic cholecystectomy. Abdom Imaging 1995; 20(3):219–221.
54. Cullis SNet al. Intraperitoneal abscess after laparoscopic cholecystectomy. Surg Laparosc Endosc 1992; 2(4):337–338.
55. Tekin A. Mechanical small bowel obstruction secondary to spilled stones. J Laparoendosc Adv Surg Tech A 1998; 8(3):157–159.
56. Willekes CL, Widmann WD. Empyema from lost gallstones: a thoracic complication of laparoscopic cholecystectomy. J Laparoendosc Surg 1996; 6(2):123–126.
57. Barnard SPet al. Cholelithoptysis and empyema formation after laparoscopic cholecystectomy. Ann Thorac Surg 1995; 60(4):1100–1102.
58. Hui TTet al. Iatrogenic gallbladder perforation during laparoscopic cholecystectomy: etiology and sequelae. Am Surg 1999; 65(10):944–948.
59. Trerotola SOet al. Percutaneous removal of ''dropped'' gallstones after laparoscopic cholecystectomy. Radiology 1993; 188(2):419–421.
60. Bulkin AJ, Tebyani N, Dorazio RA. Gallstone pancreatitis in the era of laparoscopic cholecystectomy. Am Surg 1997; 63(10):900–903.
61. Acosta JM, Ledesma CL. Gallstone migration as a cause of acute pancreatitis. N Engl J Med 1974; 290(9):484–487.
62. Edye Met al. Intraoperative cholangiography is still indicated after preoperative endoscopic cholangiography for gallstone disease. Surg Endosc 2002; 16(5):799–802.

9

Exploration of the Common Bile Duct

Koji Otsuka, Fumihiko Fujita, Luca Giordano, and Edward H. Phillips
Cedars–Sinai Medical Center, Los Angeles, California, U.S.A.

INTRODUCTION

Although the incidence of common bile duct stones (CBDS) is relatively low, the presence of CBDS increases the morbidity of biliary surgery fourfold and is potentially life-threatening. While the introduction of therapeutic laparoscopy revolutionized the surgical approach to patients undergoing cholecystectomy, it completely altered the approach to CBDS. Preoperative diagnostic endoscopic retrograde cholangiography (ERC) became the standard for patients suspected of having choledocholithiasis, in order to avoid having to operate on patients with choledocholithiasis discovered during laparoscopic cholecystectomy. Postoperative endoscopic sphincterotomy (ES) became the preferred approach to treat common duct stones encountered at surgery or discovered afterward. In some areas, ERC/ES increased by 243% [1]. In an effort to treat patients with common duct stones in one session and to avoid the potential complications of ES, several techniques of laparoscopic common bile duct exploration (LCBDE) evolved. Hopefully, the treatment of CBDS in patients who are going to need a cholecystectomy will increasingly be managed surgically by these laparoscopic techniques.

The results of LCBDE are excellent. The morbidity rate is 6–9%; mortality rate is 0.3–0.9% [2–6]. However, the success rate of LCBDE is based on the experience of the operator. The experienced surgeon knows when a specific technique has a good chance of success and when it does not. In experienced hands the transcystic duct technique will be applicable in 80% of cases and will be successful in 90%. While complications of LCBDE are infrequent, they include retained stones, CBD puncture, avulsion of the cystic duct, persistent cholangitis due to high intraductal pressure, hepatic abscess, cystic duct stump leak, delayed stricture, entrapped wire basket/stone assemblage, and pancreatitis. All of these complications can be minimized by careful attention to detail and by applying the proper technique to the appropriate situation. It is always important to keep in mind when it is not safe to proceed with the laparoscopic technique. Such situations occur when there is less than adequate instrumentation, loss of exposure, or uncontrollable bleeding or when efforts to conclude the operation have been protracted beyond a reasonable time. These problems dictate that the operation should be converted to an open technique.

TECHNIQUES

LCBDE can be divided into two major types. One is via the cystic duct (transcystic common bile duct exploration, or LTCBDE) and the other is via choledochotomy.

TABLE 1 Indications for Exploration of the Common Bile Duct

	Radiographic Fluoroscopy	Transcystic Exploration	Laparoscopic Choledochotomy
1–7 stones	+	+	+
8 or more stones	−	−	+
Stone size >10 mm	−	−	+
Common bile duct diameter	Any	Any	> 5 mm
Drain	Optional	Optional	Suggested
Contraindication	Friable cystic duct Intrahepatic stones, multiple large stones	Friable cystic duct Intrahepatic stones, multiple large stones	Small-diameter common bile duct
Advantages	No T tube, shorter hospital stay	No T-tube, shorter hospital stay	Access hepatic and distal ducts, T tube for postop.access
Disadvantages	Equipment, special baskets required	Expensive equipment, endoscopy skill required	Laparoscopic suturing, T tube

To understand and avoid the complications unique or common to both, it is necessary to understand the techniques themselves and the indications for each (Table 1). These techniques are simple lavage, fluoroscopic-guided stone extraction using special wire baskets, biliary endoscopy with wire basket stone retrieval, intraoperative endoscopic or antegrade sphincterotomy, and lithotripsy (Table 2). Most transcystic techniques require the proper method of cystic duct dilation to avoid avulsion of the duct and mucosal injury to the CBD.

Transcystic Choledochoscopy

The patient is placed on the operating table in the supine position. The operating team is positioned in the same way as for laparoscopic cholecystectomy (Fig. 1). A fifth 5-mm trocar may be helpful and should be placed just under the rib cage in the anterior axillary line to facilitate insertion of the choledochoscope at the proper angle (Fig. 2). After review of the intraoperative cholangiogram, a strategy for treatment of choledocholithiasis should take into account the number of stones and their location. If the location of the stones (distal to the cystic duct entrance

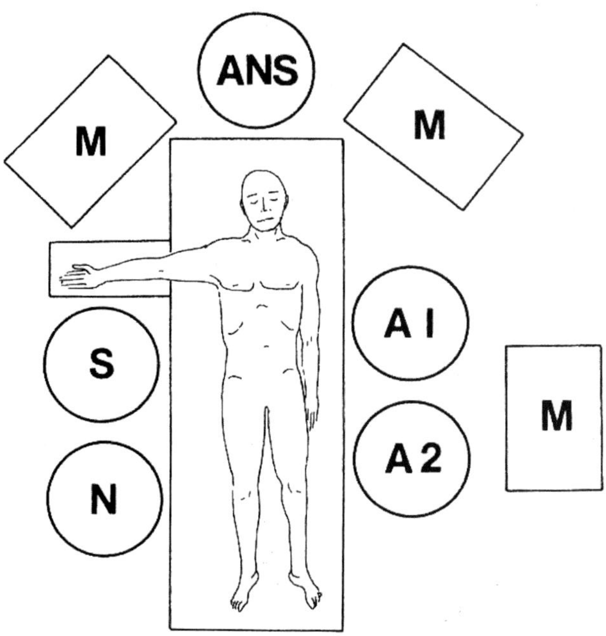

FIGURE 1 Patient positioning for laparoscopic transcystic exploration of the common bile duct. A-assistant; ANS-anesthesiologist; M-monitor; N-nurse; S-surgeon.

TABLE 2 Techniques of Common Bile Duct Exploration (CBDE)

Technique	Complications	Avoidance
Dissection of cystic duct to CBD	Avulsion of cystic duct/CBD junction Tear of cystic duct/CBD junction	1. Direct visualization 2. Do not use cautery 3. Perform blunt dissection 4. Be patient
Dilation of cystic duct	Avulsion of cystic duct Tear of cystic duct/CBD junction	1. Radial expanding balloon preferable to sequential graduated bougie 2. Pick balloon that will only attain diameter equal or less than inner diameter of CBD as estimated IOC[a] 3. Dilate under direct vision
Lavage	Retained stones	1. Completion IOC 2. Use a different technique to clear stone
Radiographic fluoroscopy-guided basket	Bile duct puncture	Special spiral basket with soft lead wire
	Entrapped basket	Proper dilation of cystic duct
Choledochoscopy	Puncture (basket or scope)	1. Do everything under direct vision 2. Irrigation forceful enough to keep visualization and avoid collapse of the duct
	Hypothermia	Warm irrigation
Choledochotomy	Stricture	1. Anterior wall incision 2. Do not devascularize 3. Do not use cautery for incision 4. Suture ligate bleeding vessels on wall of CBD
	Puncture	Instrumentation under direct vision
	Bile leak	Use biliary stent, T tube, cystic duct tube, subhepatic drainage
	Pancreatitis	Avoid unnecessary instrumentation of ampulla
	Retained stone	T tube
Lithotripsy	Puncture/bleeding	1. Perform via choledochotomy 2. Direct vision and irrigate debris

[a] Intraoperative cholangiography.

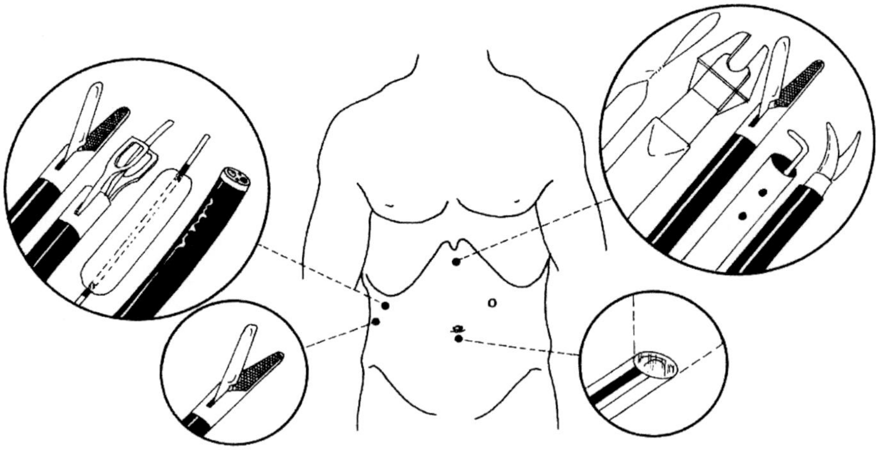

FIGURE 2 Instrument locations for laparoscopic transcystic exploration of the common bile duct.

in the common duct) and the patient's condition permit, the cystic duct should be dissected bluntly down close to its junction with the common duct. It is often necessary to make an additional incision in the portion of the cystic duct closer to the common duct so that less of the cystic duct requires dilatation. The location of the incision should allow an adequate length of cystic duct stump (~ 1 cm) for closure with an endoloop at the end of the procedure. A floppy-tipped 0.035-in. hydrophilic guidewire is inserted inside a balloon-dilating catheter and advanced to the opening of the cystic duct under laparoscopic guidance. The guidewire is inserted through the cystic duct into the common duct and its position confirmed by fluoroscopy or static radiography. The balloon-dilating catheter should have a 4-cm distal balloon with an outer diameter of 6 mm. It should be the radially dilating type of balloon, not a Fogarty type. The balloon's outer diameter should not be larger than the inner diameter of the common duct as measured on the cholangiogram. After the guidewire is inserted without resistance or after x-ray or fluoroscopic confirmation of the guidewire's location, the balloon-dilating catheter is inserted over the guidewire into the cystic and common ducts (Fig. 3). Two-thirds of the balloon should be inserted. The balloon is then inflated slowly with a LeVeen syringe attached to a pressure gauge (Fig. 4). The balloon should be inflated to the insufflation pressure recommended by the manufacturer (usually 12 atm) and held there for 3 min. It is then deflated and

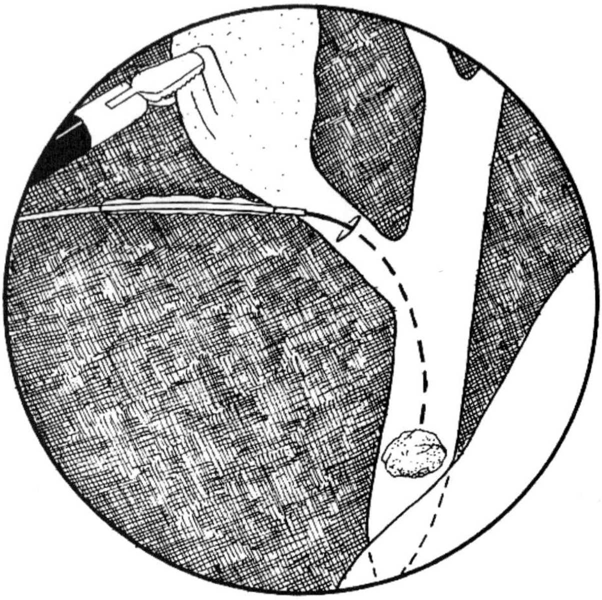

FIGURE 3 Insertion of the balloon-dilating catheter over a guidewire.

the assemblage is removed. A flexible 2.7- to 3.2-mm OD choledochoscope is introduced through a tube reducer into the opening in the cystic duct (Fig. 5). The endoscope can be inserted over a guidewire if it is 150 cm long, or it can be inserted ''freehand'' or gently guided with an atraumatic grasping instrument. The endoscope should have bidirectional deflection and a working channel of at least 1.2 mm. Once the endoscope is in the cystic duct, irrigation with warm saline should be initiated. Attention must be paid to the temperature of the irrigant, as hypothermia can occur from instillation of cold fluid. Once a stone is seen, irrigation is turned off or decreased. Always entrap the stone closest to the scope, and do not bypass any stones, as they may be irrigated up into the liver. A straight four-wire basket should be advanced beyond the stone, opened, and then pulled back to entrap it. The basket should be pulled up lightly against the end of the endoscope so that they can be withdrawn in unison (Fig. 6). This process is repeated until all the stones are removed. A completion cholangiogram is essential. At this point a decision regarding cystic duct tube drainage must be made. A latex (not silicone) tube can be placed for postoperative decompression of the biliary system in elderly or immunosuppressed patients with cholangitis. We choose latex because, unlike silicone, it will form a tract, thereby decreasing the

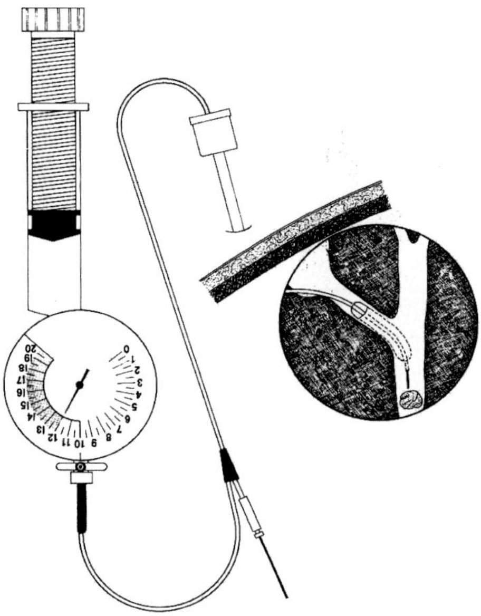

Figure 4 Balloon dilatation of the cystic duct.

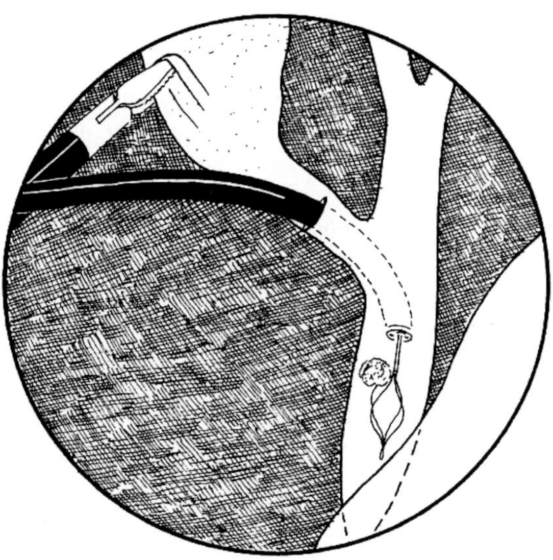

Figure 5 Transcystic choledochoscopy.

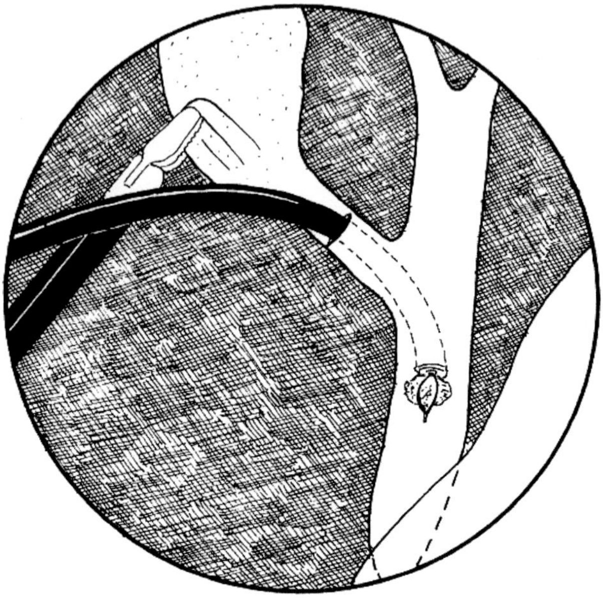

FIGURE 6 Basket extraction of common bile duct stone under direct vision with transcystic flexible biliary endoscope.

risk of an uncontrolled leak. In patients who are likely to be harboring a retained stone, it is useful to insert a cystic duct tube for postoperative cholangiography and, if necessary, percutaneous stone extraction via the tube tract. If the pre-exploration intraoperative cholangiogram shows a different number of common duct stones than that found on endoscopy, a tube should also be considered. The cystic duct stump should be closed with endoloops, as clips may slip off the thinned duct.

Fluoroscopic Wire Basket Stone Retrieval

The retrieval of stones with a wire basket under fluoroscopic guidance is feasible if fluoroscopy is available. Special spiral wire baskets with flexible leaders must be used to avoid injuring the CBD. The basket is placed into the common duct via the cystic duct. It is advanced under fluoroscopic guidance into the distal common duct and opened. Hypaque (dietrizoate muglumine and diatrizoate sodium) 25% is injected through the wire basket. The basket is then pulled back until the stone is captured. The advantage of not having to dilate the cystic duct is offset by the problem of extracting the wire basket with the captured stone through the nondilated cystic duct. In our experience, this technique is not as successful as other techniques via the cystic duct; it can lead to an impacted basket and stone requiring choledochotomy for its removal. Nevertheless, it can be an easy and successful technique in selected patients—those with relatively few common duct calculi whose size is close to the inner diameter of the cystic duct.

Choledochotomy

This procedure is more technically challenging and should not be attempted without considerable experience with laparoscopic surgery, including suturing techniques and endoscopic stone manipulation.

The procedure begins by placing cephalad traction on the cystic duct. The anterior wall of the common duct is exposed with blunt dissection. Stay sutures (4-0 chromic sutures on a genitourinary needle) are placed on the lateral and medial sides of the CBD and held. The anterior wall of the common duct is incised with a microscissors inserted through the subxiphoid trocar. A fiberoptic endoscope is then passed through that same trocar. Even an 8-mm OD flexible choledochoscope can be passed in this fashion. The larger scope permits utilization of a full-sized Segura wire basket; stones as large as several centimeters have been removed in this manner. The proximal portions of the biliary tree can then be inspected and cleared, and another 1-mm endoscope can be passed through the larger, ''mother'' scope's working channel to explore the smaller biliary radicles.

After clearing the biliary system, a T tube is placed and sewn in place—a rather demanding technical feat. The back wall of the T tube is trimmed, and it is then placed entirely in the abdominal cavity. The trimmed limb is inserted in the CBD. After the tube is secured with 4-0 chromic interrupted sutures, the side arm of the T tube is withdrawn with the lateral 5-mm trocar. Again, a completion cholangiogram must be obtained. Alternative methods of closing the choledochotomy are being developed with the hope of eliminating either placement of a T tube or the difficult intracorporeal suturing and knot tying.

Biliary Balloon Catheter Stone Retrieval

Stone retrieval with a biliary balloon catheter is occasionally helpful, especially in cases with a dilated cystic duct. A biliary balloon catheter can be passed blindly or under fluoroscopic control via the cystic duct into the distal common duct or the duodenum. The balloon is inflated gently, and the catheter is then withdrawn, modulating the pressure on the balloon. This is often successful via choledochotomy, but has the potential to pull the stone into the common hepatic duct, out of reach of an endoscope, when used via the cystic duct.

COMPLICATIONS

General

Surgical judgment is the key to selecting the proper approach to the treatment of CBD stones and, thus, to minimizing complications. Knowledge of the outcomes of the different treatments can improve the surgeon's judgment. A prospective multicenter study of endoscopic sphincterotomy (ES) in 2347 patients showed that procedure-related morbidity was 9.8%, procedure-related mortality 0.5%, and total mortality 2.3% [7]. Surgical results should be compared and therapeutic recommendations should keep in consideration these morbidity figures. The long-term sequelae of the approach, such as ampullary stricture following ES, should also be considered.

The 30-day mortality rate in laparoscopic CBD exploration is from 0–0.9% and includes cholecystectomy [3–5,8–12]. Myocardial infarction was the leading cause of postoperative mortality. Aspiration pneumonia occurred in 2% of our patients and was the cause of death in one patient.

A review of 1200 cholecystectomies on the teaching service at our hospital just prior to the introduction of LC was performed by Morgenstern and colleagues [13]. They analyzed 220 patients who underwent open CBDE and found that patients under age 60 had no mortality, but patients over 60 had a 4.3% mortality. On the other hand, we reported only two LTCBDE procedure–related complications (2%), no mortality in patients under 65 years of age, and one death in 256 LCBDEs [14]. There were no cases of delayed stricture and a 90% satisfaction rate.

Preoperative Measures for the Prevention of the Avoidable Complications

Several studies can be performed to investigate biliary anatomy and the presence of common bile duct stone(s): endoscopic retrograde cholangiography, magnetic resonance cholangiography, and endoscopic ultrasound are usually compared.

Endoscopic Retrograde Cholangiography (ERC)

Since the introduction of ERC in 1974, ERC and endoscopic sphincterotomy (ES) have become an important means of diagnosis and treatment of common bile duct stones [15,16]. The major drawback of these procedures is the potential for serious complications. The most common serious complications of ERC and ES are pancreatitis, cholangitis, hemorrhage, and perforation. ES-related complications occur in 8–16% and death results in 0.4–6% [7,17–19]. Consequently, reliance on preoperative ERCP/ES is indicated when there is a suspicion of malignant disease, worsening pancreatitis, or severe cholangitis or when patients present who are unfit for surgery [20–23].

Magnetic Resonance Cholangiography (MRC)

Over the last few years, MRC has rapidly developed as a reliable, noninvasive examination of patients with pancreaticobiliary diseases. MRC is a noninvasive technique with no known complications. The sensitivity of MRC is 88–95%, its specificity is 82–94%. Its positive predictive value is 78–97%, and its negative predictive value is 81–97% for the detection of common bile duct stones [24–26]. Therefore, MRC is a simple, noninvasive method for preoperative screening for CBD stones in high-risk patients.

Endoscopic Ultrasound (EUS)

Reports indicate that the sensitivity of EUS is 89–93%; specificity, 95–97%; positive predictive value, 80–98%; and negative predictive value, 88–97%. The morbidity rate is 4.1% [27,28]. A recent prospective cohort study suggests that EUS is more sensitive than MRC in the detection of choledocholithiasis, with similar specificity [29]. Moreover, when postoperative residual stones are suspected, EUS can be performed as an alternative to endoscopic retrograde cholangiography.

Specific Complications

Bile leakage from the liver bed, cystic duct, or accessory bile ducts is dealt with in Chapter 8. This chapter deals with problems associated with laparoscopic bile duct exploration.

Preoperative Measures to Prevent Complications

The most important preoperative decision is the timing of bile duct surgery. Elderly, frail patients with comorbid medical conditions, immunosuppressed patients, and patients with significant cholangitis should have preoperative ERCP/ES. Patients with acute infection should be given antibiotics and fluid resuscitation before surgery. Patients with mild pancreatitis who are improving should be operated on within 7 days after the resolution of their pancreatitis. In severe pancreatitis, however, especially with extended pancreatic necrosis, at least 3 weeks should elapse because of the increased infection risk [30]. These efforts will be rewarded with a decrease in operative morbidity.

One of the least appreciated measures to reduce complications is to have all the instruments, catheters, and endoscopes organized in a bile duct exploration cart or tray. It is always difficult to find the proper catheters when they are in various locations, and there is a tendency to use what is available rather than what is best. The time spent in advance of surgery organizing your operating room and educating the staff is well worth the effort.

Intraoperative Measures to Prevent Complications

The earliest and most desirable time for the diagnosis and treatment of a bile leak is at the operating table. Prompt recognition and precise localization of the site of the bile leak offers the best opportunity for the repair of a duct injury. There is no more propitious time for diagnosis and treatment than at the initial surgery. Intraoperative cholangiography (IOC) provides the best means of detecting an injury and localizing bile extravasation during laparoscopic biliary surgery [31,32]. However, the use of IOC will not help in the prevention of a biliary injury, as determined by retrospective review of 3242 consecutive laparoscopic cholecystectomies [33]. The incidence of bile duct injuries during laparoscopic cholecystectomy is reported at 0.3–0.6% [34,35].

In our series, 11 of 12 injuries (92%) were detected and successfully repaired during the initial operation [33]. Early recognition allowed for optimal repairs at the initial operation, preventing delayed complications, such as peritonitis, strictures, cholangitis, and cirrhosis. It is well known that higher injury levels, as per the Bismuth classification, and delayed recognition result in the worst outcomes [34,36]. Clearly, routine cholangiography led to lower injury levels and earlier recognition.

Leaks occur around cystic duct tubes, through closures of choledochotomies, or via punctured bile ducts. Placing a suture ligature around a cystic duct tube is not as easy as it may seem. It is important to place a closed suction drain adjacent to the cystic duct to aspirate any bile. To decrease bile leak after choledochotomy or bile duct puncture, a T tube or biliary stent should be placed. There are some instances when a primary closure of the common duct is appropriate without decompression, but a closed suction drain should be placed adjacent to the closure.

Diagnosis. Patients with large or persistent leaks will present with abdominal pain and tenderness, though some patients may have subtle presentations and complain of persistent abdominal or shoulder pain, anorexia, or low-grade fever, even at a postoperative office visit 1 to 2 weeks after the operation. If there is a possibility of a bile leak, an ultrasound examination is the best first test in looking for a fluid collection. Occasionally, cholescintigraphy using a derivative of technetium-99m hepatobiliary iminodiacetic acid (HIDA) is helpful. ERCP is sometimes needed, not only to diagnose a leak but also to place a transampullary stent in association with percutaneous drainage.

Treatment. The treatment of bile duct leaks varies depending on the site of the leak, the presence of an associated ductal obstruction, and/or evidence of a bile duct injury. Persistent symptomatic bile leaks with large or infected bilomas should be drained percutaneously. Percutaneous drainage of a biloma due to a cystic duct leak and placement of a transampullary stent will be curative in most instances and should be attempted prior to surgical intervention [37,38]. Minor bile leaks that become manifest, either as limited bilious drainage through the external drain, or as small subhepatic or intra-abdominal collections, may stop spontaneously. Most leaks cease within 24 to 72 hr. Intra-abdominal collections, generally subhepatic, are resorbed spontaneously. It has been shown that 25% of all patients will have collections of subhepatic fluid after cholecystectomy, but that 92% of these have no clinical manifestations of significance [39]. However, if the patient is symptomatic, percutaneous drainage will improve the patient's discomfort and quantitate the leak. If the leak persists for more than several days, placement of a transampullary stent should be considered.

Retained Stones

Retained stones are an important complication of CBDE. This occurs in 2–5% of CBDE [2–6]. However, this incidence can be lowered by performing drainage procedures on patients at high risk of retained stones (patients with more stones than seen on IOC and patients with 10 or more stones or intrahepatic stones). Retained stones can cause pancreatitis, obstructive jaundice, cholangitis, abscess, and pain.

Preoperative Evaluation. If patients have abnormal liver function, jaundice, and pain before operation, information about the CBD should be obtained.

Intraoperative Measures to Facilitate the Treatment of Retained Stones. The performance of a cholangiogram with 25% Hypaque is important, so that the dye will not obscure small stones. When, at the time of exploration, more stones are identified than initially seen on IOC, or when there are more than 10 stones or intrahepatic stones, a latex tube should be left in the cystic duct or a T tube left in the CBD to facilitate postoperative instrumentation or cholangiography if necessary.

Diagnosis. Patients who present with retained stones after LCBDE are usually referred for ERCP or MRC to confirm the diagnosis and to rule out other biliary and pancreatic lesions.

Treatment. Small stones (less than 3 mm) can usually pass spontaneously. However, in patients who have larger stones, ES should be offered at the time of ERCP. Surgery would be considered only if this procedure fails, either for technical reasons or when an additional drainage procedure is required.

Cholangitis/Hepatic Abscess

Obstruction and bactibilia are two essential features in the pathogenesis of cholangitis [40]. In the absence of biliary obstruction, moderate bactibilia, with bacterial concentrations in bile of up to 10^5/mL, can exist without concomitant bacteremia.

However, once the ductal pressures exceed 15 cmH_2O, reflux of radioactively labeled bacteria into bloodstream has been demonstrated [41]. *Escherichia coli*, *Klebsiella*, *Enterococcus*, and *Enterobacter* species are the most frequently cultured aerobes, while *Bacteroides* is the anaerobe most often encountered in bile cultures. This complication occurs in approximately 2% of patients with CBD stones.

Intraoperative Measures to Prevent Complications

To prevent this complication, it is most important to pay careful attention to the cystic and common ducts when any guidewires and/or balloon catheters are inserted. Cholangitis usually occurs from a stricture and retained stones. To prevent this complication, it is recommended that elderly or immunosuppressed patients have a decompressing CBD catheter placed following CBDE.

Diagnosis. The clinical presentation of cholangitis is highly variable. Symptoms of Charcot's triad are present in approximately half of the patients, with Reynolds' pentad seen in only 4–5% [42] (Table 3). Fever is the most frequent presenting sign, found in up to 92% of the patients, followed by jaundice (67%), nausea and vomiting (54%), abdominal pain (42%), and shock (4–16%) [40,43]. The pain of cholangitis tends to be diffused and not to localize to the right upper quadrant. Moreover, laboratory values are helpful. Elevation of the white blood cell count, bilirubin, transaminases, and alkaline phosphatase is typical. Sometimes the serum amylase will be also elevated. CT and US are first-line imaging studies. Both images can show biliary ductal dilation with over 90% sensitivity.

Treatment. In the treatment of these patients, it is important to remember that in cases of cholangitis and hepatic abscess, the liver still harbors many bacteria, usually for weeks after the CBD has been cleared. It is for this reason that many surgeons recommend that the gallbladder and bile specimens be cultured routinely. Elderly or immunocompromised patients should be given antibiotics, sometimes for as long as 2 weeks, especially if the CBD is not decompressed. Antibiotics can be given orally on an outpatient basis if the patient is stable.

TABLE 3 Symptoms of Cholangitis

Charcot's Triad	Reynold's Pentad
Fever	Charcot's triad
Jaundice	Mental status changes
Right-upper-quadrant pain	Shock/sepsis

However, if the patient's clinical condition progresses to manifest bacterial infection, he or she should be observed closely for clinical signs of hemodynamic compromise, with early consideration of invasive hemodynamic monitoring. Aggressive fluid resuscitation and broad-spectrum antibiotic coverage are needed. If nonoperative management fails to produce a substantial improvement soon after the initiation of the therapy, emergent biliary decompression is indicated (i.e., ERCP or PTC routes).

Stricture

Most CBD strictures occur secondary to an iatrogenic injury to the bile duct at the time of cholecystectomy and CBD exploration.

Intraoperative Measures to Prevent Complications

A stricture can stem from trauma sustained by the duct owing to the repeated passage of instruments during the operation or manipulation in the postoperative period. Cautery should never be used to make the incision in the wall of the CBD. Suture ligature is safer than cautery to control bleeding on the edge of the choledochotomy. In addition, a stricture can result from mechanical injury or thermal injury from lithotripsy. In suturing the bile duct after choledochotomy, care must be taken to ensure that as close to a watertight seal as possible is obtained without causing ischemia to this segment. It is better to have a small leak than to have a narrowed or ischemic duct.

Diagnosis. When stricture of common bile duct occurs, the most frequent presentation is jaundice, which may be constant or intermittent. Hyperbilirubinemia of 2–6 mg/dL is characteristic and should prompt further investigation with imaging studies. Precise anatomical definition of the level of the stricture and the ductal system can be obtained with MRC, PTC, or ERCP.

Treatment. In the case of a short stricture, hydrostatic balloon dilation can be performed and biliary stents placed endoscopically or percutaneously. These techniques are suggested to have a higher success rate than repeated surgical attempts in the management of anastomotic stricture [44,45]. If there is a complete stenosis due to a clip placement or to unsuccessful dilation or stent positioning, surgery would be recommended and should probably be performed after at least 3 weeks. Generally, it is felt that the longer the time interval the better (months would be ideal) to allow time for the intense inflammatory reaction to subside.

Pancreatitis

Pancreatitis can occur after any technique of CBDE. However, ampullary balloon dilation or antegrade sphincterotomy is more likely to result in pancreatitis. Ampullary balloon dilation is highly successful with stones 5 mm or less in diameter, but postoperative hyperamylasemia occurs in approximately 25% of these patients. With antegrade sphincterotomy performed during LCBDE. Some were described as transient with asymptomatic elevation in serum amylase levels immediately after surgery [46,47]. Choledochoscopy with instrumentation of the ampulla or radiographically guided instrumentation can also result in pancreatitis. In transcystic choledochoscopy, pancreatitis occurs in 0.3% [6,48].

Intraoperative Measures to Prevent Complications

Careful and judicious use of instruments inside of the bile duct is required to avoid this complication. Unnecessary instrumentation of the ampulla should be avoided. In general, instrumentation performed under direct vision (choledochoscopy) is safer.

Diagnosis. Patients with pancreatitis frequently complain of upper abdominal pain that radiates through to the back. Anorexia, nausea, and vomiting are occasionally present. The pain is frequently described as constant and either sharp or burning, only slightly relieved by lying in a knee chest position. Biochemical diagnosis of pancreatitis is based on elevations of serum amylase and lipase. Serum amylase usually exceeds 1000 IU/dL, but it is not uncommon to see amylase levels in the range of 1200–1400 IU/L or higher [49]. Average lipase values in biliary pancreatitis are greater than 8000 IU/L, in contrast to the range of 1800–2800 IU/L for nonbiliary etiologies [50]. Other serum markers noted to be elevated in pancreatitis are fibrinogen, α_1-antiprotease, C-reactive peptide, trypsinogen activation peptide, and leukocyte elastase. Imaging studies are diagnostic in most patients with pancreatitis. Plain film radiography may help confirm the diagnosis by demonstrating a dilated or sentinel loop of small bowel adjacent to the pancreas in the upper midline or left upper quadrant. The ‘‘colon cutoff’’ sign is thought to be stem from colonic spasm near the area of pancreatic inflammation. On the other hand, a CT scan will demonstrate pancreatic inflammation, peripancreatic fluid, and even the viability of the pancreas. Ultrasound is not often helpful because the intestinal gas from the associated ileus will obscure the tissues.

Treatment. The treatment of biliary pancreatitis involves the identification and removal of the obstructing stone, which is sometimes impacted in the ampulla of Vater. Eighty percent of the CBD stones causing gallstone pancreatitis will pass spontaneously within the first 24 hr [51]. Pain management is also very important. Narcotics that produce an increase in the tone of the sphincter of Oddi (i.e., morphine) should be avoided. Intramuscular administration of meperidine in doses of 75–100 mg every 3–4 hr usually avoids this problem. Fluid and electrolyte management is fundamental because of the significant volume shifts caused by pancreatic inflammation. Urinary output should be maintained at no less than 0.5 mL/hr/kg and can be used as an index of organ perfusion in patients with unimpaired renal function. Patients with severe pancreatitis showing signs of hypovolemia, hypocalcemia, or falling hemoglobin should undergo early transfer to an intensive care unit. Early invasive hemodynamic monitoring may be necessary.

Entrapment of a Common Bile Duct Stone

The bile duct stones are usually larger than the inner diameter of the cystic duct. In this situation, the stone and basket assemblage can become entrapped within the common duct so that it cannot be removed through the cystic duct opening. When this occurs, the wire must be cut and, occasionally, a choledochotomy must be performed in order to remove the basket and stone.

CONCLUSION

In the management of CBDE in the laparoscopic era, several variables have been shown to be important. The patient's age, medical condition, and comorbid illnesses, as well as preoperative studies, the presence or absence of the gallbladder, the diameter of the bile duct, and the number, size and location of stones determine the appropriate choices. The rule we recommend is do not improvise a laparoscopic common bile duct exploration, but always to take particular notice of every detail in preparing for the operation.

REFERENCES

1. Fletcher DR. Changes in the practice of biliary surgery and ERCP during the introduction of laparoscopic cholecystectomy to Australia: Their possible significance. Aust NZ J Surg 1994; 64(2):75–80.
2. Dorman JP, Franklin ME, Glass JL. Laparoscopic common bile duct exploration by choledochotomy. An effective and efficient method of treatment of choledocholithiasis. Surg Endosc 1998; 12(7):926–928.
3. Berthou JC, Drouard F, Charbonneau P, Moussalier K. Evaluation of laparoscopic management of common bile duct stones in 220 patients. Surg Endosc 1998; 12(1): 16–22.
4. Martin IJ, Bailey IS, Rhodes M, O'Rourke N, Nathanson L, Fielding G. Towards T-tube free laparoscopic bile duct exploration: a methodologic evolution during 300 consecutive procedures. Ann Surg 1998; 228(1):29–34.
5. Keeling NJ, Menzies D, Motson RW. Laparoscopic exploration of the common bile duct: Beyond the learning curve. Surg Endosc 1999; 13(2):109–112.
6. Giurgiu DI, Margulies DR, Carroll BJ, Gabbay J, Iida A, Takagi S, et al. Laparoscopic common bile duct exploration: long-term outcome. Arch Surg 1999; 134(8): 839–843; discussion 843–844.

7. Freeman ML, Nelson DB, Sherman S, Haber GB, Herman ME, Dorsher PJ, et al. Complications of endoscopic biliary sphincterotomy. N Engl J Med 1996; 335(13): 909–918.
8. Phillips EH, Rosenthal RJ, Carroll BJ, Fallas MJ. Laparoscopic trans-cystic-duct common-bile-duct exploration. Surg Endosc 1994; 8(12):1389–1393; discussion 1393–1394.
9. Berci G. Laparoscopic management of common bile duct stones. Surg Endosc 1994; 8(12):1452–1453.
10. Rhodes M, Nathanson L, O'Rourke N, Fielding G. Laparoscopic exploration of the common bile duct: lessons learned from 129 consecutive cases. Br J Surg 1995; 82(5):666–668.
11. DePaula AL, Hashiba K, Bafutto M. Laparoscopic management of choledocholithiasis. Surg Endosc 1994; 8(12):1399–1403.
12. Arvidsson D, Berggren U, Haglund U. Laparoscopic common bile duct exploration. Eur J Surg 1998; 164(5):369–375.
13. Morgenstern L, Wong L, Berci G. Twelve hundred open cholecystectomies before the laparoscopic era. A standard for comparison. Arch Surg 1992; 127(4):400–403.
14. Phillips EH, Liberman M, Carroll BJ, Fallas MJ, Rosenthal RJ, Hiatt JR. Bile duct stones in the laparoscopic era. Is preoperative sphincterotomy necessary. Arch Surg 1995; 130(8):880–885; discussion 885–886.
15. Classen M, Demling L. [Endoscopic sphincterotomy of the papilla of vater and extraction of stones from the choledochal duct (author's transl)]. Dtsch Med Wochenschr 1974; 99(11):496–497.
16. Kawai K, Akasaka Y, Murakami K, Tada M, Koli Y. Endoscopic sphincterotomy of the ampulla of Vater. Gastrointest Endosc 1974; 20(4):148–151.
17. Targarona EM, Ayuso RM, Bordas JM, Ros E, Pros I, Martinez J, et al. Randomised trial of endoscopic sphincterotomy with gallbladder left in situ versus open surgery for common bileduct calculi in high-risk patients. Lancet 1996; 347(9006):926–929.
18. Suc B, Escat J, Cherqui D, Fourtanier G, Hay JM, Fingerhut A, et al. Surgery vs endoscopy as primary treatment in symptomatic patients with suspected common bile duct stones: a multicenter randomized trial. French Associations for Surgical Research. Arch Surg 1998; 133(7):702–708.
19. Schreurs WH, Juttmann JR, Stuifbergen WN, Oostvogel HJ, Vroonhoven TJ. Management of common bile duct stones: selective endoscopic retrograde cholangiography and endoscopic sphincterotomy: Short- and long-term results. Surg Endosc 2002; 16(7):1068–1072.
20. Neoptolemos JP-, Locke DL, London NJ, Bailey IA, James D, Fossard DP. Controlled trial of urgent endoscopic retrograde cholangiopancreatography and endoscopic sphincterotomy versus conservative treatment for acute pancreatitis due to gallstones. Lancet 1988; 2(8618):979–983.
21. Leung JW, Chung SC, Sung JJ, Banez VP, Li AK. Urgent endoscopic drainage for acute suppurative cholangitis. Lancet 1989; 1(8650):1307–1309.
22. Siegel JH, Rodriquez R, Cohen SA, Kasmin FE, Cooperman AM. Endoscopic management of cholangitis: Critical review of an alternative technique and report of a large series. Am J Gastroenterol 1994; 89(8):1142–1146.

23. Pellegrini CA. Surgery for gallstone pancreatitis. Am J Surg 1993; 165(4):515–518.
24. Chan YL, Chan AC, Lam WW, Lee DW, Chung SS, Sung JJ, et al. Choledocholithiasis: Comparison of MR cholangiography and endoscopic retrograde cholangiography. Radiology 1996; 200(1):85–89.
25. Dwerryhouse SJ, Brown E, Vipond MN. Prospective evaluation of magnetic resonance cholangiography to detect common bile duct stones before laparoscopic cholecystectomy. Br J Surg 1998; 85(10):1364–1366.
26. Stiris MG, Tennoe B, Aadland E, Lunde OC. MR cholangiopancreaticography and endoscopic retrograde cholangiopancreaticography in patients with suspected common bile duct stones. Acta Radiol 2000; 41(3):269–272.
27. Prat F, Amouyal G, Amouyal P, Pelletier G, Fritsch J, Choury AD, et al. Prospective controlled study of endoscopic ultrasonography and endoscopic retrograde cholangiography in patients with suspected common- bileduct lithiasis. Lancet 1996; 347(8994):75–79.
28. Montariol T, Msika S, Charlier A, Rey C, Bataille N, Hay JM, et al. Diagnosis of asymptomatic common bile duct stones: Preoperative endoscopic ultrasonography versus intraoperative cholangiography—A multicenter, prospective controlled study. French Associations for Surgical Research. Surgery 1998; 124(1):6–13.
29. Scheiman JM, Carlos RC, Barnett JL, Elta GH, Nostrant TT, Chey WD, et al. Can endoscopic ultrasound or magnetic resonance cholangiopancreatography replace ERCP in patients with suspected biliary disease? A prospective trial and cost analysis. Am J Gastroenterol 2001; 96(10):2900–2904.
30. Uhl W, Muller CA, Krahenbuhl L, Schmid SW, Scholzel S, Buchler MW. Acute gallstone pancreatitis: Timing of laparoscopic cholecystectomy in mild and severe disease. Surg Endosc 1999; 13(11):1070–1076.
31. Morgenstern L, McGrath MF, Carroll BJ, Paz-Partlow M, Berci G. Continuing hazards of the learning curve in laparoscopic cholecystectomy. Am Surg 1995; 61(10): 914–918.
32. Phillips EH, Berci G, Carroll B, Daykhovsky L, Sackier J-, Partlow M. The importance of intraoperative cholangiography during laparoscopic cholecystectomy. Am Surg 1990; 56(12):792–795.
33. Carroll BJ, Friedman RL, Liberman MA, Phillips EH. Routine cholangiography reduces sequelae of common bile duct injuries. Surg Endosc 1996; 10(12): 1194–1197.
34. Andren-Sandberg A, Johansson S, Bengmark S. Accidental lesions of the common bile duct at cholecystectomy. II. Results of treatment. Ann Surg 1985; 201(4): 452–455.
35. Strasberg SM, Hertl M, Soper NJ. An analysis of the problem of biliary injury during laparoscopic cholecystectomy. J Am Coll Surg 1995; 180(1):101–125.
36. Chapman WC, Halevy A, Blumgart LH, Benjamin IS. Postcholecystectomy bile duct strictures. Management and outcome in 130 patients. Arch Surg 1995; 130(6): 597–602; discussion 602–604.
37. Davids PH, Rauws EA, Tytgat GN, Huibregtse K. Postoperative bile leakage: Endoscopic management. Gut 1992; 33(8):1118–1122.
38. Kozarek RA, Ball TJ, Patterson DJ, Brandabur JJ, Raltz S, Traverso LW. Endoscopic treatment of biliary injury in the era of laparoscopic cholecystectomy. Gastrointest Endosc 1994; 40(1):10–16.

39. Elboim CM, Goldman L, Hann L, Palestrant AM, Silen W. Significance of post-cholecystectomy subhepatic fluid collections. Ann Surg 1983; 198(2):137–141.
40. Lipsett PA, Pitt HA. Acute cholangitis. Surg Clin North Am 1990; 70(6):1297–1312.
41. Jacobsson KE, Rosengren B. Cholangiovenous reflux. Acta Chir Scand 1962; 123: 316.
42. Kadakia SC. Biliary tract emergencies. Acute cholecystitis, acute cholangitis, and acute pancreatitis. Med Clin North Am 1993; 77(5):1015–1036.
43. Himal HS, Lindsay T. Ascending cholangitis: surgery versus endoscopic or percutaneous drainage. Surgery 1990; 108(4):629–633; discussion 633–634.
44. Millis JM, Tompkins RK, Zinner MJ, Longmire WP, Roslyn JJ. Management of bile duct strictures. An evolving strategy. Arch Surg 1992; 127(9):1077–1082; discussion 1082–1084.
45. Lillemoe KD, Pitt HA, Cameron JL. Current management of benign bile duct strictures. Adv Surg 1992; 25:119–174.
46. Curet MJ, Pitcher DE, Martin DT, Zucker KA. Laparoscopic antegrade sphincterotomy. A new technique for the management of complex choledocholithiasis. Ann Surg 1995; 221(2):149–155.
47. DePaula AL, Hashiba K, Bafutto M, Zago R, Machado MM. Laparoscopic antegrade sphincterotomy. Surg Laparosc Endosc 1993; 3(3):157–160.
48. Paganini AM, Feliciotti F, Guerrieri M, Tamburini A, Sanctis A, Campagnacci R, et al. Laparoscopic common bile duct exploration. J Laparoendosc Adv Surg Tech A 2001; 11(6):391–400.
49. Hiatt JR, Calabria RP, Wilson SE. The amylase profile: A discriminant in biliary and pancreatic disease. Am J Surg 1987; 154(5):490–492.
50. Sadowski DC, Todd JK, Sutherland LR. Biochemical models as early predictors of the etiology of acute pancreatitis. Dig Dis Sci 1993; 38(4):637–643.
51. Acosta JM, Galli OM, Rossi R, Chinellato AV, Pellegrini CA. Effect of duration of ampullary gallstone obstruction on severity of lesions of acute pancreatitis. J Am Coll Surg 1997; 184(5):499–505.

10

Colorectal Surgery

Gustavo Plasencia and Moises Jacobs
Coral Gables, Florida, U.S.A.

Procedures performed laparoscopically offer a wide variety of advantages to the patient, including less pain, quicker recovery, shorter duration of ileus, quicker return to full function, and a decreased immunological insult. Unfortunately, a laparoscopic procedure does not isolate the patient from a series of potential complications common to laparoscopic or any other type of surgery. Laparoscopic colon surgery is among the most difficult operations that can be performed laparoscopically and requires advanced laparoscopic skills. Complications resulting from laparoscopic colon surgery may be inherent to the procedure itself or to the laparoscopic technique.

PREOPERATIVE COMPLICATIONS

Preoperative complications result primarily from either a poor choice of a surgical candidate for laparoscopic colon resection or a lack of adequate workup in the evaluation phase. Poor patient choice may occur because of multiple prior abdominal operations, the presence of a very large tumor, or adjacent organ involvement. An adequate workup should enable the surgeon to identify many of these potential problems. A patient who is a poor anesthetic risk can readily be identified either by the surgeon or the anesthesiologist in the preoperative period. Among the primary concerns in this area are patients with complex cardiovascular and pulmonary problems. These patients should be readily identified and alternative therapy instituted if indicated. On the other hand, we have found that patients who carry a high risk for an open colectomy, especially for pulmonary complications, can often tolerate a laparoscopic procedure.

Perhaps the most critical aspect of preventing preoperative complications lies in the area of preoperative planning and preparation of the operating team by the surgeon. As stated previously, colon surgery is among the most difficult operations that can be performed laparoscopically; surgeons wishing to embark on it should have advanced laparoscopic skills, including suturing and knot tying. The surgeon should also have a working knowledge of stapling techniques for division of tissue, as well as for the creation of anastomoses. A moderate amount of planning should go into each operation, including the possible necessity for colonoscopic intervention and conversion to an open procedure.

Particular attention should be paid to bowel preparation, as inadequate preparation, or preparation that is poorly planned and carried out, will often result in conversion of a procedure to open due to unexpected and unneeded contamination. Oral antibiotics (such as metronidazole), including intraoperative and perioperative broad-spectrum antibiotics with enteric coverage, are routinely used.

INTRAOPERATIVE COMPLICATIONS

The next general area of complications comprises those that occur intraoperatively. Consultations with the anesthesiologist should determine the type of anesthesia being contemplated, the expected duration of the procedure, and the various manipulations that will be needed during the surgery. The patient should be properly positioned for a given procedure: the patient's arms should be tucked in at his or her side in order to allow adequate access above the shoulders.

We approximate the procedures of open surgery in that the surgeon and assistant each use both hands; therefore we try to limit each procedure to four trocars. We like to use three 5-mm trocars for the graspers and dissectors and a 12-mm trocar for passage of the endostaplers. As a result, we let gravity become our second assistant, and we place the patient in steep positions to ensure better visualization of particular segments of the colon (steep Trendelenburg position for visualization of the sigmoid, rectum, and cecum) and to let the small bowel fall out of the way. Thus the patient should be very securely fixed to the table so as to prevent him or her from sliding off when steep positioning is required. This can be done either with a beanbag or with a series of tapes across the shoulders.

Potential intraoperative anesthesia-related complications include cardiovascular compromise and hypercapnea from the pneumoperitoneum.

In preparing for a procedure, the laparoscopic surgeon should think through a given operation and become fully aware of each step to be performed prior to actually starting the operation. A poorly prepared surgeon will have a very high rate of conversions, as well as prolonged procedures.

Instrumentation used in laparoscopic colon surgery is also very important: artraumatic graspers should be used to minimize the risk of bowel injury, even though we feel the bowel should be grasped as little as possible. Grasp the mesentery, the fat, the appendices epiploicae, create windows in the mesentery, and push up on the bowel. Angled scopes also give the advantage of looking down on the colon, as in open surgery. We use a 5-mm 30-degree laparoscope in our practice.

A number of complications are related to access to the abdominal cavity. Patients who have had prior surgery will obviously be likely to have numerous adhesions. Whether a Verress needle or Hasson trocar is to be used for insufflation, alternative-site insufflation should be performed. Proper placement of trocars is vital to successful laparoscopic surgery, and the trocars should be placed preferentially outside of the rectus abdominis muscle and away from major vascular structures, such as the superior epigastric and inferior epigastric arteries in the abdominal wall. All trocars following the initial trocar should be placed under direct vision.

One of the primary problems in laparoscopic colorectal surgery is that the colon is a four-quadrant organ (a much wider anatomic field than is seen with either laparoscopic cholecystectomy, hernia repair, or Nissen fundoplication). The requirements for identification of anatomy in each quadrant are ever-present. Lack of identification of anatomy can be the basic reason for failure and complications. Recognition of anatomy from a number of different points of view and from a wide-sweeping area is the key to successful laparoscopic colonic resection for benign or malignant disease. This often requires a more intricate knowledge of the anatomy, particularly as seen from several points of view and through various windows in the mesentery. When he or she cannot palpate vessels, the surgeon must have an intricate knowledge not only of the normal anatomy but also the abnormal anatomy, with possible vascular deviations from normal that may occur in a given segment of the colon. Key to the recognition of anatomy is having certain ''fixed'' structures to which one can always refer. Among these fixed structures are the ureter, cecum, ligament of Treitz, pancreas, liver, and spleen. These structures give the laparoscopic surgeon, in the process of performing a laparoscopic procedure, a point of view from which to begin identifying a given anatomical structure.

In our practice we follow four steps in performing colectomies:

Identification of lesion
Mobilization of involved segment
Devascularization
Resection and anastomosis

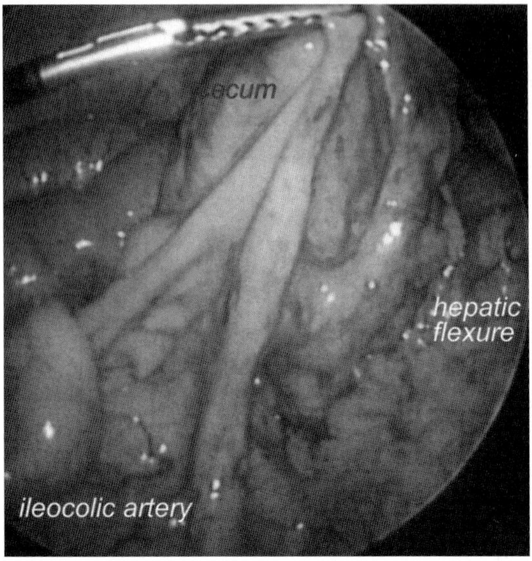

FIGURE 1 Partial cecal resection under colonoscopic control.

IDENTIFICATION OF LESION

When a disease process involves the serosa, the area in question can easily be seen; however, when the lesion does not extend to the serosa, as in the case of a small cancer or polyp, palpation may not be possible, making identification much more difficult. Therefore, preoperative tattooing of a lesion or a preoperative barium enema examination can be extremely helpful. If the lesion is to be tattoed, methylene blue should not be used, as it spreads throughout the colon wall and mesentery, making it difficult to locate the lesion with precision at the time of surgery. We normally use nonabsorbable inks, such as India ink. When in doubt, intraoperative colonoscopy (Fig. 1) may be performed; this is much more cumbersome and may cause bowel dilation, which may can lead to conversions. The colon proximal to the colonoscope must be occluded to prevent dilatation. If the colonoscopy extends to the cecum, the terminal ileum must be occluded. Early on in our experience, we removed segments of colon that proved to be without the intended pathology, thus requiring conversion to open.

MOBILIZATION OF INVOLVED SEGMENT

We want the proximal and distal margins of the segment of colon that is being removed to easily reach the anterior abdominal wall at the level of our extraction incision. Therefore, before making that incision, the surgeon must make sure that sufficient mobilization has been accomplished. If one exteriorizes the bowel without sufficient mobilization, the procedure will become difficult and the incision usually ends up being enlarged, obviating the benefits of laparoscopy.

DEVASCULARIZATION

Devascularization can be accomplished extracorporeally for benign disease, but must always be done intracorporeally in malignancies. Since we believe that intracorporeal devascularization helps to make the exteriorization process easier and the extraction incision smaller, we routinely perform intracorporeal devascularization for all our colectomies.

Named mesenteric blood vessels, such as the ileocolic, middle colic, and inferior mesenteric artery, can be identified by placing traction on the mesentery; when this is done in the appropriate segment of colon, these vessels become taut and bow out like violin strings, even in obese patients (Fig. 2). Before transecting the inferior mesenteric artery, it is imperative that the surgeon make sure where the iliac vessels are; before transecting the middle colic vessels the surgeon must be aware of the superior mesenteric artey and vein. Before transecting the ileocolic artery, the surgeon must make sure that this vessel is running into the cecum, lest the small bowel should be devascularized. Injury to these structures can cause some of the most devastating and life-threatening complications.

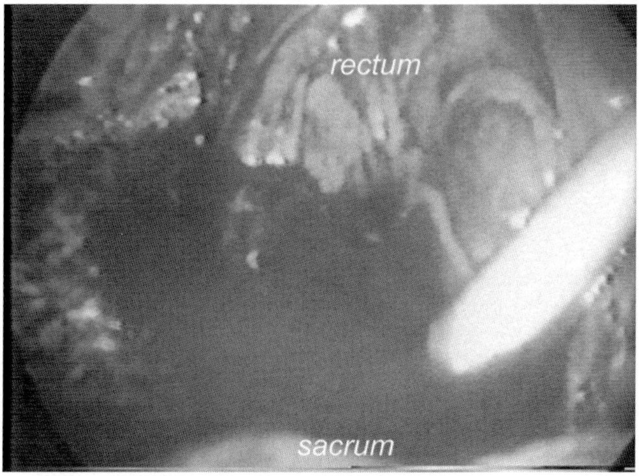

Figure 2 Identification of the ileocolic artery.

RESECTION AND ANASTOMOSIS

For right-sided lesions we usually perform extracorporeal resections and anastomosis in the standard fashion. For left-sided lesions, the resection is performed extracorporeally after dividing the bowel intracorporeally, leaving a rectosigmoid stump, and exteriorizing the proximal colon; however, the anastomosis is done intracorporeally after dropping the bowel back into the abdominal cavity. In these cases, the anastomosis is done using a transanal circular stapler.

Extraction sites are usually made by muscle splitting in benign disease and muscle cutting in malignancies. During removal, we do not want cancers to be squeezed through tight incisions. All extraction sites in cancer cases must be protected with a plastic sleeve to avoid extraction site recurrences.

Bowel injuries, including small bowel and colonic injuries, can occur in laparoscopic colon surgery. The most common injuries to the bowel occur because a portion of bowel has been grasped with a sharp instrument or grasper. Occult injuries can arise from trocar injuries and thermal burns, especially when controlling bleeding. Bleeding should be controlled as it occurs. If this is not done, the exact location of the bleeding site becomes harder and harder to recognize (Fig. 3). Second, clots that form may not be removable. As this occurs, the light begins to dim as the hemoglobin-rich blood absorbs more and more of it. When bleeding occurs, it is best to stop the procedure and control the vessel with pressure either directly from a separate trocar and a separate grasper or with direct pressure

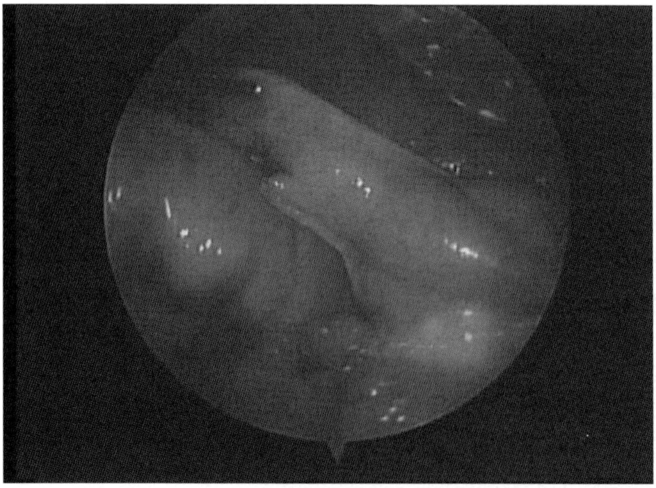

FIGURE 3 Uncontrolled pooling of blood preventing identification of the bleeding site.

from an instrument guided from the surgeon's standpoint. Then, a suction device can be brought in, all clots removed, and the exact source of bleeding visualized and subsequently controlled. There are a variety of ways to control bleeding, including the use of stapling, clipping, endoloops, the ultrasonic dissector, vascular clamps, and cautery.

POSTOPERATIVE COMPLICATIONS

A delay in ambulation can result in a multitude of problems, including thrombophlebitis, atelectasis, and delay in the return of bowel activity. Thus, ambulation should be initiated very early in the postoperative course. A common problem with laparoscopic surgery is that of trying to feed the patient too soon. We strongly recommend not feeding the patient before he or she is ready. Some patients are ready for feeding within 12–18 hr. Others need 2–3 days, depending on the extent of the procedure and the patient's individual response. We offer liquids on the first postoperative day, and then advance to solids at the patient's request or after the passage of flatus or a first bowel movement. By the third day most patients can usually tolerate solid foods.

Some later postoperative complications include trocar site implantations (Fig. 4) and hernias in trocar sites. These problems are addressed in other

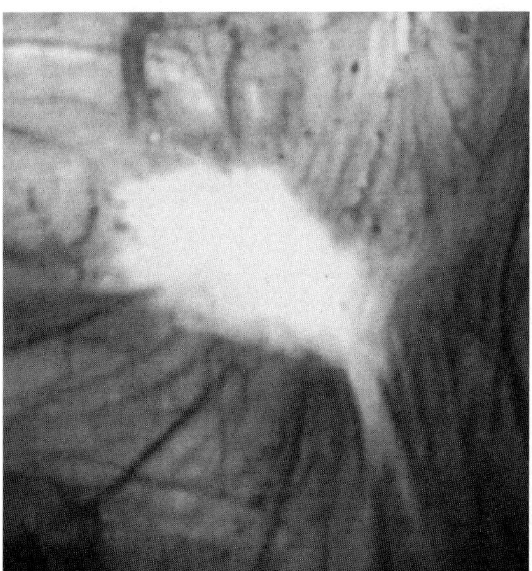

FIGURE 4 Trocar-site implant.

chapters and are not covered in detail here. Suffice it to say, however, that adequate closure of 10-mm trocar sites will help prevent hernias, and trocar site recurrences in cancer can be avoided by minimizing the manipulation of the bowel, as it is thought that cancer cells are transmitted via laparoscopic instruments to trocar sites. For that reason, we try to grasp the bowel directly as little as possible; we grasp the mesentery or the appendix epiploicae, but not the bowel.

Other delayed complications can also occur in regard to the anastomosis. Left-sided anastomosis should be checked intraoperatively with visualization, insufflation of air, or povidone-iodine through a colonoscope. A leak at the staple line must be repaired, either with intracorporeal suturing, restapling, or conversion to open. When in doubt, a diverting ostomy should be created.

SPECIFIC COMPLICATIONS

Right Colectomy

One must identify the second and third portion duodenum to avoid injury during the devascularization phase (Fig. 5). This is done by gently pushing the colonic

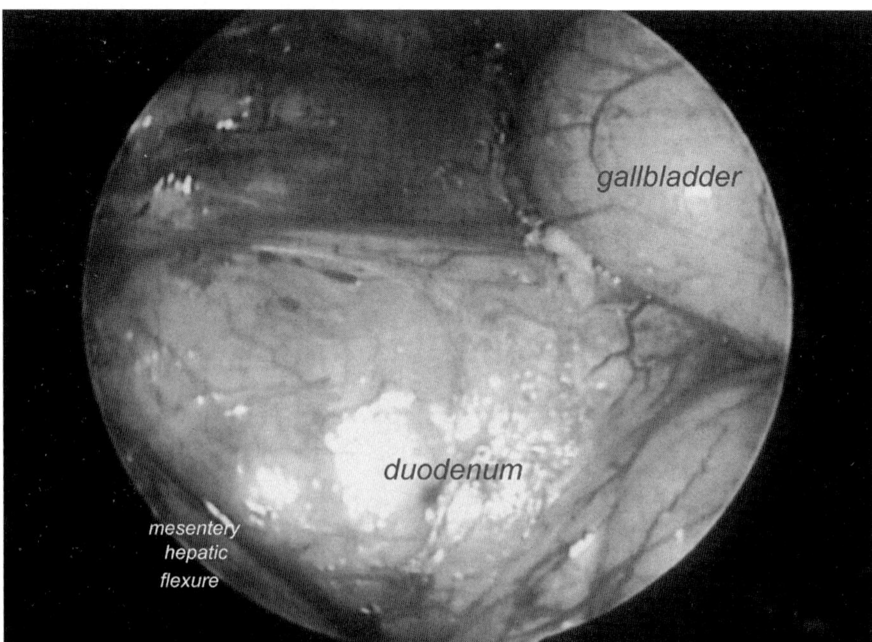

Figure 5 Exposure of duodenum in right colectomy.

mesentery down, after the gastrocolic ligament has been transected. We do not usually identify the right ureter unless we feel that it may be involved by the disease process. In taking the middle colic artery at its base, extreme care must be taken not pull up the superior mesenteric artery and mistake it for the middle colic. The bifurcation of the right left branch of the middle colic artery should be identified for appropriate localization.

One must make sure that the proximal and distal margins of resection reach the extraction site. When mobilization is limited, we prefer extraction at the umbilicus; if not, we use a right-lower-quadrant excision. When the mesentery is shortened or inflamed, it may be easier to do an intracorporeal mobilization, devascularization, resection, and anastomosis and then to extract the bowel. Because of our comfort with intracorporeal anastomosis, we are doing this more and more. In a colectomy involving the left transverse colon and descending colon, we also use this intracorporeal technique.

Left Colectomy

Ureteral Injuries

These occur much more commonly on the left than on the right. They can occur upon ligation and transection of the inferior mesenteric artery or with misidentification of the ureter as a blood vessel (Figs. 6 and 7). These injuries can also occur with staples, as the rectosigmoid colon is being transected with an endostapler and the tip catches the ureter (Fig. 8). In addition, when in closing and firing the circular stapler, the ureter can be trapped and injured.

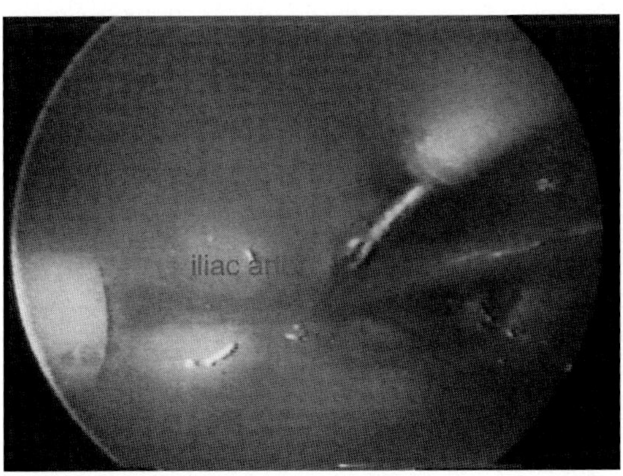

Figure 6 Transection of the left ureter after its misidentification as a blood vessel.

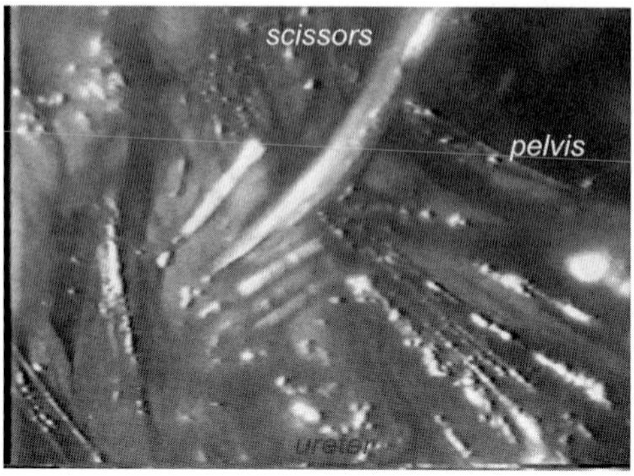

Figure 7 Completely transected left ureter.

Prevention comes from identifying the ureter on all sigmoid or lower level resections. Failure to identify the left ureter (Fig. 9) may be an indication for conversion. Ureteral stents are not helpful in identifying the ureter, as in open surgery, because of the loss of tactile sensation in laparoscopic surgery. When necessary, a repair can be done laparoscopically by an advanced laparoscopic surgeon.

Injury to the Iliac Artery/Vein

This injury (Fig. 10) can occur with aggressive and wide dissection, especially at the level of the sigmoid colon or when the anatomy is not clear to the surgeon.

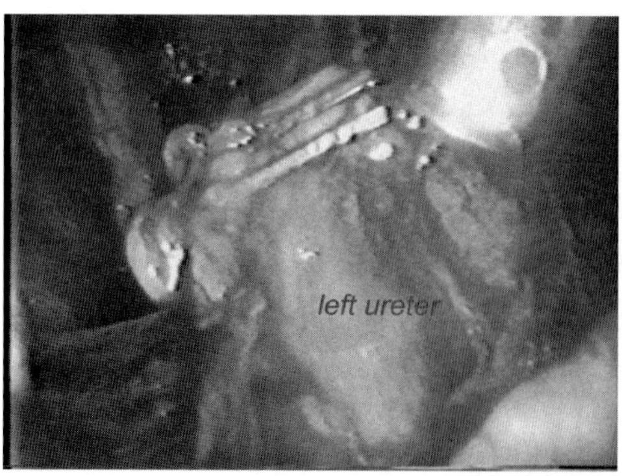

Figure 8 Transected left ureter after transection of the sigmoid colon with endostapler.

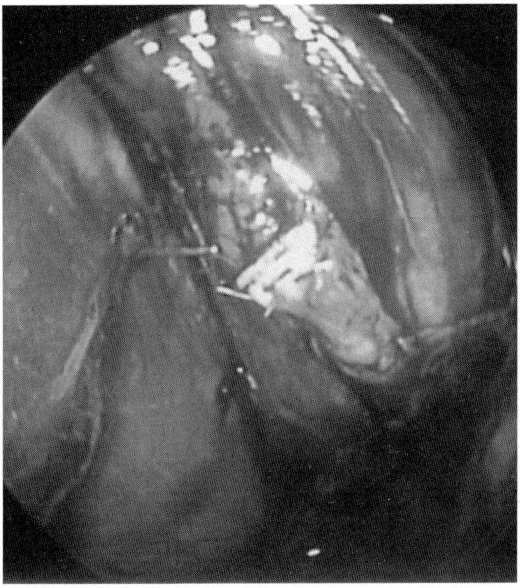

FIGURE 9 Left ureter seen crossing the iliac artery.

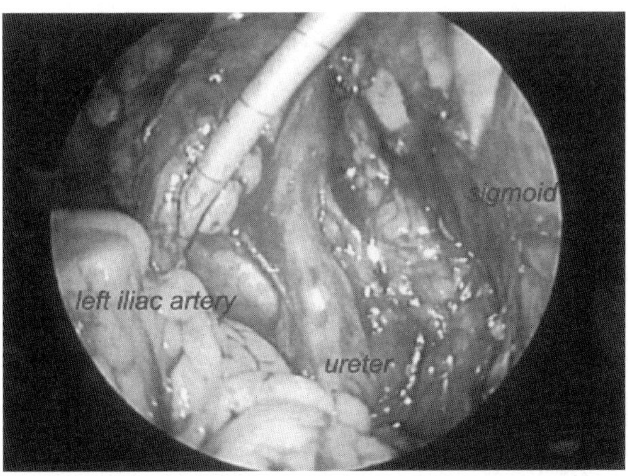

FIGURE 10 Brisk bleeding from injury to the iliac artery.

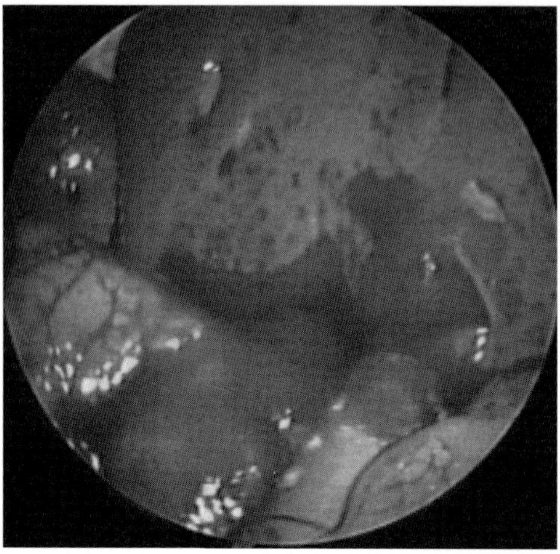

FIGURE 11 Splenic injury.

Prevention comes with knowledge of the laparoscopic anatomy. Always use the pulsation of the left iliac artery as an anatomic landmark and stay above it.

Splenic Injuries

As in open surgery, splenic injuries (Fig. 11) can occur from excessive pulling and traction. Generally, however, they occur much less in laparoscopic surgery than in open procedures because of the better visualization and more precise dissection with laparoscopy. Again, prevention is aided by a knowledge of laparoscopic anatomy and gentler dissection. Care must be taken not to dissect too much superiorly on the spleen and to devascularize the inferior pole. Dissection of the transverse colon from the omentum is suggested in benign diseases. Treatment of bleeding from a splenic injury consists of pressure, cautery, placement of clotting agents, or conversion (Fig. 12).

Anastomotic Tension

We use a suprapubic extraction site. If the distal margin of resection reaches the skin level, there should usually not be tension on the anastomosis. If there is tension on the anastomosis, proximal mobilization is needed. If mobilization is done at the splenic flexure, a monitor should be placed by the patient's left shoulder, as the working orientation of the surgeon has now changed. The surgeon should now be standing looking cephalad. We always check our anastomosis with insufflation under saline. If air bubbles are seen escaping, laparoscopic suturing is

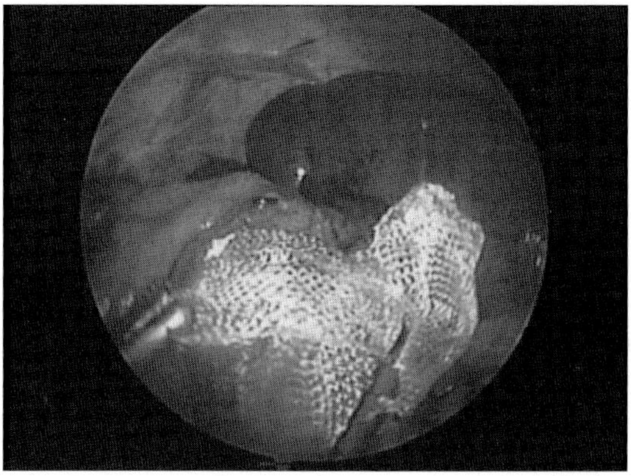

FIGURE 12 Treatment of splenic injury using Surgicel.

done; the alternative is enlargement of the extraction site and open repair. In a small number of cases, a protective ostomy may be necessary.

Small Bowel Obstructions

These can occur from adhesions, as in open surgery; but in laparoscopy, adhesions are usually less pronounced and less frequent. Small bowel obstruction can also occur from incarceration at trocar sites (Fig. 13). All trocar sites 10 mm or greater should be closed to prevent herniation. In obese patients, this may be very difficult or impossible.

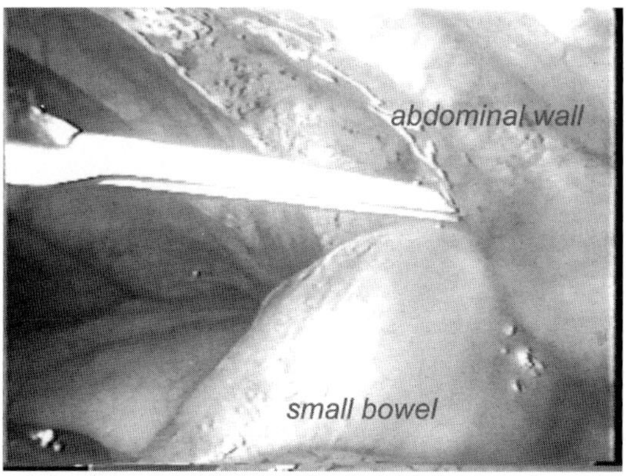

FIGURE 13 Incarcerated hernia at previously closed trocar site.

CONCLUSION

Laparoscopic colorectal surgery is safe in experienced hands. It can be economical, completed in a short period of time, and dramatically influence the postoperative phase of recovery for many patients. Each operation must be planned very meticulously and executed in a likewise meticulous manner in order to achieve maximum benefits. Learning at the table, obviously, is an ongoing experience; however, one cannot start from scratch and expect good results. Thus, being prepared for this type of surgery is most likely to lead to good outcomes in laparoscopic colorectal surgery. Many of the problems seen worldwide are direct results of inadequate preparation of the patient, of the surgeon, or of the operating team.

REFERENCES

1. Kelling G. Uber Oesophagoskopie, Gastroskopie und Coelioscopie. Munch Med Wochenschr 1901; 49:21–24.
2. Kalk H. Erfahrungen mit der Laparoskopic. Z Klin Med 1919; 111:303–348.
3. Ruddock JC. Peritoneoscopy. Surg Gynecol Obstet 1937; 65:623–639.
4. Palmer R. Instrumentation et technique de la coelioscopie gynecologique. Gynecol Obstet 1947; 46:420–431.
5. Jacobaeus HC. Endopleurale Operation unter der Leitung des Thorakoskop. Beitr Krink Tuberk 1915; 35:1–35.
6. Frangenheim H. History of endoscopy. In Gordon AG , Lewis BV, eds. Gynaecological Endoscopy. London: Chapman & Hall, 1988.
7. Muhe E. Dieerstecholecystektomie durch das Laparoskop. Langenbecks Arch Klin Chir 1986:369–804.
8. Dubois F, Berthelot G, Levard H. Cholecystectomy par coelioscopy. Nouv Presse Med 1989; 18:980–982.
9. Reddick EA, Olsen DO. Laparoscopic cholecystectomy: A comparison with mini-lap cholecystectomy. Surg Endosc 1989; 3:131–133.
10. Jacobs M, Verdeja G, Goldstein D. Minimally invasive colon resection. Surg Laparosc Endosc 1991; 1:144–150.
11. Phiffips EH, Franklin ME, Carroll BJ, Fallas M, Ramos R, Rosenthal D. Laparoscopic colectomy. Ann Surg 1992; 216:703–707.
12. Lumley JW, Fielding GA, Rhodes M, Nathanson LK, Sius B, Stitz RW. Laparoscopic-assisted colorectal surgery. Lessons learned from 240 consecutive patients. Dis Colon Rectum 1996; 39(2):155–159.
13. Leroy J. Laparoscopic colorectal resection: Technical aspects after 150 operations. Osp Maggiore 1994; 88(3):262–266.
14. Franklin ME, Rosenthal D, Abrego D, Dorman J, Glass J, Norem R, Diaz JA. Prospective comparison of open vs laparoscopic colon surgery for carcinoma. Five-year results. Dis Colon Rectum 1996; 39(10):S35–S46.

15. Lord SA, Larach S, Fenara A, Williamson P, Lago Ch, Lube M. Laparoscopic resections for colorectal carcinoma. A three-year experience. Dis Colon Rectum 1996; 39(1):148–154.
16. Trokel MJ, Bessler M, Treat MR, Whelan RL, Nowygrod R. Preservation of immune response after laparoscopy. Surg Endosc 1994; 8:1385–1387.
17. Bessler M, Whelan RL, Halverson A, Treat MR, Nowygrod R. Is Immune function better preserved after laparoscopic versus open colon resection. Surg Endosc 1994; 8:881–883.
18. AUendorf JDF, Bessler M, Whelan RL, Trokd M, Laud DA, Terry MB, Treat MR. Better preservation of immune function after laparoscopic assisted vs open bowel resection in a murine model. Dis Colon Rectum 1996; 39:567–572.
19. Larach SW, Patankar S, Fenara A, Williamson P, Perozo S, Lord A. Complications of laparoscopic colorectal surgery. Analysis and comparison of early vs latter experience. Dis Colon Rectum 1997; 40:592–596.
20. Agachan F, Sik Joo J, Weiss E, Wexner S. Intraoperative laparoscopic complications: Are we getting better. Dis Colon Rectum 1996; 39:S14–S19.
21. Geers J, Holden C. Major Vascular injury as a complication of laparoscopic surgery: A report of three cases and review of the literature. Am Surg 1996; 62:377–379.
22. Coopennan A. Complications of laparoscopic surgery. In Arregui ME , Fitzgibbons RJ , Katkhouda N , McKeman JB , Reich H, eds. Principles of Laparoscopic Surgery. New York: Springer-Verlag, 1995.
23. Diemunsch P. Anesthesie Generale pour Coelioscopie. Presented at the EITS, Seminar of Laparoscopic and Thorascopic Surgery.

11

Gastroesophageal Reflux Surgery

Todd A. Kellogg, Carlos A. Pellegrini, and Brant K. Oelschlager
The Swallowing Center, University of Washington, Seattle, Washington, U.S.A.

INTRODUCTION

Laparoscopic techniques have transformed surgery over the past decade. The utilization of laparoscopic approaches has revolutionized esophageal surgery and, in particular, operations for gastroesophageal reflux disease (GERD). As experience with laparoscopic antireflux procedures has increased, operating times, conversion rates, and perioperative complications have predictably decreased. Complication rates are currently about the same as for the open procedure (10–20%) [1,2]. Though many of these complications occur with both approaches, there are also specific complications to the laparoscopic approach. In this chapter we cover these complications with a focus on how they occur, how they are treated, and, most importantly, how best to avoid them.

CARDIOPULMONARY COMPLICATIONS

General Preoperative Evaluation

As with any operation, preoperative patient evaluation and preparation can largely diminish potential complications. Besides taking a good general medical history, an emphasis of cardiopulmonary problems is advisable because of the effect of pneumoperitoneum. Any prolonged laparoscopic operation will decrease venous return, thus affecting preload. Patients over 50 years of age or those of any age with a cardiac history should have a preoperative electrocardiogram. Any symptom or history suggestive of coronary artery disease or congestive heart failure should be thoroughly evaluated and factored into the decision to perform an antireflux operation.

CO_2 pneumoperitoneum has two basic effects on the pulmonary system. By increasing intra-abdominal pressure, it limits diaphragmatic excursion, thus compromising ventilation. The absorption of CO_2 increases the required minute ventilation; therefore patients must have adequate lung capacity and function to tolerate these procedures. Those patients with a history of significant cigarette use or pulmonary disease should have a preoperative chest roentgenogram and preoperative arterial blood gas analysis. Formal pulmonary function testing should be considered in any patient requiring bronchodilators, steroids, or supplemental oxygen.

Hypercarbia and Venous Gas Embolism

Hypercarbia may occur with all laparoscopic procedures where CO_2 pneumoperitoneum is used. Patients particularly at risk for complications of hypercarbia include those with pre-existing cardiopulmonary disease or heart failure, emphasizing the importance of careful preoperative evaluation and selection.

Anesthesia personnel should diligently assess for hypercarbia; end-tidal CO_2 monitoring is employed, in part, to monitor the effect of the CO_2 pneumoperitoneum on Pa_{CO_2}. An arterial line is not usually necessary in uncomplicated patients but should be considered in patients with significant cardiac or pulmonary disease. If CO_2 levels rise significantly, resulting in acidosis, hyperventilation is used to control Pa_{CO_2}. If this maneuver is not immediately effective, pneumoperitoneum should be reduced or discontinued until the Pa_{CO_2} can be returned to acceptable levels.

Clinically significant hypercarbia is best avoided by careful preoperative evaluation and patient selection and by diligent intraoperative monitoring. Lowering the pneumoperitoneum pressure during operation may be helpful to minimize hypercarbia and associated complications. In addition, an excessively long operative time should be avoided, especially when the patient has significant risk factors.

CO_2 venous embolism is a life-threatening complication of laparoscopic surgery, with an incidence of 0.0016–0.013% [3]. It occurs when CO_2 from the pneumoperitoneum enters veins opened during dissection. This complication can manifest itself with hypotension, tachycardia, and a sudden decrease in end-expired CO_2 partial pressures and a rapid decrease in oxygen saturations. A new cardiac murmur is typically present. Treatment begins by immediate discontinuation of the pneumoperitoneum and placing the patient in a left lateral decubitus position to trap the CO_2 away from the outflow tract in the right atrium and ventricle. A central venous catheter can then be placed to aspirate CO_2 from the atrium. Fortunately, the high aqueous solubility of CO_2 allows for rapid dissolution.

PREVENTING POOR OPERATIVE RESULTS

Proper Patient Selection

By far the most important component of successful antireflux operations is proper patient selection. Prior to operation there must be little doubt regarding the nature of the gastroesophageal pathophysiology. This depends on (1) adequate and complete preoperative evaluation, with the goals of diagnosing reflux and excluding other esophageal or gastric pathology; (2) determining the severity of the reflux; and (3) defining the anatomy. These three objectives can generally be achieved with the tests described below.

Twenty-Four–Hour pH Monitoring

Standard pH Monitoring. Twenty-four–hour pH monitoring is the ‘‘gold standard’’ for defining and quantifying gastroesophageal reflux [4,5]. It confirms the diagnosis of reflux, provides evidence of symptom correlation, and quantifies reflux severity [6].

In the absence of erosive esophagitis or Barrett’s esophagus, the diagnosis of GERD is made on the basis of symptoms. However, symptoms alone are unreliable for determining the presence or absence of reflux, and reliance on subjective evidence alone will result in inappropriate patient selection. Thus, 24-hr pH monitoring provides objective evidence of acid in the esophagus and serves to confirm the diagnosis of GERD.

Another benefit of 24-hr pH monitoring is symptom correlation. This is especially useful in cases where there is poor response to medical therapy and the diagnosis is unclear. For example, a patient with atypical symptoms and poor response to medical therapy who clearly has abnormal esophageal acid exposure is likely to benefit from surgical antireflux therapy, while a similar patient without evidence of esophageal acid exposure is not.

The severity of reflux (quantification) can also be established using 24-hr pH monitoring, allowing stratification of patients based on severity of disease [6]. This is particularly important given that endoscopic evidence of esophagitis is absent in up to half of the patients with GERD [7] and therefore cannot be relied upon to indicate the severity of disease.

Finally, pH-monitoring data obtained preoperatively serve as a baseline for comparison in the occasional patient with persistent symptoms after antireflux surgery. This is particularly important given the demonstrated poor correlation between postoperative symptoms and abnormal reflux [8,9].

Pharyngeal pH Monitoring. Respiratory symptoms—such as cough, asthma, and laryngitis—may be caused by abnormal reflux. Establishing a link between GERD and such symptoms has been difficult given there is no specific diagnostic test available. The initial approach to these patients is to first establish the diagnosis of GERD using standard 24-hr pH monitoring. However, a positive study suggests an association but does not prove causation, as this test is too nonspecific to determine a causal relationship. Pellegrini et al. were the first to consider the idea of proximal esophageal acid exposure as stronger evidence of microaspiration [10]. We have extended this idea by measuring pharyngeal reflux using a four-channel probe to perform pharyngeal 24-hr pH monitoring. We have shown that this predicts response to medical [11] and surgical [12] therapy. Further confounding the evaluation of these atypical patients is the fact that some have evidence of pharyngeal reflux with normal esophageal acid exposure [13].

Laryngoscopy is often used in conjunction with pharyngeal pH monitoring to diagnose gastroesophageal-laryngeal reflux as a cause of respiratory symptoms. Laryngeal injury is evaluated and graded, though biopsies are not generally useful [14]. Documented laryngeal injury without objective evidence of pharyngeal reflux suggests another source. The presence of both laryngeal injury and pharyngeal reflux has been found to correlate with true gastroesophageal-laryngeal reflux [15].

Stationary Esophageal Manometry

Stationary esophageal manometry provides information regarding the lower esophageal sphincter (LES) and esophageal body motility. The presence of a hypotensive LES is a strong indicator of an abnormal valve mechanism and correlates well with a significant amount of GER, though it is not a substitute for pH monitoring to confirm GERD [16]. Though a normal LES pressure signifies some preservation of sphincter function, many patients with severe GERD will have a LES pressure in the normal range and may still benefit from an antireflux operation.

Historically, measurement of the esophageal body function was considered extremely important for choosing the correct antireflux operation. It was assumed that the operation should be ''tailored'' depending on the effectiveness of peristalsis, with partial fundoplications used for patients with ineffective esophageal motility (IEM)—low amplitude of peristalsis, poorly propagated waves, etc. The idea was that a total fundoplication (e.g., Nissen) would cause too much resistance and result in dysphagia. Our experience, and that of others, has recently suggested that this is not the case [17,18]. In patients with impaired but not absent peristalsis, a properly constructed loose total fundoplication does not result in a higher incidence of dysphagia. In fact, when dysphagia is present in these patients preoperatively, we found that it resolves in all of them, likely as a result of improved esophageal motor function, which may result in better esophageal emptying. Furthermore, it appears that the biggest factor in avoiding postoperative dysphagia in patients with IEM is the resolution of GERD. Since partial fundoplications are more difficult to perform and provide an inferior reflux barrier [8], we have abandoned them except in patients with aperistalsis, such as those with scleroderma.

We still routinely perform manometry, although admittedly its importance in our minds has diminished. Perhaps the most useful aspect of manometry is the determination of the LES, so that the pH catheter can be placed accurately. The other reason is that we still occasionally diagnose primary esophageal motility disorders, such as achalasia, that were previously assumed to be GERD. In such cases we can effectively target therapy at the motility disorder (e.g., perform an esophageal myotomy) and avoid the devastating complication of performing an antireflux procedure in these patients.

It must be recognized that the presence of a primary esophageal motility disorder does not exclude GERD. In fact, motility disorders such as ''nutcracker esophagus'', diffuse esophageal spasm, and hypertensive lower esophageal sphincter may be associated with GERD. Using preoperative manometric testing, we found that of 643 patients undergoing laparoscopic Nissen fundoplication, 2.3% had high-amplitude peristaltic contractions (>160 mmHg) and 0.6% had a hypertensive LES. In this study, patients with a hypercontractile esophagus, reflux symptoms, and abnormal reflux by 24-hr pH monitoring benefited greatly from laparoscopic Nissen fundoplication [19]. Therefore, in the presence of primarily GERD symptoms, a hypercontractile esophagus should not dissuade the surgeon from performing a total fundoplication in these patients.

Upper Gastrointestinal Series

An upper gastrointestinal series (UGI) defines the anatomy of the distal esophagus, the gastroesophageal junction and its relationship to the diaphragmatic hiatus, and the stomach. Moreover, spontaneous reflux on UGI is almost always associated with abnormal reflux. Two findings may significantly influence the surgeon: (1) the presence of a peptic stricture and/or esophageal shortening and (2) a large hiatal or paraesophageal hernia.

The finding of a peptic stricture on UGI has important implications. It was once thought that patients with GERD and peptic stricture undergoing antireflux operation had an increased incidence of postoperative dysphagia and generally poorer outcomes. However, there are a number of recent studies demonstrating excellent results in this patient population [20–22]. Perhaps more germane is that, as a result of circumferential contraction from inflammation and fibrosis of the esophagus, peptic stricture is a risk factor for esophageal shortening [23].

Preoperative knowledge of esophageal shortening is beneficial in planning operative strategy, though the accuracy of UGI for diagnosing short esophagus can be as low as 50%. It has been suggested that in 3–4% of laparoscopic antireflux operations, 2.5–3 cm of intra-abdominal esophagus cannot be obtained by gastric and esophageal dissection and that the surgeon must be prepared to perform an esophageal lengthening procedure [23]. When a short esophagus is not addressed, the wrap is under tension and at increased risk of ''slippage'' or herniation [24]—a finding thought to be responsible for up to 84% of failures after open or laparoscopic antireflux procedures [25–28]. The Collis-Nissen operation is considered the gold standard esophageal lengthening procedure, but it should be used cautiously and selectively. The creation of a neoesophagus laparoscopically is technically demanding and introduces the potential for added complications. Reported complications include leaks from the gastroplasty staple line, fistulas, and acid secretion from the ectopic gastric mucosa of the neoesophagus [28,29]. Despite these potential complications, the open procedure has an established, excellent long-term success rate [30–32] and these results can apparently be duplicated using endoscopic techniques [33,34].

The presence of a large hiatal or paraesophageal hernia may change the operative strategy or approach and therefore should be looked for preoperatively by UGI. A paraesophageal hernia repair is more complex than a typical antireflux operation and requires more technical expertise. Because of the additional risks associated with this procedure, the decision to proceed with surgical repair should be carefully considered. Due to a high incidence of severe complications associated with nonoperative management it was once believed that all paraesophageal hernias should be repaired regardless of the presence or absence of symptoms [35,36]. Recent studies suggest that the risk of observation is much lower than previously thought. Rattner and colleagues showed that in asymptomatic patients, elective repair would benefit only one in five patients [37], despite the decreased morbidity associated with the laparoscopic approach. In general, our strategy has been to perform elective repair in those patients less than 60 years old and of low operative risk regardless of the presence or absence of symptoms and in symptomatic patients regardless of age.

Endoscopy

Endoscopy is important for investigating lesions and ruling out occult disease in the upper alimentary tract. For example, an esophageal stricture is often diagnostic of GERD; it can be biopsied to rule out malignancy and endoscopically dilated to relieve dysphagia. The presence of erosive esophagitis or Barrett's esophagus confirms the diagnosis of GERD and suggests severe disease. Esophagitis is not, however, an absolute indication for operation, as more than 90% of esophagitis can be relieved with medical therapy [7]. Conversely, the presence of esophagitis and complicated reflux disease despite medications is a strong indication for surgical intervention. However, the majority of patients with symptomatic reflux disease do not have evidence of esophagitis and remain candidates for antireflux [7].

Gastric Emptying and Other Studies

Other studies are occasionally used to further establish the diagnosis or to assist in determining the cause of specific symptoms. Gastric emptying studies may have a role in evaluation of the patient both pre- and postoperatively. For example, patients with vague symptoms, including abdominal pain and bloating associated with eating, are sometimes referred for antireflux surgery and are found to have gastric emptying abnormalities without GERD. Postoperatively, the study can be used to evaluate those patients with persistent severe bloating. Some still advocate a gastric emptying procedure accompanying the antireflux operation. However, it has been shown that fundoplication increases gastric emptying [38], and in our experience we have not found drainage procedures necessary. In the rare patient who has significant delayed gastric emptying postoperatively, a drainage procedure can be performed laparoscopically if necessary.

Radionuclide esophageal transit and videoesophagram, a fluoroscopic real-time evaluation focused on the esophagus, may provide insight into esophageal function. Esophageal endosonography can be used if there is suspicion of esophageal mass on routine GERD workup. Computed tomography (CT) may be helpful in chronic pain syndromes. These studies are used occasionally to better establish the diagnosis or evaluate the anatomy in atypical or complicated cases when reintervention is being considered.

Obesity

Obesity is common among patients with GERD and is an identified risk factor [39,40]. Certainly obesity makes antireflux operations technically more difficult and may decrease their efficacy. Though there are reports of equivalent results in the overweight and obese [41], morbid obesity (BMI $>$ 35) seems to be a significant risk factor for failure [42]. Therefore our approach for those that are significantly overweight has been to have them enter an aggressive weight-loss regimen before their operation. After they have lost a significant amount of weight (ideally to a BMI $\leq$ 30) we proceed with fundoplication. For the morbidly obese patient with significant reflux who has failed weight loss programs, a Roux-en-Y gastric bypass is the procedure of choice. This operation provides excellent long-term relief of GERD [43,44] and has the added benefit of long-term weight loss and the associated health benefits.

Advanced Age

There is evidence that GER is more severe in the elderly, thus supporting aggressive treatment in this patient population [45–48]. Because of the effectiveness of medical therapy and the perceived increased risks of operation, antireflux surgery is often denied to elderly patients. The question then becomes what is appropriate treatment for an elderly patient with GER refractory to medical therapy. One recent study demonstrated that elderly patients (mean age 71 years) had equivalent outcomes after antireflux surgery when compared to a younger patient group (mean age 44 years) [49]. On the other hand, morbidity and mortality after antireflux surgery increase with age. A recent study [50] examining national data reviewed 86,411 patients undergoing antireflux surgery from 1992–1997. Advancing age was associated with a significant increase in complications. The incidence of splenectomy, esophageal injury, and death all increased significantly with age. This was particularly pronounced for those patients over 60 years of age. Mortality in nearly 15,000 patients age 60–69 was 1%, or over three times the incidence for patients aged 50–59 (0.3%). In 10,000 patients aged 70–79, mortality was 2.2%. Patients aged 80–99 had a mortality of 8.3%. Therefore, although advancing age should not prevent candidacy for antireflux surgery, it should be performed only if comorbidities common to the elderly population (e.g., cardiac, pulmonary, etc.) do not preclude safe operation and the severity of disease justifies the risk.

In summary, proper patient selection is the key to excellent outcomes from antireflux operations. Each study mentioned above is important in its own way to avoid complications and poor outcomes. Some have suggested a selective approach to preoperative studies. Though most patients will not be affected by these approaches, occasionally assumptions will be made that will lead to complications. It must be remembered that GERD is not a lethal disease and has other treatment options (e.g., medications and endoscopic therapy). Thus, if antireflux operations are to continue to have a role in the treatment of GERD, they must have superior results. Such results depend on proper patient selection.

OPERATIVE TECHNIQUE

Patient Positioning

Our preference for patient position has been low lithotomy with steep reverse Trendelenburg [51]. A beanbag is used to form a seat, so as to secure the patient while in this extreme position. The video cart is placed at the head of the table. The surgeon stands between the patient's legs, allowing him or her to be in a direct line with the target tissues. We have found this to be an ergonomically superior position. The assistant holds the laparoscope and retracts while standing on the patient's left side. A self-retaining device usually holds the liver retractor, though a second assistant can perform this task while standing on the patient's right side.

Port-Site Placement

As in all laparoscopic operations, proper port-site placement is imperative. If ports are placed too close to the laparoscope, visualization of the working instru-

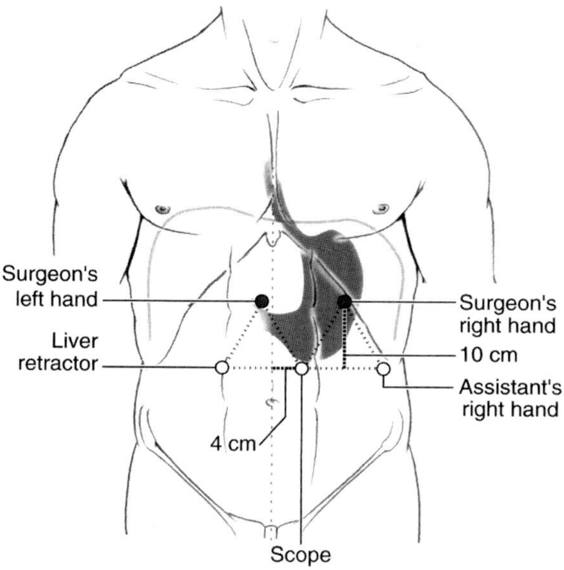

FIGURE 1 Port placement for a laparoscopic antireflux procedure. Two equilateral triangles are created by the five ports. (From Ref. 78.)

ments will be impaired, or they will ''fight'' with each other, thus compromising the operation. Ports must be placed close enough to the organ of interest (in this case the esophagus), but such that the instruments are not impeded by other organs. For example, if the left working port is placed too high, the liver will limit its use.

In general, a minimal distance of 10 cm between port sites should be observed. All ports are placed while the patient is flat prior to reverse Trendelenburg positioning. It has been our practice for the placement of the surgeon's left- and right-hand ports to be equidistant from the esophageal hiatus, forming an equilateral triangle with the laparoscope port, which is placed 2 cm left lateral to the midline and 10 cm from the costal margin (Fig. 1). The assistant's right-hand port completes an equilateral triangle with the surgeon's right-hand port and the laparoscope port, while the liver retractor port completes another equilateral triangle with the surgeon's left-hand port and the laparoscope port. Though small adjustments are sometimes necessary based on variations in body habitus, we have found that this technique produces consistently reliable port positioning.

Performing the Fundoplication

Incompetence of the cardia is caused by numerous factors including LES hypotension [52], transient LES relaxation [53], absence of a flap valve [54], gastric emptying abnormalities [55], and hiatal hernia [56]. An effective antireflux operation must address and correct each of these factors, thus restoring competence to the gastroesophageal junction. As with any operation, specific techniques have been devised that help to avoid pitfalls and postoperative failure. The following principles must be observed if the operation is to be effective:

1. The crus must be approximated posteriorly so that the diaphragmatic hiatus is gently snug when a 50–60 F bougie is in place within the esophagus.
2. The fundoplication must be constructed over the esophagus just proximal to the gastroesophageal junction and should be fixed to the esophagus to remain in that position permanently. This requires adequate mobilization of the mediastinal and intra-abdominal esophagus as well as correct identification of the gastroesophageal junction. Intraoperative endoscopy can be a useful adjunct for accurately defining the gastroesophageal junction when its location is in doubt [57].
3. The fundoplication must be constructed without tension, using the gastric fundus. The use of a 50–60 F bougie inside the esophagus assists in the performance of a ''floppy'' Nissen fundoplication.
4. A total fundoplication, such as the Nissen fundoplication, should measure 2.5–3 cm in length anteriorly. Longer fundoplications have higher rates of dysphagia without providing better control of reflux [58]. Partial fundoplications (anterior or posterior) are usually one and a half times the length of a total fundoplication.
5. The fundoplication should be constructed in a symmetrical fashion to avoid distortion. A distorted geometry can result in an ineffective fundoplication or postoperative dysphagia (Fig. 2). Symmetry is achieved by using equal portions of anterior and posterior fundus for the fundoplication.
6. The wrapped portion of the esophagus must lie below the diaphragm and be without tension.

Intraoperative Endoscopy

Intraoperative endoscopy can be very useful for examining the geometry of the fundoplication and determining the grade of flap valve. If results are suboptimal, manipulation of the wrap under direct endoscopic vision can provide the information necessary to improve the fundoplication intraoperatively [57].

Close adherence to these principles leads to excellent results, providing symptom control in 90–95% of patients. It has been demonstrated that, after properly performed fundoplication, there is significant increase in LES pressure, fewer transient LES relaxations [59,60], restoration of the flap valve [60], enhancement of gastric emptying [38], and correction of the hernia, if present

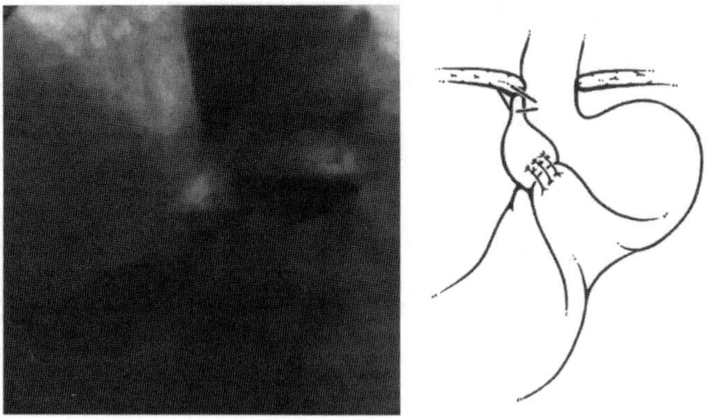

FIGURE 2 An asymmetrical fundoplication causing distorted anatomy on UGI (upper gastrointestines). Such distortion can cause recurrent symptoms of reflux or chronic dysphagia. (Adapted from Ref. 26.)

[59–61]. These changes (1) restore the physiology of the LES mechanism, (2) improve the competency of the cardia, and (3) preserve the ability to swallow normally.

SPECIFIC COMPLICATIONS AND TECHNIQUES TO AVOID THEM

Pneumothorax

Dissection of the mediastinal esophagus can result in violation of the pleura and subsequent pneumothorax. The incidence of pneumothorax during antireflux surgery ranges from 0–2% and depends on the extent and difficulty of the mediastinal dissection [1,2]. Difficulty with this dissection is often associated with inflammation from esophagitis or Barrett's esophagus and is also more common in patients undergoing reoperation. As long as there is no injury to the lung parenchyma, a CO_2 pneumothorax rarely requires treatment. The high diffusion coefficient of CO_2 allows for rapid pneumothorax resolution through absorption; thus tube thoracostomy is rarely required. When the pleura is violated, the surgeon should first discuss this with the anesthesiologist. If hemodynamic instability or pulmonary dysfunction develops intraoperatively, the pneumoperitoneum should be decompressed immediately until the anesthesiologist can stabilize the patient. Insufflation pressures can subsequently be lowered, but usually the cardiopulmonary effects can easily be treated by the anesthesiologist. If the pleural defect is seen and easily accessible for closure, it may be sutured, thereby limiting further CO_2 infiltration and hastening its resolution.

A postoperative chest roentgenogram is always performed to document the presence and size of a pneumothorax. The reason is not necessarily to treat a pneumothorax that is present, though this certainly should be done for respiratory distress. Instead, it serves as a baseline and can be used for purposes of comparison if the patient experiences symptoms such as dyspnea or hypoxia later in the postoperative course. This approach may prevent unnecessary tube thoracostomy placement.

Liver Trauma

Small liver lacerations and hematomas are fairly common during laparoscopic antireflux surgery as a result of liver retraction. These injuries are usually self-limited and uneventful. Nevertheless, attempts should be made to avoid them. Proper port positioning as described above will allow the retractor to hold the left liver lobe flat against the anterior abdominal wall rather than at an angle, which can cause lacerations or unequal compression and subsequent congestion of the liver. The color of the liver should be noted periodically for evidence of excessive congestion. An actively bleeding liver injury can often be controlled by tamponade after replacement of the liver retractor.

Occasionally, it is necessary to apply a hemostatic agent such as oxidized regenerated cellulose (Surgicel, Ethicon, Somerville, NJ). Clinically significant postoperative bleeding from liver injury can potentially be controlled with percutaneous angioembolization, although the need for this intervention is extremely rare.

Port-Site Hernia

The incidence of port-site herniation is reported to be 0.18–3% [1,63]. Though hernias at 5-mm port sites have been reported, the highest incidence is reported for 10- and 12-mm ports [63]. In general, fascial closure of any port site greater than 5 mm in diameter is recommended. A long-acting absorbable suture such as polyglycolic acid or nonabsorbable suture is used. Closure can be performed by ''open'' techniques or by way of laparoscopy. For open closure, a figure-of-eight or one to two interrupted sutures reapproximating the anterior fascia is usually adequate to close the defect. Laparoscopic closure of the fascia is performed under direct vision with a percutaneous closure device. This technique has the advantage of direct inspection of the port-site closure. In addition, visualization of the fascia is often limited during open closure because of the small size of the incision. Newer, radially dilating trocars have been shown to produce a much smaller fascial defect and may not require fascial closure [64,65].

Splenic Injury

The incidence of splenic injury and splenectomy during laparoscopic antireflux surgery has predictably decreased with surgeon experience. The incidence of injury to the spleen in most single-institution reports during primary laparoscopic antireflux surgery is 0.24%, while the incidence of splenectomy is 0.06% [1]. However, recent population studies suggest that the incidence may be much higher (2.3%) and that it is associated with surgeon experience [50]. Those surgeons having performed less than 5 operations had a splenectomy incidence of 2.9%, while those having performed 50 or more antireflux operations had an incidence of 0.18% [50]. Interestingly, the incidence of splenectomy also rises significantly with the patient's age. After 50 years of age, the incidence of splenectomy increases on average 1% per decade, to 5.4% for the 80–99-year age group [50].

Injury to the spleen most often occurs during attempts to mobilize the proximal fundus by division of the gastrosplenic ligament. The short gastric vessels in this region are often in very close proximity to the superior pole or splenic hilum and can be deep and very short. In addition, exposure in this region can be quite difficult in the patient with generous intra-abdominal fat. This is a significant benefit of the left crus approach that we have described and have used for many years [66]. With this approach, we begin the operation by dividing the phrenogastric ligament, thus exposing the left crus as far as possible toward the superior pole of the spleen. The short gastric vessels of the superior greater curvature are then divided. For this we prefer using ultrasonic shears; however, clips and the Ligasure device may also be used. With most of the fundus mobilized, a window is created between the angle of His and the left crus (connecting it with the initial dissection). The short upper pole attachments can now be safely exposed and divided without injury. In our own review of 538 consecutive patients using this approach, no splenic injury necessitating splenectomy occurred [2].

When splenic injuries do occur, they are usually capsular tears, although injuries to hilar vessels also occur. For minor bleeding, direct pressure using a broad instrument combined with a hemostatic agent such as oxidized regenerated cellulose is usually the safest approach. Severe bleeding often occurs when the surgeon is trying to coagulate or clip relatively minor bleeding. Occasionally, more significant bleeding occurs that cannot be controlled by conservative maneuvers. In these instances, electrocautery is generally not helpful and should be avoided. The first priority is adequate exposure and identification of the bleeding, since imprecise attempts at control usually worsen the situation. If bleeding cannot be efficiently controlled laparoscopically, conversion to an open approach should be performed.

Vagus Injury

The true incidence of vagus injury is not known. The incidence is highest in reoperations where adhesions are present and anatomy is distorted. Early identification of the anterior and posterior vagus nerves is the best way to avoid injury. The anterior vagus nerve is at greatest risk when the surgeon is dividing the anterior phrenoesophageal membrane, with which the vagus nerve is often intimately associated. We have found that during hiatal and mediastinal dissection, keeping the posterior vagus associated with the wall of the esophagus is the best method of avoiding injury. Because the anterior vagus lies within the gastroesophageal junction fat pad, we avoid indiscriminate retraction on this structure. When consistently observed, these techniques lead to a very low rate of vagus injury [2].

Prolonged postoperative ileus may be a sign of vagus injury. In addition, the well-known symptoms of delayed gastric emptying, early satiety, bloating, diarrhea, and dumping syndrome may be present. There are ways to determine vagal function after suspected injury [67]. Vagal secretory function can be measured by gastric acid output and pancreatic polypeptide response to sham feeding. Vagal motor function may be indirectly assessed by a technetium gastric emptying scan. Gastric reservoir function can be evaluated by measuring meal capacity. In practice, symptoms suggestive of vagal nerve injury are treated without diagnostic studies. Bloating usually resolves with time, but prokinetic agents such as metoclopramide may be effective at improving gastric emptying. If bloating persists for more than 6 weeks, it should be evaluated. If dumping syndrome occurs, it can usually be controlled with dietary manipulation (avoidance of carbohydrate-rich foods). For dumping symptoms uncontrolled by diet, there has been success using octreotide, though it is expensive and can cause unpleasant side effects. Diarrhea from vagotomy or vagal injury usually subsides after weeks to months. Dietary manipulation, fiber supplements, and cholestyramine will alleviate diarrhea in 99% of patients. The 1% with persistent diarrhea should have GI tract evaluation.

Perforation

In most published case series, the risk of gastric or esophageal perforation is 0.7–1.1% [1,2,50]. However, using population based data, Flum et al. [50] showed that the incidence is nearly 1% for inexperienced surgeons and declines to 0.17% for those surgeons who have performed 50 or more operations. There is also a significant increase in perforation with advancing age, rising to 4.5% for those over age 80 [50]. Most reports have demonstrated that the risk of esophageal perforation lies mainly with reoperations and in the passage of the bougie by anesthesia personnel [2,68,69]. To avoid bougie-related perforations, close communication with the person passing the bougie is imperative and the position of the bougie within the esophagus should be accounted for at all times. An extra monitor for anesthesia personnel allows for visual feedback during passage. The surgeon should take care not to angulate the esophagus or gastroesophageal junction and can help guide passage gently into the stomach.

Mediastinal mobilization of the esophagus can be difficult in reoperations, cases of severe esophagitis and fibrosis, or in the presence of a large hiatal or paraesophageal hernia. For these difficult cases, a lighted bougie can be used to identify the boundaries and course of the esophagus. The bougie is then pulled back for the dissection since aggressive manipulation of the esophagus with a bougie in place can lead to perforation.

Gastric perforation most commonly occurs during mobilization of the stomach and is more frequent during reoperation, when adhesions and distorted anatomy are present. Reduction of a paraesophageal hernia or a large hiatal hernia can increase the risk of perforation during mobilization of the fundus. A preoperative upper GI series is helpful to delineate the anatomy. Intraoperative endoscopy also allows for a real-time assessment of confusing anatomy and should always be available for difficult procedures.

Recognition of perforation of either the stomach or esophagus at the time it occurs may mean the difference between a relatively benign injury and an injury that is life-threatening. A small, recognized perforation of the esophagus may be repaired with suture closure. Fortunately, if the injury lies in the distal esophagus, the repair may be buttressed with the fundoplication originally described by Nissen [70]. Large defects are not amenable to simple closure and esophagectomy is often a safer albeit much more invasive procedure. The possibility should be discussed preoperatively with all patients undergoing redo or complex operations of the cardia. A gastric injury is usually easier to deal with and can be sutured or closed using a linear stapling device.

Unrecognized injuries lead to postoperative leak and sepsis. Mortality can approach 50% [71]. Early diagnosis and treatment is central to the management of these perforations. Postoperative abdominal discomfort, chest pain, fever, tachycardia, hypotension, and low urine output should all be investigated without delay. Evaluation should begin with an upper GI series, though a CT scan may be helpful, depending on local radiological support. If extravasation of contrast material is demonstrated, an immediate return to the operating room for exploration and repair is indicated. Even in the face of normal radiographic studies, persistence of symptoms is an indication to return to the operating room for exploration. Delay in the diagnosis and treatment of perforation leads to significantly increased morbidity and mortality [68,71].

Fundoplication Herniation

In a large meta-analysis, the incidence of acute wrap herniation after a primary laparoscopic antireflux procedure was 1.3% and was the most common perioperative complication [1]. In addition, wrap herniation was the most common intraoperative finding during reoperation after a failed primary minimally invasive antireflux procedure [1]. In our own study examining the causes of failure after antireflux operations, we noted that, at reoperation, the vast majority of patients (>75%) had evidence of fundoplication herniation [26].

Postoperative retching episodes, severe coughing, and excessive straining are associated with acute herniation. In the absence of technical missteps, acute herniation in this situation usually results from disruption of the fundoplication and anchoring sutures before fibrosis occurs.

Several technical factors contribute to fundoplication herniation. These include insufficient esophageal length, inadequate closure of the crus, and failure to properly anchor the fundoplication intra-abdominally. We have found that the incidence is much less when careful closure of the crus and anchoring of the fundoplication is performed. In our series of 500 patients, one episode (0.2%) of acute herniation occurred when such anchoring was performed [2]. To avoid herniation of the fundoplication, we have found the following techniques useful:

1. To adequately close the crus, we use 2–0 silk sutures placed 0.5 cm apart, being sure to take generous bites. Care is taken not to pull on the crus when tying so as to avoid damage that will weaken the closure. Adequate closure of the crus is verified by examining the hiatus with the bougie in place. Closure of very large hiatal defects can be problematic. In these cases, approximation of the crus posteriorly can result in anterior angulation of the esophagus. This may be avoided by placing one or two sutures anteriorly in addition to a moderate posterior closure.
2. Occasionally, the defect is quite large and the crus attenuated, making it difficult to close the hiatus. The following options are available in these cases: (1) a relaxing incision can be made in the right crus, allowing closure of the crus, and then using a piece of mesh to bridge the relaxing incision, or (2) direct reinforcement of the posterior crural repair with mesh can be implemented to achieve a tension-free repair [72,73]. Unfortunately, the use of mesh has resulted in esophageal injury and stricture formation [73,74]. A bioprosthesis such as small intestinal submucosa (SIS) mesh (Surgisis, Cook Surgical, Bloomington, Indiana) may provide a stronger tissue matrix and prove to be a safer alternative to synthetic material. This is performed by trimming the mesh to a U-shaped configuration and buttressing the primary repair (Fig. 3).
3. Ensure adequate esophageal length by performing substantial dissection of the mediastinal esophagus. If this does not provide at least 3 cm of intra-abdominal esophagus, a lengthening procedure should be performed.

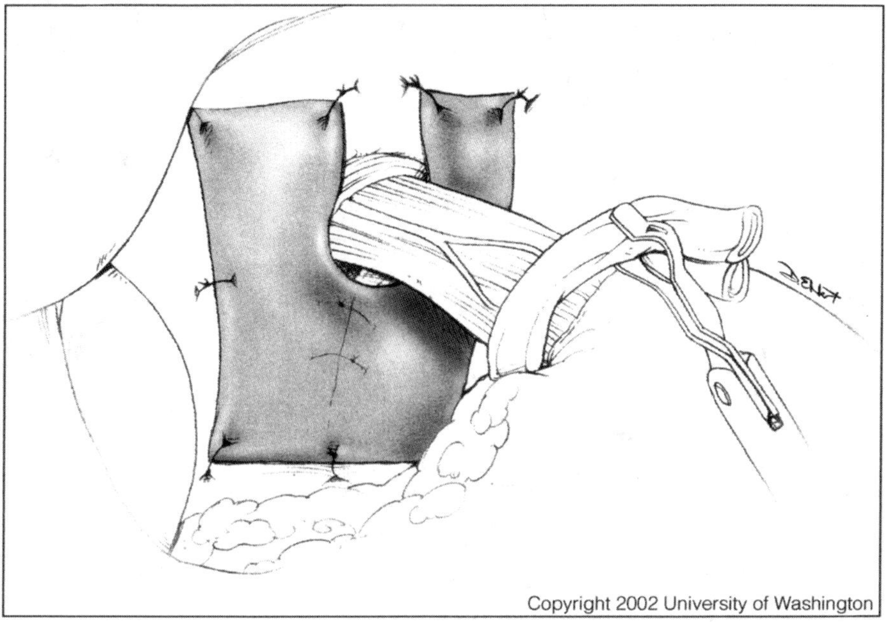

Figure 3 Reinforcement of the posterior crural repair with small intestinal submucosa (SIS) mesh.

4. Intra-abdominal anchoring of the fundoplication is achieved by placing a total of four anchoring sutures; two are placed laterally at the level of the hiatus, one on each side; these include the superior portion of the wrap, a small portion of esophagus, and crus. A third is placed from the right side of the wrap to the right crus, and a fourth is placed from the superior portion of the fundoplication midway between the first two sutures to the diaphragm anteriorly.
5. To prevent acute herniation from retching, aggressive antiemetic therapy should be instituted postoperatively and a nasogastric tube placed if severe gastric distention occurs. Stool softeners are used to prevent straining during bowel movements. Lifting of more than 10 lb is avoided for 6 weeks postoperatively.

Acute herniation should be strongly suspected when complaints of chest or epigastric pain are associated with heavy lifting or a violent coughing or retching episode. Obstructive symptoms may also be present. Patients who present with signs of obstruction require urgent reoperation.

Fundoplication herniation is the most common finding during reoperation for postoperative failure of antireflux surgery [1,25,26,75]. Patients having chronic symptoms related to fundoplication herniation should undergo thorough evaluation. Evaluation should begin with an esophagogram, which will identify an anatomical abnormality in the majority of cases. Endoscopy may be useful in some cases. Manometry and 24-hr pH monitoring may be helpful to assess the functional result of such a herniation. Reoperation should be considered when fundoplication herniation is associated with significant GERD or dysphagia.

Gas Bloat

Early gas bloat is the intragastric trapping of swallowed air resulting from the fundoplication, thus limiting the expulsion of air through belching and occurring in the face of surgically induced gastroparesis. This is most pronounced in the early postoperative period and usually lessens with time. Nevertheless, gastric distention and the inability to belch can be quite distressing. Until it resolves, patients should be advised to avoid air swallowing to the extent possible and to limit oral intake. Simethicone is sometimes effective at relieving mild or even moderate gastric distention. However, severe gastric distention may lead to primary failure of the fundoplication and thus should be treated by early placement of a nasogastric tube.

Bloating that persists beyond 6 weeks is unusual and should be evaluated. A prokinetic agent such as metoclopramide may be effective in improving gastric emptying. Upper GI and gastric emptying studies may be performed to evaluate the anatomy and function of the stomach but are rarely helpful in treatment.

Deep Venous Thrombosis and Pulmonary Embolism

The incidence of pulmonary embolism in laparoscopic antireflux surgery is 0.17% [1], which is no different than that for the open procedure. Sequential compression devices should be used throughout the operation. Subcutaneous heparin is generally safe and is sometimes used as an adjunct in patients at higher risk, such as those with a high BMI, previous deep venous thrombosis (DVT), or when prolonged surgery is anticipated.

Ileus

In our experience, postoperative ileus is the most frequent complication of antireflux surgery, occurring in 6.9% of patients [2]. The most likely etiology of postoperative ileus is surgical manipulation and the use of opiate-based pain medication. This is almost always self- limited but is difficult to differentiate from acute gastric distention and should be distinguished by abdominal x-rays. Prolonged ileus may be associated with vagus nerve injury, the avoidance and treatment of which was previously discussed.

Urinary Retention

Occurring approximately 2% of the time after laparoscopic antireflux operations, urinary retention may require reinsertion of a urinary catheter and a prolonged hospital stay [2]. Older men, especially those with benign prostatic hypertrophy (BPH), are at greatest risk. Minimizing the use of opiate-based medications postoperatively may reduce the risk of developing this complication. In general, early detection and reassurance are the most important aspects of treatment. Short-term (24–36 hr) bladder rest is usually all that is required. In instances where exacerbation of BPH is suspected, tamsulosin HCl (FLOMAX, Boehringer Ingelheim Pharmaceuticals, Inc.) can be used alone or in combination with prolonged catheterization. Follow-up with a urologist is recommended for persistent urinary retention.

Mortality

Overall mortality for primary antireflux procedures performed laparoscopically is generally reported to be between 0 and 1% [1,50]. Population studies demonstrate a substantial increase in mortality for patients over 60 years of age, rising to 8.3% for patients over age 80 [50]. In addition, with surgeon experience, mortality decreases from 1.3% (< 5 cases) to 0.0% (> 49 cases) [50]. Most deaths occur due to pre-existing comorbidities such as pulmonary and cardiac disease. The few patients who die as a direct complication of the procedure have unrecognized bowel perforation. This emphasizes the need for careful patient selection and reiterates the importance of recognizing perforation intraoperatively.

POSTOPERATIVE EVALUATION OF SYMPTOMATIC FAILURES

Symptom Recurrence

Overall, laparoscopic antireflux surgery has been shown to be effective at alleviating symptoms in 85–95% of patients, with excellent patient satisfaction. However, there are a certain number of patients in whom symptoms recur. The precise recurrence rate is difficult to determine and depends on the experience of the surgeon as well as the definition of recurrence or failure. Recurrent reflux symptoms (e.g., heartburn, regurgitation, etc.) and dysphagia are the two most common indications of the failure of antireflux surgery. Most persistent or recurrent symptoms that occur within the first 6–8 weeks after operation do not represent reflux, are self-limited, and generally require only reassurance. Significant reflux symptoms after this should be investigated with repeat 24-hr pH testing, endoscopy, UGI, and manometry, with comparison to preoperative baseline values. If an anatomical abnormality is identified in conjunction with recurrent symptoms, reoperation is often required for correction. When the anatomy is normal, medical therapy may be effective. If not, reoperation may be considered.

Postoperative Dysphagia

Current studies indicate a 2–5% incidence of postoperative dysphagia, depending on the type of antireflux procedure performed [1,76]. In the immediate postoperative period, some degree of dysphagia is expected. This is usually the result of tissue edema after esophageal and gastric mobilization and is self-limited. Dysphagia is minimized by using a specialized postoperative diet that progresses from liquids to solids in the first 4 to 6 weeks.

However, 2.5% of patients having primary antireflux procedures have dysphagia that persists for more than 2 months [1,77]. Several technical factors have been identified as important for preventing chronic dysphagia:

1. Division of the short gastric vessels has clearly been demonstrated to decrease the incidence of prolonged postoperative dysphagia by improving the mobility of the fundus, resulting in less tension on the wrap and less torsion on the esophagus [76].
2. Excessively tight closure of the crus should be avoided. Judging the size of the hiatal opening relative to the esophagus while the esophagus is empty can be difficult. Using a 60 F esophageal bougie or intraoperative endoscopy can help avoid this pitfall.
3. The fundoplication should be no more than 2–3 cm in length anteriorly and performed over a 60 F bougie. DeMeester demonstrated that by reducing the length of the wrap from 4–1 cm and performing the fundoplication over a 60 F bougie, the incidence of persistent postoperative dysphagia was reduced from 21–3% [58].
4. Avoid faulty position and geometry of the fundoplication. This can cause distortion of the fundus and torsion on the esophagus, resulting in permanent or intermittent narrowing (Fig. 2) [25,26].

If dysphagia continues for more than 6 or 8 weeks, it should be investigated. A contrast esophagogram is the first diagnostic test. The esophagogram will demonstrate whether herniation of the wrap or another geometric abnormality is present. If an anatomical abnormality is present, conservative measures can be tried, but reoperation and reconstruction of the fundoplication is usually necessary. If the esophagraphic findings are normal, endoscopy will often identify the abnormality. If endoscopic findings are normal, dilation is often successful. Patients who continue to have symptoms despite adequate trials of dilation present

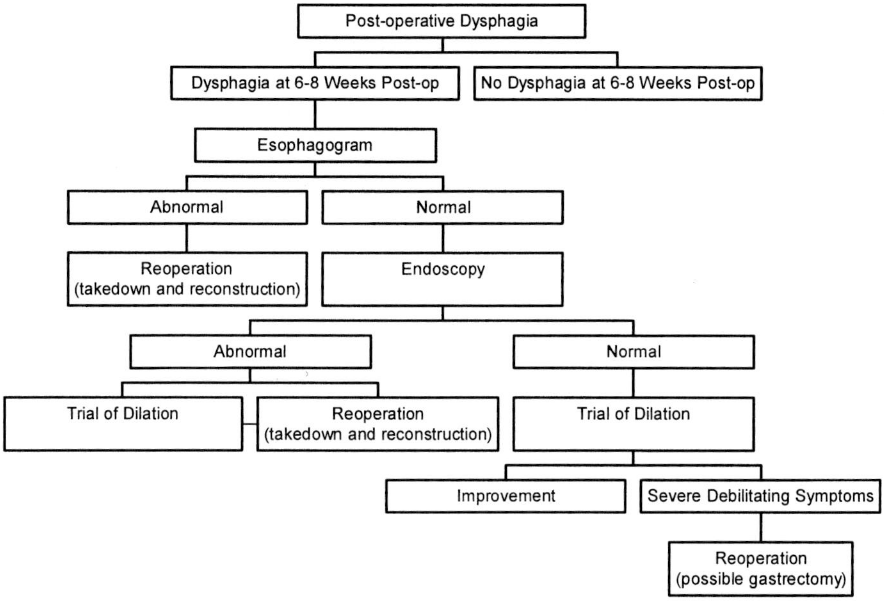

Figure 4 Algorithm for diagnosis and treatment of postoperative dysphagia after antireflux procedure.

a challenge. If symptoms are debilitating and refractory to nonoperative management, reoperation should be considered. Occasionally, if an anatomical cause cannot be identified or an appropriate dissection and reconstruction is not feasible (Fig. 4), gastrectomy becomes necessary.

SUMMARY

Laparoscopic antireflux surgery is safe and effective. The most important component of successful antireflux operations is proper patient selection. The key components of the workup include careful evaluation of symptoms, esophagogram, manometry, 24-hr pH testing, and endoscopy. Postoperative symptom recurrence, dysphagia, and acute herniation can be reduced by careful attention to technical details, including complete fundus mobilization, full esophageal dissection, meticulous closure of the diaphragmatic crura, and intra-abdominal fixation of the fundoplication. Persistent postoperative symptoms should be extensively evaluated to objectively identify abnormalities that explain the symptom. Only then should a solution be devised. Other complications are best avoided, but if they occur, they are usually treatable with a thorough knowledge of their etiology and effective interventions. Outcomes of laparoscopic antireflux procedures depend on thoroughness of the surgeon's knowledge of patient selection, technical aspects of the procedure, and the avoidance and treatment of complications.

REFERENCES

1. Carlson MA, Frantzides CT. Complications and results of primary minimally invasive antireflux procedures: a review of 10735 reported cases. J Am Coll Surg 2001; 193(4):428–439.
2. Pohl D, Eubanks TR, Omelanczuk PE, Pellegrini CA. Management and outcome of complications after laparoscopic antireflux operations. Arch Surg 2001; 136: 399–403.
3. Corwin CL. Pneumoperitoneum. In Scott-Connor CEH, ed. The SAGES Manual: Fundamentals of Laparoscopy and GI Endoscopy. New York: Springer Verlag, 1999, 37–42.
4. Stein D, DeMeester T, Peters J, Fuchs K. Technique, indications, and clinical use of ambulatory 24-hour surgery practice. Surgery 1994; 116:758–766.
5. Bremner R, Bremner C, DeMeester T. Gastroesophageal reflux: The use of pH monitoring. Curr Probl Surg 1995; 32:429–558.
6. Patti M, Diener U, Tamburini A, Molena D, Way LW. Role of esophageal function tests in the diagnosis of gastroesophageal reflux disease. Dig Dis Sci 2001; 46: 597–602.
7. Spechler SJ, Lee E, Ahnen D, Goyal RK, Hirano I, Ramirez F, Raufman JP, Sampliner R, Schnell T, Sontag S, Vlahcevic ZR, Young R, Williford W. Long-term outcome of medical and surgical therapies for gastroesophageal reflux disease: follow-up of a randomized controlled trial. JAMA 2001; 285:2331–2338.
8. Khajanchee YS, O'Rourke RW, Lockhart B, Patterson EJ, Hansen PD, Swanstrom LL. Post-operative symptoms and failure after antireflux surgery. Arch Surg 2002; 137:1008–1014.
9. Eubanks TR, Omelanczuk P, Richards C, Pohl D, Pellegrini CA. Outcomes of laparoscopic antireflux procedures. Am J Surg 2000; 179:391–395.
10. Patti MG, Debas HT, Pellegrini CA. Esophageal manometry and 24-hour pH monitoring in the diagnosis of pulmonary aspiration secondary to gastroesophageal reflux. Am J Surg 1992; 163:401–406.
11. Eubanks T, Omelanczuk P, Hillel A, Marionan N, Pope C, Pellegrini CA. Pharyngeal pH measurements in patients with respiratory symptoms prior to and during proton pump inhibitor therapy. Am J Surg 2001; 181:466–470.
12. Oelschlager BK, Eubanks T, Oleynikov D, Pellegrini CA. Symptomatic and physiologic outcomes after operative treatment for extraesophageal reflux. Surg Endosc 2002; 16:1032–1036.
13. Oelschlager BK, Chang L, Barreca M, Pope CE, Pellegrini CA. Typical GERD symptoms and esophageal pH monitoring are not enough to diagnose pharyngeal reflux: Analysis of 518 patients. Am J Gastroenterol:In press.

14. Reyes V, Yang J, Marionan N, et al. Is laryngeal biopsy useful in the diagnosis of acid pharyngitis? (abstr). Dig Dis Week: Altanta, 2001.
15. Oelschlager BK, Eubanks TR, Marionan N, Hillel A, Oleynikov D, Pope C, Pellegrini CA. Laryngoscopy and pharyngeal pH are complimentary in the diagnosis of gastroesophageal-laryngeal reflux. J Gastrointest Surg 2002; 6:189–194.
16. Zaninotto G, DeMeester T, Schwizer W. The lower esophageal sphincter in health and disease. Am J Surg 1988; 155:104–111.
17. Oleynikov D, Eubanks TR, Oelschlager BK, Pellegrini CA. Total fundoplication is the operation of choice for patients with gastroesophageal reflux and defective peristalsis. Surg Endosc 2002; 16:909–913.
18. Fernando HC, Luketich JD, Christie NA, Ikaramuddin S, Schauer PR. Outcomes of laparoscopic Toupet compared to laparoscopic Nissen fundoplication. Surg Endosc 2002; 16:905–908.
19. Barreca M, Oelschlager BK, Pellegrini CA. Outcomes of laparoscopic Nissen fundoplication in patients with the ''hypercontractile esophagus.''. Arch Surg 2002; 137:724–729.
20. Spivak H, Farrell TM, Trus TL, Branum GD, Warring JP, Hunter JG. Laparoscopic fundoplication for dysphagia and peptic esophageal stricture. J Gastrointest Surg 1998; 2:555–560.
21. Klingler PJ, Hinder RA, Cina RA, DeVault KR, Floch NR, Branton SA, Seelig MH. Laparoscopic antireflux surgery for the treatment of esophageal strictures refractory to medical therapy. Am J Gastroenterol 1999; 94:632–636.
22. Herron DM, Swanstrom LL, Ramzi N, Hansen PD. Factors predictive of dysphagia after laparoscopic Nissen fundoplication. Surg Endosc 1999; 13:1180–1183.
23. Horvath KD, Swanstrom LL, Jobe BA. The short esophagus: Patholphysiology, incidence, presentation, and treatment in the era of laparoscopic antireflux surgery. Ann Surg 2000; 232:630–640.
24. Peters JH, DeMeester TR. The lessons of failed antireflux repairs. In Peters JH , DeMeester TR, eds. Minimally Invasive Therapy of the Foregut. St. Louis: Quality Medical Pulishing, 1994, 190.
25. Hunter JG, Smith CD, Branum GD, Waring JP, Trus TL, Cornwell M, Galloway K. Laparoscopic fundoplication failures. Ann Surg 1999; 230:595–606.
26. Horgan S, Pohl D, Bogetti D, Eubanks T, Pellegrini C. Failed antireflux surgery: What have we learned from reoperations. Arch Surg 1999; 134:809–817.
27. Soper NJ, Dunnegan D. Anatomic fundoplication failure aftewr laparoscopic antireflux surgery. Ann Surg 1999; 229:669–676.
28. Jobe BA, Horvath K, Swanstrom LL. Post-operative function following laparoscopic Collis gastroplasty for shortened esophagus. Arch Surg 1998; 133:867–874.
29. Martin CJ, Cox MR, Cade RJ. Collis-Nissen gastroplasty fundoplication for complicated gastro-oesophageal reflux disease. Aust NZ J Surg 1992; 62:126–129.
30. Orringer MB, Sloan H. Combined Collis-Nissen reconstruction of the esophagogastric junction. Ann Thorac Surg 1978; 25:16–21.
31. Stirling MC, Orringer MB. Continued assessment of the combined Collis-Nissen operation. Ann Thorac Surg 1989; 47:224–230.
32. Stirling MC, Orringer MB. The combined Collis-Nissen operation for esophageal reflux strictures. Ann Thorac Surg 1988; 45:148.

33. Swanstrom LL, Marcus DR, Galloway GQ. Laparoscopic Collis gastroplasty is the treatment of choice for shortened esophagus. Am J Surg 1996; 171:477–481.
34. Johnson AB, Oddsdottir M, Hunter JG. Laparoscopic Collis gastroplasty and Nissen fundoplication: A new technique for the management of esophageal foreshortening. Surg Endosc 1998; 12:1055–1060.
35. Skinner DB, Belsey RH. Surgical management of esophageal reflux and hiatus hernia: Long-term results with 1030 patients. J Thorac Cardiovasc Surg 1967; 53:33–54.
36. Hill LD. Incarcerated paraesophageal hernia: A surgical emergency. Am J Surg 1973; 126:286–291.
37. Stylopoulos N, Gazelle GS, Rattner DW. Paraesophageal hernia: Operation or observation. Ann Surg 2002; 236:492–501.
38. Hinder RA, Stein HJ, Bremner CG, DeMeester TR. Relationship of a satisfactory outcome to normalization of delayed gastric emptying after Nissen findoplication. Ann Surg 1989; 210:458–465.
39. Beauchamp G, Duranceau AC. Diagnostic and therapeutic esophagoscopy. Indications, contraindications, and complications. Surg Clin North Am 1983; 63:801–813.
40. Barak N, Ehrenpreis ED, Harrison JR, Sitrin MD. Gastro-esophageal reflux disease in obesity: Pathophysiological and therapeutic considerations. Obes Rev 2002; 3: 9–15.
41. Fraser J, Watson DI, O'Boyle CJ, Jamieson GC. Obesity and its effect on outcome of laparoscopic Nissen fundoplication. Dis Esophagus 2001; 14:50–53.
42. Perez AR, Moncure AC, Rattner DW. Obesity adversely affects the outcome of antireflux operations. Surg Endosc 2001; 15:986–989.
43. Frezza EE, Ikramuddin S, Gourash W, Rakitt T, Kingston A, Luketich J, Schauer P. Symptomatic improvement in gastroesophageal reflux disease (GERD) following laparoscopic Roux-en-Y gastric bypass. Surg Endosc 2002; 16:1027–1031.
44. Smith SC, Edwards CB, Goodman GN. Symptomatic improvement in morbidly obese patients with gastroesophageal reflux disease following Roux-en-Y gastric bypass. Obes Surg 1997; 7:479–484.
45. Collen MJ, Abdulian JD, Chen YK. Gastroesophageal reflux disease in the elderly: More severe disease that requires aggressive therapy. Am J Gastroenterol 1995; 90: 1053–1057.
46. Mold JW, Reed LE, Davis AB, Allen ML, Decktor DL, Robinson M. Prevalence of gastroesophageal reflux in elderly patients in a primary care setting. Am J Gastroenterol 1991; 86:965–970.
47. Zhu H, Pace F, Sangaletti O, Porro Bianchi G. Features of symptomatic gastroesophageal reflux in elderly patients. Scand J Gastroenterol 1993; 28:235–238.
48. Waring JP. Management of gastroesophageal reflux disease in the elderly: More aggressive or more appropriate. Am J Gastroenterol 1995; 90:1037.
49. Khajanchee YS, Urbach DR, Butler N, Hansen PD, Swanstrom LL. Laparoscopic antireflux surgery in the elderly. Surg Endosc 2002; 16:25–30.
50. Flum DR, Koepsell T, Heagerty P, Pellegrini CA. The nationwide frequency of major adverse outcomes in antireflux surgery and the role of surgeon experience, 1992–1997. J Am Coll Surg 2002; 195:611–618.
51. Eubanks TA, Pellegrini CA. Laparoscopic Nissen fundoplication. In Cameron JL, ed. Current Surgical Therapy. 7 ed.. St. Louis: Mosby, 2001, 1411–1416.

52. Pope CE. Current concepts: acid reflux disorders. N Engl J Med 1994; 331:656–660.
53. Dodds WJ, Dent J, Hogan WJ, Helm JF, Hauser R, Patel GK, Egide MS. Mechanisms of gastroesophageal reflux in patients with reflux esophagitis. N Engl J Med 1982; 307:1547–1552.
54. Thor KB, Hill LD, Mercer DD, Kozarek RD. Reappraisal of the flap valve mechanism in the gastro-esophageal junction. Acta Chir Scand 1987; 153:25–28.
55. Lundell L, Myers JC, Jamieson GC. Is motility impaired in the entire upper gastrointestinal tract in patients with gastroesophageal reflux disease. Scand J Gastroenterol 1996; 31:131–135.
56. Patti MG, Goldberg HI, Arcerito M, Bortolasi L, Tong J, Way LW. Hiatal hernia size affects lower esophageal sphincter function, esophageal acid exposure, and the degree of mucosal injury. Am J Surg 1996; 171:182–186.
57. Chang L, Oelschlager BK, Barreca M, Pellegrini CA. Improving accuracy in the identification of the gastroesophageal junction during laparoscopic antireflux surgery. Surg Endosc:In Press.
58. DeMeester TR, Bonavina L, Albertucci M. Nissen fundoplication for gastroesophageal reflux disease. Ann Surg 1986; 204:9–29.
59. Ireland AC, Holloway RH, Toouli J, Dent J. Mechanisms underlying the antireflux action of fundoplication. Gut 1993; 34:303–308.
60. Little AG. Mechanisms of action of antireflux surgery: Theory and fact. World J Surg 1992; 16:320–325.
61. Guarner V, Martinez N, Gavino JF. Ten year evaluation of posterior fundoplasty in the treatment of gastroesophageal reflux: Long-term and comparative study of 135 patients. Am J Surg 1980; 139:200–203.
62. Jones R, Canal DF, Inman MM, Rescorla FJ. Laparoscopic fundoplication: A three year review. Am Surg 1996; 62:632–636.
63. Bowrey DJ, Blom D, Crookes PF, Bremner CG, Johansson JL, Lord RV, Hagen JA, DeMeester SR, DeMeester TR, Peters JH. Risk factors and the prevelance of trocar site herniation after laparoscopic fundoplication. Surg Endosc 2001; 15:663–666.
64. Bhoyrul S, Mori T, Way LW. Radially expanding dilation: A superior method of laparoscopic trocar access. Surg Endosc 1996; 10:775–778.
65. Bhoyrul S, Payne J, Steffes B, Swanstrom LL, Way LW. A randomized prospective study of radially expanding trocars in laparoscopic surgery. J Gastrointest Surg 2000; 4:392–397.
66. Horgan S, Pellegrini CA. Surgical treatment of gastroesophageal reflux disease. Surg Clin North Am 1997; 77:1063–1082.
67. Banki F, Mason RJ, DeMeester SR, Hagen JA, Balaji NS, Crookes PF, Bremner CG, Peters JH, DeMeester TR. Vagal-sparing esophagectomy: A more physiologic alternative. Ann Surg 2002; 236:324–336.
68. Schauer PR, Meyers WC, Eubanks S, Norem RF, Franklin M, Pappas TN. Mechanisms of gastric and esophageal perforations during laparoscopic Nissen fundoplication. Ann Surg 1996; 223:43–52.
69. Lowham AS, Filipi CJ, Hinder RA, Swanstrom LL, Stalter K, dePaula AL, Hunter JG, Buglewicz TG, Haake K. Mechanisms and avoidance of esophageal perforation by anesthesia personnel during laparoscopic foregut surgery. Surg Endosc 1996; 10: 979–982.

70. Nissen R. Eine einfache Operation zur Beeinflussung der Refluxoesophagitis. Schweiz Med Wochenschr 1956; 86:590–592.
71. Urschel JD. Gastroesophageal leaks after antireflux operations. Ann Thorac Surg 1994; 57:1229–1232.
72. Edelman DS. Laparoscopic paraesophageal hernia repair with mesh. Surg Laparosc Endosc 1995; 5:32–37.
73. Frantzides CT, Richards CG, Carlson MA. Laparoscopic repair of large hiatal hernia with polytetrafluoroethylene. Surg Endosc 1999; 13:906–908.
74. Willekes CL, Edoga JK, Frezza EE. Laparoscopic repair of paraesophageal hernia. Ann Surg 1997; 225:31–38.
75. DePaula AL, Hashiba K, Bafutto M, Machado CA. Laparoscopic reoperations after failed and complicated antireflux operations. Surg Endosc 1995; 9:681–686.
76. Patti MG, Arcerito M, Feo CV, De Pinto M, Tong J, Gantert W, Tyrrell D, Way LW. An analysis of operations for gastroesophageal reflux disease: Identifying important technical elements. Arch Surg 1998; 133:600–607.
77. Hunter JG, Swanstrom LL, Waring JP. Dysphagia after laparoscopic antireflux surgery. The impact of operative technique. Ann Surg 1996; 226:109–110.
78. Eubanks TR, Pellegrini CA. Minimally invasive treatment of achalasia and other esophageal dysmotility. In Baker RJ , Fischer J, eds. Mastery of Surgery. 4th ed.. Boston: Little-Brown, 2001.

12

Genitourinary Surgery

Sean P. Hedican and Stephen Y. Nakada
The University of Wisconsin Medical School, Madison, Wisconsin, U.S.A.

INTRODUCTION

Complex applications of laparoscopy in urology entered a new era with the report of the first laparoscopic nephrectomy by Clayman and associates in 1991 [1]. In the ensuing decade laparoscopic operations involving the kidney and other retroperitoneal and pelvic structures have become commonplace. Many of these operations may replace their open counter parts as the ''gold standard'' approach to their respective organ of interest. The pioneering work of many surgeons has helped to define the benefits of laparoscopy with respect to overall morbidity and patient outcomes. As with the introduction and development of open surgical operations, the observation and reporting of complications unique to these procedures have assisted other surgeons through avoidance and recognition.

This chapter describes the complications that have been reported during laparoscopic operations in urology that are now being performed with regularity. These include procedures on the kidney (cyst decortications; simple, radical, partial, and donor nephrectomy), prostate (radical prostatectomy), ureter (nephroureterectomy and pyeloplasty), and pelvic or retroperitoneal lymphatics (pelvic and retroperitoneal lymph node dissection).

IDENTIFICATION OF COMPLICATIONS

Intraoperative

Physiological (hypercapnia, oliguria, fluid overload, extraperitoneal gas collections)

Bleeding (abdominal wall, dissection site, and major vessel)
Bowel injuries
Solid visceral injury (spleen, liver, pancreas, adrenal)
Ureteral injuries
Tumor rupture or spillage
Diaphragm

Postoperative

Physiological (neuromuscular, renal dysfunction, congestive heart failure)
Infectious (abscess, cellulitis, peritonitis)
Bowel (ileus, obstruction, perforation)
Hernia
Pancreas (inflammation, leakage)
Bleeding
Lymphatic (chylous ascites)
Urine leakage (partial nephrectomy or pyeloplasty)

PREOPERATIVE EVALUATION TO AVOID THESE COMPLICATIONS

The preoperative assessment of patients for laparoscopic urological surgery must include a careful history and physical examination to avoid selection of patients with an unacceptably high risk of complications. Identification of these conditions also helps in counseling patients regarding their potential for a complication and ways of lowering reversible risk factors. General medical conditions that increase the risk of complications include morbid obesity, prior transperitoneal or retroperitoneal surgery, chronic obstructive pulmonery disease, and poor cardiac function.

Morbid obesity has been shown to increase the occurrence of many complications such as wound cellulitis, incisional herniation, and neuromuscular sequelae. These patients require careful and extensive padding of the operative table to prevent rhabdomyolysis from compression of their pressure points by the weight of their bodies. In addition, extra-long laparoscopic ports measuring 120 mm, instead of the standard 100-mm length, should be available for these cases to ensure the maintenance of stable and efficient access to the peritoneum. Intraoperative complication rates are as high as 22% in this patient population, with 12% requiring conversion to an open operation [2].

Chronic obstructive pulmonary disease can increase the possibility of hypercapnia and ventilation-related problems from expansion of bullous disease or spontaneous pneumothorax during laparoscopy [3,4]. Preoperative planning to insert an arterial blood gas line to enable careful CO_2 monitoring or, at minimum, an end-tidal CO_2 monitor is necessary in these patients. In severe cases, having an alternative insufflant such as helium available may be necessary, and the patient should be informed that, in case of profound hypercapnia, open conversion may be required. Kavoussi et al. reported a procedural abortion rate of 0.27% due to hypercapnia in a series of 372 laparoscopic pelvic lymph node dissections [5].

A prior history of congestive heart failure with reduced left ventricular ejection fraction will require careful management of intraoperative fluids and cardiac status. Prolonged CO_2 pneumoperitoneum at a pressure of 15 mm Hg has been shown to increase central venous pressure, systemic vascular resistance, and mean arterial pressure while having a variable effect on cardiac output, ranging from a decrease of 19% to an increase of 7% [3]. These effects, coupled with the oliguria that occurs secondary to the pneumoperitoneum and the variable amount of insensible losses induced by insufflant convection, complicate the management of intraoperative fluids. Careful preoperative consideration, including patient education, should be given to the insertion of either a central line to measure central venous pressures or, in more severe cases, a Swan-Ganz monitoring catheter to continuously measure cardiac function and filling pressures.

A discriminating preoperative assessment of the extent of tumor involvement when operating on the kidney, prostate, or retroperitoneal lymph nodes helps to avoid attempts at laparoscopic resection of tumor-bearing organs, which are best approached in an open fashion. Large tumors with adjacent organ involvement, extensive adenopathy, and tumor thrombus may require more extensive resections than can be managed via the laparoscope, including great vessel reconstruction, or lymphadenectomy.

In the case of renal malignancy, preoperative staging should include a dual-view chest x-ray to rule out metastases as well as contrast and noncontrast computed tomographic (CT) imaging to assess for adenopathy and adjacent organ involvement. In cases where a partial or donor nephrectomy is planned or in large tumors located in the hilum and extending medially toward the great vessels, it is advisable to obtain delayed images for vascular reconstruction to clearly delineate the arterial and venous anatomy of the kidney [6]. This helps prevent the inadvertent injury of accessory vessels and provides a road map for the area of dissection and resection. In cases of suspected tumor thrombus, coronal magnetic resonance imaging (MRI) with and without gadolinium is important to define the extent of thrombus involvement [7]. Tumors with thrombus extending into the renal vein or with minimal vena caval extension can be approached laparoscopically, whereas higher levels of extension are best extirpated in an open fashion [8].

The risk of positive surgical margins in laparoscopic prostatectomy specimens has been shown to be similar to that in large open prostatectomy series [9,10]. Patients with a high risk of extracapsular spread, seminal vesicle, or lymph node involvement can be predicted with accuracy based on the derived Partin nomograms determined by their preoperative prostate-specific antigen (PSA), clinical stage, and the Gleason sum of their prostate biopsy specimen [11]. High-risk patients with >15% chance of lymph node or seminal vesicle involvement based on this nomogram should undergo preoperative bone scanning to rule out metastatic disease. The prediction of locoregional spread using ultrasound, CT, or MRI imaging with endorectal coil enhancement has not proven to be of significant predictive advantage with the exception of CT scanning for gross nodal disease [12,13]. Therefore, if the bone scan is unremarkable in these patients, a CT scan of the abdomen and pelvis with and without contrast should be performed to rule out gross lymph node involvement.

In patients with a high risk of spread and no demonstrable radiographic appearance of extension, it may still be best to perform these operations via an open approach due to the improved visual and tactile information regarding the margin that can be obtained only in this fashion. Another relative contraindication to laparoscopic prostatectomy is the increased likelihood of periprostatic fibrosis observed in patients with a history of repeated prostate biopsies, transurethral resection, androgen or radiation therapy, or prostatitis. Careful assessment for the presence of a large intravesical lobular prostate extension should be performed during the ultrasound-guided prostate biopsy. This is especially important in patients with severe voiding symptoms. Flexible cystoscopy with retroflexed inspection should be performed for equivocal cases, because the presence of a large median lobe can increase the risk of leaving tissue behind at the bladder neck or of inadvertent injury of the ureters during efforts at laparoscopic resection.

Preoperative bowel preparation for all transperitoneal laparoscopic procedures is recommended to achieve several goals. In addition to placing an orogastric tube at the beginning of the procedure, mechanical preparation improves visualization by decompressing the large and small bowel. This subsequently reduces the risk of bowel injury by maximizing bowel wall thickness and improving overall definition of the planes of dissection. This is especially true during separation of the rectum from the prostate during laparoscopic prostatectomy. It has also been our observation that mechanical cleansing of the bowel speeds the return of bowel function and lessens the severity of the postoperative ileus. The final advantage of the bowel preparation is that it improves the ability to perform nondiverted laparoscopic or open surgical repair of colonic injuries, should they occur, while reducing the overall risk of their occurrence for the reasons outlined above. Patients with extensive prior transperitoneal or retroperitoneal surgery have been shown to have higher but acceptable rates of bowel or adjacent organ injury [14]. In these patients, preoperative bowel preparation is particularly important, as is the need for careful planning and the introduction of the laparoscopic trocars beginning in regions away from prior incisions.

INTRAOPERATIVE MEASURES TO PREVENT COMPLICATIONS

Physiological Complications

Judicious use of fluid replacement and anesthetic monitoring systems as outlined above is critical intraoperatively for the prevention of fluid overload. It is important to caution the anesthesiologists against chasing low urine production, as intraoperative oliguria is a common occurrence with prolonged laparoscopy. Hypercapnia can be controlled intraoperatively by lowering insufflation pressure settings and increasing tidal volumes and ventilatory rate. If these measures fail, then switching to an alternative insufflant such as helium can be performed [3,4]. There is controversy in the literature as to the impact of the transperitoneal versus retroperitoneal approach on the occurrence of hypercapnia [3,15]. Therefore the potential for hypercapnia should not guide decision making regarding the laparoscopic approach in the high-risk patient. Subcutaneous emphysema and more extensive extraperitoneal insufflant concentrations can be avoided by securing trocars at the skin level using a suture or threaded trocar. This limits ''ball valving'' of the ventilation hole above the peritoneum, which can result in significant subcutaneous emphysema and ensuing hypercapnia [3].

Avoidance of profound intraoperative oliguria, postoperative renal dysfunction, and inadvertent fluid overload is best accomplished by early fluid deficit calculation and replacement prior to initiating the pneumoperitoneum. Agents such as renal dose dopamine (2–3 μg/kg/min) and an intravenous infusion of mannitol (1 g/kg) divided over the predicted duration of the case can also be utilized to maintain a vigorous urine output. This is particularly important in performing a laparoscopic donor or partial nephrectomy. Nephrotoxic antibiotics, nonsteroidal anti-inflammatory drugs, and other medications should be avoided before, during, and in the immediate postoperative period when a significant number of the patient's functioning nephrons are being removed.

Neuromuscular complications have been reported to occur following 2.7% of prolonged laparoscopic operations in urology [16]. Patients who developed rhabdomyolysis on average weighed significantly more (mean 90 kg) than those who did not (mean 80 kg). Careful preoperative padding including the use of an axillary roll during flank positioning is paramount. This prevents excess traction on the brachial plexus of the upper extremity positioned beneath the patient. In obese patients, adequate padding should include liberal 3-in. foam with wide gel padding placed on top of a beanbag to allow supportive molding to the various bulges and creases of the individual patient. Stacks of pillows should be utilized to separate the legs or arms without excessive abduction. The head, upper shoulder and arm, hip, and legs should all be secured to the operative table with wide cloth tape to prevent shifting during air planing of patients in the flank position.

In the supine position, padded shoulder supports with the arms tucked at the side of the table enables deep Trendelenburg positioning, which is important for pelvic surgery. Careful padding of the medial and undersurface of the elbow prevents ulnar nerve injuries. The operating surgeon and assistants must also be cautioned against resting arms or equipment against the patient, which can be a temptation during extended procedures.

Doppler ultrasound studies have demonstrated a reduction in venous return from the lower extremities as a result of the increased intrabdominal pressure of the pneumoperitoneum [17]. This decreased flow results in venous stasis and increases the theoretic risk of deep venous thrombosis during prolonged transperitoneal procedures although the overall incidence of this phenomenon is unclear [3]. The use of TED stockings and sequential pneumatic compression devices on the lower extremities reduce the risk of clot formation by both improving venous return and initiating the release of plasminogen activators from the vessel walls, which stimulate the fibrinolytic system [18].

Vascular Hemorrhage

Significant vascular injury resulting in bleeding during laparoscopic urological procedures most commonly occurs during establishment of the initial entry access to the peritoneum/retroperitoneum or during dissection of the vasculature around the organ of interest. Injury to major vessels such as the inferior vena cava, aorta, iliacs, and epigastric vessels with initial entry access occurs in 0.25% of laparoscopic cases [19]. These injuries can best be avoided by careful controlled entry of the Veress needle, gripped low on the shaft, with advancement until the audible snap of the protective obturator is heard and felt by the introducing hand. In very thin patients, slight angulation inferior on insertion at the umbilicus (supine) and superior when introduced in the lower quadrant (flank position) avoids the relative proximity of the great vessels. An open access port or visual introducing cannula allows insertion of the initial trocar into the peritoneum under direct vision; both have been shown to reduce the risk of entry injuries [19]. Bleeding from the epigastric vessels is best avoided by selecting port insertion sites that lie either between the rectus bellies or lateral to them. These and other major abdominal wall vessels can usually be visualized by transillumination in thinner patients when ports are being inserted and can therefore be avoided.

Dissection-based injuries are best prevented by a clear understanding of the vascular anatomy of the organ of interest and the potential for anomalies. When a laparoscopic nephrectomy is planned, a careful road map of the arterial and vascular supply can be obtained by performing either a CT or MRI with three-dimensional vascular reconstruction [6,20]. This is standard practice for all laparoscopic donor nephrectomies but has also proven helpful for laparoscopic partial and radical nephrectomy as well as pyeloplasty when crossing lower pole vessels may be the source of ureteropelvic junction obstruction.

Common dissection errors that can result in vascular injury include ''past pointing'' of instruments when transecting structures, resulting in injury to a vessel that has not been secured. Inadvertent clip dislodgment is another cause and can be prevented by placing at least two clips on both sides of transected venous structures and three clips on major arterial vasculature. An alternative is to use locking clips (Weck Closure Systems, Research Triangle Park, NC) or the Endovascular GIA stapler to obtain more secure hemostasis. It is important to use the 2.5-mm vascular staple loads, as the larger 3.5-mm staples have proven inadequate for securing major vascular structures in animal experiments [21]. Endovascular GIA malfunction occurs during 1.7% of firings, with 50% of occurrences due to inattentive deployment over a clip or staple [22]. Careful inspection after initial closure of the device but before firing it is critical to prevent this potentially catastrophic event. Division of side branches of the renal hilar vessels up to 4-mm in size should be performed with the harmonic scalpel whenever possible so as to limit the number of clips applied to the main renal vessels. This reduces the potential risk of deploying the stapler over a clip.

Arcing of monopolar cautery to vascular structures can also result in inadvertent injury, which is why the bipolar cautery or harmonic scalpel is favored for obtaining hemostasis during laparoscopy. The harmonic scalpel, when used to transect a larger vessel approaching the size limits for its use (4 mm), should be placed on a variable setting of 2 and activated with minimal tension on the vessel to provide maximum coagulation prior to division.

Visceral or Solid Organ Injury

The risk of visceral or solid organ injury is increased in patients with previous transperitoneal surgery [14], but it does not prohibit a laparoscopic approach. In these cases it is preferable to use an open Hasson or direct vision access port to gain initial trocar entry to the peritoneum. If a Veress needle is used initially to establish the pneumoperitoneum, it should be inserted well away from sites of previous scarring. Injury to the bowel occurs in 0.13% of laparoscopic cases in urology, with 32% of these occuring during initial Veress or trocar introduction and 50% as a result of electrocautery dissection [23].

Planes of dissection should be distant to bowel when peritoneal attachments are being released with the electrocautery or harmonic scalpel. Arcing of the monopolar cautery can cause thermal injury to the bowel, as was described for vascular injuries. In one large European series looking at the incidence of complications in 2407 laparoscopic cases, 60% of the 20 visceral injuries observed were due to monopolar cautery [24]. Unattended insertion of instruments during which the pointed tips of dissectors are driven forcibly into the bowel or a solid organ can also result in serosal tears, punctures, or lacerations. These injuries can be prevented by always keeping the tips of the introduced instruments pointed up along the abdominal wall or by directly visualizing their insertion into the peritoneum. Any time the spleen or liver must be retracted to gain access to the left or right kidney, respectively, all fascial attachments must be released to prevent tearing of the fragile capsules of these organs. Blunt retractors with a wide surface area, such as the Diamond Flex Triangle retractor (Genzyme Surgical Products, Tucker, GA) should be utilized for retraction to prevent small focal points of pressure, which can lead to puncture or rupture of the organ.

Any time dissection of the planes surrounding solid organs is performed, gentle blunt dissection should precede transection of bulky tissue bundles. This will help define the extent of organs such as the pancreas, adrenal gland, sigmoid colon, and rectum, which are less clearly defined without tactile feedback. During laparoscopic prostatectomy, dissection of the plane between the posterior prostate surface and the rectum can be facilitated by insertion of a rectal bougie to provide the surgeon with some tactile feedback on palpation with the laparoscopic instruments. In older patients, dissection and release of the sigmoid colon should be done cautiously, particularly when fibrotic tissue planes are noted, due to the risk of diverticuli, which can be inadvertently amputated if overaggressive dissection is performed.

Bowel Obstruction/Herniation

Animal and clinical data demonstrate a reduced risk of peritoneal adhesion formation following laparoscopic versus open procedures [25]. Every effort should still be made to reduce the risk of inflammation in the peritoneum, which can lead to adhesion formation, by thoroughly irrigating and aspirating all blood, urine, or other secretions that may have been released during the operative procedure. Mobilization and handling of the bowel should be minimized to further reduce the risk of serosal injury or irritation, which can result in adhesions and eventual bowel obstruction. Any defects or windows that are created in the mesentery should be closed with clips or sutures to prevent internal bowel herniation with resultant obstruction. The incidence of port-site herniation in the literature is approximately 1%, and subfascial hernias can occur despite closure of the fascial defect [26,27]. Trocar manufacturers and some authors advocate not closing fascial splitting port defects due to the theoretically lower risk of herniation and an early favorable experience [26]. We recently reported a case of symptomatic port-site herniation following use of a nonbladed trocar where the fascia was not closed [28]. Therefore it is advisable to use a grasping needle closure device such as the Carter-Thomason (Inlet Medical, Eden Prairie, MN) [29] to provide secure full-thickness port site closure of all 10/12-mm trocar sites, as well as 5-mm port sites in children, to prevent these occurrences.

Tumor Rupture or Spillage

Recent reports following laparoscopic radical nephrectomy for low stage T1 and T2 disease have demonstrated similar actuarial 5-year cancer-free survival (approximately 91%) to open surgery [30]. In these cases, 90% of specimens were morcellated inside the peritoneal cavity within the confines of a LapSac (Cook Urological, Spencer, IN). This woven, double-layered plastic-and-nylon sack has been shown to be impermeable to tumor cells [31] and is among of the most resistant to mechanical perforation [32] making it the entrapment sack of choice when morcellation of a potentially malignant sample is planned. Other precautions to prevent possible tumor spillage include separate draping off of the site with a fenestrated towel and nephrotomy drape, use of an occlusive/protective drape (e.g., Ioban), and changing all contaminated gloves, gowns, and drapes following the morcellation procedure [33]. To date, the world literature contains two reported cases of port-site seeding following laparoscopic nephrectomy for malignancy [34,35]. One case involved morcellation of a high-grade lesion with no obvious breach in protocol [34], whereas the second case involved a patient with ascites, and morcellation occurred in a sack other than a LapSac [35].

Certain tumors, such as transitional cell cancer, have shown their propensity for implantation and tumor seeding. Therefore intact organ removal for specimens containing high-grade lesions of this cell type is favored over morcellation [36]. Whenever intact specimen removal is performed via a hand-assist port or separate incision, a wound protector or LapSac should be utilized to prevent the possibility of tumor rupture and spillage or disruption of the fat overlying the kidney. This is especially true of large malignant specimens. Recently, a case of diffuse carcinomatosis of renal cell cancer following extraction via a hand-port incision without entrapment or the use of a wound protector has been presented [37].

Bladder, Ureteral, or Collecting System Injury

The most important measure to prevent inadvertent injury to the bladder is intraoperative decompression by placement of a Foley catheter. When a Pfannenstiel incision is made for specimen extraction, as it is for donor nephrectomy, care must be taken not to make the incision too low near the pubis, which can result in bladder injury. During laparoscopic prostatectomy, release of the bladder and entry into the retropubic space is facilitated by distending it with 150 mL of saline. This degree of distention helps to define the planes without obscuring the space. An inverted horseshoe incision is then made in the peritoneum around the outline of the bladder from one medial umbilical ligament to the other. As the incision crosses above the dome of the bladder, the urachus is transected. This is primarily a bloodless plane. If bleeding does occur, it is usually a result of entry into the bladder wall, so further dissection should be performed in a more lateral or cephalad location.

Ureteral injury can occur during pelvic lymph node dissection and has been reported in 0.5% of cases [5]. This is a result of ligation and division of the ureter as it crosses the iliac artery, where it can be mistaken for a portion of the lymphatic chain. If a more tubular structure is noted in this region, careful observation for peristalsis and incremental dissection should be performed until it is clear that the structure does not represent the ureter. Injury can also occur during laparoscopic retroperitoneal dissection for testicular cancer when the medial border of the lymphatic packet is being defined or during dissection of the gonadal vasculature. In performing a laparoscopic prostatectomy, the ureter can be mistaken for the vas deferens during initial peritoneal incision if the upper of the two peritoneal ridges in the rectovesical pouch is opened instead of the lower ridge. If there is any doubt about the exposed tubular structure, it should be traced out to the external ring or back to the ejaculatory duct to prove that it is indeed the vas deferens prior to transection.

It is critical to leave generous amounts of soft tissue around the ureter when a kidney is being obtained for live donation, and many surgeons advocate leaving all of the tissue between the gonadal vein and the ureter to prevent devascularization injuries. Preservation of this tissue is facilitated by leaving the gonadal vein attached at its entry point into the renal vein. These modifications, which limit the amount of dissection around the ureter, have resulted in a noticeable reduction in the incidence of ureteral complications for laparoscopically harvested kidneys from 9% in initial series to approximately 1–2% [38,39].

Some authors have advocated the use of cystoscopically inserted ureteral access catheters to inject indigo carmine dye in performing laparoscopic renal cyst decortications close to the collecting system so as to prevent and/or recognize injury to this structure [40]. In these cases, wire manipulation of the collecting system can result in perforation of what can be a very thin separation between the collecting system and the cyst. A better alternative is the intravenous administration of indigo carmine prior to establishing the pneumoperitoneum in order to fill the collecting system with blue-tinged urine, which will usually remain present throughout the procedure due to the intraoperative oliguria that commonly occurs as a result of the pneumoperitoneum. A laparoscopic aspirating needle can then be utilized to confirm that no blue-tinged urine is present prior to unroofing what is presumed to be a cyst [41]. The intraoperative administration of indigo carmine can also be used to test the adequacy of the collecting system repair following laparoscopic pyeloplasty or partial nephrectomy.

Chylous Leakage

Chylous ascites or lymphoceles can result from inattentive sealing of large lymphatic channels following pelvic or retroperitoneal node dissection [5,42,43]. This can also occur following a laparoscopic nephrectomy if rapid transection of the perihilar lymphatics is performed without proper coagulation [44]. Larger lymphatic chains should be secured with clips, whereas smaller branches can be effectively closed using the harmonic scalpel to seal the lumen via coagulation.

Avoiding Vascular Thrombosis During Donor Nephrectomy

The incidence of vascular thrombotic events in the initial series of 20 laparoscopic donor nephrectomies was 10% [45]. These two cases occurred in right-sided grafts, both of which had a duplicated main renal vein. The harvest length of vein from the right side can be problematic due to the shortened distance to the vena cava and the approximate/cm of vein length consumed by the Endovascular stapler. Laparoscopic manipulation of these shortened vein segments was thought to contribute to thrombosis formation and graft loss in these two patients. The lateral attachments of the kidney should be maintained until after dissection of the branches of the main renal vein in order to prevent torsion of the pedicle [39]. Preoperative CT with three-dimensional vascular reconstructions helps to evaluate candidates for laparoscopy in whom it is almost always more desirable to remove the left kidney than the right, especially when multiple veins are present [6,39]. A right laparoscopic kidney harvest is best reserved for patients with an exceptionally long, single right renal vein and unfavorable left-sided anatomy. During the donor operation, vigorous urine output should be maintained using renal-dose dopamine, mannitol, and topical vasodilating agents (e.g., papavarine 30 mg/mL) whenever obvious main renal artery spasm is observed.

POSTOPERATIVE MEASURES TO PREVENT COMPLICATIONS

The most effective way of avoiding preventable catastrophic postoperative complications is to recognize the early signs of potential problems, thus enabling early intervention. A high degree of suspicion should arise in regard to patients who do not experience a relatively predictable return of bowel function and reasonable pain control following laparoscopic surgery. In patients with poor urine output and tachycardia, with or without labile blood pressure, a delayed bleed should be suspected and serial hematocrits obtained.

Avoidance of excessive narcotic pain medication with the substitution of nonsteroidal anti-inflammatory drugs such as ketorolac, whenever feasible, helps to limit the adverse effects on bowel motility. Early use of motility-inducing suppositories in patients developing gaseous distention in the presence of bowel sounds can assist in decompression and limit the pain of abdominal distention, especially when a focal rectal ileus is suspected. Early ambulation and incentive spirometry help to reduce the risks of deep venous thrombosis and atelectasis, respectively. Catheter removal in older male patients should be delayed until they are sufficiently recovered from anesthesia, as urinary retention is a common minor complication following laparoscopy [46]. This is especially important in all patients with a history of voiding problems.

CLINICAL SIGNS AND WORKUP FOR SUSPECTED COMPLICATIONS

Postoperative Bleeding

As mentioned above, poor urine output and tachycardia with or without labile blood pressure should raise the suspicion of postoperative bleeding. If the patient is stable, this can be further evaluated with serial hematocrits; in cases where blood losses persist, a CT scan should be obtained to help define the location of the bleeding [47]. Potential sites of postoperative hemorrhage include the vessels or vascular stumps of the organ on which surgery was performed, surrounding solid organ injury (e.g., spleen, liver, or adrenal), and injuries to abdominal wall or mesenteric vessels. In such cases it is also important to assess coagulation parameters, including the platelet count, to make sure that no component of coagulopathy is contributing to the problem.

The scenarios of prompt cardiovascular collapse, blood pressure that does not respond to fluid or blood resuscitation, or a persistently falling hematocrit despite transfusion require prompt open re-exploration. The surgeon should be prepared to handle major bleeding in this situation from large vessel stumps of the artery or vein. Reported cases of delayed clip dislodgment from the renal artery or vein following nephrectomy have resulted in these types of situations and require immediate control of the great vessels. This may require the support of a vascular surgeon [48].

Bowel and Associated Visceral Injuries

The incidence of bowel injury during laparoscopic urologic procedures is 0.87%; of these, 70% are undiagnosed at the time of surgery [23]. Unlike the typical peritoneal signs observed with most bowel injuries, perforations following laparoscopy tend to involve the unusual constellation of focal trocar-site pain, abdominal distention, diarrhea, and leukopenia [23]. These presenting signs can rapidly lead to profound sepsis and death; therefore prompt recognition and correction are paramount. If the patient's condition is relatively stable, a CT scan of the abdomen and pelvis can be very helpful in defining the problem [47]. In their review of the literature, Bishoff et al. reported that 80% of bowel injuries discovered after the time of laparoscopic surgery eventually required laparotomy [23]. If the patient is unstable or the suspicion is high for an occult bowel injury, exploration should be performed.

If significant abdominal distention and nausea with or without vomiting occur postoperatively, then an ileus, bowel obstruction, or injury must all be considered. The evaluation should start with a flat and upright plain film examination of the abdomen to look for fluid-filled loops of small and large bowel and whether or not air is present in the descending colon and rectum. If a bowel obstruction is still suspected, a CT scan of the abdomen with oral and rectal contrast to look for a transition point should then be performed. The CT scan will also reveal a possible port-site hernia, pancreatitis, or fluid collections of lymph, urine, bile, or pancreatic secretions. Cadeddu et al. demonstrated that CT imaging in the evaluation of complications after laparoscopic urological surgery provided a symptom-related diagnosis in 75% of patients [47]. Evaluation of bilirubin or amylase and lipase in the blood or aspirated fluid collections should be performed when a solid organ injury to the liver or pancreas with associated bile or pancreatic leakage is suspected.

Chylous ascites can occur following laparoscopic retroperitoneal lymph node dissection [42,43] or nephrectomy [44] and should be suspected by symptoms of enlarging abdominal girth, distention, anorexia, and vomiting. The diagnosis is made by the presence of significant ascites on CT scan, in which measured triglyceride levels are higher than serum levels. Treatment consists of a diet low in fat and medium-chain triglycerides, with total parenteral nutrition and peritoneovenous shunts reserved for refractory cases [49].

SPECIFIC MANAGEMENT OF INTRAOPERATIVE UROLOGIC COMPLICATIONS

Bleeding

In a review of 2407 laparoscopic procedures performed at four German centers, the incidence of major hemorrhage was 1.7%. This risk increased depending on the complexity of the procedure [24]. Troublesome hemorrhage can result during initial entry access to the peritoneum or retroperitoneum or during dissection around major vessels and organs. Major vascular injury that occurs as a result of Veress needle or initial trocar insertion is usually best managed with urgent conversion to reduce the risk of profound blood loss due to the lack of an adequate number of introduced ports to control the situation endoscopically.

Most venous bleeding that does not arise from the vena cava or its major tributaries can initially be controlled by compression with a sheet of surgical cellulose (Surgicel, Johnson & Johnson, Inc., Arlington, TX). The harmonic shears or bipolar cautery can be used to effectively coagulate smaller vessels up to 4 mm in diameter if they can be adequately exposed. If a sufficient stump exists, then a 10-mm clip can also be used to obtain hemostasis. In applying clips to an actively bleeding stump, it is best to attempt to pinch the end of the stump closed with a dissector while placing the vessel on slight stretch. The first clip is applied as close to the base of the stump as the surrounding tissues will allow in the hope that a second, more distal clip can then be applied. The operating surgeon should be aware of the angles of approach and introduce the clip applier via a port where good perpendicular access to the base of the vessel can be obtained.

Direct puncture or laceration of the vena cava, iliac veins, or main renal vein during dissection usually requires closure with laparoscopic suture or prompt conversion to an open approach. The pneumoperitoneum will limit the blood loss from these structures, which can be further compressed using the suction aspirator and another blunt-tipped instrument [50]. A very effective way of suturing major venous injuries involves the use of a 6-in. segment of Prolene suture on an RB-1 needle with a preapplied Vicryl clip (LapraTy; Ethicon Endo-Surgery, Inc., Cincinnati, OH) on one end. This allows rapid suture closure of large vessel lacerations without the need for intracorporeal knot-tying, as another LapraTy can simply be applied to the distal end after finishing the running stitch.

In general, arterial injuries can be managed in much the same way as venous injuries with two exceptions. These are that even small arterial injuries do not tend to seal as a result of compression alone, and the vigor of large artery bleeding from the aorta, iliac artery, and main renal artery often precludes the ability to perform suture repairs. When feasible, the application of either compressive or self-locking clips or use of an Endo-GIA stapler is preferred. Obviously these methods should only be deployed in the case of vessels supplying a structure that is being removed during the operation. A large injury to a renal artery that occurs during laparoscopic donor nephrectomy or pyeloplasty must be repaired instead of clipped, and this usually requires conversion to an open exposure [48]. One should avoid poorly defined placement of clips or staples due to the risk of injuring or occluding major adjacent vascular structures that supply organs such as the bowel. Rapid ligation of the entire renal hilum, artery, and vein together for troublesome bleeding during extirpative laparoscopic nephrectomy has been described using the Endovascular GIA stapler, and early follow-up data have not revealed the occurrence of arteriovenous fistulas [51].

Injury to a vessel of the abdominal wall may become evident at the time of trocar insertion if it involves the inferior epigastric artery. In such cases blood may run out along the shaft of the port or drip into the peritoneal cavity. More commonly, such injuries do not become evident until the port is removed and vigorous bleeding is noted at the port-site incision. The Carter-Thomason fascial closure device (Inlet Medical, Eden Prairie, MN) can be utilized in these situations to create a full-thickness figure-of-eight suture pass around the cut ends of the lacerated vessel. This device is essentially a grasping needle that allows the introduction of a closure stitch through the fascia, muscle, and parietal peritoneum of the abdominal wall [29]. As the grasped end of suture emerges on the peritoneal surface, it is held with a laparoscopic instrument and then passed back to the grasping needle after it has been inserted similarly through the fascia at the other side of the incision. This accomplishes the dual task of closing the fascial defect and ligating the bleeding ends of the vessel. If this procedure is not successful, open exploration of the port site may be required.

Minor lacerations and abrasions of the spleen, liver, or adrenal gland can occur during retraction or dissection. Bleeding can usually be controlled using compression and the application of a sheet of Surgicel. If hemorrhage persists, the argon-beam coagulator can be utilized to provide a broad coagulative spray to the area. Another effective treatment option includes the application of a fibrin sealant, which can be delivered using a double-barreled syringe and a laparoscopic extension [52]. Once applied, the coagulum should not be disturbed. This same material can also be utilized on the renal parenchyma during partial nephrectomy, cyst decortication, or cryotherapy to aid in hemostasis.

If an injury occurs to the tail of the pancreas, a consultation should be obtained of a general surgeon and resection with Endo-GIA stapling of the injured segment considered, due to the risk of persistent pancreatic leakage. In this scenario, a drain should be placed and monitored for amylase and lipase content prior to removal.

Bowel Injury

As indicated above, the majority of laparoscopic bowel injuries (70%) are not recognized at the time of surgery [23]. When a full-thickness or abrasion injury is identified during the operation, it can usually be repaired laparoscopically. Nezhat and associates reported the laparoscopic repair of 9 small bowel, 4 colon, and 13 rectal injuries in 26 patients without a resultant complication when a preoperative bowel preparation was utilized [53]. Bishoff et al. discussed the importance of oversewing even serosal abrasions, as these can lead to fistulization and abscess formation if left alone [23]. If a rectal injury occurs during laparoscopic prostatectomy, a tongue of omentum should be interposed between the double-layered rectal repair and the urethral anastamosis to prevent rectourethral fistula formation. In addition, four-finger anal dilation should be performed, as it is for an open repair, to decrease the temporal resistive tone of the anus during defecation [54].

On rare occasions, when a left-sided laparoscopic nephrectomy is being performed, the stomach may be injured along the greater curvature during release of the spleen. If this should occur, the injury can be repaired with a noncutting linear endoscopic stapler (e.g., ENDOPATH EZ45: NO-KNIFE; Ethicon Endo-Surgery, Inc., Cincinnati, OH), which fires three to four parallel rows of staples without cutting the tissues. Thereafter, 24 hr of nasogastric decompression should be performed along with antiulcer prophylaxis. Injuries to the duodenum carry an increased risk of morbidity and mortality due to the high enteric flow with elevated concentrations of pancreatic and biliary secretions. It is imperative to have an excellent closure of this portion of the bowel, which is best accomplished through an open repair unless the surgeon is exceptionally skilled at laparoscopic suturing of the bowel.

Diaphragmatic Injury

During release of the splenic attachments on the left, triangular ligaments to the liver on the right, or the cephalad extent of large upper-pole renal tumors on either side, it is possible to lacerate the diaphragm. Dissection injuries to the diaphragm and pleura occur in approximately 0.45% of laparoscopic renal surgeries [55]. The anesthesiologist should be alerted regarding the injury since the pressure and diffusion of CO_2 into the pleural cavity can result in decreased oxygen saturation, increased airway pressures, increased end-tidal CO_2, and hemodynamic instability [56]. Similarly, if these observations are made by the anesthesiologist and a diaphragmatic injury has not been noted by the surgeon, a subtle injury should be suspected and careful inspection of the area of dissection performed.

These injuries can be managed by placing figure-of-eight closure sutures at the site of injury after first inspecting the chest to make certain an injury to the lung has not occurred. Before the final suture is tied down, the suction aspirator device should be utilized to aspirate any residual CO_2 from the chest. An alternative is to give a large inspiratory breath while the sutures are tied, followed by placement of a 6F central line catheter with extra side holes into the chest via the sixth intercostal space to aspirate any residual CO_2 [55]. A postoperative chest x-ray should be obtained; small residual pneumothoraces can usually be observed due to the rapid absorption of CO_2.

Ureteral Injury

Ureteral injuries are uncommon, and the type of repair depends upon the extent of the injury and the location. The incidence of injury has been reported to be 0.5 and 0.7% for laparoscopic pelvic lymph node dissection and radical prostatectomy, respectively [5,57]. Minor nonthermal laceration to any region of the ureter can be treated with either simple stent placement with the aid of a flexible cystoscope or stent placement in addition to suture closure of the laceration using 4-0 polydioxone surgical (PDS) suture mounted on an RB-1 needle. Injuries created using heat-generating instruments should have the edges of the laceration debrided to healthy tissue prior to closure.

Complete transection of the upper or midureter can be spatulated medially on the proximal side and laterally on the distal side then reanastomosed. If created by electrocautery or harmonic scalpel dissection, the edges should be freshened.

The anastomosis can be performed using either freehand suturing techniques or a suture-assist instrument such as the Endostitch Autosuturing Device (U.S. Surgical Inc., Norwalk, CT), depending on surgeon preference. A corner stitch should be placed at each of the spatulations and tied down to approximate the two ends of the ureter. The anterior and posterior defects are then closed in a watertight fashion using a series of interrupted or two running sutures, depending again on individual surgeon preference. Following the repair, a ureteral stent is then inserted using a flexible cystoscope.

In general, due to the watershed effect on the blood supply, it is best to manage complete distal ureteral transections by reimplantation of the ureter. A psoas hitch of the bladder or Boari flap reconstruction may be required depending on the level of the injury and the distance that must be bridged by the reconstruction. Distal ureteral injuries usually require an open repair, especially in the case of a radical prostatectomy, where a careful balance of limited tension between the ureteral reimplantation and the urethrovesical anastomosis must be achieved.

Renal Collecting System Injury

Visible injuries to the collecting system that occur during laparoscopic partial nephrectomy or cyst decortication should be managed by placement of a stent and a retroperitoneal 15F round Davol drain to monitor leakage. If possible, several interrupted or short running sutures of 4–0 PDS should be utilized to close the defect prior to stent placement. A watertight closure can be confirmed by the intravenous administration of indigo carmine. A Foley catheter should be left in place for 24 to 48 hr to prevent the reflux of urine up the stent and through the area of the repair. In cases where leakage of urine remains substantial 72 hr following the operation, introduction of a nephrostomy tube into the collecting system should be considered to further maximize drainage. Only rare cases will require an open repair.

CONCLUSIONS

Careful preoperative planning, intraoperative avoidance measures, and postoperative monitoring can significantly reduce major complications associated with laparoscopic genitourinary surgery. Prompt diagnosis and management are the tenets of well-trained, experienced laparoscopic surgeons. When complications do occur, the information provided in this chapter should serve as a guide for their prompt recognition and effective management.

REFERENCES

1. Clayman RV, Kavoussi LR, Soper NJ, et al. Laparoscopic nephrectomy: Initial case report. J Urol 1991; 146:278–282.

2. Mendoza D, Newman RC, Albala D, et al. Laparoscopic complications in markedly obese urologic patients (a multi-institutional review). Urology 1996; 48:562–567.
3. Wolf JS. Pathophysiologic effects of prolonged laparoscopic operation. Semin Surg Oncol 1996; 12:86–95.
4. Wolf JS, Clayman RV, McDougall EM, et al. Carbon dioxide and helium insufflation during laparoscopic radical nephrectomy in a patient with severe pulmonary disease. J Urol 1996; 155:2021.
5. Kavoussi LR, Sosa E, Chandhoke P, et al. Complications of laparoscopic pelvic lymph node dissection. J Urol 1993; 149:322–325.
6. Pizzo JJ, Sklar GN, Wong J, et al. Helical computerized tomography arteriography for evaluation of live renal donors undergoing laparoscopic nephrectomy. J Urol 1999; 162:31–34.
7. Oto A, Herts BR, Remer EM, et al. Inferior vena cava tumor thrombus in renal cell carcinoma: staging by MR imaging and impact on surgical treatment. Am J Roentgenol 1998; 171:1619–1624.
8. Desai MM, Gill IS, Ramani AP, et al. Laparoscopic radical nephrectomy for cancer with level I renal vein involvement. J Urol 2003; 169:487–491.
9. Guillonneau B, El-Fettouh H, Baumert H, et al. Laparoscopic radical prostatectomy: Oncological evaluation after 1,000 cases at Montsouris Institute. J Urol 2003; 169: 1261–1266.
10. Epstein JI. Incidence and significance of positive margins in radical prostatectomy specimens. Urol Clin North Am 1996; 23:651–663.
11. Partin AW, Kattan MW, Subong EN, et al. Combination of prostate-specific antigen, clinical stage and Gleason score to predict pathological stage of localized prostate cancer: A multi-institutional update. JAMA 1997; 277:1445–1451.
12. Hricak H, Dooms GC, Jeffrey RB, et al. Prostatic carcinoma: Staging by clinical assessment, CT, and MR imaging. Radiology 1987; 162:331–336.
13. Bernstein MR, Wein AJ, Siegelman ES, et al. Lack of correlation of clinical and pathologic staging of capsular involvement in prostate cancer using endorectal coil magnetic resonance imaging. J Pelvic Surg 1999; 5:203–207.
14. Seifman BD, Dunn RL, Wolf JS. Transperitoneal laparoscopy into the previously operated abdomen: Effect on operative time, length of stay and complications. J Urol 2003; 169:36–40.
15. Ng CS, Gill IS, Sung GT, et al. Retroperitoneoscopic surgery is not associated with increased carbon dioxide absorption. J Urol 1999; 162:1268–1272.
16. Wolf JS, Marcovich R, Gill IS, et al. Survey of neuromuscular injuries to the patient and surgeon during urologic laparoscopic surgery. Urology 2000; 55:831–836.
17. Jorgensen JO, Hanel K, Lalak NJ, et al. Thromboembolic complications of laparoscopic cholecystectomy. BMJ 1993; 306:518–519.
18. Inada K, Koike S, Shirai N, et al. Effects of intermittent pneumatic leg compression for prevention of postoperative deep venous thrombosis with special reference to fibrinolytic activity. Am J Surg 1988; 155:602–605.
19. Chandler JG, Corson SL, Way LW. Three spectra of laparoscopic entry access injuries. J Am Coll Surg 2001; 192:478–491.
20. Smith PA, Ratner LE, Lynch FC, et al. Role of CT angiography in the preoperative evaluation for laparoscopic nephrectomy. Radiographics 1998; 18:589–601.

21. Lee B, Marcovich R, Aldana J, et al. Assessment of renal hilar and large vessel hemostasis with the laparoscopic Endo-GIA stapler in porcine model—Effect of staple size (abstr P1–3). J Endourol 2003; 16(suppl 1):A1.
22. Chan D, Bishoff JT, Ratner L, et al. Endovascular gastrointestinal stapler device malfunction during laparoscopic nephrectomy: Early recognition and management. J Urol 2000; 164:319–321.
23. Bishoff JT, Allaf ME, Kirkel W, et al. Laparoscopic bowel injury: Incidence and clinical presentation. J Urol 1999; 161:887–890.
24. Fahlenkamp D, Rassweiler J, Fornara P, et al. Complications of laparoscopic procedures in urology: Experience with 2,407 procedures at 4 German centers. J Urol 1999; 162:765–771.
25. Moore RG, Partin AW, Adams JB, et al. Adhesion formation after transperitoneal nephrectomy: Laparoscopic versus open approach. J Endourol 1995; 9:277–280.
26. Shalhav AL, Barret E, Lifshitz DA, et al. Transperitoneal laparoscopic renal surgery using blunt 12-mm trocar without fascial closure. J Endourol 2002; 16:43–46.
27. Montz FJ, Holschneider CH, Munro MG. Incisional hernia following laparoscopy: A survey of the American Association of Gynecologic Laparoscopists. Obstet Gynecol 1994; 4:143–148.
28. Lowry PS, Moon TD, D'Alessandro A, et al. Symptomatic port site hernia associated with a non-bladed trocar following laparoscopic live donor nephrectomy. J Endourol 2003; 17:493–494.
29. Carter JE. A new technique of fascial closure for laparoscopic incisions. J Laparoendosc Surg 1994; 4:143–148.
30. Cadeddu JA, Ono Y, Clayman RV, et al. Laparoscopic nephrectomy for renal cell cancer: Evaluation of efficacy and safety: a multicenter experience. Urology 1998; 52:773–777.
31. Urban DA, Kerbl K, McDougall EM, et al. Organ entrapment and renal morcellation: Permeability studies. J Urol 1993; 150:1792–1794.
32. Rassweiler J, Stock C, Frede T, et al. Organ retrieval systems for endoscopic nephrectomy: A comparative study. J Endourol 1998; 12:325–333.
33. Portis AJ, Elnady M, Clayman RV. Laparoscopic radical/total nephrectomy: A decade of progress. J Endourol 2001; 15:345–354.
34. Fentie DD, Barrett PH, Taranger LA. Metastatic renal cell carcinoma after laparoscopic radical nephrectomy: Long-term follow-up. J Endourol 2000; 14:407–411.
35. Castilho LN, Fugita OEH, Mitre AI, et al. Port site tumor recurrences of renal cell carcinoma after videolaparoscopic radical nephrectomy. J Urol 2001; 165:519.
36. Shalhav AL, Portis AJ, McDougall EM, et al. Laparoscopic nephroureterectomy—A new standard for the surgical management of upper tract transitional cell cancer. Urol Clin North Am 2000; 27:761–773.
37. Hands-On Laparoscopy: A Problem-Oriented Approach. Houston: American Urological Association Office of Education, August 11, 2002.
38. Fabrizio MD, Ratner LE, Kavoussi LR. Laparoscopic live donor nephrectomy: pro. Urology 1999; 53:665–667.
39. Cadeddu JA, Ratner L, Kavoussi LR. Laparoscopic donor nephrectomy. Semin Lap Surg 2000; 7:195–199.

40. Roberts WW, Bluebond-Langner R, Boyle K, et al. Laparoscopic ablation of symptomatic parenchymal and peripelvic renal cysts. Urology 2001; 58:165–169.
41. Hedican SP. Laparoscopy in urology. Surg Clin North Am 2000:1465–1485.
42. Janetschek G, Peschel R, Hobisch A, et al. Laparoscopic retroperitoneal lymph node dissection. J Endourol 2001; 15:449–455.
43. Janetschek G, Hobisch A, Hittmair A, et al. Laparoscopic retroperitoneal lymphadenectomy after chemotherapy for stage IIB nonseminomatous testicular carcinoma. J Urol 1999; 161:477–481.
44. Shafizadeh SF, Daily PP, Baliga P, et al. Chylous ascites secondary to laparoscopic donor nephrectomy. Urology 2002; 60:345.
45. Fabrizio MD, Ratner LE, Montgomery RA, et al. Laparoscopic live donor nephrectomy. Urol Clin North Am 1999; 26:247–256.
46. Hedican SP, Wolf JS, Moon TD, et al. Complications of hand-assisted laparoscopy in urologic surgery (abstr 91). J Urol 2002; 167(suppl):22.
47. Cadeddu JA, Regan F, Kavoussi LR, et al. The role of computerized tomography in the evaluation of complications after laparoscopic urological surgery. J Urol 1997; 158:1349–1352.
48. Hsu THS, Su L, Ratner LE, et al. Renovascular complications of laparoscopic donor nephrectomy. Urology 2002; 60:811–815.
49. Baniel J, Foster RS, Rowland RG, et al. Management of chylous ascites after retroperitoneal lymph node dissection for testicular cancer. J Urol 1993; 150:1422–1424.
50. Thiel R, Adams JB, Schulam PG, et al. Venous dissection injuries during laparoscopic urological surgery. J Urol 1996; 155:1874–1876.
51. Phelan M, Hrebinko R. En masse stapling of renal hilar vessels during laparoscopic nephrectomy does not result in arteriovenous fistula (abstr P10–16). J Endourol 2003; 16(suppl 1):A43.
52. Canby-Hagino ED, Morey AF, Jatoi I, et al. Fibrin sealant treatment of splenic injury during open and laparoscopic left radical nephrectomy. J Urol 2000; 164:2004–2005.
53. Nezhat C, Hezhat F, Ambroze W, et al. Laparoscopic repair of small bowel and colon: a report of 26 cases. Surg. Endosc 1993; 7:88–89.
54. Borland RN, Walsh PC. The management of rectal injury during radical retropubic prostatectomy. J Urol 1992; 147:905–907.
55. Pizzo JJ, Jacobs SC, Bishoff JT, et al. Pleural injury during laparoscopic renal surgery: Early recognition and management. J Urol 2003; 169:41–44.
56. Joris JL, Chiche JD, Lamy ML. Pneumothorax during laparoscopic fundoplication: Diagnosis and treatment with positive end-expiratory pressure. Anesth Analg 1995; 81:993–1000.
57. Guillonneau B, Rozet F, Cathelineau X, et al. Perioperative complications of laparoscopic radical prostatectomy: The Montsouris 3-year experience. J Urol 2002; 167: 51–56.

13

Geriatrics

Salvador Morales-Conde and Auxiliadora Cano
University Hospital Virgen Macarena, SevilleSpain

INTRODUCTION

The elderly are increasingly fit and healthy. The aging population in the western world will determine trends in health care in the following decades [1]. Currently, 40% of all surgical activities are targeted toward treating patients above 65 years of age [2]. Lifestyle issues and quality of life are thus important considerations when decisions are made regarding management of medical problems in this population. The goal in the treatment of elderly is to restore them to the best possible quality of life. Elderly patients represent a unique surgical challenge because of the associated complex comorbidity and diminished cardiopulmonary reserve. Since laparotomy is a major stress in the elderly, laparoscopic surgery may be particularly advantageous in this population. Therefore minimally invasive surgery in the elderly may have larger impact than in the younger population in terms of less postoperative pain, fewer cardiorespiratory complications, shortened hospital stay, and rapid return to physical activities [3–8].

Although the definition of the term *elderly* is arbitrary, patients over 65 years are at a higher risk of complications from surgery than are younger patients. Disorders of the digestive system requiring surgical intervention are more prevalent in this group of patients, as is the prevalence of comorbid conditions—especially that of the cardiac, respiratory, renal, and immune systems—which adversely affect the postoperative outcome. However, recent advances in anaesthesia—coupled with better patient selection, better perioperative cardiac care, and widespread adoption of minimally access surgery—have led to more complex gastrointestinal procedures being undertaken for elderly patients. However, these remains some concern as to the performance of minimally invasive surgery in the elderly [9–11].

GENERAL COMPLICATIONS IN THE ELDERLY

As the population ages and as surgical and anesthetic techniques advances, more and more elderly patients are referred for surgery. As a result, the physician must be increasingly aware of the response to surgery among the aged and the management of the geriatric surgical patient in the perioperative period. Elderly patients are prone to cardiac, respiratory, and infectous complications; thus, they must be screened for the presence of pre-existing disease. In addition, the geriatric patient must be carefully monitored postoperatively to guard against untoward sequelae.

Most of the series in the literature of elderly patients who are submitted to a laparoscopic procedure show a higher rate of complications and conversion than those series comprising younger patients. The association between various factors and the postoperative outcome has been studied especially in laparoscopic cholecystectomy, determining that factors such as advanced age increase both the postoperative morbidity and the postoperative hospital stay [12]. An increase in morbidity from 6.1% in younger patients to 16% in elderly patients has been demonstrated. Some other factors related to the postoperative outcome are longer duration of the procedure, acute cholecystitis, and history of ischemic heart disease—circumstances usually associated with advanced age.

The perioperative responsibility of the physisician lies in a meticulous examination of these sources of risk in order to maximize the likelihood of a beneficial result.

Preoperative Evaluation of Patients and Measures for the Prevention of Complications

The use of a laparoscopic approach in elderly patients may pose problems because of their often poor overall health, especially with regard to cardiopulmonary function. Patients above 65 years of age are generally expected to have an increased incidence of comorbidity. Recent reports on patients of this age affirmed this, with approximately half of such patients having coronary artery disease, 20% having cardiac arrhythmias, and 10% with congestive heart failure [13]. These comorbid conditions are comparable to those reported by other authors evaluating laparoscopic cholecystectomy in the elderly, in which hypertension and coronary artery disease are the most commonly encountered comorbid disease [14–16].

Importantly, the preoperative classification of patients over 65 years of age by the American Society of Anesthesiologists (ASA) reveals a higher risk than younger patients. However, other studies [17] show no increased risk of intraoperative hypercabia or cardiac arrhythmia in elderly patients who undergo pneumoperitoneum for a laparoscopic procedure, even when 42% of these patients had cardiopulmonary diseases, the percentage of which rises to 68% in patients above 80 years of age [18]. For these reasons, a careful preoperative assessment of cardiovascular risk factors as well as adequate monitoring of these patients during laparoscopy are necessary for the detection and treatment of possible hemodynamic complications.

In this sense, recent studies [19], and results from our own series of laparoscopic cholecystectomy in elderly patients (Table 1) demonstrate that the percentage of patients above age 75 with ASA III and IV classifications is significantly higher than that in the group below age 75 (62 vs. 33%); however, morbidity was not higher among the older patients regardless of the procedure performed. Therefore increased concern about performing elective laparoscopic operations on patients older than 75 years may be unjustified. On the other hand, some authors consider that patients above age 80 who have multiple comorbid conditions to have a worse prognosis than those below that age [13], together with a higher prevalence of nonelective procedures, a higher conversion rate to open operation, the presence of more intraoperative complications, and the percentage of complication of the disease, such as the evidence of common bile duct stone passage [20].

In general, many elderly patients are taking antihypertensive and cardiological medications. These medications should be maintained, although there is some

TABLE 1 Risk in Patients Who Underwent a Laparoscopic Cholecystectomy in Our Institution[a]

	Age	
ASA[b]	65–74	75–89
II	17.4%	0%
III	59.1%	60%
IV	23.5%	40%
	$p < 0.01$	

[a] It is observed that the percentage of patients age > 75 with ASA III and IV is significantly higher than that age < 75.

[b] American Society of Anesthesiologists Classification

controversy concerning diuretics and renin-angiotensin system inhibitors. Diuretics reduce the intravascular volume during the first 6 months of therapy, and patients treated with angiotensin-converting enzyme (ACE) inhibitors or angiotensin-receptor antagonists (ARAs) adapt poorly to reduced venous return and can experience severe hypotension and bradycardic crises during anesthesia [21,22]. Due to the difficulties in venous return that can occur during laparoscopy, discontinuation of these drugs 24 hr prior to surgery should be considered and vascular filling optimized in all cases before anesthesia is administered. Postponement of the procedure is advisable when diastolic blood pressure values are above 110–120 mmHg. Hypotensive therapy should be started—preferably without diuretics or ACE inhibitors and ARAs—and continued for several days or weeks until systemic vascular resistance is reduced and the relative hypovolemia of the hypertensive patient is offset. Preoperative consultation with the anesthesiologist may be helpful in some patients.

It should be also taken under consideration that patients with cardiac comorbidity may be undergoing treatment with heparin and warfarin, thus presenting a higher rate of bleeding (23). An evaluation of the levels of anticoagulation before surgery is necessary to avoid this complication.

On the other hand, normal physiological changes of aging increase the likelihood of renal-electrolyte disorders in the elderly surgical patient [24]. The most important of these changes include a decrease in the renal function, decreased urinary concentrating ability, and narrowed limits for the excretion of water, sodium, potassium, and acid. Because of the decrease in renal function, the elderly surgical patient is at increased risk for virtually every cause of acute renal failure—an outcome associated with a mortality of greater than 50%. Certain types of surgery—especially cardiac, aortic, and biliary tract operations—are associated with higher risk of acute renal failure than are others. A minimally invasive approach may prevent these complications, since it is a less aggressive approach to the surgical patient.

In general, advanced age, although a risk factor, cannot be considered a contraindication to surgery and to a laparoscopic approach. However, physiopathological alterations of the elderly patient should be evaluated. Treatment of any functional decline of an organ, malnutrition, dehydration, and use of adequate anesthesiologic management contribute to the minimization of postoperative morbidity and mortality.

Intraoperative Measures to Prevent Complications

There are some concerns in performing minimally invasive surgery in the elderly. The increase in intra-abdominal pressure during pneumoperitoneum can lead to an increase in systemic vascular resistance and central filling pressures with a decrease in cardiac index, which may be detrimental in elderly patients with limited cardiac reserves [25]. A high insufflation pressure may also compress the inferior vena cava, further compromising venous return and cardiac output. For these reasons, some authors use a low insufflation pressure of <8 mmHg to minimize any such cardiovascular problems [26]. It has also been demonstrated that gradual abdominal insufflation to 12 mmHg followed by a limited 10-degree reverse Trendelenburg position is associated with cardiovascular stability in elderly ASA III patients [27–29].

The limitations on thoracopulmonary distensibility imposed by increased intra-abdominal pressure is more important in elderly patients and makes the use of volume-controlled ventilation advisable, with volume adjustment based on expired CO_2 ($EtCO_2$) values. Generally an increase of 15–20% in current volume over normal figures and maintenance of the respiratory rate are sufficient, although occasionally the latter must also be increased to control hypercapnia. The CO_2 absorption rate tends to stabilize after the initial rise and does not usually represent a major problem. Nevertheless, CO_2 retention may occur in patients with severe pulmonary disease.

It has been demonstrated that the duration of surgery in elderly patients may be increased due to various factors. In order to help prevent the hypothermia observed in laparoscopic procedures of some duration [30,31], the use of closed- or semi-closed-circuit ventilation systems with low flow rates and humidifying filters is advisable.

The basic guidelines for monitoring this group of patients do not differ from those for anesthesia in general, although several special considerations may be necessary. Electrocardiography, pulse oximetry and blood pressure measurements are recommended, as well as airway and intra-abdominal pressure measurements. $EtCO_2$ measurement is effective for detecting complications, but only as a guideline. Moreover, although healthy patients maintain a good correlation with arterial CO_2 values (Pa_{CO_2}) [32], the variations in Pa_{CO_2} may not be reflected in $EtCO_2$ [33] in patients with cardiopulmonary disease. As a result, blood gas analysis should be considered in high-risk patients or in intraoperative situations of hypoxemia, elevated airway pressure, or sudden changes in $EtCO_2$. Lateral flow spirometry can be used to detect changes in lung compliance and in ventilation flow and pressure curves, parameters of use for diagnosing respiratory complications. During insufflation of the pneumoperitoneum, close monitoring of hemodynamic parameters is necessary in these patients for early detection of catastrophic complications, such as vascular puncture or gas embolism. A physical inspection should also be performed to rule out the possibility of subcutaneous emphysema. Insufflation and the changes in position must be performed gradually in patients with high cardiocirculatory risk, and hemodynamic variables must be monitored before, during, and after the changes. In patients with limited cardiac function, direct, continuous measurement of arterial and central venous pressures must be considered, possibly with the insertion of a pulmonary artery catheter to monitor hemodynamic changes [34]. During the entire procedure, one should be alert to the surgical movements and carry out regular inspections of the abdomen, since the surgeons are focused on a specific area of the monitor and may not notice a problem in another area.

Conversion rate is another dilemma associated with laparoscopic surgery in the elderly. The high conversion rate associated with elderly patients (35) appears to result primarily because of patients presenting with inflammatory processes, such as acute cholecystitis, and complication of these diseases. The incidence of acute cholecystitis in this patient population ranges from 33.7% to 49% in some series [36]. These circumstances have been demonstrated to increase the difficulty of laparoscopic cholecystectomy significantly, with reported conversions of 27–36% [36–38]. But in some series a high rate of conversion has been related to an increase in the Pa_{CO_2} in the blood produced by excessive operative time [39], since these patients usually present more difficult procedures due to inflammatory processes, as noted previously. A gasless procedure has been proposed as an alternative to avoid this type of complication in elderly patients classified as ASA class III, reducing the rate of conversion due to hemodynamic complications produced by excessive operative time.

One of the most important aspects of the avoidance of complications is to realize that conversion to open procedure, after an adequate trial by an experienced laparoscopic surgeon, should not be regarded as a complication or an operative failure but as an measure designed to prevent complications.

Postoperative Measures to Prevent Complications

Medical postoperative complications have predominated over surgical complications in reports of open cholecystectomy, and this tendency has also been demonstrated in the laparoscopic series [40]. In general, elderly patients have a longer hospital stay, reflecting a higher conversion rate and more postoperative complications than in the general population who undergo a laparoscopic procedure.

One of the concerns in the postoperative period in the elderly is that of pulmonary function after surgery. A recent report [41] has prospectively assessed pulmonary function before operation, 24 hr after surgery and on the seventh postoperative day in patients over 70 years of age, comparing these studies to younger patients in order to evaluate the safety of this approach and to identify measures to prevent such complications. Preoperative values of forced vital capacity (FVC) and forced expiratory volume in 1 sec (FEV_1) is significantly lower in older patients than in younger patients, while the value of FVC, FEV_1, and forced expiratory flow at 50% 24 hr after surgery is less depressed in older patients and also recovered more quickly in these patients 7 days after the operation. These results show that laparoscopy gives excellent results in geriatric patients and can be recommended as the treatment of choice for the elderly.

Other specific complications are also know to be associated with these type of patients, such as cardiogenic pulmonary edema [17]. This can be precipitated by excessive perioperative fluid therapy and not from the positive pressure of the pneumoperitoneum. For that reason, due to the frequent preoperative cardiovascular instability of these patients, careful management of fluid therapy is necessary in the postoperative period. Additionally, due to the decline in renal function observed in the elderly, it is important to maintain normal intravascular volume and avoid hypovolemia so as to prevent the development of acute renal failure [24]. Meticulous attention must be paid to salt and water balance and to the dosage of any drug given in the postoperative period. Should perioperative renal insufficiency occur, evaluation and management in the elderly patient are similar to the usual practices in a younger individual.

On the other hand, it is important that the patient be involved in the preoperative decision-making process to the extent possible, and also that adequate postoperative and discharge planning be part of the preoperative management of the elderly person.

SPECIFIC COMPLICATIONS OF DIFFERENT LAPAROSCOPIC PROCEDURES IN THE ELDERLY

Laparoscopic Cholecystectomy in the Elderly

The incidence of gallstones increases with age [42]. Therefore cholecystectomy is a common operation in elderly patients [43]. Age has never been a contraindication for laparoscopic cholecystectomy, although the laparoscopic approach initially was reserved for low-risk patients. This type of patient selection also occurred with some other types of situations, such as obesity, but experience has led to increased indications for laparoscopic surgery.

In the elderly, gallstone disease is associated with much higher morbidity and mortality [44]. Therefore a more aggressive approach to symptomatic cholelithiasis in the form of elective surgery is justifiable. This concept has been reinforced by the excellent results produced by laparoscopic cholecystectomy in the elderly .

Different studies have shown that elderly patients experience more complications and a longer hospital stay than younger patients after laparoscopic cholecystectomy [17]. In a recent study comparing laparoscopic cholecystectomy in patients over 75 years of age with that in younger patients, the conversion rate to open surgery was 22% in older patients versus 13% in the younger group [45]. Mortality and morbidity rates were respectively 1 and 13.7% in elderly patients versus 0 and 6.6% in younger patients. Not surprisingly, the hospital stay was shorter in the second group (4.5 vs. 6.9 days). Therefore an increase in complications is observed in older patients, but the procedure should be considered feasible

TABLE 2 Laparoscopic Cholecystectomy in Elderly Patients

Author/Year	No. of patients	Age	Hospital stay	Conversion	Mortality	Morbidity
Feldman et al., 1994 (94)	1508	>65	NS[a]	NS	0.46%	NS
Fried et al., 1994 (95)	337	>65	69.2 hr	10.4%	0.6%	11.6%
Milheiro et al., 1996 (41)	52	>69	3 days	15%	2%	14%
Lo et al., 1996 (96)	30	>65	5.9 days	23.3%	0%	26.7%
Lujan et al., 1997 (97)	264	>65	3.71 days	8.3%	0%	13.5%
Tagle et al., 1997 (13)	90	≤65	5 days	3%	2%	5%
Mayol et al., 1997 (98)	61	>70	4.3 days	NS	0%	20%
Conzalez et al., 1997 (99)	76	>80	NS	NS	11.8%	50%
Maxwell et al., 1998 (20)	105	≥80	7.9 days	16%	4.8%	13.3%
Pessaux et al., 2000 (17)	102	>75	6.9 days	21.6%	1%	13.7%
Laycock et al., 2000 (100)	5014	>65	5.5 days	NS	1.6%	NS
Ballesta et al., 2002 (26)	232	>70	3.4 days	4.3%	3.4%	10.8%
Morales et al., 2003	192	≥65	1.9 days	3.1%	0.5%	4.1%

[a] Not stated.

with a low morbidity rate, since these results are favorable when compared with open cholecystectomy in this patient population. Open cholecystectomy series in elderly patients have consistently demonstrated higher rates of morbidity and mortality and longer hospital stays [9,46–48]. Laparoscopic cholecystecomy is reported to be better tolerated than open cholecystectomy by patients aged 70 and over [49].

One point to be considered in efforts to avoid complications in these patients is that chronic cholecystitis should be managed with elective laparoscopic cholecystectomy rather than waiting for complications to develop an elderly patient probably has a long history of gallbladder disease and more acute attacks. A recent study has shown that elderly patients are significantly more likely than younger patients to present with acute cholecystitis (40 vs. 18%), gallstone pancreatitis (19 vs. 6%), and stones in the common bile duct (21 vs. 5%) [49]. For these reasons, many patients over age 80 who undergo laparoscopic cholecystectomy present via the emergency room with acute complications of cholelithiasis, since many of these patients and/or their physicians prefer to avoid surgery for their symptomatic disease. In a study by Uecker et al. (50), a retrospective review of 70 patients over 80 years of age found that of those who underwent cholecystectomy, only 17 [24.28%] presented for elective management of chronic biliary disease, while the remaining 53 patients presented via the emergency room with acute complications. While all of these patients had comorbid conditions, those who underwent surgery in an emergent setting had a higher rate of conversion

(12.5 vs. 37%), complications (19 vs. 28.3%) and mortality (0 vs. 13.2%). There are other acute complications of this disease, such as choledocholithiasis and cholangitis, which, when electively treated, can increase the quality of life and reduce the rate of morbidity and mortality related to surgery.

However, elective surgery in elderly patients is also associated with a higher rate of conversion and morbidity than in younger patients, because the procedure becomes more difficult in patients over 65 years of age. The most important factor associated with this high rate of conversion and the increase in the difficulties is the degree of inflammation and adhesions due to chronic inflammation after multiple acute attacks. These produce severe fibrosis in the elderly, which accounts for most of the conversions in the majority of the studies. Repeated inflammation results in a fibrotic gallbladder with dense adhesions to surrounding structures, rendering laparoscopic dissection difficult.

In general, elderly patients with uncomplicated gallstone disease appear to be excellent candidates for laparoscopic cholecystectomy, but most present complicated gallstone disease, thereby increasing the conversion rate, hospital stay, and preoperative morbidity. However laparoscopic procedures in the elderly can be performed with results that are superior to those reported for open cholecystectomy. We advocate earlier elective cholecystectomy for patients with symptomatic cholelithiasis before they become still older, when associated systemic disease will increase their overall risk, especially in the event of an emergency operation.

Laparoscopic Cholecystectomy in the Elderly: Our Experience

The aim of our analysis was to determine the safety of simple laparoscopic cholecystectomy in aged patients. We analyzed the outcome of patients between 65 and 74 years of age and in those over age 75 who underwent laparoscopic cholecystectomy for symptomatic gallbladder disease. All patients over 65 years of age with symptomatic gallbladder disease and without choledocholithiasis, septic shock, diffuse peritonitis, gallbladder malignancy, or contraindications for general anesthesia were selected for simple laparoscopic cholecystectomy. The conversion rate to open cholecystectomy, age, length of hospital stay, and number of complications or deaths were determined for those patients who underwent laparoscopic cholecystectomy. Complications were categorized as either medical morbidities or mortalities or surgical morbidities or mortalities.

The patients were divided into two groups: group 1, patients 65–74 years old, and group 2, patients over 75 years old. Complications and lengths of stay were determined for each group. Group 1 was compared with group 2.

From March 1997 to December 2002, a total of 192 patients aged 65 and older underwent laparoscopic cholecystectomy. The mean age was 71.31 years,

TABLE 3 Factors Associated Conversion

Causes of Conversion	FREC (%)
Cholecystoenteric fistula	2 (1%)
Plastron	2 (1%)
Common bile duct lesion	1 (0.5%)
Bleeding	1 (0.5%)
Total	6 (3.1%)

range 65–89 years. There was no difference in sex distribution between groups, but patients over 75 years of age were considered at higher risk than patients of group 1 (Table 1). Laparoscopic cholecystectomy was completed in 186 patients, for a conversion rate of 3.1% (Table 3). The mean length of hospital stay was 1.96 days. Group 1 (from 65–74 years of age) included 146 patients. Group 2 (over 75 years) comprised 46 patients.

Major complications were presented in 8 patients (4.16%). Seven of the patients (3.64%) experienced major surgical complications and 1 a major medical complication (0.52%). The mortality rate was 0.52% (1 case), due to an initial surgical complication that required emergency surgery and developed into a medical complication.

The overall morbidity rate was 4.16%, with no statistically significant increase in group 2 (2.8% for group 1 vs. 8.7% for group 2). Patients in group 1 showed a conversion rate (3.4 vs. 2.2%) to that similar of older patients. Mean length of hospital stay was significantly shorter for group 1 (1.70 vs. 2.82 days) (Table 4).

TABLE 4 Laparoscopic Cholecystectomy in Elderly Patients in Our Institution

	Age			
	65–74	75–89	Total	Significance
Cases	146	46	192	
Conversion	5 (3.4%)	1 (2.2%)	6 (3.1%)	$p>0.5$
Major surgical complication	3 (2.1%)	4 (8.7%)	7 (3.6%)	$p>0.5$
Major medical complication	1 (0.7%)	0 (0%)	1 (0.5%)	$p>0.5$
Mortality	0 (0%)	1 (2.2%)	1 (0.5%)	$p>0.5$
Hospital stay	1.70	2.82	1.96	$p<0.05$

Laparoscopic Exploration of the Common Bile Duct in the Elderly

Common bile duct stones occur more frequently with advanced age [51,52]. Operative morbidity and mortality after open cholecystectomy and common bile duct exploration are related to pre-existing cardiovascular disease rather than advanced age alone. Myocardial infarction is most commonly the leading cause of death, followed by cirrhosis [53]. Operative mortality after biliary tract surgery in the elderly, however, is associated with emergent rather than elective operations [52,54]. A recent report revealed that mortality occurred in 12.5% of elderly patients after emergency biliary tract surgery, whereas it was uncommon after elective operation [52]. The recommendation from these studies is that patients with symptomatic biliary tract disease, particularly the elderly, should be managed aggressively with early elective surgery to avoid the risk associated with emergent procedures, which are always potentially fatal in these patients [52].

The introduction of a minimally invasive approach with endoscopic and laparoscopic techniques to these situations has reduced the morbidity and mortality rate, especially in the elderly. The introduction of endoscopic retrograde cholangiopancreatography (ERCP) with endoscopic stone extraction is aimed at reducing mortality in elderly patients by relieving acute suppurative cholangitis, possibly avoiding surgery altogether by leaving the gallbladder in situ in high-risk patients. Discussion currently is focused on the advantages or disadvantages of following a double-staged procedure, combining endoscopic techniques and surgery, or a single-staged approach. A recently published randomized controlled trial [55] comparing laparoscopic single-stage and endolaparoscopic double-stage management of gallstones and common bile duct stones has reported equivalent success rates for the two options but a significantly shorter hospital stay for the single-stage approach. However, laparoscopic common bile duct exploration still is not adopted by many surgeons, possibly because it is considered a demanding technique with a long learning curve. On the other hand, ERCP must not be overutilized, since there is morbidity and mortality associated with this technique and different studies recommend performance of ERCP only in patients who have obstructive jaundice, ascending cholangitis, or both. It is not an indicated procedure in patients who present with gallstone pancreatitis [56].

In conclusion, a minimally invasive approach to common bile duct stones in the elderly has reduced the mortality and morbility related to this situation. The combination of an endolaparoscopic approach or a laparoscopic single-stage approach should be evaluated depending on the experience of the surgeon and the endoscopist and the situation of the patient. In elderly patients with acute septic cholangitis, emergency ERCP may be the treatment of choice.

Laparoscopic Antireflux Surgery in the Elderly

Gastroesophageal reflux (GER) is among the most common disorders affecting the upper gastrointestinal tract [57]. Most patients with symptomatic gastroesophageal reflux disease (GERD) can be treated effectively with medical therapy. Surgery, though a more definitive approach, is usually reserved for young patients with risk factors predictive of medical failure or those who develop recurrent or progressive disease [57]. In the 1990s, laparoscopic antireflux surgery became increasingly accepted as the preferred surgical therapy for younger patients with severe or complicated GERD.

Although symptomatic GER occurs in patients of all ages, the disease pattern and the incidence of esophageal mucosal injury are different in patients > 65 years of age [58–60]. Because the disease is often more severe in older patients, a more aggressive treatment approach has been advocated [58,60,61]. Several etiological factors that may be associated with aging have been implicated in the development of GERD in the elderly [61,62], including increased gastric acid secretion, disordered esophageal peristalsis, a decreased esophageal protective mechanism (reduced salivary bicarbonate secretion), delayed gastric emptying, increased incidence of hiatal hernia, and use of medications that can injure the esophageal mucosa or diminish lower esophageal sphincter pressure.

With the availability of modern antisecretory therapy, most patients with symptomatic GERD can be managed medically regardless of their age. Surgical intervention has been reserved for patients with complications or those whose symptoms are refractory to medications; it has also been used as an alternative to lifelong medical therapy. Despite these established indications for surgery, the role of antireflux surgery in the treatment of GERD in the elderly has not been well defined. The perceived morbidity associated with open antireflux operations has undoubtedly limited the acceptance of surgery in the past, despite one controlled trial that demonstrated a superior outcome with open Nissen fundoplication as compared with medical therapy using ranitidine [63]. Techniques for laparoscopic antireflux procedures have been consolidated in recent years.

The results of different studies suggest that laparoscopic antireflux surgery can be performed safely and with a high degree of success in the elderly population. Brunt et al. [64] found no mortality in 339 patients undergoing laparoscopic antireflux surgery. Thirty-six patients were aged 65 years or older and had a complication rate of 16.7% vs. 4.3% in 303 patients younger than age 65. These results were comparable with those of a similar-sized retrospective comparison of elderly and nonelderly patients undergoing laparoscopic antireflux surgery [65]. Although a relatively small number of elderly patients were evaluated in these studies [64–66], there were few serious complications, functional outcomes were good, and the failure rate of fundoplication was acceptably low. Differences in operative time, intraoperative blood loss, postoperative stay, and time until resumption of normal activities seem to be related to the high ASA scores and the higher proportion of mixed paraesophageal hernias in the elderly group [66]. Paraesophageal hernias are more frequent in older patients—57% of elderly patients who undergo laparoscopic fundoplication [67]; this entity is technically challenging and known to be associated with higher complication rates [68].

Laparoscopic Colonic Surgery in the Elderly

The benefit of laparoscopic cholecystectomy have been universally recognized, and this has become the procedure of choice for symptomatic cholelithiasis, but laparoscopy-assisted colectomy has not had such universal acceptance despite the fact that laparoscopic colectomy has been proven safe and feasible, with complication rates similar to those of open colectomy [69–72]. Several nonrandomized studies have found no increase in port-site recurrences or decreased survival when laparoscopic colectomy was performed for cancer [73–76]; different multicenter, prospective, randomized controlled trials are currently being conducted to definitively answer this question [77].

The incidence of both benign and malignant disease of the colon increases with chronological age and most colon and rectal operations have a high degree of complexity, making the laparoscopic approach technically challenging in this group of patients.

Advantages in laparoscopic colectomy include decreased postoperative pain, quicker return of bowel function, and shorter length of stay [69,78]. The advantages of laparoscopic colectomy may be more beneficial in the elderly [79–81], who often have more comorbid conditions, leading to greater postoperative complications and lengths of stay [82–85]. A recent study showed decreased morbidity and increased postoperative independence in elderly patients undergoing laparoscopic colectomy compared to open colectomy [81], although few data have been published on the possible selective advantage of laparoscopic colectomy in the elderly population [79]. Recent studies comparing laparoscopic and open colonic resection in patients over 75 years of age [19] and in those aged 80 years or older [86] have found decreased narcotic use, quicker return to bowel function, and shorter length of stay in the laparoscopic group, with the same rate of morbidity and mortality in both groups, although several published reports have demonstrated that morbidity is lower for laparoscopic colectomy compared to open colectomy in this group of patients [79,81,87].

One important fact is that pulmonary complications are reduced after a laparoscopic procedure compared to open colorectal resection in elderly patients [88]. However, the duration of surgery and length of stay in the intensive care unit is significantly prolonged in patients above 70 years of age, although this declines with the surgeon's experience.

In general, although several reports have documented that as age increases, morbidity and mortality increase following colorectal resections [83,84,89,90], recent studies demonstrate that elective surgery in the elderly can be done safely, with morbidity and mortality rates similar to those of younger patients [82,85,91], especially if surgery is performed on a minimally invasive basis, showing no statistically significant differences between the younger and older groups relative to the incidence of complications (11 vs. 14%, respectively), conversion (8 vs. 11%, respectively), or length of ileus (2.8 vs. 4.2 days, respectively) [91].

Laparoscopic Gastric Surgery in the Elderly

Gastric surgery is a disease of aging. Cancer surgery is safe for older patients and should not be denied on the basis of chronological age. The curability of cancer in the elderly is predicated on the individual's tolerance of major surgery. During the past two decades, studies have shown a marked reduction in operative morbidity and mortality associated with gastric surgery in the elderly. The reasons may be multifactorial and include better patient selection, better perioperative control of concomitant disease, improved attention to postoperative nutrition, improved surgical techniques, use of prophylactic antibiotics and prophylaxis against stress ulceration and thromboembolic complications. The benefits of laparoscopy-assisted gastrectomy, when compared with conventional gastrectomy, include less pain, a rapid return to gastrointestinal function, and a shorter hospital stay [5,92–94]. However, there are no published series specifically addressing the indications, contraindications, and advantages of laparoscopic gastrectomy in elderly patients. Ballesta et al. [26] have described 3 deaths among 12 gastrectomies for carcinomas. This high number of deaths may be related to the learning curve, to the nature of the disease, and to the longer operative time, which may have adversely affected the already compromised cardiopulmonary function in some of these patients. Larger series are necessary to evaluate the benefits of laparoscopic gastric resection for carcinoma—a disease usually associated with patients over 65 years of age—and to define measures for avoiding complications associated with this procedure.

CONCLUSIONS

The frail elderly patent with surgical disease presents a unique challenge to the geriatrician. Coexisting medical disease and increasing surgical risk coupled with a perceived reduction in benefit based on a limited functional capacity or life span often make the frail elderly unable or unwilling to undergo major surgery. The many recent advances in medical therapy, such minimally invasive surgery, offer a real alternative to major open surgery in this population.

The question of age as a risk factor for surgery is complicated. There are many factors that have an impact on mortality and morbidity rates in the surgical care of the elderly. The most important of these are the physiological changes of aging, underlying disease states, the type of procedures performed, and whether the procedure is performed as an emergency. Although there are many risks in performing surgery in elderly patients, there are many patients who do well and benefit from undergoing surgical procedures. Age alone should never be used as the criterion to deny indicated surgery in an elderly patient.

Regarding laparoscopic cholecystectomy, results reported indicate that since the risks of cholecystectomy performed as an emergency are higher, symptomatic elderly patients with gallstones should be considered good candidates for early elective cholecystectomy. Results from our data and from various other studies suggest that elderly patients with uncomplicated gallstone disease are excellent candidates for laparoscopic cholecystectomy, and this should be considered before complicated disease develops.

Risk assessment, decision making, and perioperative care are typically more challenging in the elderly than in younger patients. An understanding of the physiological changes of aging and their effect on surgical care is essential if the best outcomes are to be achieved.

REFERENCES

1. Murray CJ, Lopez AD. Alternative projects of mortality and disability by cause 1990–2020: Global Burden of Disease Study. Lancet 1997; 349:1948–1504.
2. Keating HJ, Lubin MF. Peroperative responsibilities of the physician/geriatrician. Clin Geriatr Med 1990; 6:459–467.
3. Barkun JS, Fried GM, Barkun AN. Randomised controlled trial of laparoscopic versus mini-cholecystectomy. Lancet 1992; 340:1116–1119.
4. Steiner CA, Bass EB, Talamani MA, Pitt HA, Steinberg EP. Surgical rates and operative mortality for open laparoscopic cholecystectomy in Maryland. N Engl J Med 1994; 330:403–408.
5. Adachi Y, Shiraishi N, Shiromizu A, Bandoh T, Aramaki M, Kitano S. Laparoscopy-assisted Billroth I gastrectomy compared with conventional open gastrectomy. Arch Surg 2000; 135:806–810.
6. Barkun JS, Barkun AN, Sampalis JS, Fried G, Taylor B, Wexler MJ, Goresky CA, Meakins JL. Randomized controlled trial of laparoscopic versus mini-cholecystectomy. Lancet 1992; 340:1116–1119.
7. Chen H, Alabaz O, Iroatulam A, Nesim A, Weiss E, Nogueras J, Wexner SD. Laparoscopic colectomy for benign disease is associated with reduction in disability compared with laparotomy. Surg Endosc 1998; 12:1397–1400.
8. Goh YG, Eu KW, Seow-Choen F. Early postoperative results of a prospective series of laparoscopic vs open anterior resections for rectosigmoid cancers. Dis Colon Rectum 1997; 40:1565–1568.
9. Margiotta SJ, Horwitz JR, Willis IH, Wallack MK. Cholecystectomy in the elderly. Am J Surg 1998; 156:509–512.

10. Shamburek RD, Farrar JT. Disorders of the digestive system in elderly patients. N Engl J Med 1990; 322:438–443.
11. Kaltic MR. Surgery in centenarians. In: Kaltic MR, ed. Geriatric Surgery. Munich. Germany: Urban & Schwarzenberg, 1990, 741–743.
12. Lyass S, Perry Y, Venturero M, Muggia-Sullan M, Eid A, Durst A, Reissman P. Laparoscopic cholecystectomy: What does affect the outcome? A restrospective multifactorial regression analysis. Surg Endosc 2000; 14(7):661–665.
13. Tagle FM, Lavergne J, Barkin JS, Unger SW. Laparoscopic cholecystectomy in the elderly. Surg Endosc 1997; 11:636–638.
14. Massie MT, Massie LB, Marrangoni AG, D'Amico FJ, Sell HW. Advantages of LC in the elderly and in patients with high ASA classifications. J Laparoendosc Surg 1993; 3(5):467–475.
15. Saxe A, Lavson J, Phillips E. Laparoscopic cholecystectomy in patients aged 65 or older. J Laparoendosc Surg 1993; 3(3):215–219.
16. The Southern Surgeons Club. A prospective analysis of 1518 laparoscopic cholecystectomies. N Engl J Med 1991; 324:1073–1078.
17. Pessaux P, Tuech JJ, Derouet N, Rouge C, Regenet N, Arnaud JP. Laparoscopic cholecystectomy in the elderly: A prospective study. Surg Endosc 2000; 14(11): 1067–1069.
18. Adducci E, De Cosmo G, Onorati F, Cataldo R, Primieri P, Villani A. Anesthesia in the elderly patient. Our experience. Minerva Anestesiol 1993; 59(7–8):351–355.
19. Sklow B, Read T, Birnbaum E, Fry R, Fleshman J. Age and type of procedure influence the choice of patients for laparoscopic colectomy. Surg Endosc 2003; 17: 923–929.
20. Maxwell JG, Tyler BA, Maxwell BG, Brinker CC, Covington DL. Laparoscopic cholecystectomy in octogenarians. Am Surg 1998; 64(9):826–831.
21. Coriat P, Ricker C, Douraki T, et al. Influence of chronic angiotensin converting enzyme inhibition on anesthetic induction. Anesthesiology 1994; 81:299–307.
22. Colson P, Ryckwaert F, Coriat P. Renin angiotensin system antagonists and anesthesia. Anesth Analg 1999; 89(5):1143–55.
23. Hazey JW, Brody FJ, Rosenblatt SM, Brodsky J, Malm J, Ponsky JL. Laparoscopic management and clinical outcome of emphysematous cholecystitis. Sur Endosc 2001; 15(10):1217–1220.
24. Beck LH. Peroperative renal, fluid, and electrolyte management. Clin Geriatr Med 1990; 6(3):557–569.
25. Harris Sn, Ballantyne GH, Luther MA, Perrino AC. Alterations of cardiovascular performance during laparoscopic cholectomy: A combined hemodynamic and echocardiographic analysis. Anesth Analg 1996; 83:482–487.
26. Ballesta López C, Cid JA, Poves I, Bettonica C, Villegas L, Memon MA. Laparoscopic surgery in the elderly patients. Experience of a single laparoscopic unit. Surg Endosc 2003; 17(2):333–337.
27. Dhoste K, Lacoste L, Karayan J, Lehuede MS, Thomas D, Fusciardi J. Haemodynamic and ventilatory changes during laparoscopic cholecystectomy in elderly ASA III patients. Can J Anaesth 1996; 43:783–788.
28. Dorsay DA, Greene FL, Baysinger CL. Haemodynamic changes during laparoscopic cholecystectomy monitored with transesophageal echocardiography. Surg Endosc 1995; 9:128.

29. Zollinger A, Krayer S, Singer TH, Seifert B, Heinzelmann M, Schlumpf R, Pasch TH. Haemodynamic effects of pneumoperitoneum in elderly patients with an increased cardiac risk. Eur J Anaesth 1997; 14:266–275.
30. Castillo V, Gutiérrez-Crespo A, Suarez F, Luis-Navarro JC, Gómez-Arguelles MA. Variación de la temperatura corporal en relación con la insuflación de CO_2 en el curso de la colecistectomía laparoscópica. Rev Esp Anestesiol Reanim 1996; 43(6): 201–203.
31. Rose DK, Cohen MM, Soutter DI. Laparoscopic cholecystectomy: The anaesthetist's point of view. Can J Anaesthesiol 1992; 39:809–815.
32. McKinstry LJ, Perverseff RA, Yin RW. Arterial and end-tidal carbon dioxide in patients undergoing laparoscopic cholecistectomy. Anesthesiology 1992; 77:108.
33. Yamanaka MK, Sue DY. Comparison of arterial-end-tidal PCO_2 difference and dead space/tidal volume ratio in respiratory failure. Chest 1987; 92(5):832–835.
34. Feig BW, Berger DH, Dougherty TB. Pharmacologic intervention can reestablish baseline hemodynamic parameters during laparoscopy. Surgery 1994; 116(4): 733–741.
35. Kama NA, Doganay M, Dolapci M, Reis E, Atli M, Kologlu M. Risk factors resulting in conversión of laparoscopic cholecystectomy to open surgery. Surg Endosc 2001; 15(9):965–968.
36. Bickel A, Rappaport A, Kanievski V, Vaksman I, Haj M, Geron N, Eitan A. Laparoscopic management of acute cholecystitis prognostic factors for success. Surg Endosc 1996; 10:1045–1049.
37. Cox MR, Wilson TG, Luck AJ. Laparoscopic cholecystectomy for acute inflammation of the gallbladder. Ann Surg 1993; 218:630–634.
38. Zucker KA, Flowers JL, Baileys RW. Laparoscopic management of acute cholecystitis. Am J Surg 1993; 165:508–514.
39. Montori A, Boscaini M, Gasparrini M, Miscusi G, Masoni L, Onorato M, Montori J. Gallstone in elderly patients: Impact of laparoscopic cholecystectomy. Can J Gastroenterol 2000; 14(11):929–932.
40. Firilas A, Duke E, Max MH. Laparoscopic cholecystectomy in the elderly. Surg Endosc 1996; 10(33):1045–1049.
41. Milheiro A, Castro Sousa F, Oliveira L, Joao Matos M. Pulmonary function alter laparoscopic cholecystectomy in the elderly. Br J Surg 1996; 83(8):1059–1061.
42. Huber FD, Martin EW, Cooperman M. Cholecystectomy in elderly patients. Am J Surg 1983; 146:719–722.
43. Reiss R, Deutsch AA. Emergency abdominal procedures in patients above 70. J Gerontol 1985; 40:154–158.
44. Reiss R, Nudelman I, Gutman C, Deutsch AA. Changing trends in surgery for acute cholecystitis. World J Surg 1990; 14:567–571.
45. Pessaux P, Tuech JJ, Duplessis R, Seicean R, Arnaud JP. Laparoscopic cholecystectomy after age 75. Chirurgie 1999; 124(4):419–422.
46. Houghton PWJ, Jenkinson LR, Donaldson LA. Cholecystectomy in the elderly: A prospective study. Br J Surg 1985; 72:220–222.
47. Pigott JP, Williams GB. Cholecystectomy in the elderly. Am J Surg 1988; 185: 408–410.

48. Smith N, Max MH. Gallbladder surgery in patients over 60: Is there an increased risk. South Med J 1987; 80:472–474.
49. Magnuson TH, Ratner LE, Zenilman ME, Bender JS. Laparoscopic cholecystectomy: Applicability in the geriatric population. Am Surg 1997; 63(1):91–96.
50. Uecker J, Adams M, Skipper K, Dunn E. Cholecystitis in the octogenarian: Is laparoscopic cholecystectomy the best approach. Am Surg 2001; 67(7):637–640.
51. Crump C. The incidence of gallstones and gallbladder disease. Surg Gynecol Obstet 1931; 53:447–455.
52. Sullivan DM, Hood TR, Griffen WO. Biliary tract surgery in the elderly. Am J Surg 1982; 143:218–220.
53. McSherry CK, Glenn F. The incidence and causes of death following surgery for non-malignant biliary tract disease. Ann Surg 1980; 191:271–275.
54. Strohl EL, Diffenbaugh WG. Biliary tract surgery in the aged patient. Surg Gynecol Obstet 1953; 97:467–470.
55. Cuschieri A, Lezoche E, Morino M, Croce E, Lacy A, Toouli j, Faggioni A, Ribeiro VM, Jakimowicz J, Visa J, Hanna GB. EAES multicenter prospective randomized trial comparing two-stage vs single-stage managements of patients with gallstone disease and ductal calculi. Surg Endosc 1999; 13:952–957.
56. Hazzan D, Geron N, Golijanin D, Reissman P, Shiloni E. Laparoscopic cholecystectomy in octogenarians. Surg Endosc 2003; 17:773–776.
57. Peters JH, DeMeester TR. Indications, principles of procedure selection, and technique of laparoscopic Nissen fundoplication. Semin Laparosc Surg 1995; 6: 140–143.
58. Mold JW, Reed LE, Davis AB, Allen ML, Decktor DL, Robinson M. Prevalence of gastroesophageal reflux in elderly patients in a primary care setting. Am J Gastroenterol 1991; 86:965–970.
59. Waring JP. Management of gastroesphageal reflux disease in the elderly: More aggressive or more appropriate. Am J Gastroenterol 1995; 90:1037.
60. Zhu H, Pace F, Sangaletti O, Porro Bianchi G. Features of symptomatic gastroesophageal reflux in the elderly patients. Scand Gastroenterol 1993; 28:235–238.
61. Collen MJ, Abdulian JD, Chen YK. Gastroesophageal reflux disease in th elderly: More severe disease that requires aggressive therapy. Am J Gastroenterol 1995; 90:1053–1057.
62. Triadafilopoulos G, Sharma R. Features of symptomatic gastroesophageal reflux disease in elderly patients. Am J Gastroenterol 1997; 92:2007–2011.
63. Spechler SJ. Comparison of medical and surgical therapy for complicated gastroesophageal reflux disease in veterans. N Engl J Med 1992; 326:786–792.
64. Brunt LM, Quasebarth MA, Dunnegan DL, Soper NJ. Is laparoscopic antireflux surgery for gastroesphageal reflux disease in the elderly safe and effective. Surg Endosc 1999; 13:838–842.
65. Trus TL, Laycock WS, Wo JM, Warning JP, Branum GD, Mauren SJ, Katz EM, Hunter JG. Laparoscopic antireflux surgery in the elderly. Am J Gastroenterol 1998; 93:351–353.
66. Khajanchee YS, Urbach DR, Butler N, Hansen PD, Swanstrom LL. Laparoscopic antirreflux surgery in the elderly. Surgical outcome and effect on quality of life. Surg Endosc 2002; 16(1):25–30.

67. Bammer T, Hinder RA, Klaus A, Libbey JS, Napoliello DA, Rodriguez JA. Safety and long-term outcome of laparoscopic antireflux surgery in patients in their eighties and older. Surg Endosc 2002; 16(1):40–42.
68. Trus TL, Bax T, Richardson WS, Branum GD, Mauren SJ, Swanstrom LL, Hunter JG. Complications of laparoscopic paraesophageal hernia repair. J Gastrointest Surg 1997; 1:221–228.
69. Dean PA, Beart RW, Nelson H, Elftmann TD, Schlinkert RT. Laparoscopic-assisted segmental colectomy: Early Mayo Clinic experience. Mayo Clinic Proc 1994; 69: 834–840.
70. Falk PM, Bear RW, Wexner SD, Thorson AG, Jagelman DG. Laparoscopic colectomy: A critical appraisal. Dis Colon Rectum 1993; 36:28–34.
71. Lumley JW, Fielding GA, Rhodes M, Nathanson LK, Siu S, Stitz RW. Laparoscopic-assisted colorectal surgery lessons learned from 240 consecutive patients. Dis Colon Rectum 1996; 39:155–159.
72. Senagore AJ, Luchtefeld MA, Mackeigan JM, Mazier PW. Open colectomy versus laparoscopic colectomy: are there differences. Am Surg 1993; 59:449–554.
73. Franklin ME, Rosenthal D, Abrego-Medina D, Dorman JP, Glass JL, Norem R, Diaz A. Prospective comparison of open vs laparoscopic colon surgery for carcinoma: Five-year results. Dis Colon Rectum 1996; 39(suppl):S35–S46.
74. Khalili TM, Fleshner PR, Hiatt JR, Sokol TP, Manookian C, Tsushima G, Phillips EH. Colorectal cancer: comparison of laparoscopic with open approaches. Dis Colon Rectum 1998; 41:832–838.
75. Leung KL, Yiu RYC, Lai PBS, Lee JFY, Thung KH, Lau WY. Laparoscopic-assisted resection of colorectal carcinoma: Five-year audit. Dis Colon Rectum 1999; 42:327–333.
76. Milsom JW, Bohm B, Hammerhofer KA, Fazio V, Steiger E, Elson P. A prospective, randomized trial comparing laparoscopic versus conventional techniques in colorectal cancer surgery: A preliminary report. J Am Coll Surg 1998; 187:46–54.
77. Stocchi L, Nelson H. Laparoscopic colectomy for colon cancer: trial update. J Surg Oncol 1998; 68:255–267.
78. Peters WR, Bartels TL. Minimally invasive colectomy: Are the potential benefits realized. Dis Colon Rectum 1993; 36:751–756.
79. Delgado S, Lacy AM, Garcia Valdecasas JC, Balague C, Pera M, Salvador L, Momblan D, Visa J. Could age be an indication for laparoscopic colectomy in colorectal cancer. Surg Endosc 2000; 14:22–26.
80. Seshadri PA, Mamazza J, Schlachta CM, Cadeddu MO, Poulin EC. Laparoscopic colorectal resection in octogenarians. Surg Endosc 2001; 15:806–811.
81. Stocchi L, Nelson H, Young-Fadok TM, Larson DR, Ilstrup MS. Safety and advantages of laparoscopic *vs* open colectomy in the elderly: matched-control study. Dis Colon Rectum 2000; 43:326–332.
82. Spivak H, Maele DV, Friedman I, Nussbaum M. Colorectal surgery in octogenarians. J Am Coll Surg 1996; 183:46–50.
83. Walsh TH. Audit of outcome of major surgery in the elderly. Br J Surg 1996; 83: 92–97.
84. Whittle J, Steinberg EP, Anderson GF, Herbert R. Results of colectomy in elderly patients with colon cancer, based on Medicare claims data. Am J Surg 1992; 163: 572–576.

85. Wise WE, Padmanabhan A, Meesig DM, Arnold MW, Aguilar PS, Stewart WR. Abdominal colon and rectal operations in the elderly. Dis Colon Rectum 1991; 34: 959–963.
86. Stewart BT, Stitz RW, Lumley JW. Laparoscopically assisted colorectal surgery in the elderly. Br J Surg 1999; 86:938–994.
87. Lacy AM, Garcia-Valdecasas AM, Pique JM, Delgado S, Campo E, Bordas JM, Taura P, Grande L, Fuster J, Pacheco JL, Visa J. Short-term outcome analysis of a randomized study comparing laparoscopic vs open colectomy for colon cancer. Surg Endosc 1995; 9:1101–1105.
88. Schwenk W, Bohm B, Witt C, Junghans T, Grundel K, Muller JM. Pulmonary function following laparoscopic or convertional colorectal resection: A randomized controlled evaluation. Arch Surg 1999; 134(1):6–13.
88. Lewis AAM, Khoury GA. Resection for colorectal cancer in the very old: Are the risks too high. Br Med J 1988; 296:459–461.
89. Waldron RP, Donovan IA, Drumm J, Mottram SN, Tedman S. Emergency presentation and mortality from colorectal cancer in the elderly. Br J Surg 1986; 73:214–276.
90. Reissman P, Agachan F, Wexner SD. Outcome of laparoscopic colorectal surgery in older patients. Am Surg 1996; 62:1060–1063.
91. Asao T, Hosouchi Y, Nakabayashi T, Haga N, Mochiki E, Kuwano H. Laparoscopically assisted total or distal gastrectomy with lymph node dissection for early gastric cancer. Br J Surg 2001; 88:128–132.
92. Azagra JS, Goergen M, De Simone P, Ibañez-Aguirre J. Minimally invasive surgery for gastric cancer. Surg Endosc 1999; 13:315–317.
93. Shimizu S, Uchiyama A, Mizumoto K, Morisaki T, Nakamura K, Shimura H, Tanaka M. Laparoscopically assited distal gastrectomy for early gastric cancer: Is it superior to open surgery. Surg Endosc 2000; 14:27–31.
94. Feldman MG, Russell JC, Lynch JT, Mattie A. Comparison of mortality rates for open and closed cholecystectomy in the elderly: Connecticut statewide survey. J Laparoendosc Surg 1994; 4:165–171.
95. Fried GM, Clas D, Meakins J. Minimally invasive surgery in the elderly patient. Surg Clin North Am 1994; 74:375–387.
96. Lo CM, Lai ECS, Fan ST, Liu CL, Wong J. Laparoscopic cholecystectomy for acute cholecystitis in the elderly. World J Surg 1996; 20:983–987.
97. Lujan JA, Sanchez-Bueno F, Parrilla P, Robles R, Torralba JA, Gonzalez-Costea R. Laparoscopic vs open cholecystecomy in patients aged 65 and older. Surg Laparosc Endosc 1998; 8:208–210.
98. Mayol J, Marttinez-Sarmiento J, Tamayo FJ, Alvarez Fernandez-Represa J. Complications of laparoscopic cholecystectomy in the ageing patient. Age Ageing 1997; 26:77–81.
99. Gonzalez JJ, Sanz L, Grana JL, Bermejo G, Navarrete F, Martinez E. Biliary lithiasis in the elderly patient: Morbidity and mortality due to biliary surgery. Hepato-Gastroenterology 1997; 44:1565–1568.
100. Laycock WS, Siewers AE, Birkmeyer CM, Wennberg DE, Birkmeyer JD. Variation in the use of laparoscopic cholecystectomy for elderly patients with acute cholecystitis. Arch Surg 2000; 135:457–462.

14

Incisional and Ventral Hernia Repair

Karl A. LeBlanc
Minimally Invasive Surgery Institute, Baton Rouge, and Louisiana State University School of Medicine, New Orleans, Louisiana, U.S.A.

INTRODUCTION

Laparoscopic incisional and ventral hernia repair (LIVH) was first reported in 1993 [1]. Since that time, this procedure has continued to be used as a method of repair of these types of hernias as well as other more complicated ones, such as parastomal and parapubic hernias [2–4]. Many events that occur during and after this operation have been reported in the literature. Many of these are commonplace with these procedures, such as the formation of a seroma, the presence of an ileus, and the postoperative pain that is experienced by these patients. These are so common that many authors do not consider them true complications but rather expected consequences of the procedure itself. Others, however, are significant problems. It is important for the surgeon to be familiar with the prevention and management of these, because despite one's best efforts, they will occur. This chapter outlines these complications as well as the methods for their avoidance, diagnosis, and management.

PREOPERATIVE EVALUATION

There are few laboratory or radiological studies that can identify and prevent the complications shown in Table 1. The preoperative evaluation of the incisional hernia patient should center on the recognition of any comorbid conditions that may make this operation too perilous. In general, these are few, but these patients

TABLE 1 Common Complications of Laparoscopic Incisional and Ventral Hernia Repair

Intraoperative
Hemorrhage
Intestinal injury
Postoperative
Nausea, vomiting
Ileus
Seroma
Pain
Infection
Recurrence

must have sufficient cardiac and pulmonary reserve to permit the use of general anesthesia (also see Chapter 5). Prevention of intraoperative and postoperative complications related to these organ systems will require consultation with the appropriate medical specialist.

The surgeon should also make sure that the patient has adequate hepatic function preoperatively. The presence of portal hypertension, while not a contraindication in all cases, may present significant hemorrhagic problems if not anticipated preoperatively. Additionally, if the patient has ascites from this or from renal disease, attempts should be made to minimize leakage of this fluid on laparoscopic entry into the abdomen. One should try to place trocars in the upper abdomen if possible, to use 5-mm trocars with a ''Z'' path of entry, and to close all trocar sites with transfascial sutures.

PROCEDURE

The methodology of LIVH has been described in numerous publications. This chapter is not meant to provide an in-depth description of the operation. However, the general concepts are noted here so as to put the complications into context. In all of these repairs, the abdomen must be entered with one of several techniques. The initial step will be the release of all adhesions that may be encountered. This can be done with or without the use of an energy source to maintain hemostasis. This is the part of the procedure that which is most fraught with the significant risk of the entire operation: enterotomy. Many surgeons believe that the risk of an unrecognized enterotomy is so great that they avoid the use of any energy source. Others, myself included, use the ultrasonic scalpel selectively. If no bowel is involved in the adhesive process, this can be done carefully. However, if the intestine must be lysed from the anterior abdominal wall, it is recommended that such procedures be avoided. This will minimize the risk of an enterotomy. One must remember that other causes of enterotomy do exist, such as traction injury. This too must be avoided.

Once the adhesions are lysed, the hernia defect is measured and an appropriately sized prosthetic biomaterial is chosen and inserted into the abdominal cavity. This is then affixed to the anterior abdominal wall with a metal fixation device of the surgeon's choosing. Transfascial sutures are then placed along the periphery of the biomaterial to maintain adequate fixation. A few surgeons feel that this step is unnecessary, but the majority believe that this additional fixation is mandatory.

SPECIFIC COMPLICATIONS AND THEIR MANAGEMENT

The majority of the complications known to occur with the laparoscopic approach are not different from those of the open repair (Table 1). A few complications, such as an unrecognized enterotomy, can lead to significant mortality. Most, however, are not reported. The complications seen with laparoscopic repair range from 5–30% (average 15.2%), while those of the open repair range from 27–34% [5–12]. One of the recognized strengths of the laparoscopic operation is that the complication and recurrence rates are lower than with the open one.

Intraoperative Hemorrhage

Intraoperative hemorrhage can occur at the insertion of one of the trocars. The exact incidence of this is not known, as this type of injury is rarely reported because it is generally of no consequence and can be readily controlled. The use of one of the noncutting trocars provides an increased margin of safety during entry through the abdominal wall. If hemorrhage does occur, it can be stopped in a variety of ways. The trocar can be removed and replaced with a larger one to tamponade the vessels that are bleeding. Alternatively, the trocar can be removed and the site cauterized, or a transabdominal suture can be placed before or after its removal.

Hemorrhage can occur during the most challenging portion of the procedure, the adhesiolysis. This will usually originate from one of the vessels within the omentum and can be managed with electrocautery or the ultrasonic shears. If this method is chosen, the surgeon must be especially cautious to make sure that there is no adjacent intestine at that site. The application of the energy necessary to eliminate the source of bleeding can produce sufficient heat to inflict a small lateral burn to the bowel wall, which may not become apparent until a few days later, when that site perforates. This is discussed in detail below and in Chapter 3. Alternatively, the use of hemoclips, looped sutures, or suture ligation can be effective for this problem.

Another common occurrence of hemorrhage is that which results during the fixation of the prosthetic biomaterial. Any of the metal devices or the transfascial sutures that are placed can puncture or lacerate the inferior epigastric vessels. This will be easily identified because either brisk bleeding will be seen or a hematoma will rapidly be formed. One must be quick to apply direct pressure at that site and then place one or more transfascial sutures with one of the devices designed for that purpose.

Intestinal Injury

This is a significant event and one that occurs with some frequency. Serosal injury occurring during the dissection of the intestine can be managed as one would during any bowel surgery. If the lumen has not been violated, one may elect to leave this injury untouched, or the surgeon can close it with either sutures or endoscopic staples. There do not appear to be any benefits or adverse events associated with any of these choices. In our series, we used all of these alternatives without any complications [9].

A recognized enterotomy was a known complication with the open operation, and it is not surprising that this is a known complication of the laparoscopic approach as well. Its incidence varies significantly. Most series report an absence of this complication, but there are many that do report this problem. The incidence of enterotomy varies up to 6 and 14.3% [13,14]. Generally the actual number of patients who have incurred an enterotomy is approximately 1–3% [9,15–18].

The management of a recognized enterotomy is currently somewhat controversial. In many centers, if this event occurs, the hernia procedure is terminated. The surgeon will repair the injury either laparoscopically or by a conversion to the open operation [19]. The hernia can then be repaired with an open method, using a tissue repair, or the repair can be deferred. In that instance, the intestinal repair is completed and the hernia repair is aborted. The patient can then be returned to the operative suite 2–4 days later and the laparoscopic hernioplasty performed. This delay will allow any contamination, to be eliminated, and this short interval of time will not allow the formation of dense adhesions subsequent to the intra-abdominal procedure. Some will delay for several weeks, but this is not recommended unless there was a significant amount of spillage of intraluminal contents.

More recently, there have been reports showing that the repair of this recognized injury to the small bowel and completion of the intended hernia repair may be safe. This enterotomy must not associated with a large amount of spillage of the intestinal contents. Many series have repaired this injury and proceeded to repair the hernia in the intended manner, including the laparoscopic insertion of a prosthetic biomaterial [17,20]. Others have resected gangrenous bowel and completed the hernia repair [21]. There does not appear to be an adverse consequence to this decision, at least at the time of this writing. However, if the intestinal necrosis that may occur with an electrosurgical injury is underestimated when the injury is oversewn, there may be an extension of the necrosis and subsequent development of an intra-abdominal abscess, which requires laparotomy, resection, and removal of the prosthesis [15].

An injury to the colon carries a much greater potential for a sinister outcome if the hernia repair is completed as planned. Therefore the majority of surgeons will simply repair the injury and repair the hernia by a laparotomy. Some, however, have carried out the hernia repair with a simultaneous colon resection as a preplanned operation with an adequately prepared colon [17].

The current recommendations for the treatment of a recognized bowel injury are as follows:

Serosal injury—no treatment or closure by any method; completion of the hernia repair as planned.

Small intestinal intraluminal injury—primary closure by any method; completion of the hernia repair as planned *if* the laparoscopic repair is secure and there has been minimal or no spillage of the intestinal contents. If there has been significant spillage and/or the surgeon is not fully familiar with the technique of laparoscopic repair, the procedure should be converted to a laparotomy and the hernia repaired with sutures alone. A return to the operating suite as a later time, following repair of the injury, can also be elected.

Colonic injury—primary closure by any method; a nonprosthetic open repair can be done simultaneously or the patient may be returned to operation at a later time for a laparoscopic prosthetic repair.

An unrecognized enterotomy can be a significant complication; it is known to occur in up to 6% of patients [10,13,15,16,20]. Such an enterotomy can occur either as a traction injury from one of the grasping instruments or may result from a burn that is incurred during the use of an energy source to lyse the adhesions. In either case, the injury will generally not be manifest in the initial hours following the procedure. The usual postoperative course of these patients calls for rapid discharge from the hospital, usually within 24–48 hr. [9,17,20,22]. Therefore increasing pain, fever, and abdominal distention should be evaluated with laboratory testing and CT scanning if the patient does not appear to exhibit an acute surgical abdomen. Following the LIVH, there should not be any significant accumulation of intraperitoneal fluid. Free air should have been resorbed before the third postoperative day [23]. Where ascites or free air is found within the abdominal cavity and there is even a slight suspicion of an unrecognized enterotomy, the patient should be laparoscoped to assess the abdomen. This can be both diagnostic and therapeutic. If the findings appear benign, then no further therapy is needed. If significant contamination is found, open laparotomy will generally be required, with resection of the involved intestine and excision of the prosthesis. The abdomen can be closed primarily with or without retention sutures. However, if there is the possibility of an abdominal compartment syndrome, the prosthesis can be left in place to allow for expansion of the abdomen. The status of the biomaterial should be closely monitored and its removal may be electively planned as the patient's condition stabilizes.

Hematoma

The incidence of hematomas varies considerably with this procedure. There are several series that have not experienced this complication [13,19,24]. Many others have seen this in 1–15% of the patients [16–18,22]. These can be due to a puncture of one of the small superficial vessels in the abdominal wall, the musculature, or an inferior epigastric vessel. Entry into the abdominal cavity with one of the cutting trocars increases the risk of such an event.

Certainly if the hemorrhage is noted intraoperatively, the surgeon can use electrocautery. If that does not contain the bleeding (e.g., the epigastric vessels) the use of either clips or suture may be required. The assistant should apply direct pressure to the bleeding site with a laparoscopic instrument and possibly external pressure. A suture-passing device can then be used to pass sutures transfascially, thus controlling the hemorrhage. This is very effective.

Late hematomas may develop at trocar sites or within the hernia sac. The former is usually due to muscular bleeding and is self-limited. Warm compresses will usually suffice to treat such a hematoma. A hematoma within the hernia itself usually represents an injury to a larger vessel that was not recognized during the operation due to the pressure effect of the insufflated abdomen, or it may represent a large seroma with a significant blood component. Again, observation and conservative management will generally be sufficient to treat this problem. The use of an abdominal binder may assist in this effort. Aspiration is not usually necessary and can increase the risk of infection.

Prolonged Ileus

This entity is not an entirely unexpected phenomenon given the degree of dissection of the intestine and intra-abdominal organs as well as the surgical hemorrhage that occurs. It is seen in an average of approximately 2% of the reported series. This ranges from 1–8% [9,15,16,24,26]. It should be treated with mobilization, antiemetics, nasogastric suction, and hydration. These measures usually result in resolution of the problem rather quickly.

The main consideration in the patient with an ileus is the possibility of an unrecognized enterotomy. This is a very significant event and one that can eventuate in mortality. The risk, of course, is that this is not acknowledged or diagnosed until several days later, at which time there is a significant incidence of sepsis and death (see above).

This entity cannot be totally avoided during this procedure. A high index of suspicion should be maintained if there has been a large dissection of the intestinal adhesions to the abdominal wall. One should be quick to evaluate the patient with an abdominal radiograph if there appears to be an ileus that lasts longer than 24–48 hr. This could indicate such an event. The presence of free air beyond 24 hr postoperatively may indicate an intestinal perforation [27]. While the initial treatment should rely on a nasogastric tube, the surgeon must be alert to this possibility.

Seroma

The development of a seroma is so common after this procedure that many surgeons do not believe it to be a real complication. This occurrence should be expected, because the peritoneum within the hernia sac is not removed. The fluid secreted by that surface will result in a fluid collection. One study reported that the incidence of this event was 100% in all the patients who were followed with ultrasonic studies [28]. In view of this, it is surprising that more such events are not reported in the literature.

This apparent disparity is related to the definition of the seroma. Many authors do not list this entity as a complication unless it persists beyond 6 weeks [11,20]. Others, such as the present author, believe that the seroma must persist beyond 8–12 weeks and be symptomatic or clinically large to be considered a complication. The incidence of seroma varies widely and can range from 0–43% [7,9–11,17,29]. An overall review of the current literature calculates the incidence of clinically significant seromas to average 4–5% of patients after LIVH.

It is virtually impossible to prevent seromas with certainty. Kirshtein attempted to pierce the biomaterial with the Veress needle but found that omitting this step did not have any appreciable effect on the incidence of seromas [30]. Others have used the DualMesh with holes (W. L. Gore & Associates, Inc., Flagstaff, AZ), but this too is associated with a postoperative seroma rate of 11.8% [17]. Therefore it does not appear that perforation of this product offers any benefit in the prevention of seromas. This is probably related to the fact that cellular ingrowth is so rapid that these small openings are sealed rather quickly while fluid production continues. Alternatively, the use of other biomaterials that are polypropylene-based does not eliminate the appearance of fluid collections [31–33].

Some have tried to use pre-emptive measures to prevent the development of seromas. The argon beam coagulator has been used to scarify the peritoneum of the hernia sac so as to diminish the seromas postoperatively. The application of electrocautery and the ultrasonic scalpel with the use of a single suture in the center of the hernia defect to fixate the prosthetic biomaterial has been used. A prospective randomized study used a central suture in one group of patients and added the application of the energy source in a second group. The seroma rate was statistically significantly different in the second group (25 vs 4%). This study, however, did not evaluate any hernias that were greater than 100 cm^2 in size, which are the hernias that are the most likely to develop notable fluid accumulations postoperatively [34]. Nevertheless, this may be a useful technique. There is a potential risk of the excessive application of the electrosurgical energy to the thin area of the hernia itself, which can result in a full-thickness necrosis of the thin subcutaneous tissue and skin. This, in turn, can lead to sloughing of the tissue and exposure of the prosthetic biomaterial, this increasing the risk of infection. This theoretical aspect has not received significant attention in the literature, however.

In an effort to inhibit or diminish the development of these known problems, many surgeons will place an abdominal binder on the patient while he or she is still on the operating table. This will be worn for 3–14 days, depending upon the initial size of the protruding hernia. The size of the binder, the length of time that its use is recommended, and whether a bulky dressing is used have not been standardized. There have been no prospective randomized trials to evaluate the effectiveness of this maneuver, but the experience of this author and others appears to suggest that there is a decrease in both the size and duration of clinically significant seromas by as much as 50% [32].

Once the seroma is confirmed, the management of this problem is controversial. Many surgeons believe that these problems will resolve, usually within 12 weeks, if given enough time to do so [19,29,30,35]. Not all authors agree, however. Carbajo aspirated all of the 11.8% of seromas that occurred in his recent series without any complication [17]. I do not attempt to aspirate seromas unless the patient remains symptomatic for longer than 6 months and the ultrasonic evidence does not reveal any significant resolution of the seroma. If the patient is obviously symptomatic and experiencing pain, this will require earlier intervention. One or two aspirations will usually suffice. However, this complication occurs in less than 1% of my patients.

Aspiration is not free of risk. Bacteria can be introduced into the fluid collection, with a resulting infection. This has been noted in a few series [7,19]. Therefore strict sterile technique is mandatory. Additionally, I prefer to obtain an ultrasonic examination of the fluid collection to make sure that a recurrent hernia is not misdiagnosed, so that bowel would be inadvertently punctured during the procedure. This test will also identify the presence of a multiloculated fluid collection, which would be difficult to aspirate. If such is found, ultrasonically directed aspiration or even incision and drainage would be needed to adequately treat the seroma. This is rarely necessary, however.

A computed tomography (CT) scan can also be used to evaluate the hernia sac. This can be another effective tool to verify whether the content of the former hernia site is a recurrent hernia or a seroma. Interestingly, one study noted that some of the postoperative fluid collections contained air as late as 6–12 days postoperatively [31]. This can mimic either a recurrent hernia or an abscess. None of the cases in which this was discovered required any intervention and all resolved. Therefore clinical and laboratory correlation is important.

Persistent Postoperative Pain

In deference to other laparoscopic procedures, LIVH can be associated with more abdominal pain than the initial laparotomy that eventuated in the incisional hernia. This is probably based on the use of the fixation devices needed to secure the prosthesis to the wall of the abdomen. Additionally, it is believed that transfascial sutures will incorporate the subcutaneous nerves as well as the muscle tissue, which increases the degree and persistence of postoperative pain. Because the average length of hospital stay after these procedures is approximately 1–2 days, it must be assumed that the acute postoperative pain is manageable with oral analgesics [9,17,20].

The problematic cases are those where the pain persists beyond 6–8 weeks, which occurs in 1–2% of patients [9,16,20]. This type of pain must not be confused with the pain associated with a large, persistent seroma. The two are usually easily differentiated by history and, if necessary, radiological testing. The latter type of pain will usually be described as sharp, intermittent, and intense. It can be exacerbated by movement, deep breathing, or a cough.

If such a condition appears to be present, one should first evaluate the hernia site with ultrasonography or CT scanning. This will be needed to affirm that there is no persistent seroma or a recurrent hernia that is actually causing the pain. If none is found, initial treatment consist of either nonsteroidal anti-inflammatory drugs or a brief course of steroids. This, of course, can be initiated at any point in the course of evaluating the problem. If it does not result in improvement, injection at the site of the pain with bupivacaine may result in the complete resolution of symptoms. This, too, can be done at the outset of this complaint. If successful, only one or two injections are usually required.

If significant pain persists, laparoscopy may become necessary. Adhesions can be lysed and any sutures (or tacks) at the site of the apparent pain can be cut and/or removed. While very seldom required, in the experience of this and other authors, this is a very effective way to eliminate the pain in nearly every patient [16]. An alternative is the direct approach through an incision over the suture site under local anesthesia. The suture can be excised, but this is usually difficult in the patients with a large amount of subcutaneous tissue.

Infection

One of the great benefits of this operation is the decrease in the frequency of wound complications in these patients [8]. Measures that have been suggested to minimize this risk include careful surgical preparation of the abdominal surface, a plastic iodine-impregnated drape, the use of prophylactic antibiotics, and the choice of a biomaterial that contains an antimicrobial agent. This complication can be seen in up to 16% of these patients [8,9,16,18,20]. The use of a biomaterial (DualMesh Plus, W. L. Gore & Associates, Flagstaff, AZ) that is impregnated with both silver and chlorhexidine has been said to decrease the rate of infection. We have not encountered a postoperative infection when this type of prosthesis was used [9].

This complication can be subdivided into minor and major infections. The minor infections are generally those that involve the sites of the trocar or transfascial suture incisions. These lesions usually present with erythema or drainage, which can be managed with local and parenteral antiobiotics providing gram-positive coverage [25,36]. They should resolve within 7–10 days of treatment. If this approach fails, there is the possibility of a major infection involving the biomaterial.

A major infection that involves the prosthesis can manifest itself by drainage from one of the trocar sites. Therefore lack of a quick response to the treatment outlined above should lead to a CT scan. An ultrasonic examination may not be helpful, as the image may be obscured by the presence of a seroma or significant intestinal gas. These patients will usually also demonstrate a leukocytosis and elevation of the sedimentation rate. If serious infection is confirmed, a short course of parenteral antiobiotics with drainage has been successful in a very few cases [16,19]. But in the majority, removal of the biomaterial will be necessary to eradicate the infection. This is particularly true if the prosthesis contains a component of expanded polytetrafluoroethylene (ePTFE) [9,18,20]. The use of a polypropylene mesh does not, however, guarantee that the mesh will not have to be removed in the face of an infection [36]. Removal of the mesh nearly always results in a recurrence of the original hernia [9,20,25,36,37].

The seldom discussed difficulty associated with an infection of the prosthetic biomaterial is the usually large defect that remains after the patch that repairing the fascial defect has been removed. Almost with certainty, the patient will be left with the original hernia. Attempts at primary tissue repair in such a case are fraught with failure because most of these hernias are larger than 4 cm and are associated with an infection at the time of removal of the patch, both of factors which increase the incidence of recurrence. In an effort to accomplish excision of the biomaterial and repair of the hernia, two other options exist. There are few, if any, reports in the literature of these procedures for this problem.

If the patient is stable and not septic, one may elect to excise the central portion of the patch sequentially. The remaining material will then be sewn together to reapproximate the prosthesis. The patient will then be returned to the operating room several days later (usually after 7–10 days) for another partial excision of the central portion of the patch. During that time local wound care, dressing changes, and parenteral antibiotics are continued. Usually, within 2–3 weeks, the fascial edges will be approximated enough that a primary repair with sutures can be accomplished without concern of an abdominal compartment syndrome. There is still a high risk of recurrence, but this may be lower and less certain than with an initial closure of the infected hernia defect. This approach has not been published to date, but I have used this technique successfully.

Another alternative for the treatment of major infection is excision of the infected biomaterial and a tension-free closure of the hernia defect with one of the collagen matrix biomaterials currently available. The potential advantages of these products are that they appear strong enough to repair the hernia defect and may be resistant to infection. A formal laparotomy can be performed during which the prosthesis is excised and replaced with one of these biomaterials, preferably placed with a Rives-Stoppa technique. Drains are then placed and the skin is closed over the prosthesis. There are anecdotal reports of the success of this method. The use of this repair in an infected setting can only be performed if there is no enteric fistula. An enteric fistula will dissolve the collagen in the product, which will render it useless as a prosthesis.

Finally, it is important for the surgeon to be aware that the skin overlying the hernia defect may actually be normal and uninfected despite the fact that there is significant erythema. This can appear after several days following the operation (Fig. 1). This condition has not been adequately described in the literature but can be a source of significant concern. It may occur in approximately 2–13% percent of the patients [8,29,30]. This can be alarming in that the surgeon may suspect that an infection exists or is developing. In my experience, this will usually be seen in obese patients, those with an incarcerated hernia, or the patients who require a large amount of tissue dissection during the operation. This condition is unassociated with fever, pain or leukocytosis. It does not require treatment and will usually resolve in 4–6 weeks (Fig. 2).

Bowel Obstruction

This is another infrequent complication of LIVH. The obvious concern with this entity is the need to ascertain the correct diagnosis. A patient with this condition may exhibit the signs and symptoms of an ileus, obstruction, or acute abdomen. Diagnosis and treatment must be rapid and accurately performed. As noted above, a significant number of patients will develop an ileus that resolves with conservative management. Those that do not resolve should be investigated further to rule out an organic obstruction or a missed enterotomy. The usual radiological tests may be sufficient for some patients, but one should be quick to obtain a CT scan

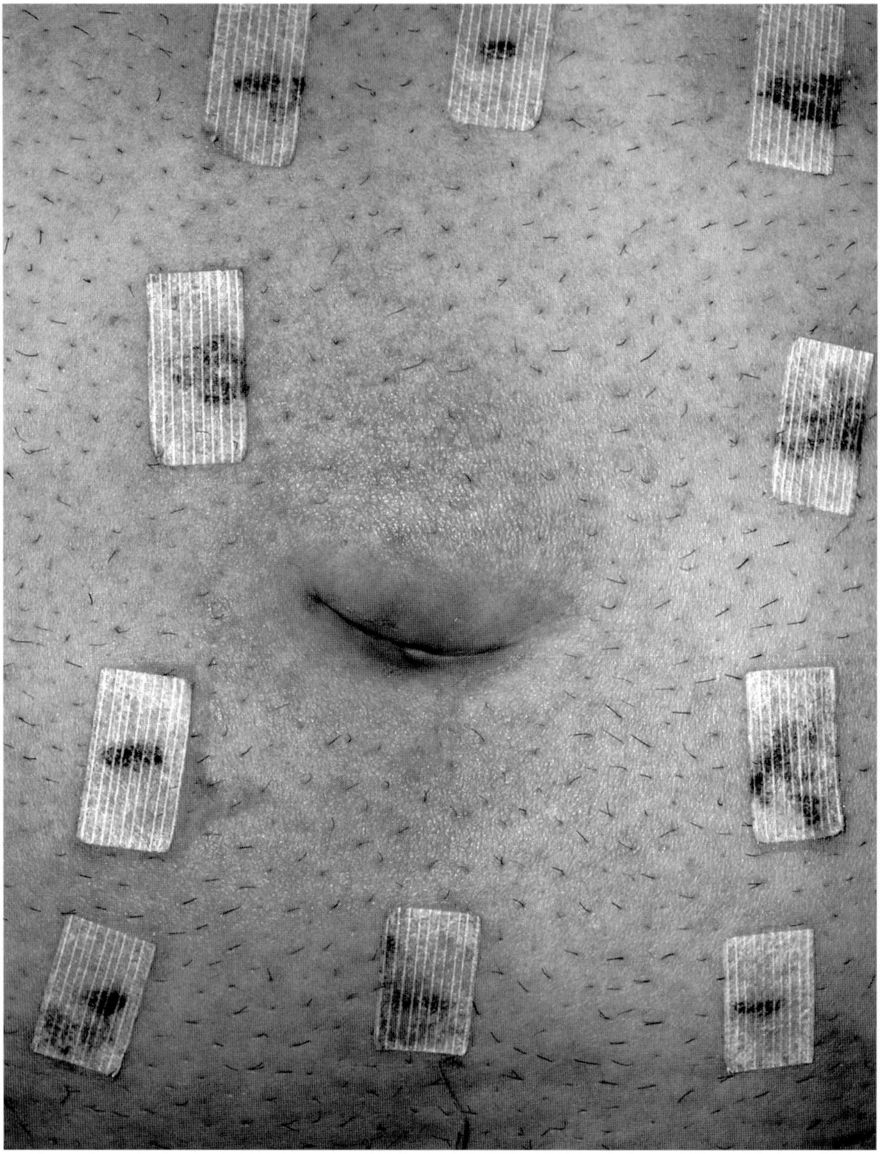

FIGURE 1 Postoperative erythema 1 week after LIVH.

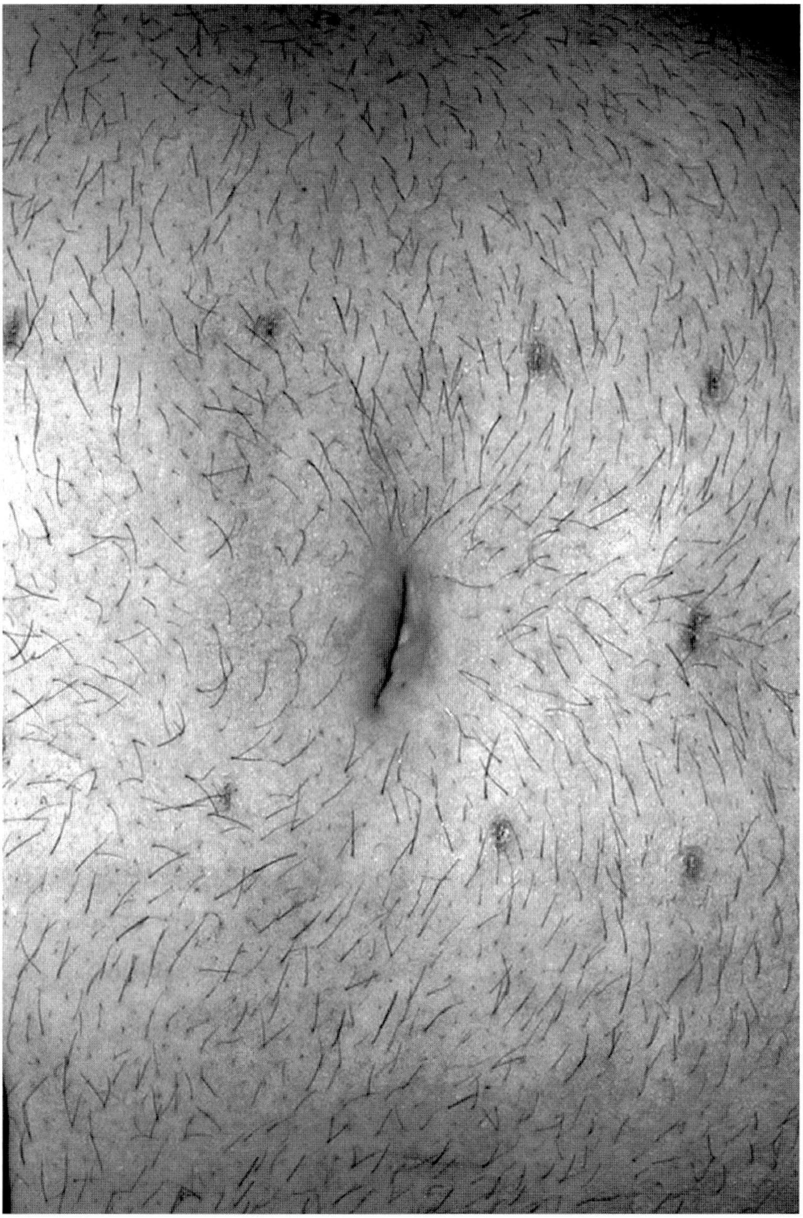

FIGURE 2 Resolution of the erythema in Fig. 1 after 4 weeks.

to investigate the appearance of the entire abdominal cavity. This may be the only test that will reveal fluid-filled, distended loops of small intestine, air-fluid levels, or significant free air in the abdominal cavity. One should also not forget that the possibility of a trocar hernia as the source of this condition (see Chapter 3.)

This complication has been reported in only a few series but has ranged from 0.3–3% in these papers [16,17,38]. These reports represent a total of six patients. Three of these obstructions were due to the migration of the small bowel between the biomaterial and the anterior abdominal wall. In these reports, the exact sites at which the fixation devices were placed were not given. One could assume, however, that these devices were too far apart to prevent this complication. This reiterates the recommendation that transfascial sutures should be placed no more than 5 cm apart and that additional tacks or constructs should be placed at 1- to 1.5-cm intervals along the periphery of the biomaterial [39,40]. The other obstructions in the six patients noted above were caused by postoperative adhesions. In one of these cases, there was associated colonic erosion due to a polypropylene mesh that was inserted 23 months prior to the event [16].

If there is no indication of a bowel injury or the presence of gangrenous obstruction, nasogastric suction and hydration is a reasonable treatment. If the condition of the patient deteriorates or does not improve, surgical intervention will be necessary. Either laparoscopy or laparotomy can be used to access the abdominal cavity.

Enterocutaneous Fistula

This is quite an unusual complication of LIVH but one that has been reported in a few series. The exact etiology has not been determined in all instances because of the rarity of this problem. At least three enterocutaneous fistulas have been noted in the literature [16,17]. This represented an incidence of 0.3 and 1.4%, respectively, in these series. These were reported both in the early and late postoperative period. Only one of these was successfully managed nonoperatively. The other two cases required open surgical resection or simple suture repair and drainage. While the causes of these fistulas were not identified in the reports, one could assume that an unrecognized enterotomy resulted in the development of the fistulas subsequent to the operation. Additionally, erosion by one of the tacks into the intestine has already been suggested as an etiological factor in the development of an intestinal fistula [7].

The workup of this complication should proceed as it would for any other enterocutaneous fistula. Examinations can include CT scans and fistulograms. From the reports in the literature, the use of nonsurgical treatment may be an option in some patients. Surgical intervention appears to be successful more often that the nonoperative option. One must be sure that the appearance of the fistula does not also represent drainage from a prosthetic infection. This, however, should not be too difficult a task, given the amount and characteristics of the drainage.

Miscellaneous Complications

Pneumonias and other pulmonary complications are common to all surgical procedures. While these can sometimes be prevented, they cannot be eliminated completely. Adequate preoperative preparation of all patients, especially those with a history of pulmonary disease, should help to minimize the risk. Factors that increase the risk include the need for general anesthesia, the placement of the fixation devices resulting in splinting of the abdominal wall, and the postoperative ileus that is often seen in these patients. Respiratory failure or pneumonia can be seen in 0.49–3.5% of patients [20,41–43]. However, most reported series have found that there are few respiratory problems with this operation. The appropriate management of these complications will be dictated by the clinical condition of the patient, as after other surgical interventions.

Although quite rare, the development of a pneumothorax has been reported. This developed after the passage of subcostal transfascial suture that traversed the pleural space [15]. It was successfully managed by closed-tube drainage.

Urinary complications such as retention or infection can be seen with some frequency following this operation, an occurrence well known to hernia repair. These events have been reported in 0.74–3.6% of these individuals, commonly male [10,16,17,43]. Given the usual age of these patients, these problems are not unexpected. The usual treatment will be given to those so affected.

Trocar hernias were more commonly seen in the early period of the development of this operation [9]. The usual site is at the insertion sites of trocars larger than 5 mm. This has been reported in 0.25–3% of these operations [9,15,20]. The larger trocars were used almost exclusively in the past, but now more of the smaller trocars are used. Some surgeons will use only the smaller trocars for the entire procedure [39]. Prevention of these hernias can be aided with the use of one of the dilating trocars rather than the cutting variety, resulting in a smaller defect. At the completion of the operation, the larger trocar sites should be closed with the same suture-passing instrument that places the fixating sutures. Additionally, any trocar sites that have been significantly manipulated during the procedure may have become larger, so that closure of these also will be prudent. Further discussion of this topic can be found in Chapter 3.

The repair of these hernias can be either with an open or a laparoscopic technique. A small hernia in a thin patient can be approached more easily from the anterior surface than a larger hernia in an obese patient. The exact sizing of the defect can be difficult or impossible in many of these cases. Whichever method is chosen, the use of a prosthetic biomaterial is recommended. These patients have demonstrated a propensity for hernia formation and may have a collagen deficiency predisposing them to hernia development. A tension-free repair will afford the best long-term result in these patients. A possible exception may be the development of a hernia in the immediate postoperative period. In that situation, the use of transfascial suturing will be easy and reliable [15,19].

Recurrence

This complication is the true measure of the effectiveness of any hernioplasty. Recurrence rates of 50% are associated with the tissue repair of incisional hernias, while the use of a prosthetic biomaterial in the open approach has lowered this to approximately 25% and less. The cumulative recurrence rate of the laparoscopic repair is about 4.4% in the current literature. It should be acknowledged that these latter series are obtained with a follow-up that usually is only about 3 years, but this is the time frame within which most recurrences with the open repair are seen [44]. In our experience with the laparoscopic approach, we have also found that a 3-year follow-up is necessary to accurately assess the recurrences seen after this procedure [19].

The recurrences that we have seen in our own patients, early in our experience, were due to inadequate size of the biomaterial and the use of a method of fixation that did not include transfascial sutures [19]. In our first 100 patients, the additional use of transfascial sutures reduced the number of recurrences from 13% to zero. Based on this experience, the use of two methods of fixation including sutures is an integral part of the procedure in all patients.

At least six studies have compared the open procedure with the laparoscopic repair. Thoman summarized five of these in 2002, and several were referenced earlier in this chapter. In all but one of these comparison studies the laparoscopic repair was associated with a lower rate of recurrence [45]. It should be noted that this paper erroneously reported a higher recurrence rate for one study for the laparoscopic group, that of Carbajo. The only report that has a higher incidence of recurrences was that of DeMaria, which represented only one patient [7]. That series represented the early experience of the surgeons. Another study compared the open repair without mesh, open repair with mesh, and laparoscopic repair. The respective recurrence rates of these patients were 9, 6, and 1% [37]. The rate of relapse of hernias has been consistently shown to decline with the use of mesh, and it declines further with the minimally invasive approach.

A summary of several large series that all comprise more than 100 patients is shown in Table 2. Several show a fairly large number of recurrences. The majority of these occurred in the learning phase of the operators' experience or were due to a complication that occurred following the hernia repair, such as an infection or a bowel fistula. In our own series, we noted that the lack of sutures, too small a prosthesis, or infection led to recurrence. The second 100 patients in our series had recurrences that were due to different etiologies than the first 100,

TABLE 2 Recurrence Rates After Incisional and Ventral Hernia Repair

Author	Number of Patients	Recurrence Rate (%)
Heniford	100	3
Rosen	100	17
Franklin	112	1
Toy	144	4
Bageacu	159	15.7
LeBlanc	200	6.5
Chowbey	202	1
Carbajo	270	4.4
Heniford	407	2
Total	**1694**	**4.4**

usually infections that required excision of the prosthesis. Two other recurrences in the latter group were due to a suture fracture or a new hernia that appeared below the prior repair. There was also a decline in the rate of recurrence from 9% to 4% between these two groups of patients [9]. As shown in this table, the average recurrence was still an acceptable 4.4%, similar to that of most reported series in the literature.

The secure repair of any hernia so that a recurrence is not seen postoperatively is the goal of all surgeons. Even in this procedure, this has not been achieved nor is it expected to eliminate any recurrence. Some risk factors—such as advanced age, obesity, pulmonary or hepatic insufficiency, and steroid usage—cannot be avoided. However, there are issues that the surgeon can address to minimize the risk of recurrence, such as provision of an adequate exposure of the defect, so that all of the prosthetic biomaterial contacts fascia rather than preperitoneal fat. It is necessary to provide a complete fascial surface to allow the biomaterial to be adjacent to it, so that maximum tissue penetration occurs. The interposition of adipose tissue will impede this process and predispose to a recurrence.

Whatever biomaterial is used, it must overlap the defect by 3 cm or more. This distance has been shown to decrease the recurrence rate [8–10,19]. Other authors believe that a 5-cm overlap should be used [13,17]. There is no argument with that figure, but it may be difficult to obtain in some cases. However, the larger overlap should be used in those hernias that are located very high or low on the abdominal wall and in significantly obese individuals. This large overlap of the biomaterial reduces the tension on the repair, which will assist in the prevention of recurrence. Additionally, the more difficult areas of fixation, such as those mentioned, will benefit from a larger surface area to allow ingrowth of fibroblasts and collagen and account for any contraction of the tissues that could result in a decrease in the surface area of the product. It is also recommended to place a large enough piece of biomaterial so that as much of the incision that developed the hernia is covered, with the intention of preventing the development of a later hernia above or below the current repair [9].

One of the most critical aspects of this repair is to make sure that the biomaterial is adequately fixed to the abdominal wall to ensure an effective repair. This fixation should include transfascial sutures. As noted earlier, we demonstrated the effectiveness of this technique in our first 100 patients by eliminating a recurrence, with an average follow-up of 51 months in these patients. My preference is to place these sutures no more than 5 cm apart along the periphery of the patch using a suture-passing instrument. Others place them 4–6 cm apart [13,20].

Not all authors share the view that there is a need for these transfascial sutures. Berger uses sutures merely to position the prosthesis and does not tie them. He believes that sutures increase postoperative pain [15]. His recurrence rate was only 2.7% but there was less than 2 years of follow-up. Carbajo shares the same view [17]. In his series spanning more than 8 years, there was a recurrence rate of only 4.4%. This type of result is uncommon, but Rosen found no difference in recurrence regardless of the methods of fixation [18]. In that series, there were many surgeons with no standardized technique; therefore it cannot be a valid assumption that fixation does not affect the recurrence rate. This is confirmed by Bageacu, in that the recurrence rate was 15.7% when only two or four transfascial sutures were used [16]. A recent experimental study confirmed the superior strength of sutures versus tacks alone to fix mesh against the abdominal wall. The results of that study indicate that the ‘‘addition of transabdominal sutures should be preferred’’ [46]. A large overlap of prostheses does not appear to be protective against recurrence because a 9-cm overlap without sutures has been followed by a recurrence [13].

Finally, the fixation by a metal device is undisputed. I prefer to place the Onux Salute constructs (Onux Medical, Inc., Hampton, NH) approximately 1–1.5 cm apart between the sutures. This is usually followed by a second row behind the first to ease the tension on the initial row (Fig. 3). This appears to provide the best fixation of the patch so that the patch is flat against the abdominal wall with no rollover [47]. Others recommend 1.5 cm [13]. Carbajo uses only tacks (ProTack, USSG/Tyco International, Norwalk, CT) placed 2 cm apart. A second row is then placed inside of this one to perform the ‘‘double-crown’’ technique. This appears to be successful in his series of patients. He uses a 1.5-mm-thick DualMesh Plus product with holes [17]. Whether or not this affects his outcomes is undetermined.

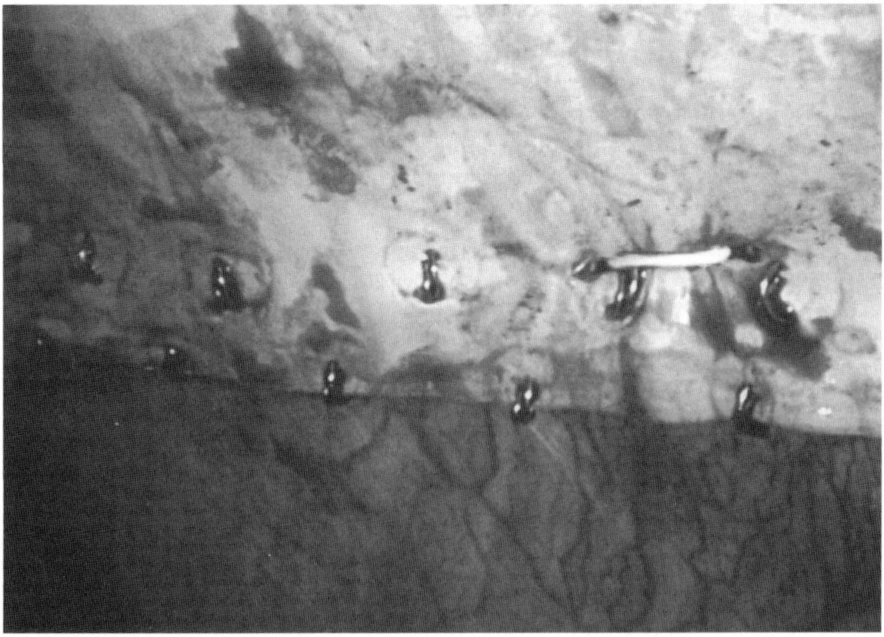

FIGURE 3 Correct positioning of the constructs and transfascial sutures along the periphery of the biomaterial.

If a recurrence is suspected, an ultrasonic examination may differentiate between this and a seroma. A CT scan is the preferred method of diagnosis even if the patient has an obvious hernia. This study will enable the surgeon to plan the necessary repair. It would be helpful if the presence of incarcerated bowel in the sac were noted preoperatively. The repair can easily be approached laparoscopically in most cases. The trocar positions may differ from those of the original procedure due to the location of the recurrence. One should uncover the entire prosthesis unless it is impossible to do so due to adhesions or bleeding. The repair can be effected with an additional biomaterial with the same fixation (including sutures). I prefer a larger overlap and more fixation for a recurrence. It must be remembered that the ePTFE patch-to-patch interface will not achieve any ingrowth of tissue. Therefore the fixation of the biomaterial is dependent upon its manner of fixation. Removal of the previously placed mesh is not recommended.

CONCLUSION

LIVH is a very successful procedure that is gaining in popularity. The majority of repairs are performed with the use of an ePTFE patch, transfascial sutures, and additional metal fixation devices. These methods decrease the rate of recurrence. The most difficult portion of the operation is the lysis of adhesions, which can result in an enterotomy. Recognition of this and other complications can be assured only with a high index of suspicion and appropriate testing, which is then followed by the appropriate treatment. Despite the most stringent care and the surgeon's best abilities, complications cannot always be avoided. The proper management of these when they occur is, therefore, of critical importance.

REFERENCES

1. LeBlanc KA, Booth WV. Laparoscopic repair of incisional abdominal hernias using expanded polytetrafluoroethylene: Preliminary findings. Surg Laparosc Endosc 1993; 3:39–41.
2. LeBlanc KA, Bellanger DE. Laparoscopic repair of paraostomy hernias. J Am Coll Surg 2002; 194(2):232–239.
3. Deol ZK, Shayani V. Laparoscopic parastomal hernia repair. Arch Surg 2003; 138: 203–205.
4. Hirasa T, Pickleman J, Shayani V. Laparoscopic repair of parapubic hernia. Arch Surg 2001; 136:1314–1317.
5. Leber GE, Garb JL, Alexander AI, Reed WP. Long-term complications associated with prosthetic repair of incisional hernias. Arch Surg 1998; 133:378–382.
6. White TJ, Santos MC, Thompson JS. Factors affecting wound complications in repair of ventral hernias. Am Surg 1998; 64(3):276–280.
7. DeMaria EJ, Moss JM, Surgerman HJ. Laparscopic intraperitoneal polytetrafluoroethylene (PTFE) prosthetic patch repair of ventral hernia. Surg Endosc 2000; 14: 326–329.
8. Robbins SB, Pofahl W, Gonzales RP. Laparoscopic ventral hernia repair reduces wound complications. Am Surg 2001; 9:896–900.
9. LeBlanc KA, Whitaker JM, Bellanger DE, Rhynes VK. Laparoscopic incisional and ventral hernioplasty: Lessons learned from 200 patients. Hernia 2003; 7:118–124.
10. Ramshaw BJ, Esartia P, Schwab J, Mason EM, et al. Comparison of laparoscopic and open ventral herniorrhaphy. Am Surg 1999; 65:827–832.
11. Park A, Birch DW, Lovrics P. Laparoscopic and open incisonal hernia repair: A comparison study. Surgery 1998; 124(4):816–822.
12. Carbajo MA, Martin del Olmo JC, Blanco JI, de la Cuesta C, Toledano M, et al. Laparoscopic treatment vs open surgery in the solution of major incisional and abdominal wall hernias with mesh. Surg Endosc 1999; 13:250–252.
13. Koehler RH, Voeller G. Recurrences in laparoscopic incisional hernia repairs: A personal series and review of the literature. JSLS 1999; 3:293–304.
14. Chari R, Chari V, Eisenstat M, Chung R. A case controlled study of laparoscopic incisional hernia repair. Surg Endosc 2000; 14:117–119.
15. Berger D, Bientzle M, Mäller A. Postoperative complications after laparoscopic incisional hernia repair. Surg Endosc 2002; 16:1720–1723.
16. Bageacu S, Blanc P, Breton C, Gonzales M, et al. Laparoscopic repair of incisional hernias. Surg Endosc 2002; 16:345–348.

17. Carbajo MA, Martín del Olmo JC, Blanco JI, Toledano M, et al. Laparoscopic approach to incisional hernia. Surg Endosc 2003; 17:118–122.
18. Rosen M, Brody F, Ponsky J, Walsh RM, et al. Recurrence after laparoscopic ventral hernia repair. Surg Endosc 2003; 17:123–128.
19. LeBlanc KA, Booth WV, Whitaker JM, Bellanger DE. Laparoscopic incisional and ventral herniorraphy in 100 patients. Am J Surg 2000; 180(3):193–197.
20. Heniford TB, Park A, Ramshaw BJ, Voeller G. Laparoscopic ventral and incisional hernia repair in 407 patients. J Am Coll Surg 2000; 190(6):645–650.
21. Voeller G. Laparoscopic repair in the emergent setting. In: LeBlanc K, ed. Laparoscopic Hernia Surgery: An Operative Guide. London: Arnold Medical Publishers, 2003, 111–113.
22. Moreno-Egea A, Castillo Bustos JA, Aguayo JI. Day surgery for laparoscopic repair of abdominal wall hernias. Hernia 2002; 6:21–25.
23. Feingold DL, Widmann WD, Calhoun SK, Teigen EL, et al. Persistent post-laparoscopy pneumoperitoneum. Surg Endosc 2003; 17:296–299.
24. Toy FK, Bailey RW, Carey S, Chappuis CW, et al. Prospective, multicenter study of laparoscopic ventral hernioplasty. Surg Endosc 1998; 12:955–959.
25. Rosen M, Brody F, Ponsky J, Walsh RM, et al. Recurrence after laparoscopic ventral hernia repair. Surg Endosc 2003; 17:123–128.
26. Holzman MD, Purut CM, Reintgen K, Eubanks S, Pappas TN. Laparoscopic ventral and incisional henioplasty. Surg Endosc 1997; 11:32–35.
27. Farooqui MO, Bazzoli JM. Significance of radiologic evidence of free air following laparoscopy. J Reprod Med 1976; 16(3):119–125.
28. Susmallian S, Gewurtz G, Ezri T, Charuzi I. Seroma after laparoscopic repair of hernia with PTFE patch: Is it really a complication. Hernia 2001; 5:139–141.
29. Parker HH, Nottingham JM, Bynoc RP, Yost MJ. Laparoscopic repair of large incisional hernias. Am Surg 2002; 68(6):530–534.
30. Kirshtein B, Lantsberg L, Avinoach E, Bayma M, et al. Laparoscopic repair of large incisional hernias. Surg Endosc 2002; 16:1717–1719.
31. Lin BHJ, Vargish T, Dachman AH. CT findings after laparoscopic repair of ventral hernias. Am J Radiol 1999; 172:389–392.
32. Chowbey PK, Sharma A, Khullar R, Baijal R, Vashistha A. Laparoscopic ventral hernia repair. J Laparoendosc Adv Surg Tech 2000; 10(2):79–84.
33. Gillian GK, Geis WP, Grover G. Laparoscopic incisional and ventral hernia repair (LIVH): An evolving outpatient technique. JSLS 2002; 6:315–322.
34. Tsimoyiannis EC, Siakas P, Glantzouissis G, Koulas S, et al. Seroma in laparoscopic ventral hernioplasty. Surg Laparosc Endosc Percut Tech 2001; 11(5):31–321.
35. Park A, Heniford BT, LeBlanc KA, Voeller GR. Laparoscopic repair of incisional hernias. Part 2: Surgical technique. Contemp Surg 2001; 57(5):225–238.
36. Franklin ME, Dorman JP, Glass JL, Balli JE, Gonzales JJ. Laparoscopic ventral and incisional hernia repair. Surg Laparosc Endosc 1998; 8(4):294–299.
37. Wright BE, Niskanen BD, Peterson DJ, Ney AL, et al. Laparoscopic ventral hernia repair: Are there comparative advantages over traditional methods of repair. Am Surg 2002; 68(3):291–296.
38. Ben-Haim M, Kuriansky J, Tal R, Zmora O, et al. Pitfalls and complications with laparoscopic intraperitoneal expanded polytetrafluoroethylene patch repair of postoperative ventral hernia. Surg Endosc 2002; 16:785–788.

39. LeBlanc KA. Current considerations in laparoscopic incisional and ventral herniorraphy. JSLS 2000; 4:131–139.
40. LeBlanc KA. The critical technical aspects of laparoscopic repair of ventral and incisional hernias. Am Surg 2001; 67(8):809–812.
41. Roth JS, Park AE, Witzke D, Mastrangelo MJ. Laparoscopic incisional/ventral herniorraphy: A five-year experience. Hernia 1999; 4:209–214.
42. Aura T, Habib E, Mekkaoui M, Brassier D, et al. Laparoscopic tension-free repair of anterior abdominal incisional and ventral hernias with an intraperitoneal Gore-Tex mesh: Prospective study and review of the literature. J Laparoendosc Adv Surg Tech 2002; 12(4):263–267.
43. Heniford BT, Ramshaw BJ. Laparoscopic ventral hernia repair. Surg Endosc 2000; 14:419–423.
44. Hesselink VJ, Luijendijk RW, de Wilt JHW, Heide R, Jeekel J. An evaluation of risk factors in incisional hernia recurrence. Surg Gynecol Obst 1993; 176:228–234.
45. Thoman DS, Phillips EH. Current status of laparoscopic ventral hernia repair. Surg Endosc 2002; 16:939–942.
46. van't Riet M, de Vos van Steinwijk PJ, Kleiniensink GJ, et al. Tensile strength of mesh fixation methods in laparoscopic incisional hernia repair. Surg Endosc 2002; 16:1713–1716.
47. LeBlanc KA, Bellanger DE, Rhynes KU, Baker DS, Stout R. Tissue attachment strength of prosthetic meshes used in vertral and incisional hernia repair: a study in the New Zealand white rabbit adhesion model. Surg Endosc 2002; 16(11):1542–1546.

15

Inguinal Hernia Repair

Guy Voeller
Memphis, TennesseeU.S.A.

INTRODUCTION

Cheatle was the first surgeon to mention the retroinguinal space of Bogros, used to perform laparoscopic inguinal hernia repair. He performed high ligation of the indirect hernia sac using a posterior preperitoneal approach. Henry ''rediscovered'' Cheatle's work in 1926 and Jennings in the United States wrote a paper in 1942 about the same approach, labeling it a ''new method.'' Many subsequent surgeons refined this autogenous approach, with Nyhus as its main proponent in the early 1960s [1].

Acquaviva, using an anterior approach, was the first to place mesh in the preperitoneal space for hernia repair [2]. Estrin, in the United States, was the first to place a unilateral piece of mesh via a posterior preperitoneal approach after repairing the hernia primarily [3]. In 1967, Rives, in France, described a similar procedure; a picture from this shows posteriorization of the cord structures. Stoppa was the first to use mesh via a posterior preperitoneal approach without first repairing the hernia defect. We place a unilateral piece of mesh laparoscopically without suturing the hernia—what we might call an Estrin-Rives-Stoppa repair [4].

In the United States, following the introduction of the laparoscopic approach to the repair of inguinal hernias, the transabdominal preperitoneal (TAPP) approach was initially the dominant laparoscopic repair. Dulucq in Europe reported a large series of laparoscopic inguinal hernia repairs using a totally extraperitoneal

(TEP) technique. From 1990 to 1995 he performed 864 repairs with no major complications and only three recurrences [5]. Many others soon followed with both TAPP and TEP series. While both the TAPP and TEP are done with equal success, the TEP is the technique that is predominantly taught today.

The procedure of laparoscopic inguinal hernia repair (LIHR) has matured so much since its introduction in the early 1990s that, when done by an experienced surgeon, serious complications are extremely rare. Minor complications (what should be more properly called ''side effects''), such as bruising and seromas, are not uncommon and are seen in the hands of even the most experienced surgeons. This chapter presents the current methods of laparoscopic inguinal hernioplasty and the complications associated with them. Most importantly, the prevention and avoidance of these events is described.

PREOPERATIVE PREPARATION TO AVOID COMPLICATIONS

The British government, as well as many ''experts,'' have stated that LIHR should be performed only for recurrent inguinal hernias or bilateral inguinal hernias. This philosophy, I believe, is certain to lead to major complications. There is a long learning curve to LIHR. Therefore, the notion that one can get past the learning curve by operating only on the two most difficult repairs (i.e., recurrent and bilateral) is foolish and dangerous. When the surgeon first approaches this operation, a properly done unilateral LIHR will take 2 hr to complete and sometimes longer. Hundreds of repairs must be done to decrease the operative time to 30–45 min. For the novice surgeon, to have to repair a bilateral groin hernia may be asking too much of both patient and surgeon. In the case of recurrent hernias, the preperitoneal anatomy is distorted, and the larger the number of previous repairs, the greater the distortion. To encounter unfamiliar anatomy that is also scarred from the prior surgery is dangerous for both patient and surgeon. For these reasons, we believe that the beginning laparoscopic surgeon must learn LIHR through the repair of primary unilateral hernias rather than more complex defects. This will avert bad results and dissatisfaction with the technique.

While LIHR can be accomplished with epidural or spinal anesthesia, general anesthesia is usually utilized. We have successfully performed LIHR on hundreds of patients with cardiac and respiratory disease without major morbidity. The key to a successful outcome is careful patient selection, preoperative evaluation by internists, and high-quality anesthesia. In our series of over 2000 TEP repairs, there has not been a death. There has been one myocardial infarction and one pulmonary embolus. Thus, the only strong contraindication for LIHR is the inability of the patient to safely tolerate general anesthesia.

The novice surgeon should generally avoid patients with previous preperitoneal surgery. The scarring from the previous surgery presents difficulty in the identification of the proper anatomy and increases the risk of complications. This was confirmed by Ramshaw, who found increased morbidity in patients with previous preperitoneal surgery [6]. We avoid LIHR in anyone who has had an open prostatectomy for the above reasons. Last, the novice surgeon should not attempt to repair large inguinoscrotal hernias. If the contents can be returned into the abdominal cavity preoperatively or with the induction of anesthesia, LIHR is possible in experienced hands. If the viscera cannot be reduced, we favor an open repair to avoid morbidity.

INTRAOPERATIVE COMPLICATIONS

For safe LIHR, a new up-to-date video system is critical. This is especially true for TEP repair. During laparoscopic cholecystectomy, the liver is a constant "backstop" that aids the surgeon in the maintenance of his or her orientation. In LIHR, this is not the case; there are several important structures within millimeters of the proper plane of dissection that can easily be injured if visualization is impaired. These potential problems mandate that the best light source, camera, and laparoscope be available for the procedure.

Access into the abdominal cavity for the TAPP repair can be with either a Verress needle or open Hasson-type technique. Basic laparoscopic training pertains to this method, in that the avoidance of visceral or vascular injury is no different than in any other laparoscopic surgical procedure. The TAPP repair poses the additional risk of injury to the inferior epigastric vessels as the lateral trocars are placed. Proper identification of these vessels with the laparoscope and placement of the trocars lateral to the rectus muscle can readily avoid this risk. If the bleeding is not profuse, one can stop it by compressing the abdominal wall between a grasper placed intra-abdominally and a hand placed on the abdominal wall. If the hemorrhage is brisk, it should be controlled by a transfascial U-stitch or figure-of-eight suture.

In TEP repair, the inferior epigastric vessels can be injured during the creation of the preperitoneal space. If the surgeon creates the space manually, the dissector can injure the vessels. If the balloon dissection is used to create the space, branches of the inferior epigastric vessels or their branches can be torn. Such injuries are usually readily controlled with clips and/or cautery, since they can be visualized with the laparoscope. The (hooked) cautery device should be insulated all the way to the tip, because this instrument is very helpful. The insulation will prevent the cautery from "grounding out" onto the other adjacent tissues in the small preperitoneal space.

Urinary bladder injury has been reported during the placement of the balloon down to the pubis. To prevent this occurrence, it is important to keep the tip of the trocar at the level of the pubic bone so that it will not go below that. If the tip of the trocar is used too forcefully, the bladder may then be injured.

Another possible injury can occur when a Foley catheter is used and the balloon for the Foley is inflated with 10–15 mL of water. As the preperitoneal distention balloon is then inflated, it compresses the Foley balloon, thereby creating a shearing type of force against the two balloons; this can tear the bladder. We use a Foley catheter in every case, but with only 4–5 mL of water in the balloon. While many surgeons simply have the patient void before surgery, we have found this to be less than satisfactory because the bladder fills up quickly and can make dissection and mesh placement less than perfect. With the technique outlined above, we have never had a bladder injury of any type in over 2000 TEP repairs.

Figure 1 is an illustration from the third edition of the Nyhus hernia textbook. All of the important structures in the preperitoneal space are depicted. The peritoneum would be covering all of the structures, and it is necessary to dissect this away from these structures to safely perform the LIHR. The two linear structures lying on the psoas muscle are nerves. To avoid serious complications during LIHR, it is critical that the surgeon understand this anatomy thoroughly. The novice can injure any of the pictured structures very quickly and easily; it is rare that the experienced laparoscopic herniologist will do so. However, injury can and does occur even in the ''best of hands.'' The cord structures can be injured with too vigorous dissection of an indirect hernia sac off of the vas deferens or testicular vessels. The iliac vessels lie below the cord structures and can be injured with inaccurate or too vigorous dissection of the cord. The iliac vein is more

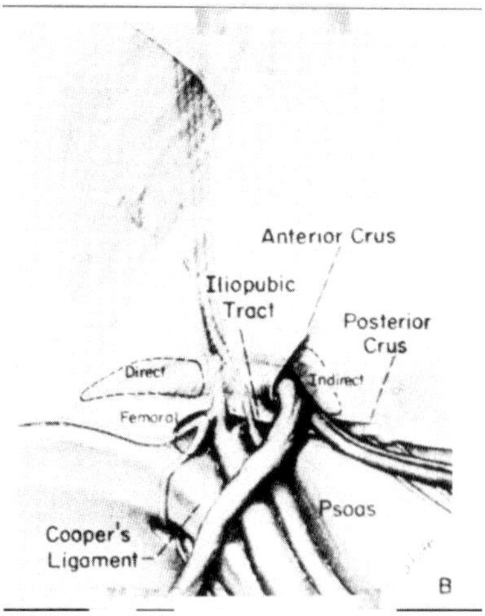

Figure 1 NO LEGEND (CIP)

susceptible to injury with a femoral hernia, since the contents of the hernia can often be incarcerated in such a way that significant force is required to reduce them completely. The vein is the lateral border of a femoral hernia, and great care should be taken to avoid injuring it. If injury does occur, the surgeon will necessarily have to resort to an open procedure, via a lower midline incision, to control and repair the injury. The small bowel and/or colon can be injured with any instrument or energy source. During a TEP repair, the bowel is covered by the peritoneum and an injury will be more easily missed than with the TAPP repair. The surgeon must always be aware of any viscera contained in an indirect or femoral hernia sac, since they can be injured readily. Injury to the cord structures is a well-known complication of all types of inguinal hernia repair. Ischemic orchitis is seen in about 3–5% of open repairs but is very rare in LIHR.

The most often discussed complications of LIHR, especially early in its evolution, were nerve related problems. It is clear from Fig. 1 that the illustrator, long before LIHR was even contemplated, was trying to point out the nerves to be avoided. Skandelakis has shown, using cadavers, that these nerves often run through the iliopubic tract and not just below it, as depicted. Nerve injury is readily avoided during LIHR if a few rules are followed. First, one must know their course along the psoas muscle and up, under, or through the iliopubic tract. The psoas muscle should be revealed by sweeping the peritoneum and fat off of the muscle. This is done so the mesh will lie on the muscle, thus preventing a lateral recurrence under the mesh. During this dissection, the nerves will be revealed. One should never use the cautery in this area. To avoid placing tacks into these nerves, one simply needs to palpate the iliac crest laterally while tacking and never place tacks or any other fixation device below this structure. As the nerves course onto the anterior abdominal wall, it is theoretically possible to place a tack into them, especially in thin patients. The nerves, however, are deep to the muscle; if one is careful about the force used to place these devices, this problem should be avoided. In addition, one should use as few fixation devices as possible. With indirect hernias, the ''funnel'' effect created by the psoas and abdominal muscles makes displacement of a large piece of mesh into the defect very unlikely. For this reason, we will place one tack into the muscle lateral to the epigastric vessels, one into the muscle medial to the epigastric vessels, and one into Cooper's ligament. For direct hernias, where mesh displacement into the defect is more likely, we anchor the mesh into Cooper's ligament with three to five tacks. When properly performed, nerve injury is much less likely with LIHR than an open repair, where the nerves can scar into the mesh, causing neuralgia or a need for neurolysis or transaction to treat any subsequent neuralgia. In over 2000 TEP repairs, we have had one patient who experienced lateral femoral cutaneous nerve irritation 2 weeks postoperatively. This resolved with 2 weeks of treatment with nonsteroidal anti-inflammatory drugs (NSAIDs)

POSTOPERATIVE COMPLICATIONS

Trocar hernias should almost never occur after TEP repair. The working ports are two 5-mm trocars that are placed into the preperitoneal space, and the 10 mm port is, likewise, only in the preperitoneal space. In over 2000 TEPs, we have yet to see a trocar hernia. The TAPP repair, however, *can* lead to trocar hernias, since the ports go into the peritoneal cavity and many surgeons use 10-mm trocars for all of their port sites. These hernias can be eliminated by using 5-mm ports or reduced by suturing all 10-mm port sites. If they are not properly repaired, trocar hernias can, in turn, lead to intestinal obstruction, with all of the risks and complications inherent in acute bowel obstructions. The physical findings can be very subtle, especially if a Richter's hernia is the problem. Therefore, careful examination and evaluation is critical.

The TAPP repair is also unique in that if there are gaps in the closure of the peritoneal incision, bowel obstruction can result. The small bowel can work its way through these defects and even lead to strangulation. For this reason, the peritoneal closure should be done so that no small holes remain. Interestingly, the idea of not closing the peritoneum after TAPP was never entertained owing to worries about adhesions of the bowel to the mesh. However, an animal study showed there were much fewer adhesions if the peritoneum were left open as compared to situations where it was closed (and thus made ischemic) after a TAPP [7]. For these reasons, we never close a hole in the peritoneum if it occurs while a TEP repair is being done. We were the first to describe placing a Verress needle into the peritoneal cavity to decompress it in the event of a tear. This allows the preperitoneal space to be maintained and the repair to be finished. We leave the Verress needle in place until the procedure is completed. It is then the final laparoscopic device to be removed from the patient once we are satisfied that all of the CO_2 carbon dioxide has been evacuated from the abdominal cavity. The peritoneal tear will appear to be a large gaping hole only when the abdomen is distended with CO_2. Once all of the CO_2 has been evacuated, the edges of the tear will oppose one another and soon seal. To support this concept, in our over 2000 TEP repairs, the peritoneum has frequently been torn and handled as above, with no patient developing a bowel obstruction as a result.

Post–hernia repair neuralgia can be seen postoperatively after LIHR, but in experienced hands it is infrequent and occurs less often than that with open repair. The most common complaint is testicular pain, due to irritation of the genital branch of the genitofemoral nerve; it is usually very short-lived. Gentle dissection in the proper planes will help keep the incidence of this problem low. The lateral femoral cutaneous nerve is vulnerable if one places any fixation below the level of the iliac crest. The patient will present with neuralgia paraesthetica, which, when severe, will require removal of the offending tack. An attempt at conservative management is occasionally warranted, because sometimes this problem is short-lived and responsive to analgesics. The ilioinguinal and iliohypogastric nerves are very susceptible to becoming involved in the scarification process following mesh implantation during an *open* inguinal hernia repair. Because of this possibility, some surgeons will transect these nerves at the time of the hernia repair. It is easier for the patient to deal with some transient numbness than with long-term pain. One big advantage of a properly performed LIHR is that these two nerves are left undisturbed. However, in a thin patient, a tack can injure these nerves as they course up onto the anterior abdominal wall. If the pain is severe, the tack will have to be removed, as nonoperative management is rarely successful. If the pain is not incapacitating, a trial of analgesia and/or blocks may cure the problem. Proper and limited use of tacks will avoid most problems. We, like others, have used fibrin glue for LIHR and found it to be effective [8]. However, this has not been widely adopted because (1) its cost is similar to that of the tacker and (2) the glue increases operative time because it must be prepared prior to use, which prolongs the procedure.

Pain from mesh, or ''meshodynia,'' is seen after both laparoscopic and open hernia repair. We havc not had to remove the mesh in any of our 2000 TEP repairs, but have had to do so in several patients referred to us. These patients present with groin pain that is not in a distribution of the nerves. All attempts to avoid surgery should be made. Referral to a pain management expert should be tried initially. If this is not successful, then removal of the mesh and tacks is the only remaining alternative. This is done through a lower midline incision. The patient should be warned that injury to visceral and vascular structures is a risk and that removal, while likely to improve symptoms, may not cure them. Over the past several years we have changed to a soft, pliable polyester mesh (Parietex, Sofradim International, Villfranche-sur-Saône, France) that, unlike polypropylene, does not shrink, contract, or stiffen readily. Klinge and others have shown that heavyweight polypropylene meshes cause loss of compliance with the abdominal wall as they shrink and stiffen [9]. We believe this may play a significant role with respect to mesh-induced discomfort.

Last, certain postoperative sequelae are inherent to LIHR. While not true complications, they need to be dealt with and understood. When a large direct hernia is repaired, fluid can accumulate in the defect after the bowel is removed. This seroma will disappear in most patients. In a small percentage, however, aspiration (in the office) will be required. We were the first to report the laparoscopic usage of the technique described by George Wantz for open repair whereby the transversalis sac is tacked up to the muscle to obliterate this space. This decreases the incidence of seroma formation. Bruising about the pubic area is also frequently seen postoperatively after the TEP repair; it disappears rapidly. The patient should be told about this preoperatively, otherwise it may cause concern that something is wrong.

SUMMARY

It is not possible to eliminate all complications that can occur during and after LIHR. The surgeon interested in performing this procedure well must be dedicated to learning the proper technique from a surgeon who has considerable experience doing LIHR. If this is done, the complication rate will be extremely low and patient satisfaction very high. While patients prefer less invasion with any surgery, we perform LIHR because we believe it is the soundest physiological way to reinforce the entire myopectineal orifice. As George Wantz said: ''When correctly performed, preperitoneal hernioplasty should prevent all hernias of the groin'' [10].

REFERENCES

1. Read RC. Preperitoneal herniorrhaphy: A historical review. World J Surg 1989; 13: 532–540.
2. Bendavid R. Introduction to tension-free repairs. Abdominal Wall Hernias: Principles and Management. New York: Springer-Verlag, 2001, 376.
3. Estrin J, Lipton S, Block IR. The posterior approach to inguinal and femoral hernias. Surg Gynecol Obstet 1963; 116:547.
4. Stoppa R, Wantz GE, Munegato G, et al. Hernia Healers. France: Arnette, 1998.
5. Dulucq J. Laparoscopic groin hernia repair. In: Darzi A, ed. Retroperitoneoscopy. Oxford: Isis Medical Media, 1996, 70–79.
6. Ramshaw BJ, Tucker JG, Conner T, et al. A comparison of the approaches to laparoscopic herniorrhaphy. Surg Endosc 1996; 10:29–32.
7. Durstein-Decker C, Brick W, Gadacz T. Comparison of adhesion formation in transperitoneal laparoscopic herniorrhaphy techniques. Am Surg 1994; 3:157–159.
8. Topart P, Vandenbroucke F, Lozac'h P, et al. Use of human fibrin tissue glue as mesh sealant in laparoscopic totally extraperitoneal (TEPP) repair for groin hernia. Hernia Repair. Tucson. AZ, 2002, 168.
9. Klinge U, Klosterhalfen B, Muller M, et al. Shrinking of polypropylene mesh in vivo: An experimental study in dogs. Eur J Surg 1998; 164:965–969.
10. SGO, 1996.

16

Hepatic Surgery

Levente J. Szalai, Archit Naik, Abtin Foroohar, and William C. Meyers
Drexel University School of Medicine, Philadelphia, Pennsylvania, U.S.A.

INTRODUCTION

The laparoscopic approach may be changing the field of hepatic surgery. Many traditional hepatobiliary procedures are now potentially feasible via the laparoscope. However, the data are not ''in'' yet. Liver surgery via the laparoscope is inherently dangerous owing to the complexity and vascularity of this organ. If one remembers back to the introduction of laparoscopic cholecystectomy and that procedure's steep learning curve [1] (and the resultant attraction of hungry lawyers), just imagine the learning curve with laparoscopic hepatobiliary procedures! If experience plays a huge role in the development of one of the most common procedures done by general surgeons, what adjective can be used to describe the role of experience in hepatic surgery?

Let us make two things clear at the outset. First, we do *not*, in general, recommend that surgeons routinely perform complex hepatobiliary laparoscopic procedures. Second, only surgeons who are very experienced in *both* hepatic and laparoscopic surgery should attempt moving into this immature field. (Additionally, we emphatically discourage general surgeons from ''cherry picking'' liver procedures, whether should be done by either the traditionally open approach or the newer, laparoscopic approach.) For example, one cannot, in general, pick out the ''easy'' lesion to remove. Experience clearly shows that the easy lesion often has a satellite lesion, detectable only by adept intraoperative ultrasonography, that should be removed by a formal French segmental resection. Similarly, most should not attempt a simple fenestration procedure on a large, apparently developmental hepatic cyst. Many of these lesions are actually cystadenomas, and recurrent cyst formation is common when minimal excision of the cyst wall is performed. Consequently, more extensive resections of hepatic cysts seem clearly the procedures of choice in appropriate patients. Therefore we intend this chapter not to be deceptive with respect to encouraging surgeons to make an aggressive entrance into the arena of laparoscopic hepatobiliary surgery. This arena needs to be developed and should now be reserved only for very experienced surgeons who can really advance the techniques. What follows are mainly some observations from a relatively large personal experience with liver surgery performed laparoscopically.

This chapter focuses on several selected hepatic laparoscopic procedures: hepatic resection, hepatic cyst excision or fenestration, ablation, and hepatic artery pump insertion.

TEN GENERAL CONSIDERATIONS (TABLE 1)

Completeness of the Laparoscopic Approach Compared to Traditional Open Operation

Probably the most important consideration before attempting any laparoscopic hepatic procedure is whether one can do the operation just as well with a laparot-

TABLE 1 Ten Considerations in Laparoscopic Hepatic Surgery

1. *Completeness of Laparoscopic Approach* — Should not be compromised as compared to the traditional open approach.
2. *Patient Safety* — The patient should not be placed at increased risk as compared to the open approach.
3. *Surgical Skill* — Surgeon should have confidence and experience in *both* hepatic *and* laparoscopic surgery.
4. *Conversion to Open Technique* — Surgical team should be prepared for quick conversion to laparotomy on account of excessive bleeding.
5. *Hemorrhage* — Surgeon should be familiar with laparoscopic moves to minimize bleeding.
6. *Vessel Clamping* — Surgeon should be familiar with various techniques for control of large blood vessels.
7. *Air Embolism* — Risk is close to zero.
8. *Liver Failure* — Potential disorientation during laparoscopic parenchymal dissection increases the risk of hepatic decompensation.
9. *Biliary Leak* — Relatively common, usually requires only simple drainage and patience.
10. *Trocar Site Metastasis* — Uncommon, but one should be aware of its possibility.

omy! One must be certain that the operation is just as safe and just as complete as could be done by the traditional open approach. For example, for resection of a malignant lesion, one must ask whether the appropriate operation can really be done laparoscopically for that particular lesion.

Patient Safety

This point is listed separately to emphasize the fact that even the most simple appearing liver lesions carry with them significant risk, particularly for an inexperienced surgeon. The important question to ask preoperatively with respect to patient safety is: Do the potential benefits of doing the laparoscopic operation outweigh the increased risks incurred by the laparoscopic approach? One must guard against the idea that newer technology is necessarily better.

Surgical Skill

In order to perform a laparoscopic hepatic procedure safely and effectively, the surgeon must not only be an experienced *laparoscopic* surgeon but also an experienced *hepatic* surgeon. A technically excellent laparoscopic surgeon cannot simply translate his or her talents to hepatic surgery. Extensive experience in hepatic surgery is a prerequisite for appropriate judgment concerning both the type of surgery to be performed and the best use of the various techniques.

Conversion to Open Technique

Since hepatic surgery, undoubtedly, comprises some of the most difficult operations that surgeons perform, particularly with respect to bleeding, one must be especially ready for conversion to the open technique. The surgeon must be prepared to convert quickly if he or she ''gets into trouble.'' The time required for conversion can truly be a matter of life or death. Therefore, the open instruments must be unpackaged and on the operative field during the laparoscopic procedure.

Hemorrhage

It is possible to believe, mistakenly, that bleeding is less risky laparoscopically because insufflation pressure actually partially tamponades venous hemorrhage. In dissecting through the liver parenchyma, the tissue and individual vessels are magnified and there really is less sinusoidal bleeding. However, the potential for significant hemorrhage is still an important risk and one must be ready for conversion.

Vessel Clamping

One must be particularly familiar with the various techniques for controlling large blood vessels during laparoscopic procedures. For example, the Pringle maneuver (portal triad clamping) can still be performed quite easily, as with modified Rumel tourniquets. There are also ways to place tapes around certain parts of the liver via minimally invasive surgical techniques to obtain hepatic venous or inferior vena caval control.

Air Embolism

An overly feared complication of laparoscopic surgery is probably the potential for air embolism. Of course, one worries about air embolism because of the CO_2 insufflation pressure above hepatic venous pressure in the presence of large, dissected hepatic veins. However, our own experience and research of case reports shows that the likelihood of air embolism during laparoscopic liver procedures is probably low. In experiments on pigs in our research laboratory, we raised intraperitoneal pressures past 40mmHg with large, open hepatic veins and did not encounter a single case of air embolism [Ricciardi and Meyers, unpublished data]. There is no clinical experience with data of this type, for obvious reasons.

Liver Failure

A dreaded complication of many hepatic procedures is liver failure. Patients with cirrhosis and tumors are at particular risk for this, even with small resections or ablations. Somehow, the remaining liver reacts adversely to the surgical trauma that it has undergone and can easily go into failure, usually for a temporary period, postoperatively. The particular reason that liver failure can be a problem with laparoscopic techniques relates to a potential disorientation during the parenchymal dissection. It is particularly easy, in working laparoscopically within the hepatic parenchyma, to lose one's visual orientation. Therefore, in working laparoscopically within the parenchyma, one must re-evaluate the operative field intermittently, perhaps with the assistance of ultrasound, to make sure the dissection is not veering off into inappropriate planes.

Biliary Leak

As with open techniques, biliary leakage commonly occurs after laparoscopic liver surgery. The patient must be warned about this event. Usually the treatment, in the absence of injury to a major bile duct, is simply simple drainage and patience. Small biliary ducts may actually be easier to identify laparoscopically. However, their occurrence remains relatively common. There is nothing special about the laparoscopic techniques that avoid this type of injury.

Trocar Site Metastasis

We are aware of several cases of trocar-site tumor implantation related to laparoscopic procedures involving malignant tumors, including metastatic colon tumors to the liver. We do not believe that port-site metastasis is a common occurrence. However, one should be aware of this possibility and that all factors accounting for its occurrence are not understood with any degree of certainty.

COMPLICATIONS OF SPECIFIC PROCEDURES (TABLE 2)

Hepatic Resection

General

Several things are important to consider in performing a laparoscopic liver resection, but the initial consideration relates to the type of resection. One can perform a small wedge resection, enucleation, formal segmentectomy, or lobectomy. The choice of resection is based on numerous criteria, such as the type and/or the extent of lesion, hepatic reserve, patient comorbidities, anatomy, and the experience of the surgeon. The location of the lesion in the posterior segments was previously thought to be a contraindication for laparoscopy. However, in experienced hands this is no longer an absolute contraindication. An additional consideration is whether to approach the surgery via straight laparoscopy or by a hand-assisted technique [2]. The latter is particularly useful for large anatomical resections. With experience, and with the use of one hand inside the abdomen, the surgeon can adopt almost precisely the same technique as with open resections.

TABLE 2 Complications of Specific Hepatic Laparoscopic Procedures

Hepatic resection	Hemorrhage Air embolism Inadequate margins
Developmental cyst removal	Inadequate degree of resection (prone to recurrence) Bleeding secondary to lack of initial decompression
Hydatid cyst removal	1. Spillage 2. Venous hemorrhage
Ablation	1. Delayed hemorrhage 2. Potential inadequacy of ultrasonographic visualization 3. Freeze injury to adjacent organs 4. Fire from combustion of radiofrequency or cautery and alcohol
Arterial pump insertion	1. Malplacement of catheter 2. GI tract injury from infusate secondary to inadequate ligation of tiny vessels to GI tract

Bleeding

For resection, the most important intraoperative complication to consider, of course, is excessive bleeding. Bleeding can occur, principally, at two points in the operation: during the initial dissection and identification of the major vessels or during the parenchymal dissection. The first objective in a laparoscopic (or open) hepatic resectional procedure is usually to gain control of the vascular inflow and outflow. The anatomy must be properly identified because the hepatic vasculature is abundant with anomalies. Also, because the laparoscopic approach limits the view and magnifies the field of vision, one can easily misinterpret the anatomy. Finally, one must be extremely careful to avoid injuring a vessel that is supplying the part of the liver to be preserved. We believe that the only way to avoid severing these vessels is through experience in the performance of the open hepatic procedures.

Another source of bleeding arises during the parenchymal division. From our experience, we have found the ultrasonic aspirator to be the best tool for dividing the parenchyma. Other options include the harmonic scalpel, the ''floating ball'' [3], and the water jet irrigator. This field is too new for a consensus on which instrument works best in limiting bleeding during laparoscopic resections. Therefore, we recommend using those instruments with which one feels most comfortable.

One way that a surgeon may manage the potential for excessive blood loss is to intermittently clamp the portal triad. We recommend intermittent clamping during major resections because the laparoscopic operative time is generally longer than that of the respective open procedure. One must, of course, also be vigilant in monitoring of the surgical field for small vessel bleeding after release of the vascular clamp [4].

Hepatic Decompensation

The highest incidence of complications after a laparoscopic liver resection occurs in patients with cirrhosis. Decompensation from cirrhosis is a major concern and leads to ascites, jaundice, and encephalopathy. There is a reliable method for preventing this complication in relation to the laparoscopic approach. Perhaps the lesser degree of physiological insult, which generally justifies a laparoscopic approach, may be the prevention of hepatic decompensation, but we have no hard evidence with respect to this.

Summary

The laparoscopic resection must not put the patient at a higher risk for complications than the respective open procedure. It is essential that the team be able to convert the laparoscopy within a matter of seconds. Major hemorrhage within the hepatic vasculature can lead to a fatality very quickly. Most other complications of hepatic resection still apply to the laparoscopic technique.

Hepatic Cyst Resection, Fenestration, or Ablation

Developmental (Nonparasitic) Liver Cysts

General. In 1968, Lin et al. suggested that superficial cysts could be fenestrated (de-roofed) and allowed to drain into the peritoneal cavity [5]. The partial excision of the cyst wall decompresses the obtunded liver without a significant compromise of hepatic function. The procedure advocated by Lin has been applied laparoscopically for various types of hepatic cysts. For large, apparent developmental liver cysts, we advocate a more aggressive resection of the cyst than has been traditionally described [6]. More of these cysts than previously realized were, following the resection, identified as cystadenomas. Despite several reports to the contrary, the recurrence rate is particularly high without an aggressive resection.

Perioperative Considerations. We prefer to use a Hasson-type cannulation of the abdomen in these patients. The reason for surgery is usually increased abdominal pressure, so it is easy to enter directly into a cyst or another organ if the closed Veress needle approach is used. We are advocates of the Hasson technique, in general, for laparoscopic procedures, but we doubly emphasize this point for resection of these lesions.

The most common, but still rare, intraoperative or perioperative complication that has been reported for solitary cyst fenestration is hemorrhage and bile leakage. In order to minimize the previous complications, the surgeon should not attempt to resect or fenestrate deeply located cysts in which the surrounding vasculature cannot be well delineated. For superficial cysts, some recommend wide deroofing [7]; however, we advocate an excision of the cyst.

The first step in the laparoscopic treatment of these cysts is hepatic ultrasonography prior to their decompression. The ultrasonic examination helps to identify the extent of the cysts and determine their proximity to major vessels, as well as to indicate tuffs of tissue that may represent neoplastic change. If a cyst is not decompressed first, portal and venous hypertension remain high, which can result in excessive blood loss. Once one decompresses a large cyst, the rapidity in which the visible veins collapse and subsequent bleeding is reduced is impressive. Excision then becomes a much easier operation. We know of two patients in whom there were disastrous complications related to failure of initial decompression of the cyst. One patient underwent a partial resection of the inferior vena cava because it blended into the cyst. Conversion was too late and the patient experienced a fatal hemorrhage. A second patient succumbed from excessive intra-abdominal bleeding from varices before the cyst was decompressed or resected.

An additional consideration for the initial decompression of a cyst is to rule out a possible choledochal cyst. Of course, this decompression would reveal the presence of bile. On the other hand, the diagnostic acumen of the treating surgeon should make this an unusual requirement. If decompression does reveal bile, one must take the appropriate steps to treat the choledocal cyst or communicating bile duct, rather than simply excising the ''developmental'' cyst.

Unfortunately, a not uncommon postoperative complication is cyst recurrence. In order to prevent this, the cyst must be resected as completely as feasible. Some cysts also have malignant potential. Therefore, the greatest margin of resection possible should be achieved. Our approach is to resect most of the wall, leaving remnants of the wall only along the dangerous areas within the hepatic parenchyma—i.e., near hepatic veins or the portal triad. There is no requirement of a radical excision, since the cyst is still likely to be benign. One can then even ablate the remaining parenchyma with electrocautery, radiofrequency, or cryosurgical techniques. One can also ablate the normal parenchyma surrounding the portions of a cyst suspected by ultrasound or direction inspection to have adenomatous tissue. Only the wall of the cyst suspected to be in contact with large vessels should be left untouched. This degree of aggressiveness highlights the need for experience in both hepatic and laparoscopic surgery. A good laparoscopic surgeon with little experience in this type of hepatic surgery faces a much higher risk of recurrence of the liver cyst.

Hydatid Cysts

Most of the management concerns mentioned with respect to developmental liver cysts also apply to hydatid cysts. However, there is an additional consideration: whether or not to decompress the cyst first. Decompression, even with the appropriate scolicidal precautions, may lead to spillage of parasitic debris into the peritoneal cavity and implantation. In order to avoid spillage, one should consider a simple excision of the entire cyst. In countries where this problem is particularly common, there has been a growing trend toward complete excision rather than decompression alone. Portal or venous hypertension is unusual with these cysts, but one does have to realize that often these cysts are quite adherent to the hepatic veins, where bleeding can be a particular problem.

Biliary leak after a pericystectomy is also a possible complication. Intraoperatively, biliary leaks can usually be identified via cholangiography or the injection of methylene blue dye through a transcystic catheter. Reported postoperative complications included hemorrhagic and infected cysts [8]. Preoperative and perioperative administration of albendazole is recommended in order to prevent the recurrence of echinococcal disease.

Polycystic Liver Disease (PLD)

General. A combination of fenestration and resection is sometimes indicated for polycystic liver disease, usually for symptomatic relief of pain. Fenestration of the numerous cysts relieves the increased pressure in the abdomen. The relief of symptoms is often temporary, because the cysts typically recur, owing to the nature of the disease. Occasionally, a patient may be identified in whom there is enough abdominal room to do this laparoscopically or via the hand-assisted technique. There are really no different potential complications here than with the traditional technique. However, the patients who can be handled in this way are rare. The technique is similar to that described below.

Preoperative Considerations. Fenestration of PLD has the largest number of reported complications. Morino et al. [9] divide PLD into two groups, according to the number, diameter, and location of the cysts. Type 1 is characterized by a large number of cysts that are in the anterior segments of the liver. Type 2 is characterized by multiple small cysts throughout the liver. Type 2 PLD is a contraindication for laparoscopic fenestration. Because of the possibility of significant postoperative ascites, patients with renal insufficiency should not undergo fenestration of cysts associated with PLD [9]. It should be noted that in PLD, the inferior margin of the liver can descend to the level of the umbilicus or below. Therefore, the use of a 30-degree viewing laparoscope placed approximately 2 to 10 cm below the umbilicus on the xiphopubic line is essential [9].

Intraoperative Considerations. As with most other hepatic laparoscopic procedures, the most common intraoperative complication of cyst fenestration for PLD is hemorrhage. Because a large majority of cysts in PLD can be deeply seated, one must be even more careful not to intrude on vascular structures. In order to delineate deep-seated cysts from nearby vascular structures, one can use a laparoscopic ultrasonic probe with color Doppler or transillumination, which will give the cysts a slightly blue appearance.

Postoperative Considerations. The development of ascites, ascitic fluid leakage via a trocar site, and pleural effusion were the three most common postoperative complications, from the highest frequency of occurrence to the lowest frequency of occurrence, for patients treated for PLD [8–10]. Patients with ascites can be treated conservatively with fluid restriction, administration of diuretics, and paracentesis. In our patients who were so treated, all reported cases of ascites resolved spontaneously after a median of 4 weeks. We believe that the single most important measure to prevent the leakage of ascites is to carefully close each trocar insertion site. A pleural effusion can be either drained via a thoracentesis or allowed to resolve on its own.

Liver Transplantation

Living-related laparoscopic donor hepatectomy for liver transplantation is a procedure currently undergoing feasibility studies in animals. We believe that the most important consideration here is adequate exposure for dissection and the size of the incision necessary to safely remove the donor piece of liver. The problem with this is the possibility of forcing the donor tissue through too small an incision, thereby injuring it. Therefore, the hand-assisted technique, as we initially used in kidney transplantation, also seems appropriate here and has been accomplished in the porcine model. Donors for child recipients are most likely to benefit from this technique once it is developed.

In Situ Ablation (Radiofrequency, Alcohol, or Cryoablation) (Figure 1)

General

In situ ablation, no matter the type, may be delivered via laparoscopy, open, or percutaneous techniques. In an attempt to elucidate the possible complications of the laparoscopic approach, one must first consider the adverse effects inherent to in situ ablation itself. The complications of cryoablation (CSA) include fracture or cracking of the liver, hypothermia, nitrogen skin burns, hemorrhage, abscess, cryoshock, other liver failure, or perforation of adjacent bowel from the cold. Particular problems with the laparoscopic technique can be inadequacy of ultraosonographic imaging due to limited degrees of freedom or a nodular liver, inade-

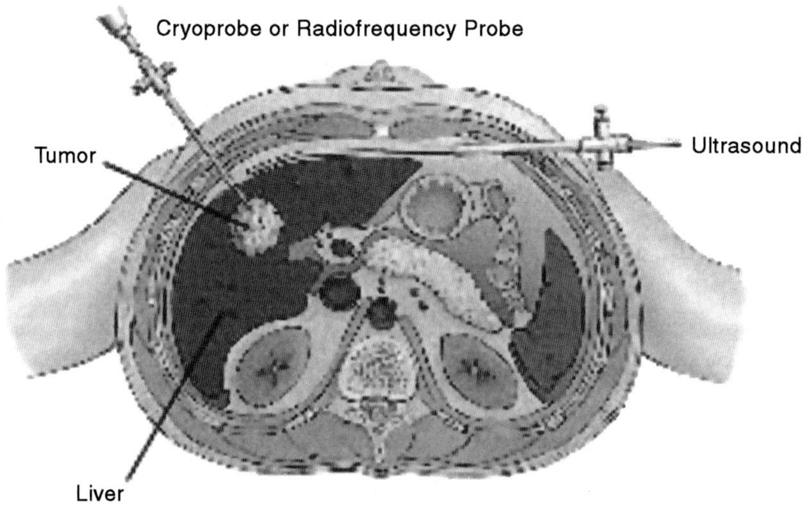

Figure 1 Laparoscopic ablation of a hepatic tumor.

quate exposure and a limited number of approaches (e.g., for lesions at the dome), and inaccuracy of trocar placement. Skin burns and bowel perforation are understandably likely to be more frequent with the laparoscopic technique, owing to the closed nature of the operation. These can be minimized by protective draping or by direct observation of the operative area for 20–30 min after completion of the ablation to make sure the bowel does not migrate to still partially frozen areas on the liver.

Lesion Recurrence

The recurrence of lesions has surfaced as a possible limitation to laparoscopic in situ ablation. Patients undergoing a laparoscopic procedure may have a shorter recurrence-free survival time than those patients who undergo an open procedure [11]. In one study, the recurrence rate is also higher in those patients who underwent CSA as compared to those who underwent radiofrequency ablation (RFA). However, these differences are probably experience-related and not specifically related to the laparoscopic approach. The latter observation—i.e., that RFA patients have lower recurrence rates—may also be due to the fact that RFA is typically used for smaller lesions. Recurrence of tumor is more likely due to an insufficient tumor ablation zone, poor tissue penetration due to patient selection, adjacent vasculature, or inaccurate ultrasonographic monitoring of the ablation process.

Hemorrhage Associated with Ablation

Bleeding is more likely with cryoablation than the other methods. Delayed hemorrhage and ''backside'' bleeding are special considerations. Delayed bleeding occurs due to a crack in the liver and desufflation after ablated tissues return to their normal temperatures. The damage occurs during the thaw or RFA, but does not become evident until after the tamponade effect of insufflation has ceased. As temperatures and perfusion normalize, vascular injuries, caused by ice crystals cutting through vessels in CSA or proximal conduction of heat during RFA, result in bleeding.

Backside bleeding refers to hemorrhage that occurs in the posterior aspect of the liver, where a freeze has occurred but was only visualized by ultrasonography. One must be aware, in using the laparoscopic technique, that cracks may occur where one does not see them. The insufflation pressure can cause a partial tamponade, whereupon the bleeding may not become apparent until after the release of the insufflation pressure and closure.

"Ice Ball" Damage

Laparoscopic in situ ablation may also be complicated by damage to parenchyma and surrounding organs including the colon, omentum, stomach, gallbladder, and

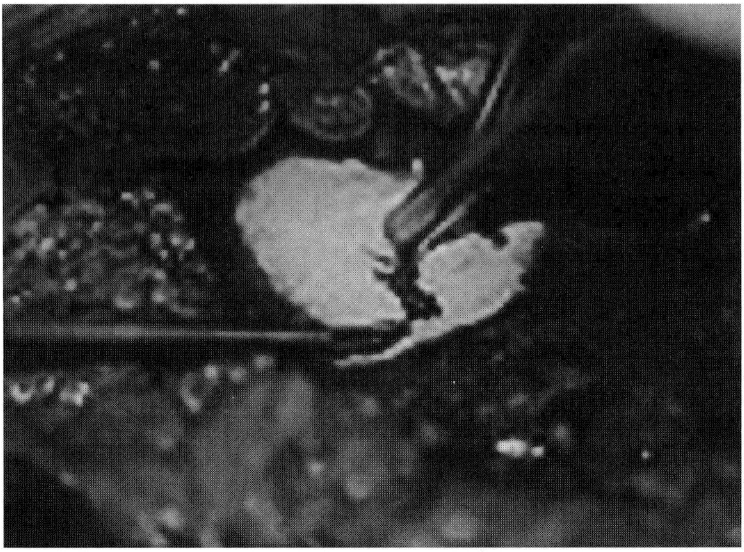

Figure 2 The "ice ball" and the surrounding tissues (e.g., omentum). It is easy to imagine the omentum or any other adjacent tissue adhering to the ice ball. Separation of tissue that is adhering to the ice ball damages the tissue or organ.

small bowel. Contact between the ablated field and adjacent loops of bowel may cause freezing or burning of the colon. Specifically, the creation of the ice ball in cryoablation produces an interesting array of complications (Fig. 2). As mentioned earlier, the ice ball may reach beyond the ablation site and cause parenchymal and/or vascular injury. The ice ball may also reach the surface of the liver and cause direct damage to the surrounding organs. When it extends to the surface, it may indirectly injure nearby loops of bowel and segments of omentum by causing them to adhere to the frozen surface of the liver. When the adherent structures are pulled away, tears will occur. Allowing the laparoscope to remain in place while continuing to maintain CO_2 insufflation may prevent this complication. Allowing the liver to return to its physiological temperature will prevent surrounding intra-abdominal contents from adhering to it.

Ablation Needles

Laparoscopic insertion of ablation needles is another source of possible bowel perforation. This can be prevented by inserting all instruments under direct vision through the laparoscope. Contact of the needles with the colon and surrounding tissues may cause burns, bowel perforation, or skin burns. The use of biodrapes will decrease these potential complications.

Lesion Location

The location of lesions may be a limiting factor in the laparoscopic management of hepatic disease. Tumors located close to vasculature, extremely deep in the liver, in the far right, or in the posterior segment, may be very difficult to access. An example is the treatment of patients with lesions adjacent to the diaphragm. Specifically, insertions of the electrode may be difficult in this location and a thoracic approach might be necessitated [12].

Laparoscopic Ultrasound

First and foremost, any ultrasound-produced image is only as accurate as the technician or surgeon operating and interpreting the ultrasound. Therefore, inexperience with laparoscopic and liver ultrasonography may be a limiting factor. Laparoscopic ultrasound may also be hindered by disease manifestations, such as a stiff, knobby liver, a cystic liver, or an enlarged liver, all of which make it more difficult to navigate the ultrasonic probe.

Other in Situ Ablation Forms (Chemical and Microwave Ablation)

In situ ablation also incorporates chemical, microwave, and alcohol mediums of ablation. Due to mixing of ablative mediums, adverse reactions such as burns and tissue damage may occur. Fire and combustion may occur when alcohol is used as an ablative medium. Combustion of the alcohol occurs from a spark from a nearby cautery device, RFA, or a hot ablative needle. Limiting the use of the previous instruments when alcohol or any other flammable medium is used can easily prevent combustion.

Laparoscopic Hepatic Artery Infusion Pump Placement

The complications of laparoscopic hepatic artery infusion pump placement (HAI) can be categorized into those associated with cholecystectomy, pump placement, or pump pocket formation and those of the laparoscopic approach. A cholecystectomy is required, since 20–30% of patients receiving HAI therapy will develop chemotherapy-induced cholecycstitis. The complications associated with general abdominal procedures—such as bleeding, postoperative pain, infection, and cardiopulmonary events—should also be kept in mind.

Pump Placement

Placement of the HAI pump requires mobilization and dissection of the gastroduodenal artery. This can be a very difficult laparoscopic dissection, exacerbated by coexisting factors, such as the maintenance of good visualization and the procurement of safe vascular control [13]. The surgeon must also recognize any aberrations in the arterial anatomy and be able to properly ligate all the appropriate vessels. It is easy to overlook ligation of tiny branches near the junction of the hepatic and gastroduodenal arteries, which cause a ''steal'' syndrome. An unligated vessel to the stomach or duodenum ''steals'' chemotherapy and causes chemotherapy damage to that organ. Of course, this complication may occur with either the open or laparoscopic technique, but it is likely to be more frequent laparoscopically, as this technique is used more widely. Laparoscopic HAI pump placement requires a truly skilled surgeon who has considerable experience in open pump placement, is familiar with the variety of abnormal anatomical presentations, and has mastered laparoscopic techniques of dissection.

REFERENCES

1. Meyers WC. Southern Surgeons Club: The learning curve for laparoscopic cholecystectomy. Am J Surg 1995; 170:55–59.
2. Meyers WC, Foley DP, Sandor A, Litwin DEM, Callery MP, Yood SM, et al. Handoscopic surgery: A prospective multicenter trial of a minimally invasive technique for complex abdominal surgery. Arch Surg 1999; 134:477–486.
3. TissueLink FB3.0™ Floating Ball, manufactured by TissueLink.
4. Cherqui D, Husson E, Hammoud R, et al. Laparascopic liver resection: A feasibility study in 30 patients. Ann Surg 2000; 232:753–762.
5. Lin TY, Chen CC, Wang SM. Treatment of non-parasitic cystic disease of the liver: A new approach to therapy with polycystic liver. Ann Surg 1968; 168:921–927.
6. Meyers WC, Jones RS. Textbook of Liver and Biliary Surgery. Philadelphia: Lippincott, 1990.
7. Klingler PJ, Gadenstatter M, Schmid T, et al. Treatment of hepatic cysts in the era of laparoscopic surgery. Br J Surg 1997; 84:438–444.
8. Kabbej M, Sauvanet A, Chauveau D, et al. Laparoscopic fenestration in polycsystic liver disease. Br J Surg 1996; 83:1697–1701.
9. Morino M, DeGiuli M, Festa V, et al. Laparoscopic management of symptomatic nonparasitic cysts of the liver. Ann Surg 1994; 219:157–164.
10. Katkhouda N, Hurwitz M, Gugenheim J, et al. Laparoscopic management of benign solid and cystic lesions of the liver. Ann Surg 1999; 229:460–466.
11. Kuvshinoff BW, Ota DM. Radiofrequency ablation of liver tumors: Influence of technique and tumor size. Surgery 2002; 132:605–612.
12. Montorsi M, Santambrogio R, Bianchi Pet al. Radiofrequency interstitial theral ablation of hepatocellular carcinoma in liver cirrhosis: Role of the laparoscopic approach. Surg Endosc 2001; 15:141–145.
13. Urbach D, Herron D, Yshodan S, et al. Laparoscopic hepatic artery infusion pump placement. Arch Surg 2001; 136:700–704.

17

Medical Malpractice Issues

Harry Rein
Longwood, Florida, U.S.A.

OVERVIEW

This chapter, dealing with medical malpractice issues in laparoscopic surgery, is designed to make you think about your own practice—how and why you perform procedures in a certain manner. It does not take an academic view of this emotionally charged issue. While it offers the thought process, you must be willing to think of newer answers. You, the reader may either have fixed opinions and responses to the risk of being sued, or you may be insufficiently informed to think objectively in terms of the months and years involved in a lawsuit. Moreover, your medical training continuously becomes more detailed, specialized, and meticulous regarding diagnostics, instrumentation, and procedures. Indeed, even the billing process and the number of diagnosis-related groups (DRGs) sometimes overwhelms. Medical malpractice is not taught as part of medical curricula. Important issues leading to injuries and lawsuits are not addressed. Each of the subjects herein would support its own series of lectures and its own text, such as I would provide when teaching and implementing malpractice and lawsuit prevention programs. But the goal here is to have you decide whether or not every one of these related but seemingly disjointed subjects apply to you individually, distinctly, and to have you change the direction of your decision-making processes enough to minimize patient harm and substantially decrease your risk of being sued.

Just a short time ago laparoscopy was primarily diagnostic. Shortly thereafter, extrauterine pelvic procedures were performed; and in the past two decades, surgery on the gallbladder, common bile duct, liver, appendix, spleen, colon, adrenal glands, or for gastroesopheageal disease, achalasia, hernias of all types, and vascular problems has become common. Each of these procedures has the same complications as exist with open surgery. In addition, trauma, mistakes, and complications peculiar to laparoscopic surgery were introduced. Postoperatively, laparoscopic surgical patients have significantly different signs and symptoms and often have only subtle changes that have the same severity as were recognized more readily with laparotomy. These are not well taught. Patients are expected to continuously improve after a laparoscopic procedure, and if they do not, the surgeon is obligated to find out why not.

The ideal laparoscopic surgeon need not worry about the medical-legal aspects or about being sued. Indeed, he or she probably should be the author of one of these chapters on preventing, understanding, and managing the complications of laparoscopic surgery. Could you be such an author? This ideal surgeon is the fulfillment of the gleam we had in our eyes in medical school and represents the role model providing us with emotional satisfaction and assuring our patients of that which they expect, deserve, and should demand. However, real life plays funny tricks, especially when medical malpractice rears its legal head. We become angry, resentful, sometimes depressed, and occasionally vengeful. What happened along the way? How should we evaluate the threat of litigation? Can many or all of the claims against us be prevented? Why is it that some physicians have never had any claims made against them while doing more difficult or complicated procedures than ours, and some of us have been sued when, from our point of view, there was no apparent justification—or what we consider a real basis—for the fear that develops when the reality of a malpractice claim against us arises. This chapter is based on some basic themes, each of which should be thought about and is repeated simply and continually here. As you evaluate the subjects developed, these themes should direct readers to understand their own work, decrease and improve their shortcomings, motivate improved procedure, and turn anxiety of litigation into a productive appropriately powerful response to such claims. The themes upon which I construct my seminars, writes papers, and litigate these cases should be considered each time you read something here which has a personal meaning to you through experience, agreement, or controversy. These themes are as follows:

Malpractice does not imply any intentional wrong doing.
A patient cannot consent to a result caused by negligence.
After laparoscopic surgery, improvement should be continuous.
Your obligation is to look for the most serious cause of a problem, not only the most common.
Your physical presence is required when the unexpected occurs.

Why are you doing that?
Was it preventable?
Was it foreseeable?
Was it avoidable?
Is it an unacceptable result? (And unacceptable to whom?)
What if···

The various authors of this book spend their lives teaching that for patient welfare and to prevent lawsuits, you are required to think and act on the following:

Identify complications early.
Proper preoperative evaluation can prevent many of complications.
There are preoperative measures that can prevent the avoidable complications.
There are intraoperative measures to prevent complications.
There are postoperative measures to prevent complications.
There are clinical signs and workups for suspected complications.
There are specific complications of all of these complications.

HOW TO THINK ABOUT MALPRACTICE

Avoiding this chapter because, as a physician, you become angry, depressed, resentful, or intimidated when you hear the words *medical malpractice* is neither helpful nor productive. Start this subject by thinking about possible bad outcomes and wondering only whether litigation will follow, and if so, what power will you have to deal with them. Give yourself the choice of having enough knowledge to be powerful instead of continuing to feel powerless unnecessarily. Knowledge is power. If you are or have been involved in a medical malpractice case, you know that the discovery process includes depositions, the worst one being yours—that is, until you hear your adversaries tell it differently. There are two sides. They are told with different emphasis and you quickly become aware that some questions raise objections because of the way they are phrased or because the subjects were raised by being asked. There are legal reasons for these and they will be discussed. In analyzing the ''bad outcome'' case, what someone would have done, should have done, or could have done is a frequent subject of discussion, and one might object that such questioning is speculation. An argument ensues as to whether or not such questions may be asked and whether an appropriate answer is forthcoming. What soon follows is a legally intended diversion from the purpose of the discovery process, which we learned during the Nixon hearings 30 years ago. ''What did you know and when did you know it?'' Most such questions intend to develop the standard of care issue and the question of legal causation. These concepts have been defined and interpreted by various judges, stated in some statutes, and then redefined, although not made simpler, in jury instructions. It will not have any real meaning to physicians until we think about purpose, how the law applies and its intent. ''That which the reasonable prudent physician would do under similar or like circumstances …'' is the incorrect nonproductive way to think. It almost requires a definition and a discussion of each of the pertinent words in that phrase. Most doctors will answer that question, whether the particular practice met that standard of care definition, determined by the side for whom they chose to testify and not by any great defining thought process. You may think ''What is the common way, what is the average way another surgeon does this,'' or simply that this complication sometimes happens. Wrong. That is not the way to empower yourself. In order for lawyers to take the offensive in developing facts, the defendants, and occasionally opinions from experts (there is a difference), one must develop the thought process that existed at the time of the ''bad outcome.''

Peer review or your personal analysis uses different language and all too often uses the faulty standard ''There but for the grace of God go I. …'' It is too subjective, sometimes intuitive, based on personal choice and bias, and rarely considers the lawful requirements to which we are all bound. Review as it should be, case evaluation prior to litigation, the medical malpractice discovery process, and preparation of the expert witness should all depend on development of a complete and similar set of facts, perhaps in simpler language, as one would train a beginning physician who has a talent and motive to succeed but has not yet been taught the necessary skills by his or her mentors.

Consider what a doctor was doing or not doing, what he was thinking, and what the direction of his task may have been. Indeed, even more fundamental than that, there must be consideration of the reason the malpractice occurred, other than ''a slip of the knife,'' which should be seen, recognized, and repaired.

The technique failure, the real damage due to a slip of the knife, is rarely the basis for a malpractice suit. It is even more rarely known or thought about by either the surgeon or the patient. Small traumatic injuries during procedures occur quite frequently and most often are repaired or heal themselves without significant further damage, residuals, or litigation. When we evaluate cases based on their fundamentals, we must ask: What are the reasons for unrecognized harm, preventable harm, foreseeable harm, or unacceptable harm?

These reasons are to be distinguished from ''the triggering factor'' of medical malpractice lawsuits. Triggering factors are those events that bring clients to a trial lawyer's office.

Fundamental fault, the reasons for the harm as distinguished from the ''triggering'' factors, frequently arises because the doctor did not know enough, remember what he or she needed to know at the time of an event, ''panicked'' in the psychological sense of the word, as children do with wishful thinking, or was too busy and hurried to take time to reverse a process in motion.

Did the doctor know what he or she was supposed to know?
Did the doctor know that he or she did not know?
Did the doctor forget what he or she did know?
Is it malpractice if you don't know what you should know?
Is it malpractice if you don't know that you don't know?

There are differences between slips, lapses, and mistakes. A slip or a lapse has been defined as an error of execution, when the action conducted was not what was intended. The difference between a slip and a lapse is that a slip is observable and a lapse is not. For example, being caught in cutting the wrong structure would be a slip; not being able to recall whether it was cut or not would be a lapse. In a mistake, the action proceeds as planned but fails to achieve its intended outcome because the planned action was wrong. The situation could have been assessed incorrectly or there simply could have been a lack of knowledge about the situation. The original intention is inadequate and a failure of planning is involved. If these definitions are used, there should be no intent to equate any of them with ''minor,'' as any of them may have serious effects. Preconditions can contribute to a large number of unsafe acts: training deficiencies, high workload, undue pressure, inappropriate perception of hazards, and motivation difficulties.

But you are more likely to be sued because of triggering factors. In jest, at times of fatigue, when a patient's questions or demands seem unreasonable, or when the schedule of the day has been compromised due to other inefficiencies, the doctor may say things that are later ''triggers'' to bring the injured patient to the lawyer and become a litigious client. I call these triggers ''words of harm'' as they become invitations to a lawsuit. The number of initial patient visits to lawyers' offices will decrease if these words are not uttered again.

These ''words of harm'' may be triggers:

I'm the doctor, you're the patient.
Just do as I tell you and···
Trust me.
It's too complicated to explain.
You should have come sooner.
Let me tell you of the common side effects.
It's obvious; you don't need another opinion.
This is the worst case I have ever seen.
I'll tell you, then you tell your family.
Let me take this call. It's from E. F. Hutton, and when···
I don't have the time right now.
That's the dumbest nurse around.
I wonder where she left her brains.
The night shift crew is always lazy.
I didn't test because I didn't want to waste your money.

Are you here again for that?
I don't treat that problem—you should find another doctor.
It's a very safe operation. I've done hundreds of them.
There's no choice—it has to be done.
The nurse should have called sooner.
It's a borderline result—don't worry about it.
His squeezing is causing the (breast) lumps.
I don't have to check that again. I know what's causing it.
Hang up the pitocin and call me when she's ready.
That's not enough bleeding to worry about.
If it bleeds again, we'll check it out.
Your (spouse) (relative) (friend) is not a doctor.
You don't need a uterus. I'll tighten up the playpen.
In every operation there are risks; you can die from anesthesia, bleeding, infection. Almost anything can happen; but others are unusual.
You'll have to learn to tolerate some pain.
There is no reason for the pain.
Just take (aspirin), there's nothing else to be done (now).
There's nothing to it.
He used an old-fashioned technique.
I can make your breasts look good.
You'll have to pay before the doctor can see you again.
The doctor is too busy to talk to you now.
The doctor is with a very sick patient; can you call back?
He has done as much as he can for you.
The cast fits fine; all fractures hurt some.
My partner will see you for a few days after surgery.
Let's wait until your surgeon gets back.
Those are not the symptoms of (internal bleeding) (infection).

DECISION MAKING

Laparoscopic surgery inherently involves repetitive demands for decision making. Surgical decisions frequently vary in their gravity and irreversibility and the surgeon is sometimes without the luxury of having all pertinent data available concerning the problem when a decision is required. Although sometimes decisions can be made with uncertainty, most of the time planning, knowing, and understanding the procedures and their consequences obviates the need for making uninformed decisions later. Physicians are often taught that judgment must take precedence over pure logic and that it is often based on past experience. However, lack of knowledge, poor past experiences, and inadequate correction of earlier errors leads to what I choose to call "incomplete decisions." I choose to have you think of ''incomplete decisions'' as distinguished from improper or wrong decisions, because another contemporary might make the same choice even though he could be more informed and experienced. The difference, therefore, would be that greater knowledge, information, experience, and planning would take into consideration all the potential risks, complications, and alternatives overlooked by ''incomplete decisions.'' Often, when the word *judgment* is used, it is postured defensively in response to the challenge of not knowing, having limited experience, or managing a surgical misadventure (another tool using language to explain an undesired happening). Even with prior planning, our profession holds enough surprises without asking for the unanticipated.

The theme remains to continuously ask the same two questions: ''Why am I doing this?'' ''What if···?''

Minimally invasive surgery generally, and specifically laparoscopy, in its infancy was unremarkable, but it has spread to almost all fields of operative management, has been adopted by most, frightened a few, is here to stay, and brings with it both new promises for patients and responsibilities for the surgeon. Laparoscopic surgery in particular has promised decreased morbidity, faster recovery, better operative vision, and precision use of smaller instruments. Patient expectations have been increased by medical advertising and promotion, and doctors themselves have come to believe in its safety and efficacy. An important but often overlooked premise of laparoscopic surgical procedures is that patients are expected to continually improve symptomatically after the end of a procedure, without regression, and if they do not do so, the surgeon must look to his or her technique and procedure for the reason. When this is overlooked, it is because of errors in technique, lack of knowledge of anatomy or procedure, a failure to understand that postlaparoscopic adverse symptoms differ from those of open abdominal surgery, or simply magical thinking. This form of thought process includes ''If I ignore it, it probably is minor and will go away,'' without any objective reason for the conclusion. This belief system, because often our body has the capacity to heal from iatrogenic injury, is also a frequent trigger to beginning a medical malpractice case. Magical thinking is the immature, unprepared medical reaction, a poor substitute for well-reasoned, objective, watchful waiting. This method was used often in previous generations when diagnostics were meager and techniques were more difficult. Today, watchful waiting and judgment must also answer the questions ''Why am I doing this'' and ''What if···?'' When laparoscopy went from diagnostic procedure to surgical intervention and correction, it was performed most often on otherwise healthy young women. That has rapidly changed. More procedures are done on more complicated patients, operating on more organs with more disease and requiring constant alterations in the training and thinking processes. It is worth redefining necessarily proper care as doing the right thing (or not doing the wrong thing) at the right time, in the right way, for the right reason, under the right circumstances, and getting the right results. If the expected result does not follow, doing the right thing at the right time in the right way to determine what caused the unexpected result or prevented the correct result from occurring.

From this we expand the premise of this presentation, which began with ''*Why am I doing this?'' and ''What if ⋯?''* We go on to ask the question *''What could have happened; when, where, how, and why⋯?''*

STANDARD OF CARE

There are simplistic and legally accurate definitions of the phrase *standard of care*. One would be ''that care which the medical community has over the course of years determined to be sufficient and adequate.'' Or ''that care which the average patient can expect to receive from well-trained physicians in an average good hospital.'' Or ''that care which is commensurate with fundamentals in diagnosis and education—and generally practiced by physicians faced with similar problems throughout the United States.''

The law, developed over centuries and called *case law*, requires the physician to possess and to exercise the degree of skill and knowledge ordinarily possessed and exercised under similar circumstances by the members of his or her profession and to use ordinary and reasonable care and diligence, along with his or her best judgment, in the application of his or her skills to the case.

A respectable minority argument is often heard that if a number of physicians use a particular manner of treatment, then the physician is not held guilty of malpractice in choosing to use it if, in his or her best judgment, it best suits the patient's needs. However, it must be considered that conformity to a faulty practice will not justify or exonerate the physician from liability. Whether the respectable minority practice is the standard of care or not could be weighed by the jury. Lack of skill and knowledge breaches the acceptable standard of care. Failure to apply possessed skill and knowledge also creates liability.

What did you know and when did you know it?
What should I have known and when should I have known it?
What should you have done or not done to act as a reasonable physician?

These questions sound simplistic but are not an attempt to mimic the Nixon era and some current Washington, D.C., attitude. They are the meaningful approach to the practice of medicine and stimulate a process that we often refer to all too casually as the differential diagnosis. Failure to recognize or acknowledge that a physician is not applying the acceptable standard of care or able to reach it is also malpractice, as is a failure to refer a patient to a specialist in such circumstances. The standard has to be applied to the facts that exist at the time, not in retrospect. Consider that there is a responsibility for total care and for future care.

A standard of care may be judicially imposed, such as the following:

> *In most cases reasonable prudence is in fact common prudence; but strictly it is never its measure; a whole calling may have unduly lagged in the adoption of new and available devices. It never may set its own tests, however persuasive be its usages. Courts must, in the end, say what is required; there are precautions so imperative that even their universal disregard will not excuse their omission. Under the facts of this case reasonable prudence required the timely giving of a pressure test to a plaintiff whose diagnosis of glaucoma was delayed by an inadequate ophthalmologic exam. The precaution of giving this test to detect the incidence of glaucoma to patients under 40 years of age is so imperative that irrespective of its disregard by the standards of the ophthalmology profession, it is the duty of the courts to say what is required to protect patients under 40 from the damaging results of glaucoma.*

This concept is being applied to other specialties and necessary interventions.

Physicians holding themselves out to be specialists and undertaking the treatment of patients within their specialized area of medicine are required to possess and employ a higher standard of skill, knowledge, and care than general practitioners. They are required to possess and use the degree of skill, care, and learning ordinarily possessed by physicians devoting themselves to the same specialized area of practice in light of the existing state of medical knowledge. This is the reasonably careful and prudent specialist standard and not the average physician standard. Thus, a specialist probably may be held negligent when a general physician would not be.

A general physician practicing with a specialty and attempting to carry out treatments, diagnoses, and procedures of a specialist, would, however, put himself or herself in the shoes of a specialist and thereby probably change the standard of care to which he or she is held.

When a doctor is careless, the term *medical malpractice* is applied. As you may have recognized, it has become an emotionally loaded phrase that causes anger, distress, and even hatred in those to whom it is applied. Think of it as professional negligence in the pure sense of the tort, with some nuances. The references are duty and the foreseeability to what was known and should have been known and to the obligations, which result from the (fiduciary) relationship between a doctor and a patient. The requisite words might be "the failure to exercise that required degree of care, skill and diligence which the ordinary prudent physician would exercise." The breach could be described as "treatment contrary to accepted rules and standards and attributed to results which flow from such a lack of skill." Failure to apply skill possessed, or a willful, ignorant, or intentional application of the wrong measures, with failure to apply the right ones, is also negligence. The deviation from the acceptable standard of care may refer to a single act or to a continued course of treatment.

Do you have to be perfect? No. A surgeon will not be required to exercise extraordinary skill, or care, or the highest degree of care available for a particular problem. Why not? It is generally considered that a general practitioner and a specialist have different levels of skill and care, but generally if they perform the same procedure, the same service, for the same type of problem, the same standard should and does apply.

Different localities had different legal standards applied to them. The locality rule is disappearing, although it still exists and is alive and well in some states. The locality rule is a defense-oriented consideration, strictly a tool to prevent outside expert witnesses, who are necessary, from participating in the litigation, and totally unrealistic in this era of communication, transportation, and flow of information.

Not much has been said or made of the contractual relationship between physicians and their patients. Physicians do impliedly contract that they possess and will use the skill of their profession and that they will apply their best judgment, objectively measured, to the treatment and care of a particular problem.

Now that you are beginning to reason the duty to perform at certain standard levels, it will be no surprise that the standards of today are different from those of yesterday. There is an obligation to keep up. Average skill and standard may no longer be acceptable. The state of medical science is progressing so rapidly that there is a continuing obligation to keep up and to know where and when to refer to the patient or with whom to consult.

When multiple physicians are involved and damages flow from breach of an acceptable standard of care, one or more or all of the practitioners may incur liability. A frequent source of difficulty is reliance by one physician on another. If this results in negligence or if negligent treatment is the result of such reliance, it is not excused. However, even under these circumstances, it is necessary to establish that the alleged act or failure to act proximately caused the damages, the injury, or the death. Knowledge is not important. A great deal of knowledge but a careless act may cause liability in one of two ways. First, there is ordinary deviation from accepted standard of care, and second, the additional knowledge level claimed or admitted may have raised the standard level.

It is not yet established legal doctrine to talk of safety or safer alternatives in medical negligence litigation. In theory, however, Is it safe to ···? or Was it safe not to ···? are becoming essential criteria in evaluating and explaining unacceptable behavior and are stated repeatedly in this chapter because you may hear them in court. There are almost always alternatives to the course of treatment chosen. These should be evaluated, not only from the informed consent point of view but also looking at the possible alternatives.

Was it safe to do what was done, in the manner in which it was done, at the time it was done, under the circumstances it was done, by the person who did it, using the tools and techniques that were used? Was it safe to delay, procrastinate, wait, not to consult, not to refer, not to test, not to operate, not to admit the patient to the hospital? If the alternative to these would have been safer, this theory must have merit.

These concepts can be used even when alleging a deviation from acceptable standard of care or breach of acceptable standard of care, and they should be considered in the evaluation and discovery process of these complicated matters. There is almost always a choice to be made by the physician and/or the patient. The question is really whether it is a deviation from the acceptable standard of care to choose one of the alternatives over the other, whether one is a better choice or not, and how these relate to safety.

The risk-benefit ratio is becoming a major consideration in product liability litigation. This standard and concept may also be applied to evaluating the quality of medical care being rendered. There is no reason not to apply it, particularly when the risk is immediate and a benefit is remote or when a risk is remote and a benefit is immediate.

A wrong diagnosis does not equal negligence. There are wrong diagnoses with fault and without fault. The procedure, skill, care, diligence, history taken, physical examination performed, and methods involved in reaching the diagnosis are what require evaluation and lead to the allegation of carelessness or not. As stated earlier, the adoption of another physician's diagnosis, which was wrong and carelessly made, is as if the same negligent commission or omission were done by the adopting physician if he or she had the opportunity to discover the true facts and failed to do so.

Once care is started, it must be properly continued until the patient discharges the physician or the physician discharges the patient under appropriate and proper circumstances. The patient may discharge the physician at any time. The physician may discharge the patient only if arrangements are made or can be made for substitute care of equal or better nature and quality. Continuing attendance as long as the case requires is a generally accepted responsibility. Abandonment means more than failure to respond when called. It may well mean the failure to remain at the bedside, the failure to respond to a nurse's request, the failure to visit (using telephone treatment and advice as a substitute), or the delegation of authority to someone less skilled. All of these actions or inactions are deviations from the accepted standard of care, and the liability is called *negligence*. Abandonment is a different count arising from the same action and inaction.

Do not assume that a daily hospital visit is always sufficient because "that is the way it is done," "everyone does it that way," or "that is my usual procedure and practice." Is it safe? What are the alternatives? It is neglect to allow too much time to elapse between visits when attention is needed? A large number of patients, a heavy office practice, and multiple other hospital responsibilities are not excuses. They are obvious jury questions.

A new standard-of-care definition should be developed. For years, the present author has taught the following and used the language in trials. It has now been accepted as part of the seminar teaching material by laparoscopic surgeons at their annual meetings. Use it:

> *Doing the right thing (or not doing the wrong thing) at the right time, in the right way, for the right reason, under the right circumstances, and getting the right results. If the expected result does not follow, doing the right thing, at the right time in the right way to determine what caused the unexpected result or prevented the correct result from occurring.*

GYNECOLOGICAL ENDOSCOPY

Gynecological laparoscopic procedures are used here as teaching aids to understand general surgical malpractice lawsuits. If we continue to recognize that most medical malpractice lawsuits involving gynecological endoscopy and laparoscopy result from either improper prevention, inadequate recognition, or delayed intervention, we can prevent many and mitigate most of such cases. We can learn much from the events and rapid progress of the last decade. While most laparoscopic improvements have been technical and instrument-driven, a basic understanding of anatomy, physiology, and diagnostics remains essential to high-quality patient care and risk prevention.

Avoidable, preventable, foreseeable, unacceptable? Was it any of the four? Each of these four must be asked when evaluating adverse events to determine how to raise the quality of care, prevent recurrences, and understand how potential litigants will have their records evaluated. I have been successfully teaching lawyers these procedural questions for over a quarter century, they learn it and use it, yet surgeons are reticent when it comes to learning thought processes that are sometimes used by lawyers against us. We should try to determine why that is so. Malpractice litigation can best be understood, managed, and controlled if we know how those suing us think, evaluate, and proceed.

Laparoscopic surgery and more particularly minimally invasive gynecological surgery has had a great impact on patient care, physician training, litigation, and the development of medical expert witnesses in our courtrooms. When diagnostic gynecological laparoscopy was begun, there was no concept as to how it would grow, spread, develop into general surgical management of many procedures, and the difficulties that would arise from its complications. Its rapid growth is exceeded only by the simultaneous advances in its technology and the appearance of different complications in a different manner, diagnosed differently, and often not included in the ''differential.'' ''Different'' and ''differential'' diagnoses are among the themes of this review, and an axiom of laparoscopic surgery must continue to be as follows: *If a patient does not continuously improve after a laparoscopic surgical procedure, promptly look for and manage a likely complication.*

Complications, errors in judgment, surgical misadventures, and *adverse effects* are terms used by health care providers to explain for themselves, to themselves and to others, injuries to patients at the hands of the laparoscopic surgeon. Such events must be divided into at least two parts, separate thought processes and each must be evaluated separately. A surgical injury is evaluated by understanding the technique used, what happened, patient positioning, instruments, and documentation.

Was it avoidable, preventable, foreseeable, or unacceptable? After asking whether a surgical injury was any of these, there is a second half to the equation. It deals with the timeliness of recognition and necessary intervention into such complications.

Was the injury part of the differential diagnosis early enough? Was the required intervention timely and was it properly managed? Each one of these thought processes is like a chain-link fence, where each and every link must be strong, continuous, and unbroken. These are all responsibilities of the operating surgeon, which, when properly understood and followed, will enhance the enthusiasm for laparoscopic procedures and continue to improve safety and outcome.

THE SHORT LIST OF COMPLICATIONS

During the first decade of laparoscopic surgery, expectations exceeded technical skills. The gap between the two is rapidly disappearing at the locations of skilled private surgeons; major teaching centers and international seminars provide continuing higher-quality education. However, if we look at the complication rate and the litigation of preventable injuries, we note a continuous disturbing pattern. Operative complications must not only be prevented but also recognized when they occur, and appropriate management must be immediately instituted for their diagnosis, intervention, and treatment. The following list of errors is well described in the literature.

Abdominal wall injury
Adhesions
Bowel obstruction
Cardiac arrest
Fistula formation
Hemorrhage
Improper informed consent
Infection
Intestinal burns
Malignancy metastases

Organ laceration
Perforation injuries
Peritonitis
Pneumoperitoneum related
Sharp injuries
Staple injuries
Thermal injury
Thromboembolism
Traction injury
Urethral injury
Vascular injury
Visceral perforation

We know them. To prevent them they can be categorized as small, media-related complications, mechanical injuries, bleeding, anesthetic effects, electrical and laser injury, infection, embolism, and nonsurgical risks.

What to look for, when to look, how to recognize problems, how to test, when to intervene, whom to call for help, and recognizing risk are inadequately taught and incompletely understood. The different laparoscopic procedures and techniques are associated with many of the same and a vast array of different problems, which require study, understanding, and a continuing re-education of the surgeon. It is not enough to be skilled at technique alone. For example, some of the risks and hazards of operative hysteroscopy are anaphylactic reactions, fluid overload, and coagulopathy—all possibly resulting from the use of dextran 70. The products used, the length of time they are used, measurement of risk, and knowledge of substitutes available are simply not understood by many physicians, who may well find themselves as defendants because they lack this information or are preoccupied with manual dexterity and other surgical skills. Propriety of intrauterine pressures, operating time as distinguished from technique, the cause and risk of open vascular channels at best get only 5 min of discussion at intense 2-day surgical courses. Yes, only 5 min—I timed them at these presentations. How many of our hysteroscopy surgeons know in detail how wound infections occur, and what better ways exist to prevent them? Why do hematomas exist and what instrument cause them? How does bowel or omentum herniate through a port site and what technique or instrument change prevents this? If vascular and bowel injury should be feared, would a small change in positioning be considered? The severe illness that can develop following bowel injury may not appear immediately. The changes in bowel sounds studied so well with general open abdominal surgery follow different patterns with laparoscopic surgery and may develop insidiously. Fever must not be ignored and should not be assigned a benign cause until it is well understood. Paralytic ileus, common after open abdominal surgery, should not follow laparoscopic surgery; if it occurs, it should make the operator think of bowel injury until there is good evidence to suggest otherwise. Pelvic and retroperitoneal hematomas may not be recognized if the intra-abdominal pressure generated by the insufflation gas is not sufficiently reduced before inspection for bleeding. Venous bleeding may well be controlled by pressure above 5 mmHg. A low index of suspicion for ureteral injury may lead to a high incidence of litigation, while vigilance and indentifying complications and surgical injuries when they occur is not only good patient care but will keep courtrooms relatively emptier.

Delayed Complications

While we rarely think of postoperative complications occurring years after the procedures are forgotten, they do occur. It is thought that women with multiple risk factors for endometrial cancer are best treated with hysterectomy instead of endometrial ablation. Postablation tubal sterilization syndrome (PTSS) is uncommon, but it occurs and can be surgically corrected but only if known, considered, and recognized. Pregnancy after operative hysteroscopy can result in uterine rupture due to the myometrial damage incurred during hysteroscopy. As more operative hysteroscopy is performed, more delayed complications will arise. As surgeons have more valuable minimally invasive options, they must not be tempted to forego meticulous preoperative evaluation, along with understanding of the procedures and the postoperative risks thereby created.

Loose Staples

It is generally believed that loose staples remaining behind are benign and should not be of great concern. This is often true, but when it is not, these small pieces of metal become easy evidence for litigation. Staples are surgical instruments—foreign bodies—and when their sharp points are demonstrated, it is easy to make them appear to be more dangerous than small sponges, for which meticulous counting is routine. A staple left behind can perforate the bowel, causing leakage, abscess formation, adhesions, obstruction, and volvulus. Every effort should be made to remove loose staples from the operative field prior to termination of a laparoscopic procedure.

It is best not to assume too much. Some discussions among leading surgeons and teachers in the "ivory tower" suggest that the combination of high-quality training and good surgical skills always leads to good results. It is true that when substantial talent and technical skill come together the rate of surgical trauma, complications and bad results drastically declines. But in reality, there are shortcomings in surgical skills and techniques, often leaving something to be desired.

Local Metastatic Implantation

Spread of cancer after laparoscopic surgery or tumor recurrence at the port site or at the abdominal wall continues to raise safety questions. It has not been determined whether the implantation of metastases reflects the laparoscopic technique or the aggressive biological behavior of the tumor. Chemotherapy adjuvants are a strong consideration. The spread of ovarian cancer, particularly after laparoscopic surgery, continues to be reported and is of great concern.

Ovarian Remnants

Much discussion herein has been about the prompt recognition of adverse effects and their proper management. Sometimes a technique itself is a major factor, such as occurred with the initial introduction of Veress needles, for those who still use them, and trocar puncture. Syndromes due to ovarian remnants remaining after laparoscopic oophorectomy are specifically related to failures of technique. With laparoscopic oophorectomy, there is a risk of ovarian remnant due to improper tissue extraction or misapplication or improper use of pretied surgical loops, linear stapler, or bipolar electrodessication of the infundibulopelvic ligament, especially in women with a history of multiple pelvic surgeries, adhesions, or endometriosis.

Sexual Dysfunction

There has been litigation alleging an adverse impact of hysterectomy on sexuality, libido, and orgasm. Most of those cases have been unsuccessful. Available evidence shows that the quality of life is improved for most women who have had a hysterectomy and that, indeed, hysterectomy does not adversely affect sexuality.

Ureteral Injury

Iatrogenic ureteral injuries constitute a serious complication of gynecological and colonic surgery with both the open and minimally invasive procedures. Indeed, ureteral injury should be less frequent with laparoscopy because magnification and visualization are better. However, this is not always the case. Indeed, these injuries are frequently undetected, but often the failure to recognize them stems from the surgeon's failure to suspect them. The types of injury that occur from laparoscopy are not any different than those from open surgery. The symptoms are flank pain, fever, and hematuria. The delayed symptoms frequently are abdominal distention, pain, tenderness, and a diffuse form of peritonitis with its varied syndromes. A large variety of injuries may cause the same symptom complex. These injuries include transection, ligation, avulsion, crush injury, devascularization, resection, fulguration, and perforation. If intraoperative injury is suspected, careful inspection, facilitated by intravenous indigo carmine, is necessary.

Air Embolization

Air embolus associated with intra-abdominal or tubal insufflation is a rare but sometimes fatal risk. It usually occurs immediately after tubal insufflation with air. It must be immediately recognized by the anesthesiologist and be followed by prompt release of pressure and/or pneumoperitoneum. It may occur after cervical dilatation, operative hysteroscopy, and direct injection of gas into the vasculature, during intrauterine laser surgery, and by any other mechanism where the gas pressure exceeds venous blood pressure. It may be caused by the penetration of blood vessels by a cannula, a Veress needle, or a Cohen cannula within the lower uterus where the distending pressure was great enough to force air into venous sinuses. Immediate action must be taken when an air embolus is suspected. Gas instillation must be abandoned, Trendelenburg reversed, and a central venous line placed. There must be no delay in cardiopulmonary resuscitation if necessary. Patient is to be placed in the left lateral decubitus position and external cardiac massage administered, which may break up the air trap. Prevention is better than cure. Methylene blue, indigo carmine, saline, or CO_2 can be insufflated rather than air. Prevention, recognition, and intervention are all crucial in these cases.

WHAT WAS THE CAUSE?

We need to learn better ways to analyze our own thought processes. What do we do routinely and why do we do so?

Are the habits that have worked for us for years the proper habits under all circumstances?

Do we need to think of the more serious complication more often than of the more common expectation?

Although most ill effects of surgical misadventure do often correct themselves because of how well the human creature was constructed, should we not take responsibility for thinking that we may have caused the injury and fix it?

Patterns used by industry to analyze fault and control damage can be applied to the evaluation of medical judgments. Sometimes thinking ''out of the box'' is fruitful. Consider the types of errors discussed herein and others you know using the following format.

Diagnostics

Error or delay in diagnosis
Failure to employ indicated tests
Use of outmoded tests or therapy
Failure to act on results of monitoring or testing

Treatment

Error in the performance of an operation, procedure, or test
Error in administering the treatment

Error in the dose or method of using a drug
Avoidable delay in treatment or responding to an abnormal test
Inappropriate (not indicated) care

Preventive

Failure to provide prophylactic treatment
Inadequate monitoring or followup treatment

Other

Failure of communication
Equipment failure
Other system failure

Why Errors Happen

The focus should be on safety, not on ‘‘getting rid of bad apples.’’ (The opposite has been the method, with its legal stumbling blocks.)

An error is the failure of a planned sequence of mental or physical activities to achieve its intended outcome when these failures cannot be attributed to chance.

Intention

Actions do not go as intended; or the intended action is not the correct one. In the first case, the desired outcome may or may not be achieved. In the second case, the desired outcome cannot be achieved.

Slips, Lapses, or Mistakes

A slip is observable, a lapse is not.
Turning the wrong knob is a slip.
Not being able to recall from memory is a lapse.
A mistake is an incorrect planned action.

Reality Testing

While, as surgeons, we are comfortable with words such as *complications, adverse effects*, and even *mistake*, we must know that failing to be careful enough may lead to litigation. Therefore be not afraid of learning how to think for yourself and how to improve your results. If we learn where, how, and why things happen, thinking of them becomes easier. Most of the time, if we process a risk or hazard with understanding, we will recognize it and know what to do.

As we enter a new millennium, we look back on a summary of literature-reported complications of the last decade. It is impossible to know how many injuries go unreported, without discussion, without litigation, and unfortunately without teaching the operator techniques and methods of prevention. The major trocar-induced injuries were abdominal wall vessel injury, major vascular injury, visceral trauma, and incisional hernia formation. It is thought that the actual rate of such injuries is at least three times the published rate. Abdominal wall vessel injury has an incidence of 0.15–10.5%. Fortunately major vascular injuries are under 0.15%. Visceral injuries occur more often, being reported up to 2.5% of the time. In such cases, deaths occur due to delayed detection. It is thought that up to one-third of all trocar injuries cause incisional hernia formation. Of the cases reported, approximately 20% of the major vascular injuries caused death. The mean settlement of such injuries was $256,539. The average cost of settlement for a bowel injury was $437,500. Additionally, almost all of these included an allegation of delayed recognition and intervention. We must, therefore, be alert not only to prevention but, as this article started, the timely recognition and prompt appropriate intervention.

The mechanics of malpractice lawsuits should be understood so that a doctor can maintain confidence in the system, keeping control of his or her practice and emotions while helping to prepare his case and position.

CHRONOLOGY AND MECHANICS OF A LAWSUIT

A lawsuit is a civil case or civil action, filed either in a state circuit court or a federal district court, seeking money damages for one or more plaintiffs from one or more defendants. It is premised on a claim of negligence, which is generally defined as the failure to act as a reasonable person would act under the circumstances of a given situation. A professional liability case is a special kind of civil action, one filed against a member of a state-licensed profession. The premise of a professional liability case is a claim of professional negligence—defined in various ways in this chapter, including the failure to comply with the accepted standard of care for the defendant's specialty field or (in the case of a nonspecialist) in the local community or similar community to the one in which he or she practices.

Pleadings are statements filed which define the issues between the parties.

Discovery is a process involving the exchange of information and documents by means of sworn oral testimony, depositions; or written means, interrogatories, requests for admission, and document production.

Investigation of the facts of the claim or facts pertaining to the parties.

The setting of a schedule by the court for the identification of witnesses, the completion of discovery, and trial.

The evaluation of the medical issues by independent expert witnesses.
The discovery of opinions of the expert witnesses named by each side.
The submission of the case to the mediation process.
Trial of the case before a jury.

The length of this process varies among different counties. It typically takes from 12 to 60 months for a professional liability case to pass through these stages and to reach the stage at which it is ready for trial.

Commencement

A lawsuit is typically started when a physician is served with process—a complaint and a summons. When you receive these items, you should immediately contact your professional liability carrier and forward to its representative a copy of everything served on you. Some states provide for a precomplaint investigation period before a medical malpractice lawsuit may be filed. In such localities, a physician will typically receive notice of the claim by letter, most often on an attorney's stationery. Again, you should immediately contact your professional liability carrier and provide its representative with a copy of everything you have received. Caution: the notice may look like an ordinary letter. During the investigation period, the claim will be handled by a representative of your professional liability carrier; an attorney may be assigned at that point or may not be assigned until a complaint is filed.

Selection of Defense Attorney

Your professional liability carrier has the right and duty to select an attorney, who will defend the claim against you. The fees charged by the attorney are paid by your carrier; that is one of the benefits you have paid for with your premium. You sometimes have the option of requesting that your carrier retain a particular attorney to defend you, so long as the attorney is one who is on the list of attorneys approved in advance by your professional liability carrier. (The number of attorneys so approved in any geographical area is quite limited, however.) The physician's requested choice among the approved attorneys is usually followed by the carrier. You always have the choice of personally employing any attorney you select, to assist your case, and exclusively represent your very private interest. This would be at your own expense. Usually, it is not necessary to do so, but on occasion the attorney retained by the physician's professional liability carrier may suggest that the physician retain his or her own attorney. When the physician has retained such an attorney, the attorney retained by the carrier will typically include the privately retained attorney on any reports that are sent. The privately retained attorney has the right to this information, just as the physician does, but he or she does not have the right to control the defense.

Pleadings

Pleadings are the papers filed with the court to set forth the issues and the parties' respective positions on these issues. The typical pleadings are as follows:

Complaint. The pleading by which a lawsuit is started. The complaint is expected to allege, in more or less a specific fashion, the facts on which the claim is based and the plaintiff's claim regarding the requirements of the standard of care and how that standard of care was breached.

Answer. The defendant's response to the complaint. Each individual allegation may be admitted, denied, or denied in part or with qualification, or the defendant may respond by stating that he or she does not have the information necessary to admit or deny the allegation.

Affirmative Defenses. Typically filed with answer, this is a statement of those matters that would constitute an affirmative defense to the claim. Affirmative defenses are those that would defeat the claim, even if the claim of negligence is true. Thus, a statement that the statute of limitations has expired would be considered an affirmative defense. The defendant's denial that he or she was negligent is not an affirmative defense; it is simply a denial of the plaintiff's claim.

Planning and Strategy

It is vital to the defense of a professional liability case that the defendant, his or her attorney, and the claim representative from the professional liability insurer work together to learn about the case, including the medical and legal issues raised by the claim, and develop a plan of action to defend against the claim.

The steps to be taken typically include the following:

- A meeting between the defendant, his attorney, and the claims representative
- Obtaining necessary medical information (including copies of records) from the defendant and from other medical providers through the discovery process
- Arranging for one or more reviews of the claim by expert witnesses
- Early evaluation of the merits of the case and decision as to whether to settle or defend the claim

It is vital to the success of your case that you deal with your attorney in the spirit of candor. A full and frank disclosure of all information pertinent to your case, positive and negative, even if it is embarrassing or personal in nature, is essential. Your attorney must have complete information about your case in order to fully advise you and represent you, just as you must have full information from your patients about their health, their habits, their activities, etc., to fully treat them. The information that you provide is maintained with the utmost confidentiality. Except for the documents and records, which are in the possession of the defendant, the defense attorney must go through the discovery process to obtain copies of records from other providers. This takes time. Typically, your attorney will not yet have these records by the time he or she first meets with you to discuss the case.

As the case proceeds, the attorney will provide reports on depositions taken, experts' opinions received, and other matters pertinent to the case. Further, many professional liability insurance companies require that reports be submitted at certain specified times, and these reports may include the attorney's opinions on the value of the case, the chances of a successful defense, and recommendations for continued defense or settlement. Your attorney should provide copies of all reports to you as they are sent to the insurer. Many insurers also now require that the physician be provided with copies of the bills for legal fees and expenses, which the attorney submits to the insurer. This helps to provide you with information about what your attorney is doing on your behalf.

There cannot be too many meetings between you and your lawyer. You cannot be too informed. You must participate in the process and remain to the medical interpretation of others.

Confidentiality

The attorney-client privilege acts much like the physician-patient privilege. Information provided by the client to his attorney, and by the attorney to the client, is privileged and may not be disclosed to others. Both the attorney and the client must safeguard that confidentiality, however, since the law provides that a disclosure to an outside person waives the privilege and makes the information fully discoverable by an opposing party. Thus, the physician must take the following steps during the course of the litigation:

1. Reports from your attorney, any documents generated or compiled by the physician, and any documents pertaining to the litigation must not be placed in the patient's chart. Rather, they should be maintained in a separate, secure location, such as the physician's desk or a location at his or her home.
2. The physician must refrain from a discussion of the substance of the case while it is pending. Conversations with colleagues, friends, etc., are discoverable, and it is quite common for a physician to be asked in a deposition whether he or she has about spoken the case with anyone. Any information you give to an outsider is fair game. You may, if you choose, give your colleagues objective information, such as

that a lawsuit is pending, that a deposition is to be taken, etc., but no information about substance, strategy, or plan of action should be disclosed.

3. The persons who are within the scope of confidentiality and protected by the privilege include the physician, the attorney, and the claims representative handling the case for the professional liability carrier. Others may include partners or shareholders in your professional corporation if it is also a party. Those are the only people to whom confidential and sensitive information may be disclosed.
4. Often, a professional liability carrier or a hospital to which a physician has applied for medical staff privileges will request information about past or current lawsuits or even potential claims. All such inquiries should be referred to your attorney for a response while the lawsuit is pending. It is also a good idea to refer such inquiries to the attorney even after the litigation has been resolved.

Discovery

Discovery is a formal exchange of information among the parties to a lawsuit. The process involves the exchange of information and documents by means of sworn oral testimony—depositions; or through written means—interrogatories, requests for admission, document production, requests for production of medical information. These requests are made in writing, and copies are provided to all attorneys. The answers, likewise, are provided to all attorneys.

Interrogatories and Document Requests

These are the written discovery requests most commonly sent to defendants. When these requests are received, you will be contacted by your attorney to provide information to prepare the answers. The answers are given under oath, just as at a trial or in a deposition, and therefore the truthfulness of the answers must be ensured. Each request has a period of time within which the answers must be provided, although procedures are available to extend the time within which the answers are due (through a motion filed with the court or simply an agreement between parties to extend the time).

A ''request for admission'' is particularly important, since the request is deemed automatically admitted if it is not denied or otherwise appropriately answered within the time specified. Discovery requests may be simple or complex, and sometimes they may be burdensome. If a set of requests is sent to you, without any direction from your attorney as to which ones should be answered and which ones need not be answered, you should feel free to discuss them with your attorney before expending much time preparing answers.

Normally, these requests are expected to cover only the information that is known to or available to a party. They do not normally require that the party take steps to obtain this information from others (except employees of the party providing the answers). Thus, for instance, an interrogatory may request a physician to state the number of certain surgical procedures she has performed. This information may be in the possession of the hospital where she works but not in her own possession. Even though she knows that the hospital keeps those records, she is not obliged to obtain this information from the hospital to provide an answer to this question. If she has her own records reflecting this information, she is obligated to provide an answer.

Further, if the request is extremely detailed, so that it would take an inordinate amount of time to gather the information, your attorney may ask you to provide more limited information in response to the request. Again, speak with your attorney if the request appears to you to be overly detailed. Sometimes the court is asked, by the filing of a motion, to make a ruling on the sufficiency of the answers supplied. If the court so orders, more detailed responses may have to be submitted.

Request for Production of Medical Information

This is a request directed to the plaintiff, and is the means by which copies of medical records may be secured. After the submission of the request, the plaintiff has a period of 28 days to respond. The response will include one or more of the following: Providing the defendant's attorney with copies of those records in the possession of the plaintiff's attorney. Providing the defendant's attorney with a written medical authorization to provide evidence to treating doctors or hospitals that the attorney is entitled to obtain copies of their records. After the authorization is received, it is sent to treating physicians or hospitals with a request for copies of the records. This may take a few weeks. Sometimes, the provider, typically a hospital, will require a more detailed form of authorization, and this will have to be sent to the plaintiff's attorney to have it signed by his or her client. It thus sometimes occurs that copies of medical records may not be received by your attorney for a few months after the request for production of medical information is first submitted to the plaintiff. The law provides for another possible response to the request for production of medical information: a claim of privilege. This is virtually never asserted, however, since the law also provides that a party who claims privilege is thereafter barred from offering evidence as to the medical condition as to which the privilege is claimed. Since that would usually prevent the plaintiff from being able to prove his case, it is rarely invoked.

Depositions

The method of discovery most familiar to physicians is the deposition. This is a session in which a witness provides testimony in a question and answer format, under oath, similar to testimony provided in open court during a hearing or a trial. There are some important differences:

During a deposition, the presiding judge is not present and therefore cannot immediately make a ruling on an objection or on a point of evidence.

The parties are not rigidly bound by the rules of evidence. Information may be requested and must be provided, even though it may not be admissible into evidence, so long as the information is relevant or is reasonably calculated to lead to relevant information.

All attorneys for the parties have the right to appear and to question the witness. The questions and answers are recorded by a court reporter, who will then transcribe them and provide a copy of the transcript to all attorneys who order it from him or her.

You, as a party to the action, have the right to be present for any deposition that is taken in your case. Often, your attorney will suggest that you be present, to assist him or her as the questioning takes place.

Your deposition will be one of the most important in the case. There are a number of suggestions and instructions that your attorney should provide to you, in advance, to prepare you for the deposition and to assist in giving your testimony.

Motions

A motion is a request to the court, usually made in writing, for an order to require a party to a lawsuit to take certain action or to provide certain information. On occasion, a motion will ask for similar relief as to a nonparty. Motions do not usually require your appearance at court. Your attorney will advise you if a motion or a court's order requires any action on your part.

Scheduling/Pretrial Conferences

These are hearings held by the court, with the attorneys. The parties are not expected to attend. At these conferences, matters such as the setting of times for disclosure of witnesses, deadlines on pretrial discovery, mediation, and a trial date may be discussed. Your attorney should advise you of the dates that have been set.

Mediation

Mediation is a special pretrial procedure that is used in some states. A few other states have somewhat similar pretrial procedures, but the details of each are different.

A mediation hearing is a process in which a panel of three attorneys will receive written submissions from the attorneys for the parties (called mediation summaries or mediation briefs). They will hear an oral presentation on the case and the issues it presents, ask questions of the attorneys, and then provide an evaluation of the case as to each defendant. This evaluation is the figure that the panel believes represents a reasonable settlement value of the case. It is not binding on the parties, and it thus may be considered to be a recommendation as to a settlement value. Either the plaintiff or the defendant may reject it. If both sides accept it, the case is settled for that figure. Physicians are given the opportunity to participate in the mediation process as well. Each side—plaintiff and defendant(s)—may designate a health care provider in an appropriate field to sit on the panel and to participate. This is participation by physicians in the pretrial evaluation process.

Expert Witnesses

Expert witnesses are witnesses who are found by the court to have a particular expertise in a field of training or discipline, and they are allowed to testify if the court finds that their testimony will be helpful to the jury in considering the issues in the case. In a professional liability case, expert testimony is typically required on both sides except in those rare situations in which a lay jury could find a deviation from the standard of care without the use of expert testimony. An example would be leaving a surgical instrument within the patient's body after an operation.

Expert witnesses differ from lay witnesses in that they are permitted to offer specialized information, known to practitioners in their fields, and to offer opinions in areas within their area of expertise. Commonly, an expert is offered to establish, by opinion testimony, what the standard of practice required of a physician in a given situation and whether the actions of the physician did or did not comply with that standard.

It is not necessary that an "expert" have special qualifications or expertise, beyond those that the ordinary practitioner in his or her field would have. It is not necessary that an expert witness be regarded by other physicians as an "expert" in a particular area. It is simply necessary that the witness be shown to have the minimum qualifications to establish familiarity with the specialty or issue in question. Under the law, any practicing general surgeon may be qualified as an expert witness in the field of general surgery, no matter how ordinary or even mediocre a practitioner he may be. An expert witness need not be board-certified in a specialty field if he or she in fact practices that specialty as a regular part of his or her practice.

The court makes the determination of whether a proposed expert witness is, in fact, qualified to testify before the witness is allowed to testify. The issue of how convincing his or her testimony is and whether it should be believed is one for the jury to resolve.

Settlement

The majority of litigated cases are settled before they reach the point at which they are ready for trial. Most cases, that are not dismissed (voluntarily or by order of the court) are resolved by the payment of some amount of money to the plaintiff. Depending on the severity of the injury, a settlement for a fairly limited amount of money can be considered a favorable outcome, though many defendants find that concept difficult to accept. More professional medical liability cases go to trial than other types of cases. This should not be the case, but it is so. One reason is that professional liability cases are handled somewhat differently and many physicians refuse to settle until it is too late to agree to an amount, which could have settled the case sooner. Many policies of professional liability insurance provide a ''consent clause,'' under which a case cannot be settled without the specific agreement of the insured. Further, most companies insuring physicians follow a policy under which cases are not settled for ''nuisance value'' (a cheap settlement of a nonmeritorious case) if there has been no criticism of the defendant physician's actions by a reviewing expert witness or the company's claims committee. An important second reason is the unfounded fear of a federal reporting statute. This is too complicated too explain here, but suffice it to say that it is unlikely to have any of its feared impact on a doctor's future professional practice.

Physicians take lawsuits involving their professional practice very seriously, and many do not simply dismiss them as a cost of doing business, as do product manufacturers and other corporate defendants. The result is that more professional liability cases are defended as a matter of principle than are other types of cases. You should also be aware that a case might be settled at any point—before trial, during trial, or during the course of posttrial appeals. Some cases have been settled while the jury was deliberating its verdict.

Insurance Policy Limits

Typically, the professional liability insurance policy provides a ''per-occurrence'' policy limit, which represents the maximum that the insurer will pay on a single claim involving a treatment or a course of treatment and an ''aggregate'' limit, which represents the maximum that it will pay for all claims during the policy year. Since a plaintiff's recovery will include items beyond a simple award of compensatory damages, you should be aware of what is and what is not covered under your policy.

Excess Verdicts. Your policy will not pay the portion of a jury verdict that exceeds the per-occurrence policy limit. In the event of such a verdict, the plaintiff can seek to recover the excess amount from the insured physician's personal assets. In most cases, he or she will be satisfied with the policy limits, plus interest and mediation sanctions and will not attempt to recover beyond that figure.

Prejudgment Interest. In some states, the court will add to the recovery an amount representing interest from the date that the complaint was filed to the date that the judgment was entered. Your policy covers such interest, even if the total amount exceeds the policy limit, but the amount of interest covered is limited to an amount proportional to the $200,000 policy limit. Thus (assuming a $200,000 policy limit), if there is a $400,000 gross jury verdict and $30,000 in interest is added, the policy will pay the $200,000 limit and half of the interest, or a total of $215,000. If there is a gross jury verdict of $195,000 and $30,000 in interest is added, the policy will pay $225,000. There are exceptions to this rule.

Mediation Sanctions. Typically covered under the policy. Check your policy to be certain.

Appeal Bonds. The policy covers any bonds that must be filed in order to take an appeal. Again, however, the amount is limited to the per-occurrence policy limit. The policies typically do not provide reimbursement to the physician for time away from his or her practice, loss of income, etc. Check your policy or talk with your claims representative.

Limitations on Coverage

Some policies place an additional risk on the exercise of the insured's rights under the ''consent clause'' described above. These limitations clauses provide that, if the insurer has an opportunity to settle a case for a specific dollar amount and the insured physician declines to provide consent to a proposed settlement, the per-occurrence policy limit will be reduced to the amount for which the case could have been settled. For example, if a physician refuses to consent to settle a case and if the case could be settled for $50,000, then the per-occurrence limit under the policy will be reduced to $50,000, significantly limiting the protection provided by the policy. Fortunately, invocation of this clause is very rare, but it would be prudent to investigate your own policy if the question of consent arises.

Special Policy Provisions

Virtually all policies will specifically exclude coverage for intentional acts of wrongdoing. A common example of such acts in the professional liability context involves claims for sexual exploitation of patients by physicians.

Most policies also have a co-operation clause, which provides that the coverage is conditioned on reasonable cooperation by the physician with the company's claims representative and with the attorney designated to defend the physician. A physician who refuses to appear at a deposition or at the trial of his or her case or who refuses to comply with discovery requests, might, on the basis of this clause, wind up without coverage for the claim.

Role of the Defense Attorney

In the vast majority of cases, both the physician and his or her insurance company have identical interests. In those rare situations where their interests diverge, the physician must be aware of the role the attorney must play under law. Despite the fact that his or her bills are paid by the insurer, the attorney is at all times required to consider the physician as client. It may seem that sometimes the attorney does not appear to do so. The doctor must make his or her observations and wishes known to the lawyer clearly and promptly. The attorney is ethically bound to act in the best interest of the physician, even if that interest is at odds with the interests of the insurer. If a dispute arises, the assigned attorney will remain neutral; he or she will not be able to represent either the insurer or the physician in connection with the disputed matter. The attorney may not take any action during the course of his or her representation that would place the physician at a disadvantage with respect to any actual or potential dispute with his insurance carrier. This means that he may not advise the insurer on questions of coverage under the policy. The carrier will usually respect the ethical and legal principles governing the attorney's role and will not ask the attorney to do anything contrary to those principles.

Trial

The trial of a case before a jury is the culmination of all the efforts of the defendant and his or her attorney over the many months of the pretrial discovery process. This is the opportunity for all parties to present their cases to a jury and to have the factual and medical issues resolved. During a trial, the judge is to decide questions of law (including admissibility of evidence) and the jury is to decide all issues of fact. The issues of what the standard of care was, whether it was breached, and what relationship the breach had to the damages claimed are all considered matters of fact. They are, however, technical issues of medical opinion, and thus the courts require that they be proven with the aid of expert testimony. There are several stages of a trial, and they can be described only briefly here.

1. Jury selection is the first process, under which the court and the attorneys will have an opportunity to question the prospective members of the jury in order to evaluate them as potential judges of the facts and the medical issues.

2. Opening statements are given by the attorneys to provide a description of their respective positions and the testimony and evidence that will be offered to support those positions.
3. *Plaintiff's proofs*. The plaintiff's witnesses are called and documentary evidence is introduced. This will include evidence (offered through the testimony of expert witnesses) of the standard of care, the breach of the standard of care, the way in which the breach caused damages, and the extent of damages alleged to have been suffered as a result of the claimed negligence. The plaintiff must prove each of these elements by a preponderance of the evidence standard—i.e., a standard of medical probability.
4. *Defendant's proofs*. The defendant then calls witnesses and offers documentary and other evidence. This may include evidence (also offered through the testimony of expert witnesses) of the standard of care, compliance with the standard of care, the lack of a causal relationship between the treatment at issue and the damages claimed, or the extent of the damages.
5. *Closing arguments*. These give each attorney the chance to summarize the evidence and to make arguments on the evidence and how it bears on the issues the case presents.
6. *Jury instructions*. These are a series of statements on the jury's function and on the law the jury is to apply to the evidence it has heard.
7. *Jury deliberations and verdict*. The members of the jury then have the chance to discuss the case among themselves and to arrive at their decision on the issues. A verdict, if in favor of the plaintiff, is rendered for an amount of money intended to provide compensation to the plaintiff for the injury sustained. The verdict is most often provided in detailed form, separating past and future damages as well as economic and noneconomic damages. If the jury has found that there was negligence on the part of the plaintiff that also contributed to the injury, or if there are multiple defendants whose negligence may have contributed to the injuries in different degrees, the degrees of such negligence are specified.

The court has the opportunity to adjust the figure after the verdict, in order to:

- Reduce the economic damages by the amounts covered by insurance less the cost of premiums paid
- Limit the amount of noneconomic damages under statutes capping such awards, if any, in professional liability cases

In posttrial proceedings, the losing party also has the opportunity to make a motion for a new trial or to ask that the verdict be set aside as contrary to the great weight of the evidence. The amount of damages may also be challenged, and the court may (in rare cases) adjust the figure upward or downward if it finds that the law so requires. The postverdict proceedings also permit the prevailing party to request the imposition of costs and mediation sanctions where applicable.

Appeal

Once a judgment has been entered, the losing party may file an appeal. Appeals are most often filed on legal grounds—i.e., on issues of law—because the appellate courts give great deference to the findings of the jury on issues of fact. If an appeal is filed, it may take 18–24 months for a decision to be issued by a court of appeals and another 1–3 years or so for a final resolution by the state supreme court. A losing party may appeal to the Court of Appeals by right. Appeal is usually granted after the losing party has demonstrated to the court that a legal issue is indeed involved.

WARNINGS ABOUT BAD OUTCOMES

Now that you understand a little about the mechanics of malpractice litigation, medical thought process and language can be explained from the perspective of case evaluation, preparation, and pursuit. In addition to ''bad outcomes,'' surgeons rationalize technique failures and simply careless misuse of instruments as surgical misadventures. In some circles the term *surgical misadventure* has become an acute, less than critical, but excusable explanation of ''sometimes bad things happen to good people.'' To lawyers in a courtroom, interpreted for and before jurors, ''misadventure'' often means:

> *''You should not have been there.''*
> *''You should not have tried that.''*
> *''That was simply bad technique.''*
> *''Surgery should not be an adventure but a skilled scientific technique in well trained hands.''*

Explaining injury based on ''varied training'' may be a medical reason but is not a lawful excuse. Most of the time when a major vessel is injured during a laparoscopic procedure it is due to inadequate training, incomplete training, improper positioning, or an unacceptable distraction at a critical time. ''Varied training'' suggests that the range of such training, from outstanding to mediocre and cavalier, is acceptable. Patients are becoming more knowledgeable about advanced endoscopy because of physician advertising, education, and promotion of these procedures. It should be, but often is not, that those who advertise and promote also teach quality. Sometimes it is said of trial lawyers that today are ''rapidly becoming savvy.'' This suggests less than a complete understanding of how and what high-quality trial lawyers do. Actually, it sounds a little derogatory and thereby masks the significance of available general knowledge. Good lawyers stay up to date with new procedures, surprisingly read a great deal more than many practicing physicians, and their goal is not to catch up but to "stay ahead." Concentration must be on protecting the patient, and the medical literature should not speak as much of what we can do to protect self. If the patient is protected and properly treated, there will automatically be much less risk to all concerned. The concept remains:

> *Do the right thing, at the right time, in the right way, depending on the particular circumstances at that time, and if the anticipated response is not immediately obtained, investigate why it was not the result anticipated. There is a tendency to teach that proper documentation is a substitute, or can be used as a substitute for bad results, improper technique, untimely or improper intervention, or simply not being there with the right answers when needed.*
> *Was the procedure needed, not just wanted?*
> *Did he know how to do it or was he still on a learning curve?*
> *Was it done carefully enough or was there a little unnecessary risk?*
> *Could help have been readily available?*
> *Not every tool requires that it be used.*
> *Not every procedure requires that it be done frequently or in the next patient.*

Physicians have not yet implemented that which industry uses on a daily basis. There are techniques for proper identification and problem solving that are generic and then are specifically refined and implemented for the purposes intended. Such techniques are not taught in medical school; they should be taught in residency training programs but do not exist as such. Instead, "judgment" is a phrase frequently heard, without further explanation, by young physicians. It is no wonder that "I used my judgment" is a frequent defense when an explanation during a medical malpractice case is required. It no longer has any validity when properly examined, because we now recognize that there are both good and bad judgments. Problem identification and problem-solving techniques depend on known facts, scientific principle, and processes of inclusion and elimination. Good judgment requires accumulating all available relevant facts accurately, understanding them, sorting out those that are significant, and then acting according to what they mean and what can be expected by either action, incorrect action, or inaction. Problem recognition and problem-solving techniques are required in the previously described peer review process; simply relying on a reviewer's instinct would be inadequate. There must be a conscious development of error investigation techniques, recognition of improper surgical technique, and where, when and how intervention procedures are required.

Many physicians attempt to use the informed consent process as a prophylaxis against medical malpractice litigation. Let us assume that there was an adequate, complete, and detailed explanation of complications, risk of injury, and even alternative procedures. Let us assume that there was a bad outcome and that the patient had been warned, informed, and gave consent to the possibility of such an injury. Many doctors believe that such a patient cannot sue. Wrong. It is unlawful for a patient to consent to negligence. It must be clearly understood that there is no consent and there can be no permission granted by a patient to negligence, to a breach of the acceptable standard of care, the deviation from the acceptable means of surgical entry, to doing it wrong, to the kind of mistake such as to a misdirection of the entry needle or trocar. All these mean the same. The concept of an unintentional injury by the surgeon who tried to do it correctly, satisfying some criterion, is fallacious. Good surgical care requires doing it the right way, at the right time, for the right reason, in the right position, with the right precautions, in the right patients, under the right circumstances. If not done this way, the burden is on the doctor to prove if not, why not. Many events can be cited. For example, if a patient's body habitus creates an increased risk, doctors must stop using "risk" as suggesting a reason and excuse. *Risk* means that something needs to be avoided or prevented, and that failing to do so is unacceptable. A known risk requires even greater care, and a failure to do so creates a hazard in surgical injuries. Most litigation over the kinds of injuries created by needle and trocar entries is due to improper postoperative management, including not only delayed recognition but the failure to consult, incorrect intervention, and an incompletely or inadequately informed family about the events causing the patient not to improve as expected. Occasionally it is said that a surgical injury is "devastating for the surgeon." This is an unnecessary statement. It sounds too much like "I feel your pain, and I have some too." Feeling badly when this happens to a patient is a very good mood to display in front of a jury but has nothing to do with risk prevention, recognition, correction, and education. The event and its environment can lead to a malpractice lawsuit. A vascular injury to a great vessel during laparoscopic entry is, according to most leading surgeons, due to improper penetration or misdirection of the instrument, which includes incorrect positioning of the patient prior to instrument introduction. A rationalization that scar caused trocar introduction to be different or that it had anything to do with forcing a change in the direction or in the angle of insertion is unrealistic. The iliac vessels, for example, are injured by a medial-to-lateral misdirection. Legal action usually does not follow if damages are minimal and there is proper recognition, intervention, and timely repair with an uncomplicated postoperative recovery. In such cases litigation is usually not begun, most often fails, and is frequently dismissed. The key words are *prompt recognition*, *timely intervention*, and *proper management*. When an entry occurs with a second trocar, the question must be asked whether anyone was looking through the first. Someone should have been.

There is no excuse if there was not. The fact that injuries from a secondary trocar are hard to explain clearly implies that they should not happen. They are almost always due to carelessness. Even when smaller amounts of blood are seen, an accurate explanation is required, not be the implication that a little bit is acceptable. Great oaks from little acorns grow. When a surgeon notices dripping from a subumbilical puncture site and the patient subsequently goes into shock due to blood loss, the quality of the surgeon's inspection must be questioned. One must look for the most serious and not the most benign cause of unexpected bleeding. Just because something bad happens after instrumentation does not necessarily mean that there was any negligence. The evidentiary rule of res ipsa loquitur is generally misunderstood. Some may say that the occurrence of bleeding from the insertion side of an instrument must be negligence. That was a ruling in Canada. It would not be so in the United States, as there would probably be an expert witness for the defense indicating that this kind of thing can happen even without negligence, and under those circumstances most judges would refuse to apply the rule. We emphasize, however, that delayed recognition of significant bleeding causes severe patient injury and leads to successful litigation. Delay is a definite problem. Additionally, it should be emphasized that the direction of the must be kept in the needle and trocar midline. Whenever bleeding occurs, whenever symptoms exist, whenever the complaints are greater than the doctor likes or expects, the surgeon must look at the surgical procedure, the technique, and the events as being responsible. It is with prompt recognition, proper intervention, and correct management that patient complications are corrected and that litigation is frequently avoided.

ATTITUDES CREATE RISK

Medical malpractice happens—just like some bumper stickers exclaim—most often on weekends and holidays. It is more common when doctors are overworked and anxious to get to their hobbies or faced with treating a patient they really may not like. When these conditions occur in combination with tasks that offer doctors no immediate economic reward—telephone consultations, checking on a hospitalized patient for a colleague, or giving telephone orders to the intensive care unit for a postoperative patient who is experiencing problems—a fertile environment for malpractice incidents is created. We hear of doctors who are unable to obtain malpractice insurance and therefore refuse to deliver obstetric care to indigent or Medicaid patients because they believe these patients are at high risk for delivering brain-damaged babies and therefore for filing malpractice lawsuits. The same prejudices can be applied to laparoscopic surgery.

In the course of reviewing 12,000 medical insurance claims and malpractice lawsuits, which I do as a routine part of discovery and trial preparation, I found them to involve a substantial number of patients who are poor and uneducated;

these are the patients, often unpleasant to deal with, who fail to develop a functioning relationship with the doctor.

It is clear that such patients are frequently the fault of malpractice suits, though they are not legally *at fault*. There is a difference between being the fault and being "at fault." To be "at fault" for an injury is to negligently have caused harm, the basis for a lawsuit. Although patients who are disliked or "undesirable" may be "the fault" of a lawsuit, these are the very patients who should be treated with even greater care by doctors, perhaps because no one has ever cared enough for them. Moreover, it is for these patients that malpractice may be the most preventable of all.

Medical malpractice suits are encouraged by the fact that quality assurance and peer review committees, as well as risk-management organizations, often fail to do what they are charged to do. They do not deal with attitudes of physicians and with the nature of personal relationships between doctors and patients—what industry calls "public relations." Not only are the proceedings of peer review committees barred from use in the court, they cannot even be discovered except under extreme circumstances. These committees are composed of doctors who themselves might be at risk for criticism. Such in-hospital committees react vigorously to doctors they do not like but rarely criticize or reprimand respected physicians who just are not careful enough on weekends, on holidays, with patients in whom they have lost interest, or with families who are too inquisitive or too demanding.

Hospitals do not do enough to prevent medical malpractice because they do not believe they can exert control over physicians and because administrators need to preserve the bottom line while maintaining peace. Hospitals depend on doctors to keep the beds full and to perform more and more procedures. Many doctors see too many patients per day and perform too many procedures per week. Others fail to provide proper preoperative evaluations or to provide postoperative hands-on bedside care for more than 2–3 min per day. The postoperative surgery patient with an iatrogenic reaction needs her or his doctor for frequent revisits. That was the way it used to be; it no longer is.

To prevent malpractice events, doctors must recognize the risks, give each patient a little more attention, practice early intervention, thank nurses instead of criticizing and ignoring them, and listen to patients, even if patients do not couch their medical complaints in educated language.

The importance of warmth, compassion, caring, and listening to the patient is being written back into medical practice. Doctors are learning the importance of public relations and communication skills because the patient is making consumer demands. However, in the event that a malpractice claim is filed and a case goes to trial, juries may be less likely to award general damages—compensation for physical and psychic pain and suffering—if they perceive the doctor as "caring."

Measures to prevent malpractice will improve the quality of medical care. Quality medical care requires earlier intervention. Intervention requires recognition of problems by physicians before there is a chance to become careless.

PREVENTIVE SOLUTIONS DO EXIST

There are substantive ways to decrease laparoscopic malpractice. There is even more assurance that recurrent bad outcomes—because the correct thing was not done at the right time in the right way—can be minimized. Of the techniques available, mandatory videotaping is one. This—that is, videotaping of each and every laparoscopic procedure for purposes of ''peer review''—should be done. It must not be feared that it will be used against a physician in subsequent litigation. Even if that is an unjustified fear, it by itself may be an incentive for correction. However, peer review would create a legal privilege in most states and allow such videotapes to be used for the correction of past mistakes as well as the prevention of future harms and to be kept from litigants. Every videotape on which a patient has an adverse reaction, needs immediate additional surgery, has a significant visceral injury, needs readmission for additional medical care within 14 days of discharge, or dies should be evaluated individually by members of a skilled surgical committee. Such reviews must be nonpunitive. Faulty surgical technique, errors, or criticisms are to be reported anonymously. Fault, surgical misadventures, surgical mistakes, or poor technique are to be looked for liberally and should readily require mentoring, monitoring, or additional retraining of the surgeon being reviewed. Information about findings, not people, is to be shared among all the surgeons, and recommendations for prevention and improved techniques are to be readily made. These procedures should not be feared but should provide incentives to health care providers to demonstrate continuously improving patient safety. Surgeons whose adverse reactions are evaluated in this manner should have any subsequent laparoscopic procedure again reviewed in a similar fashion, looking for recurring errors in technique or expected improvements. Collaboration between same and similar organizations in a community is to be encouraged. This attention to safety should be strong, clear, and visible. The system is to be nonpunitive and should be reported and analyzed within the larger organization. Expectations should be consistent with current medical knowledge and surgical technique. This system, among others created by the author, works. When correctly done, it will save hundreds of thousands of dollars for the surgeons, hospitals, and insurance companies involved within a very short time, in addition to preventing the emotional upheaval associated with being sued.

A hospital administration with the approval of medical staff and sometimes contrary to the staff's desire must be required to ''***have and put in place a clear, definitive, and objective goal to identify, confront, and prevent recurrences.***''

The medical staff, as the basic organizational unit of the hospital, was, in the past, regarded as capable of effectively evaluating and controlling the practice of practitioners within the institution. That is the way it was taught. It is no longer true. It has not worked. It does not work well. A new perspective is necessary.

The movie *Dead Poets' Society* was popular some years ago. In one scene, the students in an English class were asked to stand on their desks and look at the class—their environment—and see the commonplace from a different perspective. We can learn from that approach. The way we always did it is not necessarily the best way. Constructive criticism can indeed come from without. It is there without being solicited. Fault finding can be done by a blue ribbon panel that is not swayed and preoccupied by pre-existing prejudices and fears. It is the way it is done in successful industry and efficient government and it has often resulted in some of the finest ''white paper'' reports of modern time. A special prosecutor needs no particular skill in the area being investigated, and a constructive critic need not have the goal of punishing a wrongdoer. What about a special prosecutor whose job it is to find fault and prevent it? Then, instead of suggesting punishment, he or she would improvise a solution of prevention.

While implementing preventive techniques, hospitals must continue to be careful about new appointments, properly review their credentialing procedure, rigorously adhere to applicant evaluations, institute probation periods, which have some meaning, and carry out the spirit of bylaws in addition to their perfunctory granting of privileges. Every hospital should have a bylaw suggesting the following:

> Except as otherwise determined by the board, all initial appointments to any category of the staff shall be subject to a period of observation of 6 months. Each appointee shall be assigned initially to a department where his or her performance shall be observed by the chair of the department or such chair's designee. The purpose of this observation is to determine the appointee's eligibility for continued staff membership in the staff category to which he or she was initially appointed and for exercising the clinical privileges initially granted in that department. His or her exercise of clinical privileges in any other department shall also be subject to observation by that department's chair or his or her designee. An initial appointee shall remain subject to observation until he or she has furnished to the credentials committee (or the medical executive committee) and to the chief executive officer a statement signed by the chairman of the department to which he or she is assigned. This statement should verify that the appointee meets all of the qualifications, has discharged all of the responsibilities, and has not exceeded or abused the prerogatives of the staff category to which he or she is appointed. The committee must also receive a statement signed by the chairman of the

departments in which the appointee will exercise clinical privileges that he or she has satisfactorily demonstrated his or her ability to exercise the clinical privileges initially granted to him or her.

Personal proctoring has come and gone. Bring it back. The proctors must be hand-picked and carefully selected to use their best skills and talents with proper direction. The skilled surgeon may need to polish his or her public relations. The busiest doctor in town may not have adequate time for postoperative evaluations. The anesthesiologist may not wish to postpone a case, fearing the surgical team.

These procedures all include the evaluation of medical records. They must be evaluated for substance, not form. A timely signature and a daily progress note are important but insignificant inadequate faulty measures of quality. The determination how the working diagnosis or impression fits the patient and how, when, and why procedures were done require a critical "horizontal review of medical records analysis." This technique is detailed elsewhere. It helps answer questions of greater significance than those with which medical records committees waste their time to meet the easy review standards of most hospital inspections. The more important questions to prevent malpractice and to recognize those aspects of patient care that need improvement include the following:

Was the right thing done at the right time?
Under the circumstances, was the correct course of events outlined?
Was the action implemented at the proper speed?
Was the result obtained the result expected?
Was the result obtained the result desired? If not, what was done about it?
Is the progress note consistent with expectations and with previously recorded nursing observations?

When avoidable fault is found, when foreseeable injury is recognized, when a recurrent liability is identified, checklists are necessary.

Checklists work well for airline pilots and the Nuclear Regulatory Commission. Both deal with minute-to-minute critical situations. Checklists are not a substitute for thinking or for experience, but they do serve as reminders for smart people and awaken thought processes. Tough ones should be put in place even though they may be resented by practitioners.

Checklists are avoided, rejected, and not traditional among physicians.
Checklists are necessary.
Checklists must be developed for high-risk procedures and specific indications.
Checklists are resisted by physicians.

Checklists are not a threat. They serve as reminders of what the physician knows, should know, has forgotten, or is too busy to consider.
Checklists are a form of damage control to promote zero defects.
Checklists are easy to develop.
Checklist fear is a prejudice, which must be overcome.
Checklists work and are necessary; but they are never a substitute. They must be designed to make you think more, evaluate more carefully, understand more fully, and suggest what might be overlooked.

Outside consultants must be used to critique, to find fault, to suggest the elimination of certain practices and the development of others. They must be given the specific task of elevating the quality of care, of performing individual case-management evaluations and developing specific preincident procedures. When employed for the short term in the narrow capacity for the specific purpose outlined, the consultants should have carte blanche to search records, interview nurses, discuss complaints with patients and families, observe physicians and surgical procedures, and listen in on consultations without prior notice to the medical or nursing staff. In short, *you should be a catalyst to implement quality improvement and prevention practices.*

18

Oncology

Rodrigo Gonzalez and Bruce J. Ramshaw
Emory University School of Medicine, Atlanta, Georgia, U.S.A.

INTRODUCTION

The laparoscopic approach for general surgery has had widespread acceptance since its introduction in the late 1980s. The success of this technique for procedures such as cholecystectomy, Nissen fundoplication, splenectomy, and adrenalectomy has led to its application for a wide variety of more complex surgical procedures. When laparoscopy was initially used for the treatment of patients with cancer, concerns arose as to whether the oncological principles that are considered fundamental during open surgery would be compromised.

Published data have shown through pathological examination that laparoscopically resected specimens can achieve appropriate lymph node excision and ample tissue margins [1]. However, not long after the introduction of laparoscopic surgery for patients with colorectal cancer, authors started reporting cases of port-site metastases [2,3]. Over the following 2 years, at least 35 cases of port-site recurrences following laparoscopic and thoracoscopic procedures were documented in the literature [4], raising the possibility that the curative intent of minimally invasive techniques for cancer might actually compromise cure.

Fear of port-site metastases hindered the initial enthusiasm for using laparoscopy for resection of colorectal and other cancers. This later culminated at the beginning of the last decade, when the American Society of Colon and Rectal Surgeons recommended that curative resection of colorectal cancer should not be performed laparoscopically unless it were part of a prospective, controlled clinical trial [5]. Most experts agreed with this cautious approach and recommended that for colorectal cancer, the laparoscopic approach be limited to either palliative resection of advanced lesions or curative resection of early lesions. Moreover, many surgeons have limited their laparoscopic practice to benign conditions, where outcomes after colorectal resections have improved as experience was gained, even in more complicated patients. It is expected that the use of the laparoscopic approach for colorectal diseases will continue to increase over the next few years.

The use of laparoscopy in patients with colorectal cancer is increasing despite earlier concerns regarding this use. According to a recent review of our experience during the last decade, we found that laparoscopy for the treatment of colorectal disease in almost 900 patients consistently increased from 48% of all cases in 1992 to 80% in 2001 except between 1993 and 1996, when concern was raised in the literature about port-site recurrences. Following the publication of reports showing the adequacy of laparoscopic resections for cancer, the percentage of colorectal resections rapidly increased.

Although port-site metastasis is not unique to laparoscopic colorectal surgery, it has had a major impact on its use for cure of colorectal cancer. Consequently, the vast majority of the information in the literature, and therefore included in this chapter, is derived from extensive investigation of colorectal cancer. Although controversial results have been rendered and many of the preventive measures are yet to be proven, most of the information derived from these studies is being extrapolated to cancer in other organs.

COMPLICATIONS

Colorectal Cancer

Overall morbidity after laparoscopic colectomy ranges between 6.8 and 22.3% [6,7], and is more common in patients with large tumors fixed to adjacent structures. The conversion rate reported in the literature is between 5 and 12.7% [6,7]. According to Agachan et al., the most significant variable affecting intraoperative complication rates is surgical experience [8]. Operative complications during colorectal resections include bleeding secondary to injury of the mesenteric vessels (2.3%), bowel perforation (1.9%), and injury to the ureter (0.3%) [7]. The placement of indwelling catheters during open colorectal surgery has been recommended for the prevention of ureteral injuries. Since intraoperative tactile localization of the ureters is impossible in laparoscopic surgery, the role of preoperative placement of lighted ureteral stents, placed selectively, has been recognized as a valuable adjunct to laparoscopic colectomy to safeguard ureteral integrity. Complications related to the stents occur infrequently and include transient hematuria and reflux anuria, both reversible without further intervention [9,10].

Wound infections following elective colorectal resections vary between 2.5 and 33%, according to the procedure performed [6,11–13]. Cancer is the presenting diagnosis in 66% of patients with postoperative wound infections. Use of both suprapubic and perineal closed suction drains yield infection rates from 8–18% and 7–31%, respectively [14]. Factors increasing the risk of wound infection include immunocompromised host and direct contact of bowel and skin [6]. The lengths of stay and costs are significantly increased in patients who develop wound infections.

Anastomotic leaks following colorectal resection are usually associated with technical error or inadequate vascularization. The leak rate from the anastomosis also varies according to the underlying diagnosis and the procedure performed [7,11]. The leak rate after a laparoscopic colorectal resection with primary anastomosis is between 0.8 and 4.3% [6,7,11,12]. Cancer is the most common underlying disease (64%) associated with anastomotic leaks. Leaks range from 1.5% after sigmoid resection to 5% following a left hemicolectomy. This compares favorably with the 2–8% rate reported for open colectomy [15]. The incidence of postoperative intra-abdominal abscess formation is 1% and is associated with intraoperative complications in over 80% of the cases. Milder cases of both leaks and abscesses can be managed conservatively with intravenous antibiotics and drainage, sometimes, guided by computed tomography (CT). Köckerling et al. reported successful conservative management in 63% of cases [7]. Nevertheless, urgent surgical treatment is frequently necessary in septic patients. Sepsis is among the most common causes of death in patients following colorectal resection [7,11]. In an attempt to avoid its occurrence, it is vital to perform a tension-free anastomosis, ensure an adequate blood supply, and verify the presence of an intact doughnut in the specimen retrieved from the stapler. However, leaks cannot be completely avoided and may still occur even after these preventive measures [6].

Other complications reported in the literature following laparoscopic resections for colorectal cancer include anastomotic stenosis (3.5%), pneumonia (1.2%), internal hernia (0.8%), rotation of the anastomosis (0.8%), and urinary tract infections (0.6–6%) [6,11,12].

The current oncological standards for performing a curative resection for colon cancer include "en bloc" resection, the "no touch" technique, proximal lymphovascular ligation, and complete lymphadenectomy [16]. In the performance of a laparoscopic resection, right and transverse colon cancers pose difficulties during lymph node dissection and high ligation of the middle colic vessels, respectively. Hand-assisted laparoscopic surgery (HALS) has been reported to work as a bridge between the open and laparoscopic techniques. Consequently, for surgeons in their learning curve and for more difficult resections, HALS can allow a successful colon resection without the need to convert to a formal open operation.

Complications inherent to the laparoscopic approach include trocar-site hernias (1.2%) and trocar injuries to intra-abdominal structures (0.8%) [6]. Trocar-site hernias can be minimized by closing the fascia of all trocar sites $\geq$10 mm. Trocar injuries become less as surgeons gain experience in laparoscopic techniques, and their incidence may be further decreased using the Hasson technique for initial access in patients with previous abdominal surgeries.

Gallbladder Cancer

Gallbladder carcinoma is the fifth most common cancer of the gastrointestinal tract. It is found in 0.35–2% of all biliary tract operations. Preoperative diagnosis is possible in less than 10% of cases; therefore diagnosis is usually determined only after histological examination of the gallbladder [17–19]. Frozen-section diagnosis is effective in cases with lesions of stage T2 or greater and has been recommended to prevent tumor dissemination following laparoscopic cholecystectomy for unsuspected gallbladder carcinoma [20]. In case of intraoperative diagnosis of carcinoma, most experts recommend conversion to open radical surgery. Radical hepatic resection has been proven to improve survival for patients with stage T2 gallbladder carcinoma that is first discovered after laparoscopic cholecystectomy [21].

Some retrospective series report that laparoscopic surgery is associated with acceleration of intraperitoneal dissemination in previously unrecognized gallbladder cancer, especially in stage T3, but also in patients with *in situ* carcinoma. In addition, contemporary standard preoperative diagnosis and preventive measures are inadequate to avoid this complication [22,23]. Consequently, concerns arise that an unsuspected gallbladder carcinoma can be missed when minimally invasive techniques are used, because there is no palpation feedback during the operation. The first case of port-site metastasis from an unsuspected gallbladder carcinoma was reported in 1991 [24]. Subsequently, other authors have also reported this complication [18,25–27], some even as early as 18 days after surgery [28].

In a recently published survey of almost 120,000 laparoscopic cholecystectomies, Paolucci et al. [29] reported a 0.35% incidence of gallbladder carcinoma on histological examination. Of these patients, 17% developed port-site metastases at a median of 3 months. In 13% of the patients, the tumor was classified as stage T1. The port used for gallbladder extraction was the most common site of recurrence [29], and there is usually only one implant at the time of diagnosis [19].

Wound metastases following laparoscopic cholecystectomy for unsuspected gallbladder carcinoma are rare but are more frequently encountered than with the open technique. They are known to recur following wide local excision, wide local excision with omentectomy, and radical hepatic resection [18,28]. The overall 2-year survival rate is 18.5%. The longest disease-free period following radical hepatic resection and excision of port-site metastases is 3 years [30]. With the aid of adjuvant chemotherapy alone or a combination of radiotherapy and chemotherapy, with or without excision of the wound metastases, results of disease-free survival of up to 10 months have been published [17,24,31,32].

In conclusion, most experts recommend conversion of the laparoscopic procedure in case of suspicion or documentation of gallbladder carcinoma. If the diagnosis is made postoperatively, a subsequent open hepatectomy is the current standard treatment. In case of developing port-site metastases, the patient should be offered aggressive treatment, including wide local resection and chemotherapy, with or without radiotherapy.

Hepatic Cancer

Laparoscopic partial liver resections were reported in the early 1990s [33]. However, the first anatomical liver resection (a left lateral segmentectomy) was reported by Azagra et al. in 1996 [34]. An increasing number of publications have been reported since, especially laparoscopic treatment of benign liver tumors by resection or ablation. However, laparoscopic resection of liver malignancies has not been widely accepted.

For laparoscopic resection of liver malignancies, the same oncological techniques as for the open procedures should be applied. These include the ''no touch'' technique, R_0 radical resection, and achievement of a 1-cm free surgical margin. For this purpose, the use of the laparoscopic ultrasound is of invaluable aid, since it allows the surgeon to determine tumor margins and the adjacent vascular and biliary structures. This facilitates the surgeon's choice of location of the liver transection. Other instruments and technologies have been developed to facilitate laparoscopic hepatectomies. We recently published our experience in using currently available technology (i.e., laparoscopic ultrasound, ultrasound coagulator, ultrasonic dissectors, CUSA®, the TissueLink Floating Ball, and endoscopic staplers) in an animal model of laparoscopic living-donor hepatectomy [35]. In our experience, available technology allows surgeons to compensate for the loss of tactile feedback by positively identifying major vessels and biliary anatomy, therefore decreasing bleeding and other complications.

There are numerous reports of excellent outcomes after laparoscopic hepatectomies for cancer; however, only one has reported long-term follow-up. In a multicenter European study of 37 patients, Gigot et al. reported adequate operative results with a conversion rate of 13.5%, postoperative complication rate of 22%, and reoperation rate of 5%. The surgical margin was less than 1 cm in 30% of patients. A 2-year survival rates of 44% in patients with hepatocellular carcinoma and 53% in patients with hepatic metastases from colorectal cancer was reported. No port-site metastases were reported at a mean follow-up of 14 months [36].

Despite deleterious effects of pneumoperitoneum associated with the Pringle maneuver in animal studies [37,38], Gigot and colleagues [36] reported that five patients in their series tolerated the maneuver well, which varied from 15 to 50 min. However, portal triad clamping was used for liver resections, which would not have been used during an open surgery. Furthermore, when the Pringle maneuver is used for radiofrequency ablation of liver tumors in animal studies, the ablation volume has been reported to increase the peripheral volume to almost twice in a significantly shorter time than when the maneuver is not employed, without endothelial damage or thermally induced intravascular thrombosis of the hepatic or portal veins [39].

The use of radiofrequency energy to coagulate liver tumors has gained popularity over recent years. Although not widely accepted as an alternative for surgical therapy in resectable cancers, it has a role for the focal treatment of inoperable liver tumors. It is most frequently performed percutaneously under ultrasound guidance, but some cases require liver mobilization to place the probe accurately. This is where the laparoscopic approach has gained popularity over the open technique, since it provides all the advantages of a minimally invasive approach in a debilitated patient in whom it is desired to avoid a large incision. However, it still results in complication rates similar to those of percutaneous and open techniques. In a review of 3670 cases, Mulier et al. reported complication rates of 7.2% with the percutaneous, 9.5% with the laparoscopic, and 9.9% with the open techniques [40].

Gastric Cancer

Gastric cancer remains one of the leading causes of cancer death worldwide. The experience obtained by surgeons in suturing and stapling and the development of new techniques and instruments have helped achieve adequate results following gastric resections for benign diseases. Only recently have minimally invasive techniques been explored as an alternative to traditional open surgery. The use of laparoscopically assisted distal gastrectomy was first reported by Kitano and colleagues in 1994 [41], and subsequently reported by other investigators to be safe and effective, even along with an extended lymphadenectomy.

Seeding of the abdominal wall has also been reported following minimally invasive procedures in patients with gastric cancer. However, due to the relatively small number of patients with gastric cancer approached laparoscopically, they are reported only sporadically. In a recent review of 43 patients undergoing laparoscopically assisted distal gastrectomy for early gastric cancer, Fujiwara et al. reported no port-site metastases at a mean follow-up of 37 months [42].

Gynecological Cancer

Childers et al. reported a 1% rate of trocar-site metastasis in 105 laparoscopic procedures performed, of which 80% were for ovarian cancer. Abdominal wall metastases from early-stage ovarian adenocarcinoma have been reported [43,44]. Rieger and McIntosh even reported port-site metastases from colon and ovary primaries at incisions other than the site of extraction following a laparoscopic cholecystectomy for cholecystitis [45].

Bacha et al. reported a case of port-site metastasis after a laparoscopically assisted hysterectomy and salpingo-oophorectomy in a patient with unsuspected adenocarcinoma of the fallopian tube [46].

Urological Cancer

The phenomenon of port-site metastasis has not eluded the urologists, although only sporadic cases have been reported even after more than 400 radical nephrectomies, 200 retroperitoneal lymph node dissections, and thousands of radical prostatectomies [47–49]. Contributing factors published for port-site metastasis in urology include biological aggressiveness of the tumor (high state or high grade), violation of the tumor boundaries, no use of a specimen removal bag, or ripping of the bag, specimen morcellation, and ascites [50].

PALLIATIVE LAPAROSCOPIC SURGERY

A major operation in a patient with advanced, complicated cancer has the potential for a relatively high incidence of operative morbidity and mortality; moreover, it is a highly stressful event requiring a substantial recovery in a chronically ill and often already debilitated patient. Coexisting factors such as advanced patient age and comorbid conditions may also affect these outcomes. The reported morbidity and mortality rates of patients undergoing elective open palliative surgery for primary colorectal cancer range from 18–24% and 8–9%, respectively [51,52]. Patients undergoing a palliative resection have a mean survival time of 10–12 months [51–53]. Those with less than 50% of liver involved by metastasis are reported to have longer survival time after a palliative resection [52]. Among the advantages of the laparoscopic as compared to open technique is an attenuated acute phase of the inflammatory response and reduced postoperative pain, both of which can be beneficial in patients with advanced cancer.

Port-site metastasis, probably the most compelling argument against the use of laparoscopy for patients with cancer, should be of much less concern for palliative procedures. However, patients with complicated colorectal cancer may have the added difficulty of poor visibility due to large bowel obstruction, frail tissue due to the acute inflammatory process following a perforation, or acute bleeding. Therefore we recommend that the minimally invasive approach in these patients be attempted only by surgeons adequately trained in laparoscopic techniques, experienced in complicated laparoscopic cases, and having an appropriate threshold for conversion to an open procedure when indicated.

Up to 85% of acute colonic obstructions are due to malignancy, and between 10 and 30% of the patients with colon cancer present with obstructive symptoms [54]. As an alternative to performing a colostomy in obstructed patients with nonresectable cancer, nonsurgical management modalities include balloon dilation, decompression tubes, electrocoagulation, and laser photocoagulation [55]. These therapies used in distal tumors have resulted in variable outcomes, significant morbidity, and the need to repeat the procedure. The use of stents for decompression prior to surgery or as a palliative treatment in patients with advanced colorectal cancer has recently been introduced. Reported complications include perforation (4%), pain (5%), bleeding (5%), reobstruction (10%), and stent migration (10%) [56,57]. Stents can also cause anorectal pain and tenesmus when placed in patients with rectal tumors. It is our practice to use stents when appropriate, but in cases of difficult placement, complications, or suspicion of vascular compromise of involved bowel, a surgical decompression is performed. Our experience in 5 patients includes 3 having undergone unsuccessful stent placement, 1 with suspected bowel ischemia, and 1 with perforation as a complication of the stent placement.

Laparoscopic surgery has been described to be safe and effective for palliation of patients with incurable colorectal cancer [53]. We have recently reviewed patients who underwent laparoscopic palliative surgery for acute complications of colorectal cancer, such as perforation, obstruction, and bleeding. One of the most encouraging findings in our study was the lack of operative mortalities among these patients, which compares favorably with mortality rates reported after open (8–10%) [58,59] and laparoscopic (7%) [53] elective palliative surgeries.

There is still controversy regarding the management of patients presenting with obstructed colorectal cancer, especially when the left side is involved. Emergency surgical treatment for left-sided malignant obstruction has morbidity and mortality rates of 4–60% and 3–11%, respectively [51,60,61]. Primary resection with on-table lavage and immediate anastomosis in the management of this condition has reported advantages over resection and fecal diversion [54,60]. The creation of a colostomy has reported morbidity rates of up to 34% and, according to some series, only 60% undergo stoma reversal [54]. However, the on-table lavage and primary anastomosis is an extremely time-consuming procedure and is not indicated in all patients. A recent survey showed that only 53% of surgeons select a one-stage procedure in obstructed ''good-risk'' patients, and less than half of these procedures included an on-table lavage. A proximal colostomy was recommended for all ''high-risk'' patients and for 88% of patients with perforation associated with local peritonitis [62].

In conclusion, the feasibility, safety, and efficacy of the laparoscopic approach has been demonstrated in patients with advanced and unresectable colorectal cancer, even when associated with acute complications such as perforation, obstruction, and bleeding. Since the minimally invasive approach may result in a diminished inflammatory reaction compared to the open technique in this group of already immunosuppressed and debilitated patients, surgeons experienced in laparoscopic colorectal resection should consider it a part of the armamentarium in the palliative management of advanced, complicated colorectal cancer.

PORT-SITE METASTASES

There are several reports of tumor implantation at port sites for a variety of abdominal malignancies, including gallbladder [63,64], stomach [65], pancreas [66], and ovaries [67]. However, most of these reports involve laparoscopic surgery for colorectal cancer.

Table 1 summarizes the incidence of port-site metastases following laparoscopic surgery for colorectal cancer reported in large series during the last decade. The incidence ranges between 0 and 2.5%, with a mean of 0.7% in over 3000 patients. It is interesting to note that a linear regression analysis showed a significant decline in the number of cases reported over time ($p=0.01$; $r = -0.5296$; 95% CI: -0.7776 to -0.1389). It is therefore reasonable to presume that surgeons' experience might contribute to the decreased incidence of this complication. This seems to confirm that limited experience in laparoscopic colorectal surgery may correspond to an increased risk of trocar-site recurrences.

According to a recently published review [89], port-site metastases can occur as the only site of recurrence, but this is an extremely rare event. Furthermore, the incidence does not appear to be significantly different from that reported for open surgery for malignancy. Although thoroughly studied, the exact mechanism of tumor cell seeding in the abdominal wall is unknown. The following is a summary of the proposed mechanisms, some of which have been proven to influence the risk of developing port-site metastases following laparoscopic surgery. As previously stated, most of the information is derived from results of experimental studies investigating colorectal cancer specifically.

Proposed Mechanisms

The mechanism of port-site recurrences, first noted in thoracoscopic surgery without CO_2 insufflation, is unclear. Several combinations of factors have been proposed to increase risk, including direct tumor manipulation, failure to isolate the tumor, and forceful extraction of the surgical specimen [16,88].

The Role of the Immune System

It is now well established that surgery results in decreased host resistance to tumor growth. Other experiments have shown that operative stress actually increases the tendency of tumors to metastasize. Mechanical manipulation of the primary tumor

TABLE 1 Incidence of Port-Site Metastases Reported in Recent Published Clinical Series of Laparoscopic Resections for Colorectal Cancer

Authors	Year	Number of Patients	Number of Port-Site Metastases	Percent of Port-Site Metastases
Guillou et al. [68]	1993	59	1	1.7
Boulez et al. [69]	1996	117	3	2.5
Lord et al. [70]	1996	41	0	0
Franklin et al. [71]	1996	191	0	0
Gellman et al. [72]	1996	58	1	1.7
Kwok et al. [73]	1996	83	1	1.2
Hoffman et al. [74]	1996	130	1	0.8
Vukasin et al. [75]	1996	451	5	1.1
Fleshman et al. [76]	1996	372	4	1.1
Lacy et al. [6]	1997	106	0	0
Fielding et al. [77]	1997	149	2	1.3
Larach et al. [78]	1997	108	0	0
Croce et al. [79]	1997	134	1	0.9
Khalili et al. [80]	1998	80	0	0
Bouvet et al. [81]	1998	91	0	0
Kawamura et al. [82]	1998	67	0	0
Bohm et al. [83]	1999	63	0	0
Pearlstone et al. [84]	1999	93	0	0
Leung et al. [85]	1999	217	1	0.65
Melotti et al. [86]	1999	163	2	1.2
Poulin et al. [87]	1999	172	0	0
Schiedeck et al. [88]	2000	399	1	0.25
Total		**3284**	**23**	**0.7**

can give rise to blood-borne tumor emboli, a process known as seeding, which causes distant metastatic implants. Tumor embolization begins during or immediately after the operation. Such tumor embolization along with decreased immune surveillance can result in local tumor recurrence as well as port-site and/or distant metastases.

There is evidence that stressful events, such as a surgical procedure and postoperative pain, can compromise host resistance to infectious and malignant diseases in experimental and clinical settings [90,91]. Moreover, the extent to which the immune system provides tumor surveillance in humans is unknown. Among the immune mechanisms known to recognize and kill tumor cells are the natural killer (NK) cells. Findings indicate that stress-induced suppression of NK activity is the primary mediator enhancing tumor development and may increase the patient's susceptibility to tumor metastasis during or shortly after surgery [90,91]. NK-cell cytotoxicity is significantly depressed after laparotomy compared to both anesthesia alone and laparoscopy for 24 to 96 hr after the operation [91]. NK-cell cytotoxicity is also depressed after laparoscopy but returns to near normal levels by postoperative day 4. It has also been suggested, based on animal models, that the incidences, rates, and sizes of the metastases are proportional to the surgical stress [91]. Although in a lower proportion, CO_2 has also been shown in vitro to depress peritoneal macrophage function [92] and to cause systemic immune disturbances [93]. Also, adequate postoperative pain control has been reported to attenuate immunosuppression and metastatic dissemination [94,95]. Compared to open colectomy for colorectal cancer, the laparoscopic approach results in less postoperative pain, an earlier return of bowel activity, and a shorter length of hospital stay [96–98].

Continuous pH recording in the abdominal cavity reveals a consistent fall in intraperitoneal pH to less than 6 some 45 min after CO_2 insufflation [98]. There is a significant in vivo reduction in tumor necrosis factor alpha (TNF-α) and interleukin-1 (IL-1) production and an increase in IL-10 production from intra-abdominal macrophages after exposure to CO_2 pneumoperitoneum. This effect is not seen following gasless laparoscopy, helium pneumoperitoneum, or anesthesia alone [93,99,100].

In a study of intrahepatic tumor spread following laparoscopic surgery, gasless laparoscopy showed a significantly lower degree of tumor cells, a better-preserved Kupffer cell function, and a significant reduction of the expression of cell adhesion molecule CD44v5,v6 compared to CO_2 pneumoperitoneum and laparotomy [101]. Another study by the same group of authors revealed that CO_2 pneumoperitoneum seems to stimulate the growth of tumor cells into overt liver metastases. Also, gasless laparoscopy may have a protective effect against metastatic disease of the liver [102].

The Role of CO_2

Both open and laparoscopic operations increase the risk of primary tumor growth. While tumor growth after blunt manipulation is greater following laparotomy, wound metastases after tumor laceration are five times more likely following laparoscopy [103]. Animal studies have implicated CO_2 pneumoperitoneum and direct seeding of the abdominal wall with contaminated instruments containing tumor cells after manipulation of the tumor. Compared to anesthesia control, open minilaparotomy, or helium pneumoperitoneum, CO_2 pneumoperitoneum has been found to be associated with a significantly higher incidence of port-site metastases [91,104–107]. Jones et al. demonstrated a significant increase in port-site metastases after just 10 min of pneumoperitoneum [106]. Furthermore, it has been demonstrated that metastases occur even when no laparoscopic procedure is actually performed [105,106].

Cytological examination of peritoneal washings, instruments, suction devices, and trocars has revealed the presence of tumor cells during staging laparoscopy for pancreatic cancer in humans. Only sporadically has tumor cell implantation been encountered on the camera [108]. However, CO_2 contains only very low levels of free-floating tumor cells, even in the presence of massive peritoneal tumor implants. When outgoing CO_2 was examined by means of a suction trap in 35 patients undergoing laparoscopic surgery, including 20 for benign diseases and 15 for noncolorectal cancers, malignant cells were found in only 2 of the patients with peritoneal carcinomatosis. The authors concluded that malignant cells are aerosolized, but only during laparoscopy in the presence of carcinomatosis, and that it is unlikely that tumor cell aerosolization contributes significantly to port-site metastasis [109]. In a similar study evaluating patients undergoing staging laparoscopy for pancreatic cancer, no free-floating tumor cells could be demonstrated in the CO_2, but they were retrieved on several of the instruments used [110]. Therefore tumor-site recurrences are unlikely to result from aerosolization of tumor cells [110,111].

Recurrences have been reported after thoracoscopy [112,113], mediastinoscopy [114], and abdominal lifting [115] where no CO_2 is used. It has also been demonstrated with the use of filters that cells move throughout the peritoneal cavity during laparoscopy via contaminated instruments, with local contamination of the port by water vapor dispersion remaining a possibility. This suggests that the incidence of port-site metastases might be reduced if mechanical contamination of the incisions with instruments or with the specimen can be avoided.

Scanning electron microscopic studies show that CO_2 pneumoperitoneum is associated with diffuse damage to the peritoneum [116,117]. Volz et al. found that the cellular borders of individual mesothelial cells become visible and the intercellular clefts increase in size, leaving large portions of the basal membrane exposed and sometimes denuded [116]. Following injection of tumor cells, recognizable metastases with diffuse distribution become visible after 48 hr. The entire peritoneum, including the injection site, is covered by confluent metastases 72–96 hr after the procedure. After injection of tumor cells without CO_2 insufflation, the peritoneum remains intact for up to 48 hr, followed by invasion of the basal membrane and small tumor cell clusters in the form of micrometastases. In another study, Hirabayashi et al. found that the peritoneum is peeled away and the muscular layer destroyed at the port site immediately following CO_2 insufflation, after which free cancer cells attach, developing port-site metastases [117].

Circulating tumor cells in the portal system cause metastatic spread of colorectal cancer to the liver. During laparoscopic surgery, there is a significant reduction in microcirculatory splanchnic blood flow when the pressure of the pneumoperitoneum is increased from 10–15 mmHg [118]. The resulting ischemia may render the peritoneum more susceptible to tumor ingrowth. Therefore intra-abdominal pressure has been a subject of interest regarding physiological changes during pneumoperitoneum. It is known that tumor growth, instrument contamination, and tumor recurrence at midline and port-site incisions are promoted after laparoscopy using any pressure between 5 and 15 mmHg [119,120]. However, in evaluating whether tumor growth is influenced by the amount of pressure, animal experimentation has resulted in contradictory findings. Wittich et al. reported significantly higher intra-abdominal tumor growth when the abdomen was insufflated to 16 mmHg than when it was insufflated to 4 mmHg [121]. Others have found that increasing pneumoperitoneum pressures have a limited impact on tumor growth [120,122]. Furthermore, Jacobi et al. reported an *in vitro* suppression of abdominal tumor growth after laparoscopy using CO_2 at 10 and 15 mmHg compared to pressures of 0 or 5 mmHg, and an *in vivo* suppression of tumor growth with intraperitoneal pressure of 15 mmHg compared to lower pressures [119].

Abdominal lifting (gasless procedure) has demonstrated favorable results compared with CO_2 pneumoperitoneum in terms of tumor growth and abdominal wall metastases in animal studies. Ishida et al. demonstrated that the growth of liver metastases increased following laparotomy and CO_2 pneumoperitoneum compared to abdominal lifting and to the experience with control animals (without any procedure other than tumor inoculation), whereas there was no difference between abdominal lifting and controls [123]. Bouvy et al. reported greater peritoneal tumor growth following laparotomy than in CO_2 pneumoperitoneum, which also resulted in greater tumor growth and incidence of port-site metastases compared to the group with the gasless laparoscopic approach [104]. Watson et al. found that even though growth of the primary tumor was equal in CO_2 pneumoperitoneum and gasless laparoscopy, wound metastases were less likely in the latter group [124].

Conclusion

Both the hematogenous and lymphatic routes of spread seem highly unlikely sources for abdominal wall recurrences. Studies have demonstrated that after manipulation or resection of the bowel during use of CO_2 pneumoperitoneum or an abdominal wall lifter, the instruments and ports are often contaminated with tumor cells. In contrast, CO_2 leak or desufflation-related transport of cells is infrequent [88,125]. Therefore most experts agree that spillage of cells from the primary tumor and direct seeding of the wound with viable tumor cells perioperatively are the most likely mechanisms.

However, the vast majority of published animal studies concerning port-site metastases have utilized the cell suspension model, which involves an intraperitoneal injection of a liquid suspension of tumor cells prior to the assessment of free tumor cell spread within the abdomen. This constitutes a major drawback, since it does not simulate true clinical scenarios. Furthermore, probably due to the large number of tumor cells injected, cell suspension studies usually report unrealistically high incidences of port-site metastases. Consequently it is unknown whether these findings reflect what actually occurs in clinical practice.

Preventive Measures

Measures proposed to prevent port-site metastases include suturing the ports in place to avoid displacement during the operation; handling the tumor as little as possible—utilizing the ''no-touch'' technique, in which the tumor is manipulated by grabbing adjacent structures and not the tumor itself; using an impermeable bag for specimen retrieval to minimize the risk of direct seeding from the port site and wound extraction site; and deflating the abdomen before removing the trocars to prevent contact between neoplasic cells and the skin while the CO_2 is extracted.

In a recently published experimental, randomized, single-blinded study investigating the influence of the quality of surgery on the incidence of port-site recurrences, it was demonstrated that protective surgical measures used during laparoscopic sigmoid resections resulted in a significantly lower incidence of tumor recurrences [126]. The protective measures used were the following: trocar fixation, prevention of gas leaks, rinsing of instruments with povidone-iodine, minilaparotomy protection, rinsing of trocars before removal, peritoneal closure, and rinsing of all wounds with povidone-iodine.

It is believed that direct tumor cell seeding occurs in large part when the tumor is extracted through the wound. Consequently most surgeons have implemented the use of specimen retrieval bags and wound protectors in the effort to avoid direct contact between the tumor and the skin wound. These methods decrease the risk; however, trocar-site metastases occur despite their use [127].

Experimental studies have shown that modification of the physical environment of the pneumoperitoneum might have a beneficial effect in reducing tumor growth. The use of heated and humidified CO_2 has been proven to significantly reduce trocar contamination in an in vitro experimental model [128]. Experimental use of alternative gases has resulted in contradictory findings. While some models indicate less tumor growth using helium and room air [106], others demonstrate no difference [129], and some reveal a decrease in tumor growth using CO_2 rather than air or nitrogen dioxide [130].

Another approach for the reduction of tumor cell implants consists of the use of different chemotherapy agents. Both heparin and taurolidine cause inhibition of tumor growth and tumor cell implantation compared to control animals (with only tumor inoculation) but have maximum effects when used simultaneously [131]. Intraperitoneal instillation of a povidone-iodine solution in a rat model prevented wound recurrence compared with instillation of isotonic sodium chloride solution, methotrexate, aqueous chlorhexidine acetate, and intramuscular injection of methotrexate. Based on their results, the authors recommended routine peritoneal washings with diluted povidone-iodine solution during laparoscopic colorectal resections for cancer [132]. A similar study reveals greater efficacy with 5-fluorouracil compared to water, isotonic sodium chloride solution, and heparin [133]. Port-site metastases were prevented by taurolidine irrigation but not by ocreotide irrigation in an animal model of pancreatic cancer [134]. In another experimental study, heparin and Gly–Arg–Gly–Asp–Ser (GRGDS) pentapeptide showed a trend toward decreased number and size of tumors compared with the tumor-only groups, although the differences were not statistically significant [135].

The use of intraperitoneal chemotherapy at the time of laparoscopic colorectal resection for cancer or in the early postoperative period has been suggested. The rationale for this therapeutic approach is that isolated intraperitoneal tumor cells are the ideal targets for locoregional chemotherapy. In an experimental study, doxorubicin was found to be most effective if administered intraperitoneally before postoperative day 3, and intraoperative administration of recombinant tissue plasminogen activator (rt-PA) significantly increased the efficacy in both early and delayed intraperitoneal chemotherapy with doxorubicin [136].

These findings imply that prophylactic irrigation with different substances may decrease cell adherence and prevent tumor implantation to the wound site after accidental intraoperative tumor cell spillage. However, it is important to remember that these modalities are still under investigation; they are not proven and are sometimes not accepted in the clinical setting.

Wound recurrences in Open Surgery

There is evidence that recurrences at the level of the wound incision also occur following open resections for colorectal cancer. Although more frequent in cases of advanced primary disease at the time of surgery, they have also been described in early-stage tumors. The incidence of wound recurrences in two large reviews of over 3000 open colectomies for cancer was reported between 0.6 and 1% [137,138]. Hughes et al reported a 1% recurrence rate following open surgery for primary tumors classified as Dukes stage B [137].

In a prospective, nonrandomized study, Santoro et al. compared 50 open versus 50 laparoscopic resections for colorectal cancer. They reported similar 5-year disease-free survival rates and found recurrences at the trocar-site and wound incision in the laparoscopic and open cases, respectively [139]. Feliciotti et al. reported a 2% wound-site recurrence rate in the laparoscopic group (including a recurrence at the laparotomy incision in a patient converted to open) and none in the open group in 158 patients with a minimum follow-up of 3 years [140].

There are three prospective, randomized trials reported to date evaluating the incidence of wound recurrences following laparoscopic and open colorectal surgery. Stage et al. reported no recurrences at 14 months follow-up in 18 patients who underwent laparoscopic and 14 patients who underwent open colorectal resections [141]. In a series of 44 laparoscopic and 47 open resections for colorectal cancer, Lacy et al. reported no wound metastases in either group, with similar local recurrence rates after a mean follow-up of 21 months [142]. Finally, Milsom et al. reported two wound recurrences at a median of 20 months after open resections in 42 patients. Conversely, they did not find recurrences at a median of 18 months after laparoscopic resections [143]. Despite the fact that the small sample size of these series limits the significance of their results, they provide reassurance that acceptable oncological results after laparoscopic colorectal surgery are feasible and comparable to those of open surgery.

Although tumor growth is enhanced through CO_2 laparoscopy compared to anesthesia alone, there is less tumor growth than after conventional laparotomy [103,144,145]. This reduced tumor growth after laparoscopic surgery might be explained by the reduced postoperative acute-phase response and the decreased consequences in the immune system.

CONCLUSION

As with benign abdominal pathology, the laparoscopic approach has been used to diagnose, treat, and manage essentially all types of abdominal cancers. With the laparoscopic approach, the basic principles of oncological surgery can and should be employed. This seems to be more important than the questions of gasless versus CO_2 laparoscopy and hand-assisted versus total laparoscopic approaches for the prevention of complications, specifically port-site metastases. With attention to good technique, there are now numerous reports suggesting that laparoscopy for abdominal cancer can result in equal or less wound metastasis when compared to the open approach. The potential to have a less deleterious effect of a patient's immune system has been proposed as one possible advantage of the laparoscopic approach when a curative resection is attempted. Continued attention to the technique and improvement in training advanced laparoscopic procedures will help to minimize complications related to the learning curve. Ongoing prospective studies will add to our knowledge of the appropriate role for laparoscopy in the cancer patient.

REFERENCES

1. Alexander RJT, Jacques BC, Mitchell KG. Laparoscopically assisted colectomy and wound recurrence (letter). Lancet 1993; 341:249–250.

2. O'Rourke N, Price PM, Kelly S, Sikora K. Tumor inoculation during laparoscopy (letter). Lancet 1993; 342:368.
3. Goh YC, Eu EW, Seow Choen F. Early postoperative results of a prospective series of laparoscopic versus open anterior resection for rectosigmoid cancer. Dis Colon Rectum 1997; 40:776–780.
4. Johnstone PA, Rohde DC, Swartz SEet al. Port-site recurrences after laparoscopic and thoracoscopic procedures in malignancy. J Clin Oncol 1996; 14:1950–1956.
5. The American Society of Colon and Rectal Surgeons. Practice parameters for the treatment of rectal carcinoma. Dis Colon Rectum 1993; 36:989–1006.
6. Lacy AM, García-Valdecasas JC, Delgado Set al. Postoperative complications of laparoscopic-assisted colectomy. Surg Endosc 1997; 11:119–122.
7. Köckerling F, Rose J, Schneider Cet al. Laparoscopic colorectal anastomosis: Risk of postoperative leakage. Results of a multicenter study. Surg Endosc 1999; 13: 639–644.
8. Agachan F, Joo JS, Weiss EG, Wexner SD. Intraoperative laparoscopic complications. Are we getting better? Dis Colon Rectum 1996; 39(10 suppl):S14–S19.
9. Chahin F, Dwivedy AJ, Paramesh Aet al. The implications of lighted ureteral stenting in laparoscopic colectomy. JSLS 2002; 6:49–52.
10. Senagore AJ, Luchtefeld M. An initial experience with lighted ureteral catheters during laparoscopic colectomy. J Laparoendosc Surg 1994; 4:399–403.
11. Poulin EC, Schlachta CM, Seshadri PAet al. Septic complications of elective laparoscopic colorectal resection. Surg Endosc 2001; 15:203–208.
12. Bokey E, Chapuis P, Fung Cet al. Postoperative morbidity and mortality following resection of the colon and rectum for cancer. Dis Colon Rectum 1995; 38:480–487.
13. MacArdle C, Morran C, Pettit Let al. Value of oral antibiotic prophylaxis in colorectal surgery. Br J Surg 1995; 82:1046–1048.
14. Lumley JW, Fielding GA, Rhodes Met al. Laparoscopic-assisted colorectal surgery: Lessons learned from 240 consecutive patients. Dis Colon Rectum 1996; 39: 155–159.
15. Lazorthes F, Chiotassol P. Stapled colorectal anastomosis: Perspective integrity of the anastomosis and risk of postoperative leakage. Int J Colorect Dis 1986; 1:96–98.
16. Fujita J, Uyama I, Sugioka Aet al. Laparoscopic right hemicolectomy with radical lymph node dissection using the no-touch isolation technique for advanced colon cancer. Surg Today 2001; 21:93–96.
17. Gornish AL, Averbach D, Schwartz MR. Carcinoma of the gallbladder found during laparoscopic cholecystectomy: A case report and review of the literature. J Laparoendosc Surg 1991; 1;361–367.
18. Sandor J, Ihasz M, Fazekas Tet al. Unexpected gallbladder cancer and laparoscopic surgery. Surg Endosc 1995; 9:1207–1210.
19. Reddy YP, Sheridan WG. Port-site metastasis following laparoscopic cholecystectomy: A review of the literature and a case report. Eur J Surg Oncol 2000; 26: 95–102.
20. Aoki T, Tsuchida A, Kasuya Ket al. Is frozen section effective for diagnosis of unsuspected gallbladder cancer during laparoscopic cholecystectomy? Surg Endosc 2002; 16:197–200.

21. Wakai T, Shirai Y, Hatekeyama K. Radical second resection provides survival benefit for patients with T2 gallbladder carcinoma first discovered after laparoscopic cholecystectomy. World J Surg 2002; 26:867–871.
22. Wysocki A, Krzywon J. Does the laparoscopic cholecystectomy accelerate the intraperitoneal dissemination of previously unrecognized gallbladder cancer? Int J Surg Invest 2000; 2:313–317.
23. Wibbenmeyer LA, Wade TP, Chen RCet al. Laparoscopic cholecystectomy can disseminate *in situ* carcinoma of the gallbladder. J Am Coll Surg 1995; 181: 504–510.
24. Drouard F, Delamarre J, Capron JP. Cutaneous seeding of gallbladder cancer after laparoscopic cholecystectomy (letter). N Engl J Med 1991; 325:1316.
25. Jacobi CA, Keller H, Monig S, Said S. Implantation metastasis of unsuspected gallbladder carcinoma after laparoscopy. Surg Endosc 1995; 9:351–352.
26. Copher JC, Rogers JJ, Dalton ML. Trocar-site metastasis following laparoscopic cholecystectomy for unsuspected carcinoma of the gallbladder. Surg Endosc 1995; 9:348–350.
27. Sailer M, Debus S, Fuchs KH, Thiede A. Peritoneal seeding of gallbladder cancer after laparoscopic cholecystectomy. Surg Endosc 1995; 9:1290–1300.
28. Kim HJ, Roy T. Unsuspected gallbladder cancer with cutaneous seeding after laparoscopic cholecystectomy. South Med J 1994; 87:817–820.
29. Paolucci V, Schaeff B, Schneider M, Gutt C. Tumor seeding following laparoscopy: International survey. World J Surg 1999; 23:989–997.
30. Wade TP, Comitalo JB, Andrus CHet al. Laparoscopic cancer surgery. Surg Endosc 1994; 8:698–701.
31. Pazet D, Fondrinier E, Rotman Net al. Parietal seeding of carcinoma of the gallbladder after laparoscopic cholecystectomy (letter). Br J Surg 1992; 79:230.
32. Lomis KD, Vitola JV, Delbeke Det al. Recurrent gallbladder carcinoma at laparoscopy port-sites diagnosed by positron emission tomography: Implications for primary and radical second operations. Am Surg 1997; 63:341–345.
33. Gagner M, Rheault M, Dubuc J. Laparoscopic partial hepatectomy for liver tumor (abstr). Surg Endosc 1992; 6:99.
34. Azagra JS, Goergen M, Gilbart et al. M. Laparoscopic anatomical (hepatic) left lateral segmentectomy: Technical aspects. Surg Endosc 1996; 10:758–761.
35. Lin E, Gonzalez R, Venkatesh KRet al. Can current technology be integrated to facilitate laparoscopic living donor hepatectomy? Surg Endosc 2003; 17:750–753.
36. Gigot J-F, Glineur D, Azagra JSet al. Laparoscopic liver resection for malignant liver tumors. Preliminary results of a multicenter European study. Ann Surg 2002; 236:90–97.
37. Haberstroh J, Ahrens M, Munzar Tet al. Effects of the Pringle maneuver on hemodynamics during laparoscopic liver resection in the pig. Eur Surg Res 1996; 28:8–13.
38. Takagi S. Hepatic and portal vein blood flow during carbon dioxide pneumoperitoneum for laparoscopic hepatectomy. Surg Endosc 1998; 12:427–431.
39. Shen P, Fleming S, Westcott C, Challa V. Laparoscopic radiofrequency ablation of the liver in proximity to major vasculature: Effect of the Pringle maneuver. J Surg Oncol 2003; 83:36–41.

40. Mulier S, Mulier P, Ni Yet al. Complications of radiofrequency coagulation of liver tumors. Br J Surg 2002; 89:1206–1222.
41. Kitano S, Iso Y, Moriyama M, Sugimachi K. Laparoscopy-assisted Billroth I gastrectomy. Surg Laparosc Endosc 1994; 4:146–148.
42. Fujiwara M, Kodera Y, Kasai Yet al. Laparoscopy-assisted distal gastrectomy with systemic lymph node dissection for early gastric carcinoma: A review of 43 cases. J Am Coll Surg 2003; 196:75–81.
43. Childers JM, Aqua KA, Surwit EAet al. Abdominal-wall tumor implantation after laparoscopy for malignant conditions. Obstet Gynecol 1994; 84:765–769.
44. Baron MA, Ladonne JM, Resch B. Abdominal wall metastasis from ovarian cancer after laparotomy. A case report. Eur J Gynaecol Oncol 2002; 23:561–562.
45. Rieger N, McIntosh N. Port-site metastasis from synchronous primaries of the colon and ovary following laparoscopic cholecystectomy. Eur J Surg Oncol 1998; 24: 144–145.
46. Bacha EA, Barber W, Ratchford W. Port-site metastases of adenocarcinoma of the fallopian tube after laparoscopically assisted vaginal hysterectomy and salpingo-oophorectomy. Surg Endosc 1996; 10:1102–1103.
47. Tsivian A, Sidi AA. Port-site metastases in urological laparoscopic surgery. J Urol 2003; 169:1213–1218.
48. Portis AJ, Elnady M, Clayman RV. Laparoscopic radical/total nephrectomy: A decade of progress. J Endourol 2001; 15:345–354.
49. Janetshek G. Laparoscopic retroperitoneal lymph node dissection. Urol Clin North Am 2001; 28:107–120.
50. Sulser T, Guillonneau B, Vallancien Get al. Complications an initial experience with 1228 laparoscopic radical prostatectomies at 6 European centers (abstr). J Urol 2001; 165:150.
51. Liu SK, Church JM, Lavery IC, Fazio VW. Operations in patients with incurable colon cancer—Is it worthwhile? Dis Colon Rectum 1997; 40:11–14.
52. Mäkelä J, Haukipuro K, Laitinen S, Kairalouma MI. Palliative operations for colorectal cancer. Dis Colon Rectum 1990; 33:846–850.
53. Milsom JW, Kim SH, Hammerhofer KA, Fazio VW. Laparoscopic colorectal cancer surgery for palliation. Dis Colon Rectum 2000; 43:1512–1516.
54. Deans GT, Krukowski ZH, Irwin ST. Malignant obstruction of the left colon. Br J Surg 1994; 81:1270–1276.
55. Oz MC, Fonde KA. Endoscopic alternatives in the management of colonic strictures. Surgery 1990; 108:513–519.
56. Carmäñez F, Echenagusia A, Simö G, et al. Malignant colorectal obstruction treated by means of self-expanding metallic stents: Effectiveness before surgery and palliation. Radiology 2000; 216:492–497.
57. Saida Y, Sumiyama Y, Nagao J, Takase M. Stent endoprosthesis for obstructing colorectal cancers. Dis Colon Rectum 1996; 39:552–555.
58. Hasegawa H, Kabeshima Y, Watanabe Met al. Randomized controlled trial of laparoscopic versus open colectomy for advanced colorectal cancer. Surg Endosc 2003; 17:636–640.
59. Khot UP, Wenk Lang A, Murali K, Parker MC. Systematic review of the efficacy and safety of colorectal stents. Br J Surg 2002; 89:1096–1102.

60. Arnaud J-P, Bergamaschi R. Emergency subtotal/total colectomy with anastomosis for acutely obstructed carcinoma of the left colon. Dis Colon Rectum 1994; 37: 685–688.
61. Smothers L, Hynan L, Fleming Jet al. Emergency surgery for colon carcinoma. Dis Colon Rectum 2003; 46:24–30.
62. Goyal A, Schein M. Current practices in left-sided colonic emergencies. A survey of US gastrointestinal surgeons. Dig Surg 2001; 18:399–402.
63. Clair DG, Lautz DB, Brooks DC. Rapid development of umbilical metastases after laparoscopic cholecystectomy for unsuspected gallbladder carcinoma. Surgery 1993; 113:355–358.
64. Fong Y, Brennan MF, Turnbull Aet al. Gallbladder cancer discovered during laparoscopic surgery: Potential for iatrogenic tumor dissemination. Arch Surg 1993; 128: 1028–1032.
65. Cava A, Ronian J, Gonzalez Quintala Aet al. Subcutaneous metastasis following laparoscopy in gastric adenocarcinoma. Eur J Surg Oncol 1990; 16:63–67.
66. Delcastillo CF, Warshaw A. Peritoneal metastases in pancreatic carcinoma. Hepatogastroenerology 1993; 40:430–432.
67. Gleeson NC, Nicosia SV, Mark JEet al. Abdominal wall metastases from ovarian cancer after laparoscopic surgery. Am J Obst Gynecol 1993; 169:522–523.
68. Guillou PJ, Darzi A, Monson JR. Experience with laparoscopic colorectal surgery for malignant disease. Surg Oncol 1993; 2:S43–S49.
69. Boulez J. Chirurgie du cancer colo-rectal par voie celioscopique. Ann Chir 1996; 50:219–230.
70. Lord SA, Larach SW, Ferrara Aet al. Laparoscopic resections for colorectal carcinomå: A 3-year experience. Dis Colon Rectum 1996; 39:148–154.
71. Franklin ME, Rosenthal D, Abrego-Medina Det al. Prospective comparison of open vs laparoscopic colon surgery for carcinoma: Five-year results. Dis Colon Rectum 1996; 39:S35–S46.
72. Gellman L, Salky B, Edye M. Laparoscopic-assisted colectomy. Surg Endosc 1996; 10:1041–1044.
73. Kwok SP, Lau WY, Carey PDet al. Prospective evaluation of laparoscopic-assisted large bowel excision of cancer. Ann Surg 1996; 223:170–176.
74. Hoffman GC, Baker JW, Doxey JBet al. Minimally invasive surgery for colorectal cancer: Initial follow-up. Ann Surg 1996; 223:790–796.
75. Vukasin P, Ortega AE, Greene FLet al. Wound recurrence following laparoscopic colon cancer resection. Dis Colon Rectum 1996; 39:S20–S23.
76. Fleshman JW, Nelson H, Peters WRet al. Early results of laparoscopic surgery for colorectal cancer: Retrospective analysis of 372 patients treated by Clinical Outcomes of Surgical Therapy (COST) Study Group. Dis Colon Rectum 1996; 29: S53–S58.
77. Fielding GA, Lumley J, Nathanson Let al. Laparoscopic colectomy. Surg Endosc 1997; 11:745–749.
78. Larach SW, Patankar SK, Ferrrara Aet al. Complications of laparoscopic colorectal surgery: analysis and comparison of early vs latter experience. Dis Colon Rectum 1997; 40:592–596.

79. Croce E, Azzola M, Russo Ret al. Laparoscopic colectomy: The absolute need for a standard operative technique. JSLS 1997; 1:217–224.
80. Khalili TM, Fleshner PR, Hiett JRet al. Colorectal cancer: Comparison of laparoscopic with open approaches. Dis Colon Rectum 1998; 41:832–838.
81. Bouvet M, Mansfield PF, Skibber JMet al. Clinical, pathologic, and economic parameters of laparoscopic colon resection. Am J Surg 1998; 176:554–557.
82. Bohm B, Schwenk W, Muller JM. Langzeitergebnisse nach laparoskopischer Resektion colorectaler Carcinome. Chirurgie 1999; 70:453–455.
83. Pearlstone DB, Mansfield PF, Curley SAet al. Laparoscopy in 533 patients with abdominal malignancy. Surgery 1999; 125:67–72.
84. Leung KL, Yiu RY, Lai PBet al. Laparoscopic-assisted resection of colorectal carcinoma: Five-year audit. Dis Colon Rectum 1999; 42:327–333.
85. Melotti G, Tamborrino E, Lazzaretti MGet al. Laparoscopic surgery for colorectal cancer. Semin Surg Oncol 1999; 16:332–336.
86. Poulin EC, Mamazza J, Schlachta CMet al. Laparoscopic resection does not adversely affect early survival curves in patients undergoing surgery for adenocarcinoma. Ann Surg 1999; 229:487–492.
87. Schiedeck TH, Schwandner O, Baca Iet al. Laparoscopic surgery for the cure of colorectal cancer: Results of a German five-center study. Dis Colon Rectum 2000; 43:1–8.
88. Allardyce RA. Is the port-site really at risk? Biology, mechanisms and prevention: A critical view. Aust N Z J Surg 1999; 69:479–485.
89. Pearlstone DB, Feig BW, Mansfield PF. Port site recurrences after laparoscopy for malignant disease. Semin Surg Oncol 1999; 16:307–312.
90. Ben-Eliyahu S, Page GG, Yirmiya R, Shakhar G. Evidence that stress and surgical interventions promote tumor development by suppressing natural killer cell activity. Int J Cancer 1999; 80:880–888.
91. Da Costa ML, Redmond HP, Bouthier-Hayes D. The effect of laparotomy and laparoscopy on the establishment of spontaneous tumor metastases. Surgery 1998; 124:516–525.
92. Watson RW, Redmond HP, McCarthy Jet al. Exposure of the peritoneal cavity to air regulates early inflammatory responses to surgery in a murine model. Br J Surg 1995; 82:1060–1065.
93. Jacobi CA, Wenger R, Sabat Ret al. The impact of laparoscopy with carbon dioxide versus helium on immunologic function and tumor growth in a rat model. Dig Surg 1998; 15:110–116.
94. Gaspani L, Bianchi M, Limiroli Eet al. The analgesic drug tramadol prevents the effect of surgery on natural killer cell activity and metastatic colonization in rats. J Neuroimmunol 2002; 129:18–24.
95. Page GG, Ben-Eliyahu S, Liebeskind JC. The role of LGL/NK cells in surgery-induced promotion of metastasis and its attenuation by morphine. Brain Behav Immunol 1993; 8:241–250.
96. Hasegawa H, Kabeshima Y, Watanabe Met al. Randomized controlled trial of laparoscopic versus open colectomy for advanced colorectal cancer. Surg Endosc 2003; 17:636–640.

97. Braga M, Vignali A, Gianotti Let al. Laparoscopic versus open colorectal surgery. A randomized trial on short-term outcome. Ann Surg 2002; 236:759–767.
98. Dennis H, Jeanine T, Mehran A. Laparoscopic vs open resection for colorectal adenocarcinoma. Dis Colon Rectum 2001; 44:10–19.
99. Neuhaus SJ, Watson DI, Ellis Tet al. Influence of gases on intraperitoneal immunity during laparoscopy in tumor-bearing rats. World J Surg 2000; 24:1227–1231.
100. West MA, Hackam DJ, Baker Jet al. Mechanism of decreased in vitro murine macrophage cytokine release after exposure to carbon dioxide: Relevance to laparoscopic surgery. Ann Surg 1997; 226:179–190.
101. Gutt CN-, Schemmer Pet al. Impact of laparoscopic and conventional surgery on Kupffer cells, tumor-associated CD44 expression, and intrahepatic tumor spread. Arch Surg 2002; 137:1408–1412.
102. Gutt CN, Reimber V, Kim ZGet al. Impact of laparoscopic surgery on experimental hepatic metastases. Br J Surg 2001; 88:371–375.
103. Mathew G, Watson DI, Rofe AMet al. Wound metastases following laparoscopic and open surgery for abdominal cancer in a rat model. Br J Surg 1996; 83: 1087–1090.
104. Bouvy ND, Marquet RL, Jeekel H, Bonjer HJ. Impact of gas(less) laparoscopy and laparotomy on peritoneal tumor growth and abdominal wall metastases. Ann Surg 1996; 224:694–701.
105. Jacobi CA, Sabat R, Bartholomaus Bet al. Pneumoperitoneum with carbon dioxide stimulates growth of malignant colonic cells. Surgery 1997; 121:72–78.
106. Neuhaus SJ, Watson DI, Ellis Tet al. Wound metastasis after laparoscopy with different insufflation gases. Surgery 1998; 123:579–583.
107. Ng WT, Yeung HC, Koh GH, Ng WF. Mechanisms of port-site metastasis after laparoscopic cancer surgery (letter). Br J Surg 1996; 83:1478.
108. Ikramuddin S, Lucus J, Ellison ECet al. Detection of aerosolized cells during carbon dioxide laparoscopy. J Gastrointest Surg 1998; 2:580–583.
109. Reymond MA, Wittekind C, Jung Aet al. The incidence of port-site metastases might be reduced. Surg Endosc 1997; 11:902–906.
110. Whelan RL, Sellers GJ, Allendorf JDet al. Trocar site recurrence is unlikely to result from aerosolization of tumor cells. Dis Colon Rectum 1996; 39:S7–S13.
111. Collard JM, Reymond MA. Video-assisted thoracic surgery surgery (VATS) for cancer: Risk of parietal seeding and of early local recurrence. Int Surg 1996; 81: 343–346.
112. Downey RJ, McCormack P, LoCiero J. Dissemination of malignancies following video-assisted thoracic surgery. J Cardiovasc Thorac Surg 1996; 111:954–960.
113. Sullivan WD, Passamonte PM. Mediastinoscopy incision site metastasis: Response to radiation therapy. South Med J 1982; 72:172–177.
114. Kawamura YJ, Sawada T, Sunami Eet al. Gasless laparoscopic-assisted colonic surgery. Am J Surg 1999; 117:515–517.
115. Volz J, Köster S, Spacek Z, Paweletz N. The influence of pneumoperitoneum used in laparoscopic surgery on an intraabdominal tumor growth. Cancer 1999; 86: 770–774.
116. Hirabayashi Y, Yamaguchi K, Shiraishi Net al. Development of port-site metastasis after pneumoperitoneum. A scanning electron microscopy study. Surg Endosc 2002; 16:864–868.

117. Schilling MK, Redaelli C, Krähenbähl Let al. Splanchnic microcirculatory changes during CO_2 laparoscopy. J Am Coll Surg 1997; 174:378–382.
118. Jones DB, Guo WL, Reinhard MKet al. Impact of pneumoperitoneum on trocar site implantation of colon cancer in a hamster model. Dis Colon Rectum 1995; 38: 1182–1188.
119. Jacobi CA, Wenger FA, Ordemann Jet al. Experimental study of the effect of intra-abdominal pressure during laparoscopy on tumour growth and port-site metastasis. Br J Surg 1998; 85:1419–1422.
120. Moreira H, Yamaguchi T, Wexner Set al. Effect of pneumoperitoneal pressure on tumor dissemination and tumor recurrence at port-site and midline incisions. Am Surg 2001; 67:369–373.
121. Wittich P, Steyerberg EW, Simons SHPet al. Intraperitoneal tumor growth is influenced by pressure of carbon dioxide pneumoperitoneum. Surg Endosc 2000; 14: 817–819.
122. Agostini A, Robin F, Jais JPet al. Impact of different gases and pneumoperitoneum pressures on tumor growth during laparoscopy in a rat model. Surg Endosc 2002; 16:529–532.
123. Ishida H, Hashimoto D, Takeuchi Iet al. Liver metastases are less established after gasless laparoscopy than after carbon dioxide pneumoperitoneum and laparotomy in a mouse model. Surg Endosc 2002; 16:193–196.
124. Watson DI, Mathew G, Ellis Tet al. Gasless laparoscopy may reduce the risk of port-site metastases following laparoscopic tumor surgery. Arch Surg 1997; 132: 166–168.
125. Hewitt PJ, Thomas WM, King G, Eaton M. Intraperitoneal cell movement during abdominal carbon dioxide insufflation and laparoscopy: An in vivo model. Dis Colon Rectum 1996; 39(suppl):S62–S66.
126. Schneider C, Jung A, Reymond MAet al. Efficacy of surgical measures in preventing port-site recurrences in a porcine model. Surg Endosc 2001; 15:121–125.
127. Montorsi M, Fumagalli U, Rosati Ret al. Early parietal recurrence of adenocarcinoma of the colon after laparoscopic colectomy. Br J Surg 1995; 82:1036–1037.
128. Texler ML, King G, Hewett PJ. Tumour cell movement during heating and humidification of insufflating CO_2: An in vitro model. Aust N Z J Surg 1998; 68:740–742.
129. Dorrance HR, Oien K, O'Dwyer PJ. Effects of laparoscopy on intraperitoneal tumor growth and distant metastases in an animal model. Surgery 1999; 126:35–40.
130. Farrell TM, Johnson AB, Metreveli REet al. Choice of insufflating gas influence wound metastasis (abstr). Surg Endosc 1999; 13(suppl):S33.
131. Jacobi CA, Ordemann J, Bohm Bet al. Inhibition of peritoneal tumor cell growth and implantation in laparoscopic surgery in a rat model. Am J Surg 1997; 174: 359–363.
132. Neuhaus SJ, Watson DI, Ellis Tet al. Efficacy of cytotoxic agents for the prevention of laparoscopic port-site metastases. Arch Surg 1998; 133:762–766.
133. Eshraghi N, Swanstrom LL, Bax Tet al. Topical treatments of laparoscopic port-sites can decrease the incidence of incision metastases. Surg Endosc 1999; 13: 1121–1124.
134. Wenger FA, Kilian M, Braumann Cet al. Effect of taurolidine and ocreotide on port-site and liver metastasis after laparoscopy in an animal model of pancreatic cancer. Clin Exp Metast 2002; 19:169–173.

135. Goldstein DS, Lu ML, Hattori Tet al. Inhibition of peritoneal tumor-cell implantation: A model for laparoscopic cancer surgery. J Endourol 1993; 7:237–241.
136. Pacquet P, Sutart OA, Dalton Ret al. Effect of intraperitoneal chemotherapy and fibrinolytic therapy on tumor implantation in wound sites. J Surg Oncol 1996; 62: 128–134.
137. Hughes ES, McDermott FT, Poliglase AI, Johnson WR. Tumor recurrence in the abdominal wall scar tissue after large-bowel cancer surgery. Dis Colon Rectum 1983; 26:571–572.
138. Reilly WT, Nelson H, Schroeder Get al. Wound recurrence following conventional treatment of colorectal cancer. Dis Colon Rectum 1996; 39:200–207.
139. Santoro E, Carlini M, Carboni F, Feroce A. Colorectal carcinoma: Laparoscopic versus traditional open surgery. A clinical trial. Hepatogastroenterology 1999; 46: 900–904.
140. Feliciotti F, Paganini AM, Guerrieri Met al. Results of laparoscopic vs open resections for colon cancer in patients with a minimum follow-up of 3 years. Surg Endosc 2002; 16:1158–1161.
141. Stage JG, Schulze S, Moller Pet al. Prospective randomized study of laparoscopic versus open colonic resection for adenocarcinoma. Br J Surg 1997; 84:391–396.
142. Lacy AM, Delgado S, García-Valdecasas JCet al. Port-site metastases and recurrence after laparoscopic colectomy. A randomized trial. Surg Endosc 1998; 12: 1039–1042.
143. Milsom JW, Bohm B, Hammerhofer KAet al. A prospective, randomized trial comparing laparoscopic versus conventional techniques in colorectal cancer surgery: A preliminary report. J Am Coll Surg 1998; 187:46–54.
144. Allendorf JD, Bessler M, Kayton MLet al. Increased tumor establishment and growth after laparotomy vs laparoscopy in a murine model. Arch Surg 1995; 130: 649–653.
145. Bouvy ND, Marquet RL, Lambert SWJet al. Laparoscopic bowel resection in the rat: Earlier restoration of IGF-1 and less tumor growth (abstr). Surg Endosc 1996; 10:567.

19

Pancreatic Surgery

Federico Cuenca-Abente and Michel Gagner
Mount Sinai School of Medicine, New York, New York, U.S.A.

INTRODUCTION

In 1911, Bernheim [1] published the first laparoscopic visual examination of the pancreas. Until the early 1990s, little information regarding the minimally invasive approach to the pancreatic gland was available [2]. After these reports, the procedure gained slower acceptance than other laparoscopic procedures [3].

Given its anatomical relationships and location, laparoscopic access to the pancreas is reserved for well-trained surgeons who also have access to the required technology to perform these kind of procedures [4,5]. Due to the difficulties that a surgeon can face during these demanding operations, surgical complications threaten even the most skilled surgeons. Hemorrhage, pancreatic fistula, and peripancreatic fluid collections top the list of postoperative problems. Other complications, such as splenic infarct and splenic abscess, must be mentioned, but considering their low incidence in laparoscopic surgery, they are described only briefly.

This chapter describes each procedure and focuses on the different ways of preventing and managing complications of laparoscopic distal pancreatic resection, enucleations, hand-assisted laparoscopic pancreatic surgery, and the various laparoscopic procedures used in the treatment of pancreatic pseudocysts.

TECHNICAL ASPECT OF LAPAROSCOPIC PANCREATIC RESECTION

Less than 150 cases of laparoscopic pancreatic resection have been reported in the English literature. Of these, 79.2% were distal pancreatectomies, sparing the spleen in approximately half of the patients. The overall conversion rate was 13.3% and the average length of hospital stay 7.4 days. Below, we describe several different techniques used for laparoscopic pancreatic procedures.

Spleen- and Splenic Vessel–Preserving Distal Pancreatectomy

Spleen-sparing techniques are particularly indicated for patients with benign diseases, since lymph node sampling is expected to be insufficient for curative intent in malignancy [6].

Dissecting and clipping the vessels emerging from the splenic vein and artery, at the superior edge of the pancreas, is the most commonly performed splenic preservation technique (Fig. 1). This technique requires longer operative time and laparoscopic surgical expertise. Unless delicate maneuvers are used to dissect along the upper margin of the pancreas, significant vascular damage may occur.

Distal Pancreatectomy with En Bloc Splenectomy

Distal pancreatectomy is one of the most commonly performed laparoscopic pancreatic resective procedures. As opposed to laparoscopic pancreatoduodenectomy, laparoscopic distal pancreatectomy seems to provide benefits to the patient [7] (Fig. 2).

The literature reports several different disease processes amenable to this technique. These include serous and mucinous cyst adenomas, endocrine tumors, cystic lymphangioma, chronic pancreatitis, and simple cysts.

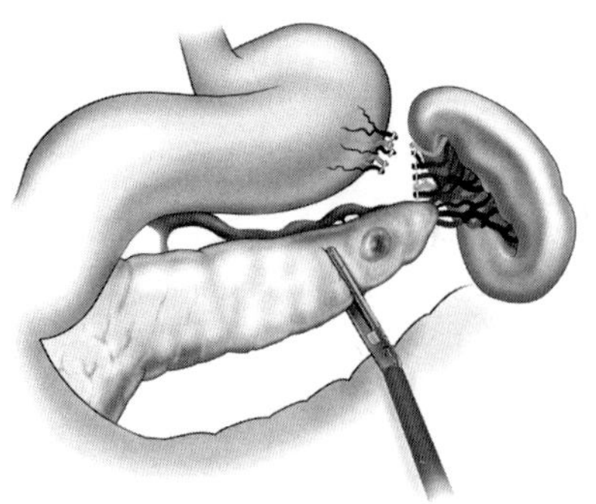

FIGURE 1 Spleen-preserving distal pancreatectomy. Only the pancreatic vessels emerging from the splenic artery and vein have been transected.

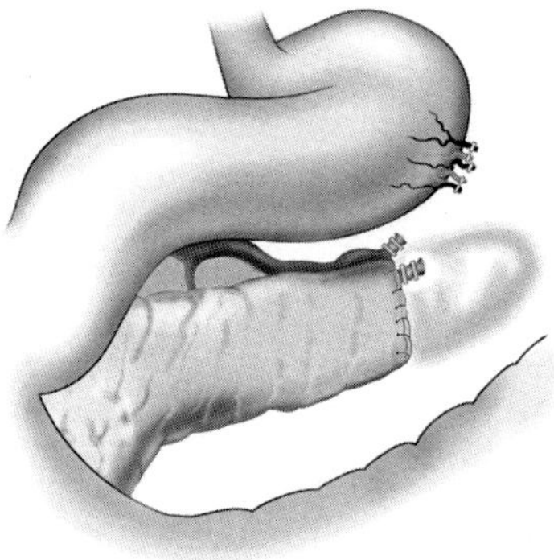

Figure 2 Distal pancreatectomy with en bloc splenectomy. The short gastric vessels have been sectioned and the distal pancreas is being divided with a stapler.

Few surgeons have described this technique, but the available data suggest that it is feasible, safe, and beneficial. Patients experience shorter hospital stays, decreased pain, faster return to normal activities, and better cosmesis [2,8–12]. On the other hand, morbidity and mortality rates [4] and operative time [2] are not better than with the open approach [2] (Fig. 3).

Spleen-Preserving Pancreatectomy with Splenic Vessel Ligation

This technique involves transection of the splenic vessels at the level of the pancreatic section. The short gastric vessels are left to perfuse the spleen. The

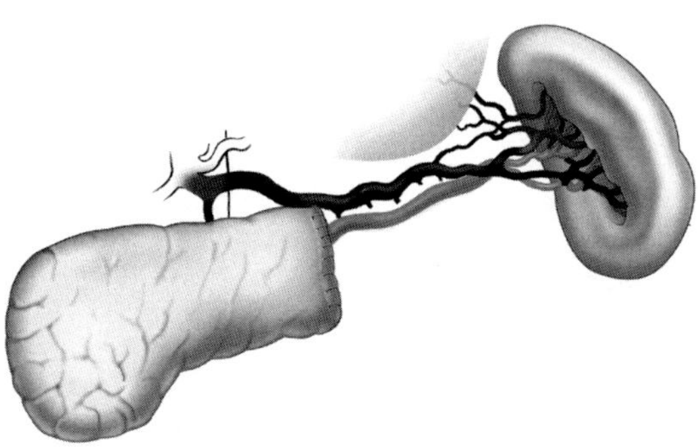

Figure 3 Distal pancreatectomy with en bloc splenectomy. The distal pancreas has been removed along with the spleen.

surgeon must keep this in mind from the beginning of the procedure to avoid inadvertent ligation of these vessels. If the surgeon plans a spleen-preserving distal pancreatectomy, these vessels may be needed for splenic salvage. If either the splenic artery or vein needs to be ligated to control hemorrhage (as this usually cannot be managed adequately with sutures or clips), the short gastric vessels will maintain spleen perfusion.

Enucleations

Islet cell tumors are the most common indication for enucleation. Of these, benign insulinomas account for the majority of cases. They are usually small, solitary lesions (<1.5 cm) located in the body or tail of the pancreas [13]. All these characteristics make the laparoscopic approach attractive.

After the tumor has been localized, it is excised using electrocauthery, sharp dissection, or ultrasonic shears (Fig. 4). Laparoscopic ultrasonography is necessary to localize the tumor and avoid injury to the splenic or mesenteric vessels and pancreatic duct.

Drainage Procedures for Pancreatic Pseudocysts

Laparoscopic surgery for pancreatic pseudocysts is mostly described in relation to internal drainage procedures. These include cyst gastrostomy by the lesser sac approach, cyst gastrostomy by the anterior approach, transgastric cyst gastrostomy, and Roux-en-Y cyst jejunostomy. Indications for a cyst gastrostomy require a symptomatic pseudocyst >5–6 cm in diameter, of greater than 6 weeks duration, and in contact with the posterior gastric wall (head or body of the pancreas) [10]. Utilization of a laparoscopic approach relies on the expertise of the surgeon.

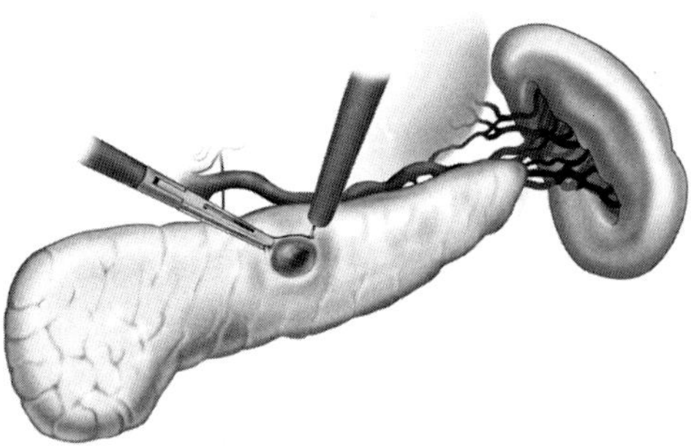

FIGURE 4 Enucleation. The tumor is dissected from the pancreatic tissue.

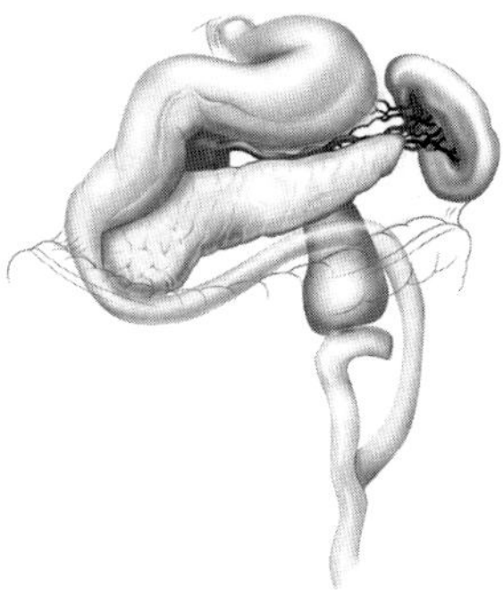

FIGURE 5 Roux-en-Y cyst jejunostomy.

Laparoscopic Roux-en-Y Pancreatic Cyst Jejunostomy

Laparoscopic Roux-en-Y cyst jejunostomy is reserved for cysts not in contact with the posterior gastric wall. In order to reach the jejunum and perform the anastomosis, the patient must be placed in a supine position. The transverse colon is retracted cephalad and the ligament of Treitz identified. The jejunum is measured and transected. Intestinal continuity is recreated with a Roux-en-Y technique (Fig. 5).

Cyst Gastrostomy by the Lesser Sac Approach

The lesser sac approach was described by Morino et al. [9]. In this technique, access to the lesser sac is achieved and an internal drainage with a linear stapler established. This results in direct communication of the posterior gastric wall with the anterior wall of the pseudocyst (Fig. 6).

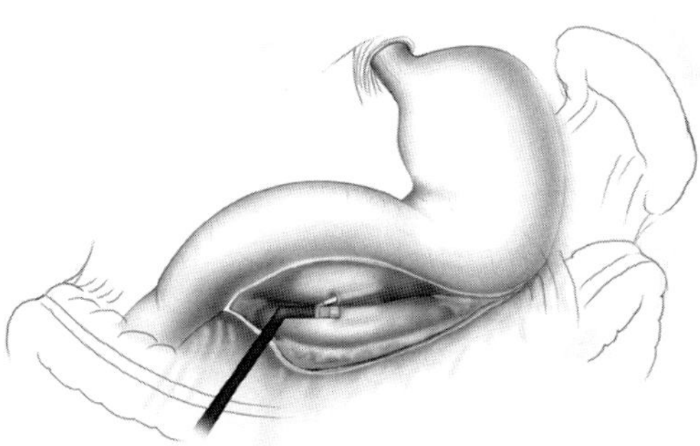

FIGURE 6 Cyst gastrostomy: lesser sac approach.

Transgastric Cyst Gastrostomy

Transgastric cyst gastrostomy involves direct insufflation of the stomach with an endoscope; then, under endoscopic guidance, laparoscopic trocars are introduced into the gastric lumen. Under direct laparoscopic transgastric vision, the cyst is treated in a similar manner as with the anterior approach.

Gagner et al. [12] and Way et al. [12] described this procedure in 1994 using a radially expanding 5-mm trocar. Trias et al. [12] described it using 12-mm cannulas with a balloon, allowing transgastric introduction of a stapler device.

Gagner has recently modified the technique with needlescopic instruments [12], achieving less operative trauma and avoiding the need for pneumoperitoneum and closure of the anterior gastric puncture sites (Fig. 7).

Cyst Gastrostomy by the Anterior Approach

A gastrotomy is created on the anterior gastric wall. After access to the gastric lumen is gained, the protruding pseudocyst is identified on the posterior gastric wall. Communication between the cyst and the stomach is created with a linear stapler, electrocauthery, or ultrasonic shears (Fig. 8).

Reinforcement of the anastomotic site may be done with running sutures if the walls are not adequately fused. The anterior gastrostomy may be closed with either a stapler or sutures.

Hand-Assisted Laparoscopic Pancreatectomy

Conventional laparoscopy has proved to be difficult in cases involving large tumors, massive intraoperative bleeding, dense adhesions, malignancy [15], and obesity [8]. Hand-assisted laparoscopic surgery may have an advantage in these groups of patients [15]. This technique basically provides assistance from the surgeon's nondominant hand while still performing a minimally invasive proce-

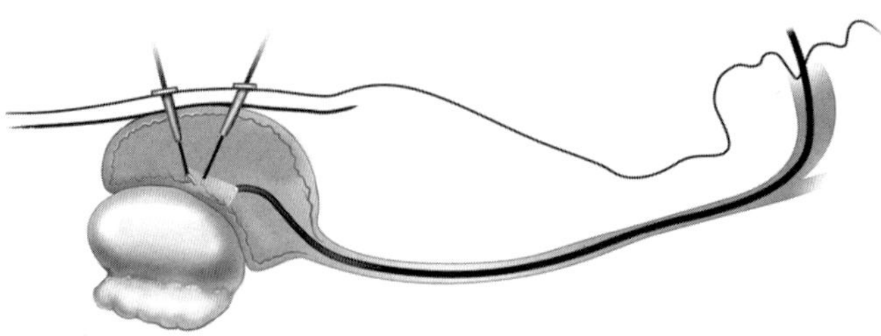

FIGURE 7 Needlescopic transgastric cyst gastrostomy with endoscopic guidance.

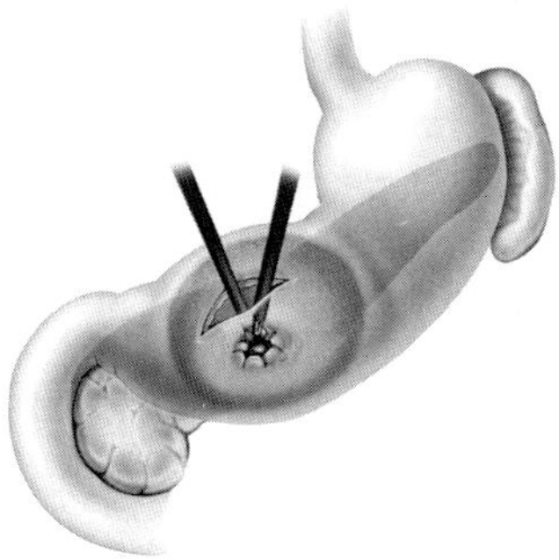

FIGURE 8 Cyst gastrostomy: anterior approach.

dure. It can be used at the outset or as an intermediary step, when the surgeon faces technical difficulty [2] (Fig. 9).

Although few cases have been reported, the advantages include assistance of the hand for dissection (to palpate and identify tissues) [8,16], mobilization of large organs [16], accessing instruments [8], and protecting the wound during extraction of malignant specimens [8]. This technique also reduces operative time. Finally, the fingers may be used to rapidly stop unexpected bleeding.

Laparoscopic Pancreatoduodenectomy

Gagner and Pomp described the first laparoscopic pancreatoduodenectomy in 1994 [17]. The procedure begins with transection of the common bile duct with a stapler, 2–3 cm above the superior pancreatic border. The duodenum is divided

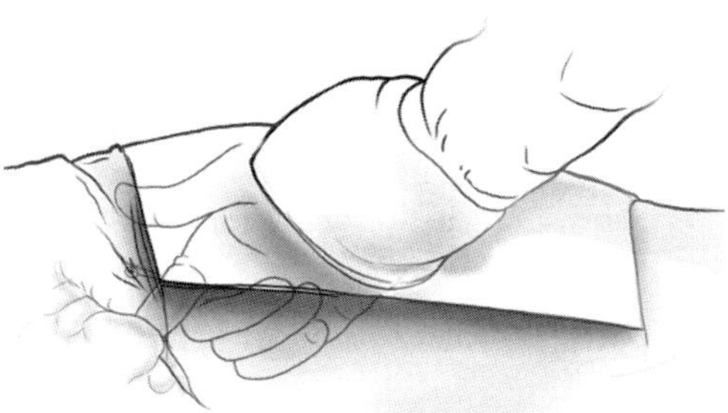

FIGURE 9 Hand-assisted distal pancreatectomy.

and the gastroduodenal artery double clipped and transected. The posterior aspect of the pancreas is separated from the portal vein with blunt dissection and the pancreas transected. The specimen is placed in a nylon bag (Cook-Surgical, Bloomington, IN) for later extraction. The three anastomoses are created with an intracorporeal technique, and a 5F pediatric tube is used to serve as a stent for the pancreaticojejunostomy. A feeding jejunostomy (T tube, 14F) is inserted through one of the trocar sites.

The procedure is demanding both technically and in terms of time, and the results do not show benefit for the patient's outcome, which may be accompanied by increased morbidity [7,17–20].

Palliation of Unresectable Pancreatic Cancer

Palliative procedures for unresectable pancreatic cancer include cholecystojejunostomy and choledochojejunostomy (biliary decompression) and gastrojejunostomy (gastric outlet decompression).

The cholecystojejunostomy can be performed using either a stapler or an intracorporeal suture technique and requires a minimum distance between the upper edge of the tumor and the cystic duct of 1.5 cm. This can be achieved with preoperative cholecystocholangiography [21].

For the choledochojejunostomy, an adequate length of the hepatic duct is exposed (2.5 cm) [7]. This anastomosis is done with intracorporeal suturing but is contraindicated in patients with portal hypertension (distended veins near the anastomotic site) [22].

A gastrojejunostomy is performed in those patients with duodenal obstruction. A jejunal limb is placed in an antecolic fashion. The anastomosis is made between the anterior, lower greater curvature of the stomach and the loop of jejunum (40–50 cm from the Treitz angle) [7]. Either a stapler or a hand-sewn technique can be used to perform this operation.

COMPLICATIONS

Hemorrhage

The incidence of bleeding in open pancreatic resections is 4.8% [23]. Bleeding can have either an acute or chronic course, and it can arise from the splenic artery, the splenic vein, or the spleen itself.

Preoperative Considerations

In planning a laparoscopic pancreatectomy, it is important for the surgeon to identify those patients who carry a higher risk of vascular (splenic pedicle) injury (Table 1).

TABLE 1 Clinical Status Associated with a High Risk of Complications

Chronic pancreatitis (bleeding)
Soft pancreas (fistula formation)
Obese patients
Previous pancreatic surgery
Tumors

There are two situations that deserve special consideration. First, the spleen-sparing technique poses a greater risk of bleeding. In such cases, the surgeon must dissect the splenic artery and vein from the upper pancreatic edge [24]. In a pancreas with dense adhesions between the gland and the vessels (e.g., chronic pancreatitis) [5,25], the incidence of intraoperative hemorrhage is increased.

Second, in cases where the tumor (or cyst) is in close proximity of the splenic hilum, bleeding is also a concern. The topography of the lesion makes the dissection at this level very risky.

These particular situations represent cases in which it would be more judicious to perform an en bloc pancreaticosplenectomy, thus avoiding vascular dissection and the subsequent risk of bleeding.

Intraoperative Maneuvers

With those patients who carry a higher risk of vascular injury, an option to prevent bleeding is to first ligate the splenic artery as close as possible to its origin. This maneuver reduces the risk of major bleeding and can reduce the size of the spleen [26], thus facilitating the subsequent steps of the operation.

Also, transection of the splenic artery and vein with endoscopic staplers (45 mm in length, 2.5 mm in height, Tyco Healthcare, Norwalk, CT) is a consideration. The section line can be reinforced with sutures, loops, or titanium clips [2] to prevent further bleeding.

In performing tumor enucleation, one must consider the vascular supply of the tumor itself. Endocrine neoplasms generally have a deep or posterior blood supply. Therefore the main vascular pedicle must be identified. Establishing its proximity to the main pancreatic vessels, using laparoscopic ultrasonography, may prevent inadvertent bleeding and help position the hemostatic clips [2].

Established Intraoperative Bleeding

When intraoperative bleeding occurs, the surgeon must remain calm and efforts must be made to identify the site of origin.

Arterial hemorrhage is characterized by a bright red appearance and the visualization of pulsatile bleeding. In this situation, the surgeon must try to identify the exact site of bleeding and proceed to control it with a vascular clamp (Karl Storz, Tutlingen, Germany). Once this has been achieved, hemostasis is obtained with titanium clips or sutures. As a last lifesaving maneuver, the vessel can be transected with a vascular stapler used to achieve hemostasis.

Even more threatening is bleeding arising from the splenic vein. Typically, the operative field quickly fills with blood. As the surgeon attempts to identify the exact source of bleeding, the fragile vein may tear further, increasing the amount of hemorrhage. As in the case of arterial bleeding, vascular control must be obtained. Vascular clamps are placed after the tear has been identified, and, if needed, the patient is resuscitated with normal saline solution once vascular control has been achieved. For definitive hemostasis, clips, intracorporeal sutures, or vascular staplers are used.

After finishing the pancreatic resection, the surgeon must check the previous site of bleeding and confirm that the patient is normotensive. A low blood pressure at this time may mask potential bleeding sites during the final examination.

If bleeding occurs from splenic trauma, gentle compression is applied and a laparoscopic argon beam coagulator is used (ConMed, Utica, NY). Wrapping the spleen with an absorbable mesh and even partial splenectomy may be attempted for treatment of grade I or II injuries [27] so as to avoid splenectomy.

In using the argon coagulator, specific recommendations to minimize the risk of gas embolism must be considered [28]. The initial setting should be ''manual'' mode with the argon kept at the lowest level and one cannula vent open. The electrode should be removed from the peritoneal cavity when coagulation is not actually being performed. Also, laparoscopic insufflators with audible and visual overpressurization alarms should be used. Finally, staff should be trained to detect and manage gas embolization during laparoscopic procedures.

Hand-assisted laparoscopic pancreatectomies offer the possibility of using the fingers directly to stop an otherwise life-threatening hemorrhage [16,29,30] without loss of pneumoperitoneum. Hinder et al. reported that it can be safe, quick, and effective [16]. This technique can be used by those who are performing their first laparoscopic pancreatectomies (or difficult cases) as a way of decreasing the possibility of complications.

Last but not least, trained surgeons must use these laparoscopic maneuvers while always remembering that conversion to laparotomy may be the best choice.

Postoperative Bleeding

Hemorrhage is a threatening complication that can also occur postoperatively. It will manifest itself as a serosanguinous fluid coming from the drain. If bleeding is severe, the drainage may be accompanied by hemodynamic instability. Reoperation is the rule for the latter patients. However, a conservative approach may benefit those in whom bleeding is light. Selective angiography and embolization is an alternative to surgery in hemodynamically stable patients. However, angiographic embolization after laparoscopic pancreatic resection has not been reported in the literature.

Fistula

Pancreatic fistula is a notorious complication of both distal pancreatectomy and pancreatic enucleation, but pancreatic enucleations carry the higher incidence.

Pancreatic fistula is the most common complication reported in laparoscopic series (17.9%). Moreover, its incidence appears to be higher than in the reported open series—10.4% [23] vs. 5% [31]. Symptoms from this complication depend primarily on the amount of enzymatic fluid draining from the pancreatic duct. This can vary from small peripancreatic collections to high outputs from fistulas. Accordingly, treatment may vary from observation to total parenteral nutrition with administration of somatostatin analogues, followed by reoperation.

Conditions that Favor Fistula Formation

The conditions that predispose patients to develop pancreatic fistulas are consistency of the gland and relation of the tumor to the pancreatic duct (enucleations).

Distal pancreatectomy for chronic pancreatitis usually carries a lower incidence of pancreatic fistula or leak due to the firm consistency of the gland as opposed to a normal, soft pancreas [2].

The macroscopic characteristic of endocrine tumors gives the surgeon the opportunity to enucleate them. Distal pancreatectomy must be considered when the tumor is in close proximity to the main pancreatic duct, when it is located in the posterior aspect of the gland, or when multiple pancreatic tumors are present.

Prevention

There are several maneuvers for the prevention of fistula formation that have been described and that warrant discussion [Table 2].

Preoperatively, it is important to determine the relation of the (endocrine) tumor with the main pancreatic duct [2], the number of tumors present, and their location. For this purpose, magnetic resonance imaging (MRI), endoscopic pancreatography, selective angiographies with calcium stimulation, and endoscopic ultrasound have been used. Intraoperative laparoscopic ultrasound can assess these characteristics [2,13] as well. The sensitivity of this method compares favorably with that of open surgery (range, 75–100%) [32–34], particularly concerning the localization of a neoplasm. Certain technical considerations are important with regard to dividing the pancreas. It is usually transected using a linear stapler (45 mm in length, 2.5 or 3.5 mm in height; Tyco Healthcare, Norwalk,

TABLE 2 Relation Between Intraoperative Precautions and Maneuvers and the Avoidable Complications Related to Each

Intraoperative Maneuver	Complication
Low implantation of the stapler	Pancreatic disruption
Running suture in pancreatic stump	Pancreatic fistula
Fibrin glue	Pancreatic fistula
Ligation of splenic artery	Bleeding
Ligation clips in the vascular staple line	Bleeding
Selective ligation of pancreatic duct	Pancreatic fistula
Ligation of pancreatic stump or application of clips	Pancreatic fistula
Observation of the spleen (coloration)	Splenic ischemia-abscess formation
Suture anastomotic line (cyst gastrostomy, anterior approach)	Bleeding
Avoidance of enucleations in tumors near the pancreatic duct and its location with laparoscopic ultrasound	Pancreatic fistula

CT). As previously stated, the pancreas is divided either alone or along with the splenic vessels [15]. The surgeon must place the stapler though the trocar that is as far as possible from the pancreas [2], left paramedian at the level of the umbilicus. This helps avoid disruption of the gland, which can occur if the stapler approaches the pancreas in a perpendicular fashion. A running suture on the edge of the pancreatic stump to secure the stapler line has been described [11,13,15], but this maneuver has not been proven to decrease the rate of fistula formation.

Some authors favor the application of fibrin glue (Baxter AG, Vienna, Austria) [13,35] as an additional method to prevent fistula formation. However, there is no strong evidence that this may decrease the rates of pancreatic leakage here either.

The surgeon should also search for leakage before completion of the procedure. During this maneuver, if the pancreatic duct is visualized, it can be clipped or sutured [2,13,35].

There is a consensus that the surgeon should place a closed suction drain near the pancreatic stump and leave it in place until it stops draining fluid. This helps manage a pancreatic fistula and prevents pancreatic ascites.

The utilization of somatostatin analogues (Sandostatin, Novartis AG, Schweizerhalle, Switzerland) has been proposed by some authors as a method of preventing the occurrence of a fistula or accelerating the closure of one. Inconsistent outcomes from different trials have not confirmed the success of this treatment [23].

Diagnosis

Drainage of fluid with a high content of amylase (>10,000 IU) confirms the diagnosis of a pancreatic fistula. This is the most common form of presentation. It can also progress to a localized collection of fluid in the resection bed. This should be confirmed with a computed tomography (CT) scan or an abdominal ultrasound.

Management

External pancreatic fistulas are managed conservatively with continuous aspiration from the drain, clinical surveillance, octreotide, and enteral or even parenteral nutrition. Over 80% of these fistulas have a successful outcome and close [36].

Reoperation may be required in cases where there is no response to conservative medical management [36]. Fortunately, based on the literature, these fistulas rarely occur after a laparoscopic resection.

Localized Collections of Pancreatic Fluid

Occasionally a fistula will manifest itself as a fluid collection near the pancreatic stump or surgical field. Due to the high morbidity and mortality associated with reoperation, these fluid collections are best treated with percutaneous drainage [37].

Inadequate clearance of blood by the drain placed during surgery may lead to the slow accumulation of blood and the formation of a hematoma. Abdominal pain, fever, and leukocytosis are the most common presenting symptoms. Hematomas may resolve spontaneously or evolve into an abscesses. In such a case, percutaneous drainage is mandatory in addition to the administration of antibiotics [38]. The success rate for percutaneous drainage in infected postoperative pancreatic collections is 75%, according to Cinat et al. [38]. Surgery must be strongly considered when a second attempt at percutaneous drainage fails [38].

Complications Related to the Treatment of Pancreatic Pseudocysts

Pseudocysts are a common complication of chronic pancreatitis, occurring in approximately 20–40% of cases. They are less likely to resolve spontaneously than pseudocysts arising from acute pancreatitis [39].

Different types of treatment are available, including CT-guided drainage, endoscopy, and surgery. The traditional surgical open approach has a recurrence rate of 5.4%, while CT-guided drainage and endoscopic treatment have a relapse incidence of 10 and 6.6%, respectively [40]. Cyst gastrostomy by an anterior approach, cyst gastrostomy by the lesser sac approach, transgastric cyst gastrostomy, and laparoscopic pancreatic cyst jejunostomy are the different laparoscopic surgical procedures reported in the literature. Each is associated with specific complications.

Cyst Gastrostomy by the Anterior Approach

During this procedure, the surgeon must prevent bleeding from the anastomotic site, particularly when the communication is established with the use of electrocautery. Park et al. [14] reported 2 of 11 patients in whom this complication occurred. Suture placement was required to ensure hemostasis in the subsequent procedures. Fabre et al. [9] performed this procedure with an endoscopic stapler device in four patients and had no complications.

The anterior approach also carries the risk of gastric leakage into the peritoneal cavity [11], although this complication has not been described in the English literature.

Cyst Gastrostomy by the Lesser Sac Approach

The only complications described with this procedure [14] include one mortality due to myocardial infarction after the patient was discharged (day 4) and one case of necrotizing pancreatitis 3 weeks after discharge.

This technique avoids performing an anterior gastrotomy, thus abolishing the risk of complications related to it.

Transgastric Cyst Gastrostomy

No specific complications have been described with this technique. However, Park et al. [14] have suggested that insufflation of the stomach must be maintained by a flexible endoscope or low-pressure pneumoperitoneum (5–8 mmHg) in order to prevent excessive gastric distention.

Laparoscopic Pancreatic Cyst Jejunostomy

In Park's recent series, three cases of pseudocysts treated with a Roux-en-Y pancreaticojejunostomy were described. Mouiel et al. [41] described the utilization of fibrin glue to secure the anastomotic site [9]. Both had no complications but stated that it was the most technically challenging procedure for the treatment of pseudocysts [14].

Other Complications

Sepsis

As splenectomy carries the risk of overwhelming postoperative sepsis with encapsulated microorganisms [42] and thrombotic events due to high blood viscosity

TABLE 3 Reported Complications

Author	Number of Cases	Surgery	Complication (no.)	Treatment
Cuschieri, *1996*	5	5 DP+S	Pancreatic fistula (1)	Resolved spontaneously
Gagner, *1996*	7	3 E	Major bleeding (splenic vein) (1)[a]	Multiple titanium clips
		4 DP	Small infected collection[a]	Percutaneous drainage
Vezaquis, *1999*	4	4 DP	Pancreatic fistula (2)	Percutaneous drainage and PN
Ueno, *1999*	1	1 DP	Small splenic infarct (1 month)	Resolved spontaneously
Cuschieri, *2000*	4	2 HADP+S	Intraop bleeding (1)	Conversion
		1 HACG	–	–
		1 HACJ	–	–
Patterson, *2001*	17	10 DP+S	Intraop bleeding (1)	Conversion
			Pancreatic fistula (1)	CT guided
		3 DP	Pancreatic fistula (2)	percutaneous
		4 E	Pancreatic fistula (1)	drainage and PN
Fabre, *2001*	13	13DP	Intraop bleeding from splenic vein (2)	Conversion (1 splenectomy)
			Pancreatic fistula (1)	Conservative
			Liquid cysts (2)	
			Bleeding from trocar (1)	Re-operation
Fernandez-Cruz, *2001*	11	5DP	Perforated duodenal ulcer	Re-operation
		2 LIGD	–	–
		4 TCG	–	–
Park, *2002*	28	9CGLSA	Myocardial infarction (1)	Death
			Necrotizing pancreatitis (1)	Multiple (open) debridement
				–
		5MLIGCG	–	
		11TCG	Postop bleeding (2)	Transfusion
		3LCJ	–	–
	23	21DP	Intraop bleeding (2)	Transfusion
			Pancreatic fistula (1)	Percutaneous drainage
		2HADP	Wound infection (1)	NR
Gramatica, *2002*	9	4E	Pancreatic fistula (1)	Resolved
		4DP	Pleural effusion (1)	spontaneously
		1DP+S	Fluid collection (1)	
Mahon, *2001*	3	2DP	Urinary retention	Catheterization
		1DP+S		
Fernandez-Cruz, *2002*	16	4 E	Pancreatic fistula (2)	Drainage
		12 DP	Pancreatic fistula (3)	Drainage
			Splenic abscess (1)	Splenectomy
			Intraop bleeding (1)	Controlled with stapler

Abbreviations: DP, distal pancreatectomy; S, splenectomy; CGLSA, cyst gastrostomy by the lesser sac approach; MLIGCG, minilaparoscopic intragastric cyst gastrostomy; TCG, transgastric cyst gastrostomy; LCJ, laparoscopic cyst jejunostomy; HADP, hand-assisted distal pancreatectomy; HACG, hand-assisted cyst gastrostomy; HACJ, hand-assisted cyst jejunostomy; E, enucleation; NR, nonreferred; PN, parenteral nutrition; LIGD, laparoscopic intragastric drainage.
[a] Surgery not specified.

[6,25,43], there is general agreement on making special efforts to avoid splenic resection.

Preoperative vaccination against encapsulated bacteria is mandatory, since the surgeon cannot guarantee spleen preservation—the most frequent reason for conversion [9].

Splenic Abscess

This complication often follows the spleen-preserving procedures (ligating vessels distal to the pancreas). In his original description, Warshaw identified one splenic abscess in 22 patients. He also mentioned that splenomegaly is a relative contraindication to this procedure, since large spleens require a greater vascular supply and the short gastric vessels alone may not adequately perfuse the organ.

Splenic abscesses present with abdominal pain and fever, a technetium-99m sulfur colloid spleen scan will show an abnormal uptake, and a CT scan will indicate sufficient or insufficient blood flow [44]. Depending on each particular case, either drainage [6] or splenectomy [10] can be performed.

Splenic Infarction

Infarction of the spleen can follow pancreatic resection. It occurs more commonly after a spleen-preserving procedure (ligating vessels distal to the pancreas) but can also occur after a conventional spleen-sparing distal pancreatectomy. We recommend a close inspection of the spleen before finishing the procedure. Evaluate the need for splenectomy. Ischemia can lead to abscess formation or severe postoperative pain. Patterson et al. [2] described one patient in whom the organ appeared to be ischemic after a spleen-sparing distal pancreatectomy, and as a result the spleen was removed.

In some situations, the spleen undergoes hypertrophy in an attempt to compensate for inadequate perfusion, as Ueno et al. reported in 1999 [45]. This requires close follow-up and analgesic.

Wound Dehiscence, Infection, and Ventral Hernia

Concerning hand-assisted techniques, potential complications include the usual ones following pancreatectomy and those related to the incision made to introduce the device (Dexterity Pneumosleeve, Pillin-Weck, Research Triangle Park, NC). These include wound infections, dehiscence, and ventral hernia.

Delayed Gastric Emptying

This complication is described in patients following pancreatoduodenectomy. In his series, Gagner described one patient with this complication who required total parenteral nutrition for a 2-week period [19].

CONCLUSION

Laparoscopic pancreatectomy is safe and effective in trained hands. There are no complications, other than the common ones, specifically related to the laparoscopic approach. Laparoscopic techniques can treat intraoperative complications and prevent them. We believe that the minimally invasive approach is preferred in patients with nonmalignant diseases and low surgical risk. However, these procedures should be done in centers with expertise in advanced laparoscopic techniques. Published data favor the utilization of laparoscopic pancreatectomy, although prospective randomized trials are needed to compare the results of the laparoscopic approach with those of open surgery.

REFERENCES

1. Bernheim B. Organoscopy: Cystoscopy of the abdominal cavity. Ann Surg 1911; 53:764–767.
2. Patterson EJ, Gagner M, Salky B, Inabnet WB, Brower S, Edye M, Gurland B, Reiner M, Pertsemlides D. Laparoscopic pancreatic resection: Single-institution experience of 19 patients. J Am Coll Surg 2001; 193:281–287.
3. Mahon D, Allen E, Rhodes M. Laparoscopic distal pancreatectomy. Three cases of insulinoma. Surg Endosc 2002; 16(4):700–702.
4. Fernandez-Cruz L, Saenz A, Astudillo E, Martinez I, Hoyos S, Pantoja JP, Navarro S. Outcome of laparoscopic pancreatic surgery: Endocrine and nonendocrine tumors. World J Surg 2002; 26(8):1057–1065.
5. Gagner M, Pomp A, Herrera M. Early experience with laparoscopic resections of islet cell tumors. Surgery 1996; 120(6):1051–1054.
6. Warshaw A. Conservation of the spleen with distal pancreatectomy. Arch Surg 1988; 123(5):550–553.
7. Cuschieri A. Laparoscopic surgery of the pancreas. J R Coll Surg Edinb 1994; 39(3): 178–184.
8. Cuschieri A. Laparoscopic hand-assisted surgery for hepatic and pancreatic disease. Surg Endosc 2000; 14(11):991–996.
9. Fabre JM, Dulucq JL, Vacher C, Lemoine MC, Wintringer P, Nocca D, Burgel JS, Domergue J. Is laparoscopic left pancreatic resection justified?. Surg Endosc 2002; 16(9):1358–1361.
10. Fernandez-Cruz L, Saenz A, Astudillo E, Pantoja JP, Uzcategui E, Navarro S. Laparoscopic pancreatic surgery in patients with chronic pancreatitis. Surg Endosc 2002; 16(6):996–1003.
11. Park A, Schwartz R, Tandan V, Anvari M. Laparoscopic pancreatic surgery. Am J Surg 1999; 177(2):158–163.
12. Trias M, Targarona EM, Balague C, Cifuentes A, Taura P. Intraluminal stapled laparoscopic cystogastrostomy for treatment of pancreatic pseudocyst. Br J Surg 1995; 82(3):403.

13. Gramatica L Jr, Herrera MF, Mercado-Luna A, Sierra M, Verasay G, Brunner N. Videolaparoscopic resection of insulinomas: Experience in two institutions. World J Surg 2002; 26(10):1297–1300.
14. Park A, Heniford T. Therapeutic laparoscopy of the pancreas. Ann Surg 2002; 236(2): 149–158.
15. Shinchi H, Takao S, Noma H, Mataki Y, Iino S, Aikou T. Hand-assisted laparoscopic distal pancreatectomy with mini-laparotomy for distal pancreatic cystadenoma. Surg Laparosc Endosc Percutan Tech 2001; 11(2):139–143.
16. Klinger P, Hinder R, Menke DM, Smith S. Hand-assisted laparoscopic distal pancreatectomy for pancreatic cystadenoma. Surg Laparosc Endosc 1998; 8(3):180–184.
17. Gagner M, Pomp A. Laparoscopic pylorus-preserving pancreatoduodenectomy. Surg Endosc 1994; 8(5):408–410.
18. Gagner M, Pomp A. Laparoscopic pancreatic resection: Is it worthwhile?. J Gastrointest Surg 1997; 1(1):20–26.
19. Jossart GH, Gagner M. Pancreaticoduodenal resection. J Hepatobil Pancreat Surg 2000; 7(1):21–27.
20. Gentileschi P, Gagner M. Laparoscopic pancreatic resection. Chir Ital 2001; 53(3): 279–289.
21. Shimi S, Banting S, Cuschieri A. Laparoscopy in the management of pancreatic cancer: Endoscopic cholecystojejunostomy for advanced disease. Br J Surg 1992; 79(4):317–319.
22. Underwood RA, Soper NJ. Current status of laparoscopic surgery of the pancreas. J Hepatobil Surg 1999; 6:154–164.
23. Halloran CM, Ghanch P, Bosennet L, Hartley MN, Sutton R, Neoptolemos JP. Complications of pancreatic cancer resection. Dig Surg 2002; 19(2):138–146.
24. Vezakis A, Davides D, Larvin M, McMahon MJ. Laparoscopic surgery combined with preservation of the spleen for distal pancreatic tumors. Surg Endosc 1999; 13(1): 26–29.
25. Aldridge M, Williamson R. Distal pancreatectomy with and without splenectomy. Br J Surg 1991; 78(8):976–979.
26. Cuschieri A, Jackimowicz J, van Spreeuwel J. Laparoscopic distal 70% pancreatectomy and splenectomy for chronic pancreatitis. Ann Surg 1996; 3:280–285.
27. Uranus S, Mischinger H, Pfeifer J, Kronberger L, Rabl H, Werkgartner G, Steindorfer P, Kraft-Kirz J. Hemostatic methods for the management of spleen and liver injuries. World J Surg 1996; 20:1107–1112.
28. Kono M, Yahagi N, Kitahara M, Fujiwara Y, Sha M, Ohmura A. Cardiac arrest associated with use of an argon beam coagulator during laparoscopic cholecystectomy. Br J Anaesth 2001; 87(4):644–646.
29. Gorey T, Bonadio F. Laparoscopic assisted surgery. Semin Laparosc Surg 1997; 4: 102–109.
30. O'Reilly MJ, Saye WB, Mullins SG, Pinto SE, Falkner PT. Technique of hand-assisted laparoscopic surgery. J Laparoendosc Surg 1996; 6(4):239–244.
31. Lillemoe KD, Kaushal S, Cameron JL, Sohn TA, Pitt HA, Yeo CJ. Distal pancreatectomy: Indications and outcomes in 235 patients. Ann Surg 1999; 229(5):693–700.
32. Berends FJ, Cuesta MA, Kazemier G, van Eijck CH, de Herder WW, van Muiswinkel JM, Bruining HA, Bonjer HJ. Laparoscopic detection and resection of insulinomas. Surgery 2000; 128(3):386–391.

33. Lo C, Lo CM, Fan S. Role of laparoscopic ultrasongraphy in intraoperative localization of pancreatic insulinoma. Surg Endosc 2000; 14(12):1131–1135.
34. Pietrabissa A, Shimi S, Vander Velpen G, Cuschieri A. Localization of insulinoma by laparoscopic intragastric inspection of the pancreas and contact ultrasonography. Surg Oncol 1993; 2(1):83–86.
35. Matsumoto T, Kitano S, Yoshida T, Bandoh T, Kakisako K, Ninomiya K, Tsuboi S, Baatar D. Laparoscopic resection of a pancreatic mucinous cystadenoma using laparoscopic coagulation shears. Surg Endosc 1999; 13:172–173.
36. Ridgeway MG, Stabile BE. Surgical management and treatment of pancreatic fistulas. Surg Clin North Am 1996; 76(5):1159–1173.
37. McLean TR, Simmons K, Svensson LG. Management of postoperative intra-abdominal abscesses by routine percutaneous drainage. Surg Gynecol Obstet 1993; 176(2): 167–171.
38. Cinat M, Wilson S, Din A. Determinants for successful percutaneous image-guided drainage of intra-abdominal abscess. Arch Surg 2002; 137(7):845–849.
39. Byrne MF, Mitchel RM, Baillie J. Pancreatic pseudocysts. Curr Treat Options Gastroenterol 2002; 5(5):331–338.
40. Soliani P, Dell'Abate P, Del Rio P, Franzini C, Piccolo D, Sianesi M. Therapy of post-necrotic pancreatic pseudocysts: Invasive treatments and their results. Chir Ital 2002; 54(4):477–486.
41. Mouiel J, Crafa F. Pancreatic cyst treated by laparoscopic cysto-jejunal anastomosis on a Roux-en-Y loop. Surg Endosc 1995; 9:625.
42. Cooper M, Williamson R. Splenectomy: Indications, hazards and alternatives. Br J Surg 1984; 71(3):173–180.
43. Mellemkjaer L, Olsen JH, Linet MS, Gridley G, McLaughlin JK. Cancer risk following splenectomy. Ugeskr Laeger 1995; 11;157(37):5097–5100.
44. Watanabe Y, Sato M, Kikkawa H, Shiozaki T, Yoshida M, Yamamoto Y, Kawachi K. Spleen-preserving laparoscopic distal pancreatectomy for cystic adenoma. Hepatogastroenterology 2002; 49(43):148–152.
45. Ueno T, Oka M, Nishihara K, Yamamoto K, Nakamura M, Yahara N, Adachi T. Laparoscopic distal pancreatectomy with preservation of the spleen. Surg Laparosc Endosc Perc Tech 1999; 9(4):290–293.

20

Pediatric Minimal-Access Surgery

Marion C. W. Henry and Craig T. Albanese
Stanford University Medical Center and Lucille Salter Packard Children's Hospital, Stanford, California, U.S.A.

INTRODUCTION

Minimally access surgery (MAS) has gained an important place in pediatric surgery, with more than three-quarters of pediatric surgeons performing laparoscopic cases [1]. Just as in adult MAS, the degree of benefit from these techniques will vary from procedure to procedure and patient to patient.

Present minimal-access techniques and tools have inherent limitations that, when combined with small patient size and confined working spaces, make for difficult operations with the potential for complications. These inherent limitations include two-dimensional images, minimal haptic feedback, confined spaces in small children, operating at a distance, motion parallax, and poor ergonomics, such as limitations in directional movement and mobility of the instrumentation.

Complications that occur during pediatric MAS must be considered in two separate categories: (1) those that are case-specific intra- and postoperative complications which can occur during both open and closed procedures (and are not addressed herein) and (2) those that are unique to minimal-access technology, such as those related to abdominal, thoracic, and retroperitoneal access, positioning, trocar insertion, instrumentation, and gas (CO_2) insufflation.

The safety of minimally invasive surgery in children has raised much concern and yielded multiple studies. Studies have shown variable rates of complications, from 1–5%, including bowel perforation, abdominal wall hematomas, pneumothorax, iliac vessel lacerations, liver lacerations, stomach perforation, bladder perforation, trocar site herniation, and gas embolism [2–7]. However, careful attention to the selection of patients, patient postioning, anatomy, trocars, instruments, and the physiological changes associated with gas insufflation can minimize the occurrence of these complications.

PATIENT SELECTION

Children with pre-existing cardiac and pulmonary disorders may not be able to tolerate the physiological stress of the reduction in functional residual capacity and hypercarbia associated with gas insufflation or one-lung ventilation during thoracoscopy. A child with a coagulopathy may not be a good candidate, as bleeding may limit visibility in the abdominal cavity, since the blood absorbs the xenon light. Prior open surgery is a relative contraindication, since safe access to the thoracic or abdominal cavities can be achieved with either an open technique or Veress needle insertion at a site remote from the previous incision. Whether or not the proposed procedure can be carried out is solely a function of the anatomy and the surgeon's experience in dealing with adhesions using minimal access techniques.

POSITIONING

Proper positioning of the child during pediatric MAS is integral to the success of the procedure. As in open surgery, the surgeon usually stands facing the structure to be operated on with the monitor ''in line'', directly in front of the surgeon. Given the requirement in advanced laparoscopic procedures for the surgeon to be able to use both hands for dissection and suturing, this often requires the surgeon to be positioned at the feet of the patient. This manner of positioning can be accomplished in multiple ways.

Low lithotomy positioning using stirrups is appropriate for children over the age of 8. Attention must be paid to careful positioning and padding of the legs in order to avoid peroneal nerve injury or stretch injury to the femoral nerves. In smaller children, the head of the bed can be removed in order to minimize the distance this position places between the child's head and the anesthesiologist. Even with this technique, the child will still be at a distance from the anesthesiologist, so additional care should be taken to ensure that the endotracheal tube is well secured, so as to avoid dislodgement [8,9].

In children under the age of 8, a supine, frog-leg position is more suitable than lithotomy. Placing the child near the foot of the bed or turning him or her 90 degrees on the bed, which is most applicable for neonates, may achieve this positioning. Removing the head of the bed or lowering the foot of the bed will bring the anesthesiologist into the closest proximity possible to the child [8,9].

If a child is going to be placed in reverse Trendelenburg position so that gravity can reduce the bowel from the surgical field—as is often the case for fundoplication, cholecystectomy, and splenectomy—the use of a beanbag molded in such a way that there is a "seat" is recommended, so that a steep tilt will not cause the child to slide on the table. It is important, when using a beanbag, that the bag itself be secured to the table, so that it does not slide with table movement.

Improper positioning during thoracoscopy can lead to complications and poorly performed or even technically impossible procedures. As with all thoracic procedures (regardless of technique), all bony prominences and the axilla must be padded to avoid pressure ulcers or brachial plexus injury. Access to the anterior mediastinum is best gained by positioning the patient supine and elevated 30 degrees. Procedures such as lung biopsy or lobectomy are best accomplished with the full lateral decubitus position.

Procedures involving structures in the posterior mediastinum are approached with the patient prone and elevated 30 degrees. In this way, anterior and posterior nonpulmonary structures can easily be accessed without the use of a lung retractor, since the combination of gas insufflation, single-lung ventilation, and gravity will keep the lung out of the operative field, necessitating the use of no more than three trocars for most procedures.

ANATOMICAL CONSIDERATIONS

The foremost anatomical consideration is the smaller surface area for access in smaller children and the smaller operating field within the abdominal, thoracic, and retroperitoneal spaces. Additionally, the small child's abdominal wall tends to be thinner and more compliant compared to that in adolescents and adults. This fact must be remembered when gaining trocar access with a Veress needle. Though the Veress needle technique is gaining increasing acceptance, an open technique is preferred by many surgeons in order to minimize risks of bowel perforation. However, the trocar insertion technique is dictated mainly by the surgeon's experience and comfort level rather than the technique itself. In either situation, attention should be paid to the possibility that the umbilical vessels and urachus may still be patent and that the epigastric vessels are easily injured, given the small cross-sectional area available for trocar access [2,7,12–16]. The liver margin is well below the rib cage in small children; the abdominal viscera are closer to the abdominal wall in children; and the bladder lies in an intra-abdominal position rather than in the pelvis [10]. The stomach should be deflated with a gastric tube. The bladder can be emptied using either an indwelling catheter or by manual pressure, called Credé's maneuver [9,11,12]. These anatomical considerations affect the choice of trocars, their route of insertion, and their location [9,11–13]. In addition, the retroperitoneoscopic approach for nephrectomy, ureteropelvic junction obstruction, and adrenalectomy—as opposed to transperitoneal MAS—is limited by a smaller working space, crowding of trocars, and a relative lack of anatomical landmarks.

Thoracosopic procedures in small children are complicated by the small, rigid chest wall with minimal intercostal space. It is often necessary to collapse the ipsilateral lung, which can be challenging if not impossible in small children. The available methods for one-lung ventilation, depending on the patient's size and the anesthesiologist's expertise, are the double lumen endotracheal tube (reserved for children older than 12 years), selective mainstem intubation (sometimes requiring the aid of fiberoptic bronchoscopy), and intratracheal intubation with mainstem occlusion by a bronchial blocker. The balloon on the blocker can deflate or burst. With all these methods, it is desirable to add 4–6 torr of CO_2 pressure to maximize lung collapse. This minimal pressure rarely results in hemodynamic or respiratory compromise.

TROCARS AND TECHNIQUE OF INSERTION

The nature of the abdominal wall in children can influence the surgeon's choice in trocar type and method of insertion. The open or Hasson technique is widely performed due to the compliant abdominal wall and short anteroposterior distance in the thorax and abdomen. The Veress needle technique is quick and easy but can injure blood vessels, bowel, urinary bladder (for laparoscopy) and heart, lungs, and diaphragm (for thoracoscopy). Gas embolism due to inadvertent puncture of a large vessel is extremely rare [16], and subcutaneous emphysema can occur by improper positioning of the needle or when a trocar is displaced into the abdominal or thoracic tissue space. This is rarely of clinical significance, although it can hinder port reinsertion or create pneumothorax or pneumomediastinum.

The most common trocar used in pediatric MAS, most notably as the first trocar inserted, is the radially expanding Step trocar (U.S. Surgical). These access devices come in two lengths, 75 and 100 mm. They are inserted with a Veress technique to allow a snug fit when they are bluntly expanded, or they can be placed with an open technique. The expandable sleeve starts at 1.7 mm in diameter and can be increased to 3, 5, 10, or 12 mm. It fits snugly and thus minimizes the chance of gas leak and dislodgement from the thin abdominal/chest wall [7,12,17,18]. When the device is removed, the tissues contract, leaving only a series of small slits with a fascial defect about half the size required for other types of trocars. With smaller defects, the risk of trocar-site herniation decreases and the cosmetic results are improved. Although most surgeons do not close 5-mm port sites in adults, these sites do present a risk for herniation in the pediatric population. It is generally advocated that the fascia of a 5-mm port, and even a 3-mm umbilical port, be closed [13,15].

Other trocars come with a sharp pyramidal tip. These are quite traumatic and may lead to gas leakage and dislodgement. Given the smaller volume of the pediatric abdominal cavity, gas leakage poses a more significant problem than in adult patients. A sharp conical trocar is less traumatic on insertion, as it stretches the tissues, resulting in a smaller opening and tighter fit in the tissues, which minimizes the risks of gas leakage or dislodgement. However, the insertion of such a trocar requires the use of great force.

Other attempts to decrease gas leakage and slippage have utilized sand-blasted cannulas and cannulas with a screw-like structure. The latter cannulas, however, actually enlarge the diameter of the entrance hole.

INSTRUMENTATION

Proper instrumentation is the key to successful pediatric MAS. Instruments for adults are frequently too long (32–36 cm) and too large in diameter (5–10 mm) for most children. An adult-length instrument leaves 75–80% of the instrument outside of the child and only 20% inside. This leads to awkward manipulation and imprecise movements. The ideal position of endoscopic instruments is to have two-thirds of the instrument inside the body cavity and the other one-third outside of the body in order to prevent motion parallax. Instrumentation that is shorter (18–22 cm) and thinner (2–3.5 mm) has been developed for pediatric procedures [11,17–19]. Similarly, nondisposable trocars that are thin (e.g., 3.5 mm), short (50–75 mm), and can be purchased with or without a gas insufflation port (the latter leading to a lower profile) have been developed.

Laparoscopes are also available in short, thin sizes. For the small patient, the most commonly used laparoscope is the 4-mm 30-degree lens that is 18 cm long [11,17,18]. There are laparoscopes copes as small as 1.2 mm, but they have poor light-gathering quality, which results in a dim, less colorful picture on the monitor, principally because any laparoscope 2 mm or less in diameter is a fiberoptic rather than a rod lens.

Electrosurgical complications leading to an inadvertent burn of adjacent structures are most commonly due to monopolar electrocautery. The noninsulated tip of the cautery device should always be under full endoscopic vision and away from any metal cannulas [12–14,17]. Other devices, such as the ultrasonic scalpel, can generate significant heat on their tips and must also be used with caution.

GAS INSUFFLATION

Pneumoperitoneum causes respiratory and cardiovascular changes in children, which can also lead to complications. Increasing the intra-abdominal pressure (IAP) has been shown to modify venous return and systemic vascular resistance. These changes can be significant and lead to an increase in arterial pressure of

20–25%. Particularly in children with limited cardiac reserve, the combination of elevated systemic vascular resistance and decreased venous return can be problematic. When IAP is less than 10 mmHg, venous return is increased, leading to an increased cardiac output. However, if the IAP is increased to 20 mmHg, the inferior vena cava becomes compressed, which results in a decrease in venous return and a subsequent decrease in cardiac output. Similarly, an increase in IAP above 20 mmHg will also cause a decrease in renal blood flow due to increased renal vascular resistance. Intra-abdominal pressures less than 15 mmHg appear to be tolerated in otherwise healthy children larger than 5 kg, while neonates should be limited to an IAP of less than or equal to 12 mmHg [8,16,20,21].

Pneumoperitoneum can also lead to displacement of the diaphragm toward the head, leading to a decrease in lung volume. This movement can lead to a reduction in lung compliance and an increase in airway resistance, which leads to an increased risk of barotrauma [16,20,21]. Restricting the mobility of the diaphragm also leads to an uneven distribution of ventilation, resulting in a ventilation perfusion mismatch, which can lead to hypercarbia and hypoxia. In addition, CO_2 insufflation of the peritoneal cavity results in systemic absorption of the gas, together with diaphragmatic splinting and a reduction in tidal volume. The end-tidal CO_2 monitor must be closely watched by the anesthesiologist and the venitilatory settings adjusted accordingly. Hypercarbia can have undesirable physiological consequences, such as tachycardia, dysrhythmia, a high cardiac output, and low systemic vascular resistance. The position of the patient can also add to these effects, as respiratory function will be less compromised when the patient is in the reverse Trendelenburg position and increased in a steep Trendelenburg position [16].

EQUIPMENT FAILURE

Paralleling the complexity of cases now being performed is the complexity of the room setup, instrumentation, and peripheral equipment. On the ''tower,'' the xenon bulbs have a fixed life span and should be periodically checked. The amount of gas in the tanks should be checked before every case. Fuses can blow, wires between monitors can become loose or disconnected, and any number of connectors can be lost or broken. Light and monopolar cords can be mismatched. Not infrequently, the small, delicate telescopes develop cracks or bends after processing. The newer instruments have handles that are interchangeable and insulating tubes that come off. These can be broken, misplaced, or put together incorrectly. The reusable trocars have valves with fixed life spans and they can leak as they get older.

CONCLUSION

MAS is rapidly becoming more pervasive in the practice of pediatric surgeons as training and familiarity increase. As technological advances bring smaller, better instruments, more procedures will lend themselves to MAS techniques. Safety considerations must be borne in mind as the feasibility of procedures increases. Above all, the learning curve must be accepted and overcome as an obstacle to these operations.

REFERENCES

1. Firilas AM, Jackson RJ, Smith SD. Minimally invasive surgery: The pediatric surgery experience. J Am Coll Surg 1998; 186(5):542–544.
2. Lobe TE. Pediatric laparoscopy: General considerations. In Scott-Conner CEH, ed. The SAGES Manual: Fundamentals of Laparoscopy and GI Endoscopy. New York: Springer-Verlag, 1999, 386–388.
3. Esposito C, Ascione G, Garipoli V, De G, Esposito G. Complications of pediatric laparoscopic surgery. Surg Endosc 1997; 11:655–657.
4. Peters C. Complications in pediatric urologic laparoscopy: Results of a survey. J Urol 1995; 155:1070–1073.
5. El Ghoneimi A, Valla JS, Limonne B, Valla V, Montupet P, Chavrier Y, Grinda A. Laparoscopic appendenctomy in children: Report of 1379 cases. J Pediatr Surg 1994; 29:786–789.
6. Little DC, Custer MD, May BH, Blalock SE, Cooney DR. Laparoscopic appendectomy: An unnecessary and expensive procedure in children?. J Pediatr Surg 2002; 37(3):310–317.
7. Rothenberg SS, Georgeson K, DeCou JM, Downey EC, Lelli JL, Raschbaum G, Moores D. A Clinical evaluation of the use of radially expandable laparoscopic access devices in the pediatric population. Pediatr Endosc Innov Techn 2000; 4(1): 7–12.
8. Siedman L. Anesthesia for Pediatric Minimally Invasive Surgery. In Lobe TE, ed. Pediatric Laparoscopy. Georgetown. TX: Landes Bioscience, 2002.
9. Ostlie DJ, Holcomb GW. Laparoscopic fundoplication and gastrostomy. Semin Pediatr Surg 2002; 11(4):196–204.
10. Georgeson KE. Laparoscopic-assisted pull-through for Hirschsprung's disease. Semin Pediatr Surg 2002; 11(4):205–210.
11. Sanfilippo JS, Lobe TE. Laparoscopic surgery in girls and female adolescents. Semin Pediatr Surg 1998; 7(1):62–72.
12. Najmaldin AS, Grousseau D. Basic technique. In Bax NMA , Georgeson KE , Najmaldin A , Valla JS, eds. Endoscopic Surgery in Children. Berlin: Springer-Verlag, 1999, 14–34.
13. Bax NMA, van der Zee DC. Complications in laparoscopic surgery in children. In Bax NMA , Georgeson KE , Najmaldin A , Valla JS, eds. Endoscopic Surgery in Children. Berlin: Springer-Verlag, 1999, 357–370.
14. Lobe TE. Pediatric laparoscopy: complications. In Scott-Conner CEH, ed. The SAGES Manual: Fundamentals of Laparoscopy and GI Endoscopy. New York: Springer-Verlag, 1999, 399–406.
15. Chen MK, Schropp KP, Lobe TE. Complications of minimal-access surgery in children. J Pediatr Surg 1996; 31(8):1161–1165.

16. Pennant JH. Anesthesia for laparoscopy in the pediatric patient. Anesthesiol Clin North Am 2001; 19(1):69–88.
17. Bax NMA. Instrumentation in pediatric endoscopic surgery. In Lobe TE, ed. Pediatric Laparoscopy. Georgetown. TX: Landes Bioscience, 2002.
18. Georgeson KE. Instrumentation. In Bax NMA , Georgeson KE , Najmaldin A , Valla JS, eds. Endoscopic Surgery in Children. Berlin: Springer-Verlag, 1999, 8–13.
19. Bax NMA. Ergonomics in (pediatric) endoscopic surgery. In Lobe TE, ed. Pediatric Laparoscopy. Georgetown. TX: Landes Bioscience, 2002.
20. Gentili A, Pigna A, Pasini L, Iannettone C, Libri M, Lima M. Anesthesia during pediatric laparoscopy: Are there changes related to the intra-abdominal pressure and the duration of peritoneal insufflation?. Pediatr Endosurg Innov Techn 1999; 3(3): 107–116.
21. Sfez M. Basic Physiology and Anesthesia. In Bax NMA , Georgeson KE , Najmaldin A , Valla JS, eds. Endoscopic Surgery in Children. Berlin: Springer-Verlag, 1999, 53–72.
22. Tagge EP, Hebra A, Goldberg A, Chandler JC, Delatte S, Othersen HB. Pediatric laparoscopic biliary tract surgery. Semin Pediatr Surg 1998; 7(4):202–206.

21

Prosthetic Biomaterials

Alfredo M. Carbonell, Kent W. Kercher, Brent D. Matthews, and B. Todd Heniford
Carolinas Medical Center, Charlotte, North Carolina, U.S.A.

INTRODUCTION

Historically, the treatment of hernias first consisted of simple suture repair. Unsatisfactory recurrence rates with simple approximation forced surgeons to search for better techniques. These failures bred the concept of using a biomaterial to bridge the fascial gap. Several metallic mesh biomaterials were developed over a 60-year period beginning with silver wire in 1900. Because of corrosion and metal fatigue, these metallic biomaterials were abandoned in favor of polymer blends. Francis Usher first introduced a woven monofilament polypropylene mesh in 1959 [1]. The newer permutations of polypropylene and expanded polytetrafluoroethylene (ePTFE), which were introduced in the 1970s, are the most common biomaterials used for herniorrhaphy in the United States today. Current data have clearly demonstrated the superiority of mesh-based hernia repair and its association with lower recurrence rates [2–5]. Despite their widespread use and relative safety, prosthetic biomaterials are still associated with troublesome complications.

WOUND INFECTION

In 1999, the Centers for Disease Control developed guidelines to accurately define a surgical site infection [6]. Superficial incisional infections must occur within

30 days of surgery, involve only the skin and subcutaneous tissue with associated purulent drainage or a positive culture of aseptically obtained subcutaneous fluid, and be associated with erythema, pain, or swelling of the incision. Deep incisional infections must also occur within 30 days of surgery or up to 1 year if a biomaterial has been implanted. These conditions are diagnosed by the presence of an abscess or spontaneous dehiscence of the wound with subsequent purulent drainage.

Several factors appear to contribute to the development of wound complications. In a retrospective review of 250 ventral hernia repairs, White and colleagues [7] identified a defect greater than 10 cm and the use of mesh as factors that affected overall wound complications. Additionally, wound infection rates significantly increased with the use of drains placed subcutaneously—a practice thought to help prevent seroma formation and hence to obliterate the dead space associated with the dissection of tissue flaps. A preoperative dose of an antibiotic, typically a first-generation cephalosporin, has been shown to decrease the incidence of wound infection from 26% to 13% in ventral hernia repair [8] and from 9% to as low as 2% in inguinal hernia repair [9–14]. When a patient develops a postoperative superficial surgical-site infection, removal of the mesh may be required; however, treatment with oral antibiotics will normally suffice.

DEEP PROSTHETIC INFECTION

The infection of a prosthetic biomaterial is a dreaded complication. Mesh infections may present immediately after surgery or be significantly delayed [15,16]. Such delayed infections appear, on average, 4.5 months following mesh implantation [17]. A distinction should be made between the superficial wound infection previously described and a true deep prosthetic infection. Mesh infections tend to occur late in the postoperative period and are characterized by acute inflammatory changes of the overlying skin and often the spontaneous development of a sinus tract draining purulent material. Occasionally the mesh may be exposed and visible in the wound bed. Factors that contribute to mesh infections differ from those of superficial infections and are distinguished by the size of flaps created, tissue viability, and the interaction between the host tissue, biomaterial, and bacterial organism. The host tissue reacts differently to different biomaterials. Polyester mesh induces a greater inflammatory and foreign-body response than polypropylene or ePTFE mesh. Polypropylene induces a stronger fibroblastic inflammatory reaction, with resulting tissue incorporation within 2 weeks of implantation, compared with the older ePTFE meshes [18]. Whether a biomaterial is multifilamented or not influences the degree of inflammation. Several investigators have shown that multifilamented polypropylene, although softer and more pliable outside the body, induces a greater foreign-body reaction and promotes persistence of bacteria in the wound bed compared with monofilament polypropylene controls [19,20]. Amid [21], on the other hand, states that macroporous biomaterials (polypropylene) deter the housing or growth of bacteria within the interstices by allowing the influx of macrophages and rapid angiogenesis, while microporous biomaterials (ePTFE) do not allow the influx of macrophages and therefore may be more susceptible to infection. Theoretically this seems plausible; however, Brown's [22] work demonstrates the superior ability of ePTFE to resist infection compared with polypropylene. In vitro and in vivo animal models in our laboratory have clearly shown the superior resistance to infection of ePTFE coated with silver/chlorhexidine compared with polypropylene [23]. It appears that bacterial colonization of the chronic fluid collections caused by the inflammatory reaction to the mesh may play a role in delayed infection of prosthetic biomaterials [24]. Additionally, colonization of the biomaterial with *Staphylococcus epidermidis*, a slime-producing skin flora, may also contribute to these late-onset infections.

The effectiveness of prophylactic antibiotics in the prevention of ePTFE vascular graft infection has been clearly shown and is dependent on maintaining an adequate antibiotic level in the perigraft tissues for the duration of the procedure [25]. We use this reasoning during lengthy hernia repairs and often administer repeat doses of antibiotics during the operation. To prevent infection, we minimize the intraoperative handling of the biomaterial and often use an iodine-impregnated adhesive drape on the patient's abdomen to reduce exposure of the mesh to the local skin flora. In the event of a prosthetic infection, the question arises of whether or not to remove the biomaterial. There is no simple answer to this. Amid [21] believes that removal of ePTFE is required, while polypropylene does not necessarily have to be removed to completely treat a deep infection. A national inquiry of 19,700 inguinal hernia repair patients from the Hernia Center of Rome found 12 (0.06%) late plug-related infections, all of which required plug removal. Petersen [17] found 8 (7%) deep prosthetic infections in 125 patients undergoing ventral hernia repair with several different biomaterials; ePTFE (3), polypropylene (3), and polyester (2). After a mean of 44 unsuccessful days of conservative wound debridement, the 3 patients with infected ePTFE mesh required its removal, while the other patients recovered without the need for mesh removal. We have treated four patients with infection of ePTFE mesh using antibiotics and a V.A.C. wound closure device (KCI Therapeutic Services Inc., San Antonio, TX) [26]. This vacuum-assisted closure device removes infectious material and fluid, thus promoting tissue granulation and contraction of wound edges by uniformly applying negative pressure to the wound margins and wound cavity. Stoppa [27] in a review of 751 patients undergoing ventral hernia repair with polyester mesh, found 2.5% early infections and 0.2% late infections, without the need for polyester mesh removal in any. Although infection can usually be controlled without removal of the mesh [18], the decision to remove a prosthetic material must be made on an individual basis after conservative measures consisting of wound debridement and antibiotic therapy have proven futile.

SEROMA

A major consequence of any ventral hernia repair procedure can be the formation of a seroma. The dissection of subcutaneous tissue flaps during open hernia repair disrupts dermal lymphatic flow, devitalizes the subcutaneous fat, and leaves a large potential space for fluid to accumulate. Concurrently, the local tissue trauma of surgery stimulates a cascade of inflammatory mediators, such as histamines, kinins, and prostaglandins. These mediators increase the permeability of surrounding vascular channels and also serve as chemoattractants for the inflammatory cells of the body, which ultimately perpetuate the capillary leak phenomenon and seroma formation [28]. Although it is clear that seroma in open ventral hernia repair is caused by extensive tissue dissection, the pathway by which seroma formation arises in the laparoscopic ventral hernia repair is less clear.

The peritoneum is a highly specialized membrane composed of polyhedral squamous cells and serves as an envelope that invests the intra-abdominal viscera. The major function of this semipermeable membrane is to maintain peritoneal fluid balance [29]. The peritoneum also contains inflammatory cells such as mast cells, macrophages, polymorphonuclear cells, and peritoneal mesothelial cells. When it is irritated, an inflammatory cascade ensues, resulting in vasodilation and contracture of the peritoneal endothelium, with the subsequent flow of protein-rich fluid into the peritoneal cavity [29]. When a foreign body such as a prosthetic biomaterial is affixed to the peritoneal surface, it can be surmised that the inflammatory reaction thus incited causes the transudation of peritoneal fluid. Because the biomaterial is now covering the potential hernia space, a large volume of seroma fluid can collect within the hernia sac, anterior to the mesh.

Susmallian et al. [30], using ultrasound, detected seroma formation in 100% of their patients undergoing laparoscopic ventral hernia repair, although only 35% were apparent clinically. This can be troublesome for both the clinician and the patient. Such a fluid collection may cause pressure below the attenuated skin and subcutaneous tissue of the hernia and serve as a nidus of infection. As demonstrated by Heniford et al. [31] in a study of more than 400 patients, nearly all seromas resolve within 2 months of surgery, and infection of the seroma was rare. If needed, a seroma can often be treated by needle aspiration. This must be done with care, as it may introduce bacteria into the fluid collection. The secondary infection of a seroma is a catastrophic complication that must be avoided. Additionally, the blind placement of needles into this area risks bowel injury, since it is sometimes difficult to differentiate a fluid collection from underlying bowel associated with a postoperative hernia recurrence [32]. The most effective way of treating a seroma is to prevent its formation. While an ideal method for preventing seroma has not been developed, Chowbey [33] stated that his rate of seromas after laparoscopic ventral hernia repair was reduced by 50% simply by using an abdominal binder.

In mastectomy and myocutaneous flap models, several investigators found that fibrin glue, composed of human fibrinogen and bovine thrombin, significantly reduces seroma volumes when compared with controls [28,34–36]. Zieren and colleagues [37] found that when fibrin sealant–coated polyglycolic mesh patches were fixed to the abdominal wall in rats, there was an increase in the concentration of fibroblasts, collagen, and hydroxyproline and perhaps improved ingrowth. Missing from the current literature are experimental studies investigating the treatment of seroma after laparoscopic ventral hernia repair. We are conducting a pilot study assessing the feasibility of reproducing seroma formation after an intraperitoneal mesh repair of a ventral hernia in New Zealand white rabbits and will proceed with an experimental study to determine the effect of fibrin sealant and the instillation of other ablative agents to prevent and treat seromas.

At present, our approach focuses on conservative management of seromas after laparoscopic ventral hernia repair. Preoperatively we inform all of our patients that they will develop a seroma that may take 6–8 weeks to resolve. In the event of a clinically evident seroma, we employ a practice of watchful waiting and do not perform an aspiration unless the seroma causes significant discomfort. Thus far, we have not had to reoperate on any patient due to a seroma. Some investigators believe that the use of drains in subcutaneous procedures appears to expedite wound healing [38], while others believe they may potentiate wound complications [39]. The incidence of drain-tract infection, however, might be reduced with the use of prophylactic antibiotics [8,40]. With the large open Stoppa hernia repair, we typically place flat, closed suction drains at the time of operation and remove them after they are draining less than 30 mL/day.

SINUSES

A sinus represents a chronic drainage tract that is not connected to an epithelium-lined organ. A large review of incisional hernias by Morris-Stiff and Hughes [18] found the incidence of wound sinus to be 0.6% for ePTFE, 1.2% for polyester, and 1.6% for polypropylene. These problems typically develop because of a chronic foreign-body reaction to a prosthetic biomaterial or suture and may be associated with an underlying infection. Molloy [41] reviewed 50 patients who underwent repair of massive incisional hernias with polypropylene mesh and found a 12% incidence of chronic wound sinus. Four patients required surgical intervention but none necessitated mesh removal. We usually use permanent monofilament suture for all our hernia applications, be it a primary suture repair or for mesh fixation. Braided sutures may be associated with an increased risk of foreign-body reaction and sinus formation [42,43]. A period of conservative management with antibiotics and wound cleansing can lead to resolution of a wound sinus. Should prolonged conservative management fail, re-exploration with suture removal alone may be all that is necessary, since it is often a suture that is the culprit [21].

FISTULAS

Enteric drainage from a wound that occurs weeks to years after a prosthetic-based hernia repair is a sentinel sign that the mesh has eroded into the intestine. There have been reports of colovesical, ileocutaneous, and colocutaneous fistulas presenting up to 15 years after incisional hernia, preperitoneal inguinal hernia, and paracolostomy hernia repair [44–50]. The true incidence of fistulas is probably underreported but ranges from 0.08–9% [18,51].

Two important factors seem to influence the development of enteric fistulas: the composition of the biomaterial itself and the anatomical space in which it is placed. Fistulas are more commonly reported after the use of polypropylene or polyester-based biomaterials [44–48,50]. In a retrospective study of 200 patients undergoing open incisional hernia repair with intraperitoneal mesh placement, Leber [52] found that multifilamented polyester mesh had a significantly higher fistula rate (16%) compared with polypropylene (1.7%), and ePTFE (0%). Additionally, he found that when omental interposition was effected between the mesh and bowel, the fistula rate was 0%, compared with 3.7% when the mesh had direct bowel contact. Karakousis [53] found a 26% enterocutaneous fistula rate when tissue was not interposed between the bowel loops and mesh, compared with 0% with tissue interposition. Vrijland [54], in an analysis of 136 patients who underwent intraperitoneal placement of polypropylene mesh for incisional hernia repair, found no fistulas after a 34-month follow-up, despite direct contact between the mesh and the underlying bowel in 42% of the patients. Although case reports of ePTFE-associated enterocutaneous fistulas are reported in the literature, all appear to be caused by an intraoperative technical error, such as enterotomy, and none appear to be caused by the mesh itself [55–57]. Therefore it appears that ePTFE is the safest biomaterial to place adjacent to exposed viscera, while polypropylene and polyester should not be used in this way.

In the event that a fistula is suspected, establishing a diagnosis is usually very straightforward. A computed tomography (CT) scan, upper GI contrast study with small bowel follow-through, or fistulogram with a water-soluble contrast material will help to confirm the diagnosis. Treatment can be complicated and usually consists of partial or complete mesh removal and bowel resection with the risk of recurrent hernia formation [58].

MESH MIGRATION

The migration of prosthetic biomaterials is rare; however, there are reports of fragments from metallic mesh migrating into the bowel, causing small bowel obstruction and erosion 30 years after the initial ventral hernia repair [59,60]. It appears that the fragments become encapsulated by loops of bowel and a foreign-body reaction ensues, causing granulation, intestinal wall necrosis, and intraluminal migration. The majority of prosthetic biomaterials rarely move, but a new trend of migration has been seen with the newer polypropylene prosthetics fashioned into a plug. They have been reported to migrate into the scrotum, intraperitoneally, or into the bladder if not properly sutured in place [61–63]. A more alarming potential complication of the patch-plug technique of hernia repair appears to be vascular compression near the femoral canal, which was reported by Cristaldi [64] after plug migration in a patient who underwent a femoral-popliteal bypass procedure. The theory of long-term mesh contracture and scar formation causing vascular compromise in the femoral vessels was investigated by Taylor [65]. He found that after a median of 3 years following either a laparoscopic or open inguinal hernia repair, no difference in femoral or testicular blood flow was seen on ultrasound between the operated and nonoperated side regardless of surgical approach.

The method of mesh fixation appears to have an impact on migration and subsequent recurrence. Some investigators believe that the fixation of mesh with staples or tacks is unnecessary in the laparoscopic repair of groin hernias [66,67]. On the other hand, mesh fixation, particularly with transabdominal sutures, is paramount to the success of the laparoscopic repair of ventral hernias. In a series of 100 laparoscopic ventral hernia repairs by LeBlanc [68], all 9 recurrences were the direct result of mesh migration due to fixation with tacks or staples alone. Heniford [31] reported similar results, with 42% of his recurrences due to the omission of transabdominal sutures. Most mesh biomaterials are approximately 1 mm thick. Therefore if the tacks are placed appropriately, only 3 mm of the tack penetrates into the peritoneum, fat, and possibly posterior fascia. These data support the argument against the practice of using tacks or staples alone, and we believe that combining suture fixation and helical tacks is a more reliable method of mesh fixation in the laparoscopic repair of ventral hernias.

When mesh migration occurs, it may present as a recurrent hernia with or without incarceration or with symptoms of obstruction or fistula. The difficulty with diagnosis of this problem is the fact that the biomaterials are not radiopaque, making them difficult to see on plain radiographs. Treatment consists of repair of the recurrence with or without mesh removal, as indicated. While most surgeons would not advocate the use of mesh in a potentially contaminated field, mesh implantation after bowel strangulation may, according to a report of 20 emergent inguinal and ventral hernia repairs for incarceration, be safe [69].

MESH FAILURE

Polypropylene mesh can shrink as much as 54% after implantation. The amount of shrinkage is less pronounced in the case of biomaterials with lower polypropylene content [70]. The shrinking and contraction of the mesh is a concern, since it can lead to hernia recurrence. This underscores the importance of adequate mesh/defect overlap. Although lightweight mesh products are marketed as more pliable and possibly more comfortable, there are no long-term data on their durability compared with the traditional heavyweight polypropylene biomaterials. Langer [71] reported a patient who experienced central mesh failure and a hernia recurrence through the polypropylene mesh. Although this was a heavyweight product, the concern is that forces act differently at the fascia/mesh interface, whereby the fascia acts as a fulcrum for the mesh to ''snap,'' causing failure.

Short-term data concerning lightweight polypropylene from Schumpelick's group in Germany show improved patient outcomes with regard to abdominal wall compliance and pain without an increase in the hernia recurrence rate, although follow-up in this study was only 8 months [72].

ISCHEMIC ORCHITIS

There has been concern that prosthetic biomaterials, particularly polypropylene plugs, placed in contact with the spermatic cord can cause scar formation and contracture of the vas deferens, with subsequent low sperm counts or ischemic orchitis and testicular atrophy. Although the incidence can be higher in recurrent hernia surgery, this appears to be related to extensive cord dissection during the hernia repair [73]. Rutkow and Robbins [74], in their review of 407 patch-plug repairs for recurrent groin hernia, did not experience any cases of ischemic orchitis. In an animal study comparing polypropylene and ePTFE mesh placed intraperitoneally over the porcine inguinal ring, LeBlanc [75] found a significantly more pronounced adhesive process to the polypropylene mesh, with ossification, necrosis of soft tissue, and venous congestion of the testes. This congestion is believed to be the pathophysiology behind ischemic orchitis. Others, however, have shown no difference in testicular blood flow regardless of the operative approach or method of mesh fixation in inguinal hernia repair [65,76].

Ischemic orchitis is probably a rare complication of prosthetic-based inguinal hernia repair; nevertheless, surgeons should avoid overzealous dissection of the spermatic cord. If the patch-plug technique is being used, suture fixation of the mesh plug appears to aid in the resolution of migration problems.

ADHESIONS

Adhesions are known sequelae of any surgery. With the intraperitoneal implantation of prosthetic biomaterials, however, the incidence rises. Many studies have been performed investigating the adhesion-forming properties of various prosthetics used for hernia repair [75,77–79]. The two factors that seem to influence adhesion formation to mesh are the composition of the biomaterial and the anatomical location of mesh placement. The macroporous (larger than 75 μm) structure of polypropylene and polyester allow the adherence of the underlying viscera to the mesh surface when the material is placed in the abdomen, while ePTFE's microporous surface reduces adhesion formation [21]. The pore size of the nonvisceral side of ePTFE averages 20 μm or less, while the visceral side measures 3 μm [18]. However, work by Pourdeyhimi [80], using a new image processing system reported that the pore size of ePTFE mesh might be twice as large as previously thought. Therefore the lack of adhesion formation might be the result of the chemical nature or hydrophobicity of the ePTFE biomaterial. Novel techniques using bioresorbable membranes—such as hyaluronate or regenerated oxidized cellulose attached to polypropylene—have been shown to reduce adhesions compared with polypropylene alone [81–84]; however, we have not found this to be the case [85]. Clinically, many investigators have reported a significant decrease in adhesions to ePTFE when compared with polypropylene or polyester mesh in both animals and humans [75,79,86,87]. The adhesions that form to the visceral or "no stick" side of ePTFE tend to be thinner, less vascular, and easier to remove from the mesh [79]. Regarding the anatomical placement of mesh, Attwood [77], found no difference in adhesion formation between the intraperitoneal onlay and the transabdominal preperitoneal placement of a polypropylene mesh in a porcine model. Farmer [78], on the other hand, found significantly more adhesions when polypropylene mesh was placed intraperitoneally as opposed to extraperitoneally in rats.

Adhesions to mesh are typically not clinically relevant unless they are encountered at repeat laparotomy or if a patient presents with bowel obstruction or fistula. When encountered, adhesions are gently lysed using sharp dissection and avoiding the use of cautery or ultrasonic shears.

PERSISTENT PAIN

Pain occurs commonly after both incisional and inguinal hernia repair. A randomized trial of primary suture repair, polypropylene mesh, or autodermal skin graft for the repair of incisional hernias found a 61% incidence of pain 1 year after repair when mesh was used compared with 22% with the autodermal graft and 17% with suture [88]. Investigators believe that the current polypropylene-based biomaterials may be unnecessarily thick and rigid, leading to an intense fibrous reaction with the formation of a large scar plate. This may cause immobility and pain in the abdominal wall. It appears that as the polypropylene content of the biomaterial decreases, abdominal wall mobility increases [89]. Welty [72], in a large prospective trial of incisional hernia repair, compared heavyweight polypropylene mesh to a second heavyweight and a third lightweight polypropylene biomaterial. Using three-dimensional stereography, he demonstrated a considerable decrease in abdominal wall mobility from increased wall stiffness. Wall stiffness increased with mesh weight and decreased with a larger pore size. The heavyweight biomaterials caused a greater number of abdominal wall paresthesias even 4 months after implantation.

With the advent of the retrorectus or Stoppa repair and the laparoscopic repair of ventral hernias, surgeons are seeing an increasing number of patients complaining of pain from the transabdominal sutures used for mesh fixation. The explanation for the localization of pain to suture sites has not been well described, but it is speculated to be caused by nerve entrapment or muscle ischemia. In a study of laparoscopic ventral herniorrhaphy, we reported a 2% incidence of prolonged suture-site pain (greater than 8 weeks in duration) in 407 patients. Their pain typically resolved with nonsteroidal anti-inflammatory drugs or injections of local anesthetic [31]. At present, postoperative patients who present to our office with prolonged suture-site pain are offered treatment with an injection just deep to the anterior fascia, circumferentially around the suture site with 25–30 mL of 0.25% bupivacaine and 1% lidocaine with 1:100,000 epinephrine. We have a success rate of greater than 96% with this treatment modality [90]. When local treatment fails, we recommend referral to an anesthesia pain service for a nerve block. If this fails, removal of the offending suture is offered.

Recent data demonstrate that tension-free inguinal hernioplasty may not be as painless as once thought. In a questionnaire sent to members of the American Hernia Society soliciting information on the complications of the patch plug technique, LeBlanc [91] discovered that more than 9% of the respondents' patients had pain that interfered with their lifestyle. In a questionnaire study by Bay-Nielsen [92], 1166 patients responded 1 year after unilateral inguinal hernioplasty with complaints of pain in the area of the hernia (28.7%) or pain that impaired work or leisure activities (11%). Only 4.5% had sought medical care for this. In an effort to elucidate the mechanism of pain in transperitoneal laparoscopic hernia repair, Leibl [76] compared the placement of a slit polypropylene mesh to a nonslit mesh fixated with sutures or with staples. There appeared to be no difference between the groups with regard to pain up to 1 year after surgery as measured by the visual analogue scale.

Inguinal pain encountered after hernia repair is not difficult to diagnose but may present a challenge in treatment. Attempts should be made to characterize and quantify the pain. Although diagnostic studies are of limited value, ultrasound or CT may help identify the location of the biomaterial and detect any major complications from its migration or scarification. If it appears that the pain is neural in origin, referral to an anesthesia pain service for a nerve block may be successful. If the pain persists, remedial surgery must be considered. Mesh removal and neurectomy of the ilioinguinal or iliohypogastric nerve has shown favorable results over mesh removal alone [93]. If it appears that the pain may be from a staple or tack used to fix the mesh in laparoscopic hernia repair, staple or tack removal may be helpful, and a combined fluoroscopic and laparoscopic technique to identify and remove the offending tack/staple has been described [94]. By limiting fixation of the mesh only to Cooper's ligament and above the iliopubic tract, neuralgia from staples and tacks can be minimal.

CONCLUSIONS

We have presented an overview of the complications associated with the use of biomaterials in hernia repair. As biomaterial science continues to evolve, it is hoped that the problematic effects associated with the use of such materials will be eliminated. As surgeons working with these new tools, we have a responsibility to critically evaluate the prosthetics we implant into our patients.

REFERENCES

1. Usher F. A new plastic prosthesis for repairing tissue defects of the chest and abdominal wall. Am J Surg 1959; 97:629–633.
2. Luijendijk RW, Hop WC, van den Tol MP, de Lange DC, Braaksma MM, JN IJ, Boelhouwer RU, de Vries BC, Salis MK, Wereldsma JC, Bruijninckx CM, Jeekel J. A comparison of suture repair with mesh repair for incisional hernia. N Engl J Med 2000; 343(6):392–398.
3. Friis E, Lindahl F. The tension-free hernioplasty in a randomized trial. Am J Surg 1996; 172(4):315–319.
4. Lichtenstein IL, Shulman AG. Ambulatory outpatient hernia surgery. Including a new concept, introducing tension-free repair. Int Surg 1986; 71(1):1–4.
5. Lichtenstein IL, Shulman AG, Amid PK, Montllor MM. The tension-free hernioplasty. Am J Surg 1989; 157(2):188–193.
6. Mangram AJ, Horan TC, Pearson ML, Silver LC, Jarvis WR. Guideline for prevention of surgical site infection, 1999. Hospital Infection Control Practices Advisory Committee. Infect Control Hosp Epidemiol; 1999; 20(4):279–280.
7. White TJ, Santos MC, Thompson JS. Factors affecting wound complications in repair of ventral hernias. Am Surg 1998; 64(3):276–280.
8. Rios A, Rodriguez JM, Munitiz V, Alcaraz P, Perez. Flores D, Parilla P. Antibiotic prophylaxis in incisional hernia repair using a prosthesis. Hernia 2001; 5(3):148–152.
9. Gilbert AI, Felton LL. Infection in inguinal hernia repair considering biomaterials and antibiotics. Surg Gynecol Obstet 1993; 177(2):126–130.
10. Abramov D, Jeroukhimov I, Yinnon AM, Abramov Y, Avissar E, Jerasy Z, Lernau O. Antibiotic prophylaxis in umbilical and incisional hernia repair: A prospective randomised study. Eur J Surg 1996; 162(12):945–948; discussion 949.
11. Lazorthes F, Chiotasso P, Massip P, Materre JP, Sarkissian M. Local antibiotic prophylaxis in inguinal hernia repair. Surg Gynecol Obstet 1992; 175(6):569–570.
12. Yerdel MA, Akin EB, Dolalan S, Turkcapar AG, Pehlivan M, Gecim IC, Kuterdem E. Effect of single-dose prophylactic ampicillin and sulbactam on wound infection after tension-free inguinal hernia repair with polypropylene mesh: The randomized, double-blind, prospective trial. Ann Surg 2001; 233(1):26–33.

13. Taylor EW, Byrne DJ, Leaper DJ, Karran SJ, Browne MK, Mitchell KJ. Antibiotic prophylaxis and open groin hernia repair. World J Surg 1997; 21(8):811–814; discussion 814–815.
14. Platt R, Zaleznik DF, Hopkins CC, Dellinger EP, Karchmer AW, Bryan CS, Burke JF, Wikler MA, Marino SK, Holbrook KF, et al. Perioperative antibiotic prophylaxis for herniorrhaphy and breast surgery. N Engl J Med 1990; 322(3):153–160.
15. Thorbjarnarson B, Goulian D. Complications from use of surgical mesh in repair of hernias. N Y State J Med 1967; 67(9):1189–1192.
16. Slim K, Pezet D, Le Roux S, Chipponi J. Mesh infection after laparoscopic herniorrhaphy. Eur J Surg 1996; 162(3):247–248.
17. Petersen S, Henke G, Freitag M, et al. Deep prosthesis infection in incisional hernia repair: Predictive factors and clinical outcome. Eur J Surg 2001; 167(6):453–457.
18. Morris-Stiff GJ, Hughes LE. The outcomes of nonabsorbable mesh placed within the abdominal cavity: Literature review and clinical experience. J Am Coll Surg 1998; 186(3):352–367.
19. Beets GL, Go PM, van Mameren H. Foreign body reactions to monofilament and braided polypropylene mesh used as preperitoneal implants in pigs. Eur J Surg 1996; 162(10):823–825.
20. Klinge U, Junge K, Spellerberg B, Piroth C, Klosterhalfen B, Schumpelick V. Do multifilament alloplastic meshes increase the infection rate? Analysis of the polymeric surface, the bacteria adherence, and the in vivo consequences in a rat model. J Biomed Mater Res 2002; 63(6):765–771.
21. Amid PK. Classification of biomaterials and their related complications in abdominal wall hernia surgery. Hernia 1997; 1(1):15–21.
22. Brown GL, Richardson JD, Malangoni MA,, Tobin GR, Ackerman D, Polk HC, Jr. Comparison of prosthetic materials for abdominal wall reconstruction in the presence of contamination and infection. Ann Surg 1985; 201(6):705–711.
23. Carbonell AM, Dreau D, Foster M, Austin C, Matthews BD, Kercher K, Sing RF, Heniford BT. An in vitro study of the susceptibility to infection of various prosthetic mesh biomaterials. 2nd International Hernia Conference. London. England: American Hernia Society, 2003.
24. Mann DV, Prout J, Havranek E, Gould S, Darzi A. Late-onset deep prosthetic infection following mesh repair of inguinal hernia. Am J Surg 1998; 176(1):12–14.
25. Bergamini TM, Peyton JC, Cheadle WG. Prophylactic antibiotics prevent bacterial biofilm graft infection. J Surg Res 1992; 52(2):101–105.
26. Kercher KW, Sing RF, Matthews BD, Heniford BT. Successful salvage of infected PTFE mesh after ventral hernia repair. Ostomy Wound Mgt 2002; 48(10):40–2, 44–45.
27. Stoppa R. Long-term complications of prosthetic incisional hernioplasty. Arch Surg 1998; 133(11):1254–1255.
28. Kulber DA, Bacilious N, Peters ED, Gayle LB, Hoffman L. The use of fibrin sealant in the prevention of seromas. Plast Reconstr Surg 1997; 99(3):842–849; discussion 850–851.
29. Schecter W. Peritoneum and Acute Abdomen. In Norton J, ed. Surgery: Basic Science and Clinical Evidence. New York: Springer-Verlag, 2000, 413–415.

30. Susmallian S, Gewurtz G, Ezri T, Charuzi I. Seroma after laparoscopic repair of hernia with PTFE patch: Is it really a complication. Hernia 2001; 5(3):139–141.
31. Heniford BT, Park A, Ramshaw BJ, Voeller G. Laparoscopic ventral and incisional hernia repair in 407 patients. J Am Coll Surg 2000; 190(6):645–650.
32. Lin BH, Vargish T, Dachman AH. CT findings after laparoscopic repair of ventral hernia. Am J Roentgenol 1999; 172(2):389–392.
33. Chowbey PK, Sharma A, Khullar R, Mann V, Baijel M, Vashistha A. Laparoscopic ventral hernia repair. J Laparoendosc Adv Surg Tech A 2000; 10(2):79–84.
34. Lindsey WH, Becker DG, Hoare JR, Cantrell RW, Morgan RF. Comparison of topical fibrin glue, fibrinogen, and thrombin in preventing seroma formation in a rat model. Laryngoscope 1995; 105(3 Pt 1):241–243.
35. Lindsey WH, Masterson TM, Spotnitz WD, Wilhelm MC, Morgan RF. Seroma prevention using fibrin glue in a rat mastectomy model. Arch Surg 1990; 125(3): 305–307.
36. Eroglu E, Oral S, Unal E, et al. Reducing seroma formation with fibrin glue in an animal mastectomy model. Eur J Surg Oncol 1996; 22(2):137–139.
37. Zieren J, Castenholz E, Baumgart E, Muller JM. Effects of fibrin glue and growth factors released from platelets on abdominal hernia repair with a resorbable PGA mesh: Experimental study. J Surg Res 1999; 85(2):267–272.
38. Fox JWT, Golden GT. The use of drains in subcutaneous surgical procedures. Am J Surg 1976; 132(5):673–674.
39. Simchen E, Rozin R, Wax Y. The Israeli Study of Surgical Infection of drains and the risk of wound infection in operations for hernia. Surg Gynecol Obstet 1990; 170(4):331–337.
40. Dougherty SH, Simmons RL. The biology and practice of surgical drains. Part 1. Curr Probl Surg 1992; 29(8):559–623.
41. Molloy RG, Moran KT, Waldron RP, Brady MP, Kirwan WO. Massive incisional hernia: Abdominal wall replacement with Marlex mesh. Br J Surg 1991; 78(2): 242–244.
42. Kon ND, Meredith JW, Poole GV, Jr., Martin MB, Kawamoto E, Myers RT. Abdominal wound closure. A comparison of polydioxanone, polypropylene, and Teflon-coated braided Dacron sutures. Am Surg 1984; 50(10):549–551.
43. Sahlin S, Ahlberg J, Granstrom L, Ljungstrom KG. Monofilament versus multifilament absorbable sutures for abdominal closure. Br J Surg 1993; 80(3):322–324.
44. Rieger N, Brundell S. Colovesical fistula secondary to laparoscopic transabdominal preperitoneal polypropylene (TAPP) mesh hernioplasty. Surg Endosc 2002; 16(1): 218–219.
45. Miller K, Junger W. Ileocutaneous fistula formation following laparoscopic polypropylene mesh hernia repair. Surg Endosc 1997; 11(7):772–773.
46. DeGuzman LJ, Nyhus LM, Yared G, Schlesinger PK. Colocutaneous fistula formation following polypropylene mesh placement for repair of a ventral hernia: Diagnosis by colonoscopy. Endoscopy 1995; 27(6):459–461.
47. Fernandez Lobato R, Martinez Santos C, Ortega Deballon P, Fradejas Lopez JM, Marin Lucas FJ, Moreno Azcoita M. Colocutaneous fistula due to polypropylene mesh. Hernia 2001; 5(2):107–109.

48. Chew DK, Choi LH, Rogers AM. Enterocutaneous fistula 14 years after prosthetic mesh repair of a ventral incisional hernia: A life-long risk. Surgery 2000; 127(3): 352–353.
49. Bothra R. Late onset small bowel fistula due to tantalum mesh. Am J Surg 1973; 125(5):649–650.
50. Aldridge AJ, Simson JN. Erosion and perforation of colon by synthetic mesh in a recurrent paracolostomy hernia. Hernia 2001; 5(2):110–112.
51. Francioni G, Ansaldo V, Magistrelli P, Pari AM, Rinaldi P, Sani C, Rafaeli W, Pari G. The use of prosthesis in abdominal and thoracic wall defect, 15 year experience: Evaluation of tissue reactions and complications. Chir Ital 1999; 51(1):21–30.
52. Leber GE, Garb JL, Alexander AI, Reed WP. Long-term complications associated with prosthetic repair of incisional hernias. Arch Surg 1998; 133(4):378–382.
53. Karakousis CP, Volpe C, Tanski J, Colby ED, Winston J, Driscoll DL. Use of a mesh for musculoaponeurotic defects of the abdominal wall in cancer surgery and the risk of bowel fistulas. J Am Coll Surg 1995; 181(1):11–16.
54. Vrijland WW, Jeekel J, Steyerberg EW, Den Hoed PT, Bonjer HJ. Intraperitoneal polypropylene mesh repair of incisional hernia is not associated with enterocutaneous fistula. Br J Surg 2000; 87(3):348–352.
55. Monteforte CA, Queirazza R, Franceschetti P, Herbst TJ. Fistula formation after implanting an ePTFE membrane. A case report. J Reprod Med 1997; 42(3):184–187.
56. Bauer JJ, Harris MT, Kreel I, Gelernt IM. Twelve-year experience with expanded polytetrafluoroethylene in the repair of abdominal wall defects. Mt Sinai J Med 1999; 66(1):20–25.
57. Balen EM, Diez-Caballero A, Hernandez-Lizoain JL, Pardo F, Torramade JR, Regueira FM, Cienfuegos JA. Repair of ventral hernias with expanded polytetrafluoroethylene patch. Br J Surg 1998; 85(10):1415–1418.
58. Losanoff JE, Richman BW, Jones JW. Entero-colocutaneous fistula: A late consequence of polypropylene mesh abdominal wall repair: Case report and review of the literature. Hernia 2002; 6(3):144–147.
59. Majeski J. Migration of wire mesh into the intestinal lumen causing an intestinal obstruction 30 years after repair of a ventral hernia. South Med J 1998; 91(5): 496–498.
60. Deligne E, Faucompret S, Louis C, Arigon JP, Breda Y. [Intestinal obstruction by migration of wire mesh into the intestinal lumen following hernia repair]. Ann Chir 2001; 126(6):590–593.
61. Dieter RA. Mesh plug migration into scrotum: A new complication of hernia repair. Int Surg 1999; 84(1):57–59.
62. Chuback JA, Singh RS, Sills C, Dick LS. Small bowel obstruction resulting from mesh plug migration after open inguinal hernia repair. Surgery 2000; 127(4): 475–476.
63. Hume RH, Bour J. Mesh migration following laparoscopic inguinal hernia repair. J Laparoendosc Surg 1996; 6(5):333–335.
64. Cristaldi M, Pisacreta M, Elli M, Valgo GL, Danelli PG, Sampietro GM, Taschieri AM. Femoro-popliteal bypass occlusion following mesh-plug for prevascular femoral hernia repair. Hernia 1997; 1:197–199.

65. Taylor SG, Hair A, Baxter GM, O'Dwyer PJ. Does contraction of mesh following tension-free hemioplasty effect testicular or femoral vessel blood flow? Hernia 2001; 5(1):13–15.
66. Beattie GC, Kumar S, Nixon SJ. Laparoscopic total extraperitoneal hernia repair: Mesh fixation is unnecessary. J Laparoendosc Adv Surg Tech A 2000; 10(2):71–73.
67. Khajanchee YS, Urbach DR, Swanstrom LL, Hansen PD. Outcomes of laparoscopic herniorrhaphy without fixation of mesh to the abdominal wall. Surg Endosc 2001; 15(10):1102–1107.
68. LeBlanc KA, Booth WV, Whitaker JM, Bellanger DE. Laparoscopic incisional and ventral herniorraphy: Our initial 100 patients. Hernia 2001; 5(1):41–45.
69. Wysocki A, Pozniczek M, Krzywon J, Bolt L. Use of polypropylene prostheses for strangulated inguinal and incisional hernias. Hernia 2001; 5(2):105–106.
70. Klinge U, Klosterhalfen B, Muller M, Ottinger AP, Schumpelick V. Shrinking of polypropylene mesh in vivo: An experimental study in dogs. Eur J Surg 1998; 164(12):965–969.
71. Langer C, Neufang T, Kley C, Liersch T, Becker H. Central mesh recurrence after incisional hernia repair with Marlex—Are the meshes strong enough. Hernia 2001; 5(3):164–167.
72. Welty G, Klinge U, Klosterhalfen B, Kasperk R, Schumpelick V. Functional impairment and complaints following incisional hernia repair with different polypropylene meshes. Hernia 2001; 5(3):142–147.
73. Fong Y, Wantz GE. Prevention of ischemic orchitis during inguinal hernioplasty. Surg Gynecol Obstet 1992; 174(5):399–402.
74. Rutkow IM, Robbins AW. The mesh plug technique for recurrent groin herniorrhaphy: A nine-year experience of 407 repairs. Surgery 1998; 124(5):844–847.
75. LeBlanc KA, Booth WV, Whitaker JM, Baker D. In vivo study of meshes implanted over the inguinal ring and external iliac vessels in uncastrated pigs. Surg Endosc 1998; 12(3):247–251.
76. Leibl BJ, Kraft B, Redecke JD, Schmedt CG, Ulrich M, Kraft K, Bittner R. Are postoperative complaints and complications influenced by different techniques in fashioning and fixing the mesh in transperitoneal laparoscopic hernioplasty? Results of a prospective randomized trial. World J Surg 2002; 26(12):1481–1484.
77. Attwood SE, Caldwell MT, Marks P, McDermott M, Stephens RB. Adhesions after laparoscopic inguinal hernia repair. A comparison of extra versus intraperitoneal placement of a polypropylene mesh in an animal model. Surg Endosc 1994; 8(7): 777–780.
78. Farmer L, Ayoub M, Warejcka D, Southerland S, Freeman A, Solis M. Adhesion formation after intraperitoneal and extraperitoneal implantation of polypropylene mesh. Am Surg 1998; 64(2):144–146.
79. Matthews BD, Pratt BL, Backus CL, Kercher KW, Heniford BT. Comparison of adhesion formation to intra-abdominal mesh after laparoscopic adhesiolysis in the New Zealand White rabbit. Am Surg 2002; 68(11):936–940; discussion 941.
80. Pourdeyhimi B. Porosity of surgical mesh fabrics: New technology. J Biomed Mater Res 1989; 23(A1 suppl):145–152.
81. Baptista ML, Bonsack ME, Delaney JP. Seprafilm reduces adhesions to polypropylene mesh. Surgery 2000; 128(1):86–92.

82. Szabo A, Haj M, Waxsman I, Eitan A. Evaluation of seprafilm and amniotic membrane as adhesion prophylaxis in mesh repair of abdominal wall hernia in rats. Eur Surg Res 2000; 32(2):125–128.
83. Hooker GD, Taylor BM, Driman DK. Prevention of adhesion formation with use of sodium hyaluronate-based bioresorbable membrane in a rat model of ventral hernia repair with polypropylene mesh—A randomized, controlled study. Surgery 1999; 125(2):211–216.
84. Naim JO, Pulley D, Scanlan K, Hinshaw JR, Lanzafame RJ. Reduction of postoperative adhesions to Marlex mesh using experimental adhesion barriers in rats. J Laparoendosc Surg 1993; 3(2):187–190.
85. Matthews BD, Mostafa G, Kercher KW, Austin CE, Norton JA, Heniford BT. Evaluation of adhesion formation to ePTFE mesh and biosurgical composties. Society of American Gastrointestinal and Endoscopic Surgeons. Los Angeles. CA, 2003.
86. Bleichrodt RP, Simmermacher RK, van der Lei B, Schakenraad JM. Expanded polytetrafluoroethylene patch versus polypropylene mesh for the repair of contaminated defects of the abdominal wall. Surg Gynecol Obstet 1993; 176(1):18–24.
87. Murphy JL, Freeman JB, Dionne PG. Comparison of Marlex and Gore-tex to repair abdominal wall defects in the rat. Can J Surg 1989; 32(4):244–247.
88. Korenkov M, Sauerland S, Arndt M, Bograd L, Neugebauer EA, Troidl H. Randomized clinical trial of suture repair, polypropylene mesh or autodermal hernioplasty for incisional hernia. Br J Surg 2002; 89(1):50–56.
89. Klosterhalfen B, Klinge U, Schumpelick V. Functional and morphological evaluation of different polypropylene-mesh modifications for abdominal wall repair. Biomaterials 1998; 19(24):2235–2246.
90. Carbonell AM, Harold KL, Mahmutovic A, Hasan R, Matthews BD, Kercher KW, Sing RF, Heniford BT. Local injection for the treatment of suture site pain after laparoscpic ventral hernia repair. Am Surg 2003; 69(8):688–691; discussion 691–692.
91. LeBlanc KA. Complications associated with the plug-and-patch method of inguinal herniorrhaphy. Hernia 2001; 5(3):135–138.
92. Bay-Nielsen M, Perkins FM, Kehlet H. Pain and functional impairment 1 year after inguinal herniorrhaphy: A nationwide questionnaire study. Ann Surg 2001; 233(1): 1–7.
93. Heise CP, Starling JR. Mesh inguinodynia: A new clinical syndrome after inguinal herniorrhaphy. J Am Coll Surg 1998; 187(5):514–518.
94. Wong J, Anvari M. Treatment of inguinodynia after laparoscopic herniorrhaphy: A combined laparoscopic and fluoroscopic approach to the removal of helical tackers. Surg Laparosc Endosc Percutan Tech 2001; 11(2):148–151.

22

Robotic and Telerobotic Surgery

Garth Ballantyne
Hackensack University Medical Center, Hackensack, New Jersey, U.S.A.

Richard M. Satava
University of Washington Medical Center, Seattle, Washington, U.S.A.

INTRODUCTION

Surgeons first attempted to introduce robotics into the operating room in the early 1990s. Orthopedic surgeons developed the first clinically successful robot, ''Robodoc,'' used in total hip replacement [1,2]. In general surgery, two concepts motivated robotics research. Once video laparoscopic surgery became commonplace in the operating room, surgeons realized that a robot might easy replace the camera holder. Simultaneously, the U.S. Department of Defense envisioned military surgeons in remote places operating on wounded soldiers on the battlefields using telerobots [3]. Both robotic camera holders and telerobotic surgical systems have recently achieved approval from the U.S. Food and Drug Administration (FDA) for use in general surgery procedures. As a result, their use in American operating rooms has been rapidly escalating and surgeons are reporting a wide range of clinical experience.

THE ROBOTIC CAMERA HOLDER

A number of surgeons have developed robotic camera holders. Moran of the University of California at Davis first described a passive, electronically regulated, pneumatically controlled camera holder in 1993 [4]. Buess and colleagues in Tubingen, Germany, developed a prototype of a robotic camera holder called the FIPS Endoarm [5], where the surgeon controls the robot with a finger ring that clips to one of the surgical instruments. The FIPS Endoarm moves with four degrees of freedom and maintains a constant relationship with the horizon. Two robotic camera holders have achieved routine clinical use in many hospitals in Europe and the United States. Armstrong Healthcare Ltd. recently obtained FDA clearance for Endoassist [6,7], where the surgeon controls the robot's movements with his or her forehead, on which he wears an infrared emitting device. The surgeon directs the infrared beam at the point on the video monitor that he or she wishes to see. The robot then tracks the position of the infrared beam on the monitor and moves the camera view to this position.

AESOP (Computer Motion Inc., Santa Barbara, CA) has achieved the greatest clinical use of any robotic device (Fig. 1). (AESOP stands for ''automated endoscopic system for optimal positioning.'') Gagner and colleagues at the Hotel-Dieu de Montreal Hospital first reported the actual clinical use of a prototype of AESOP. They described successful completion of three laparoscopic cholecystec-

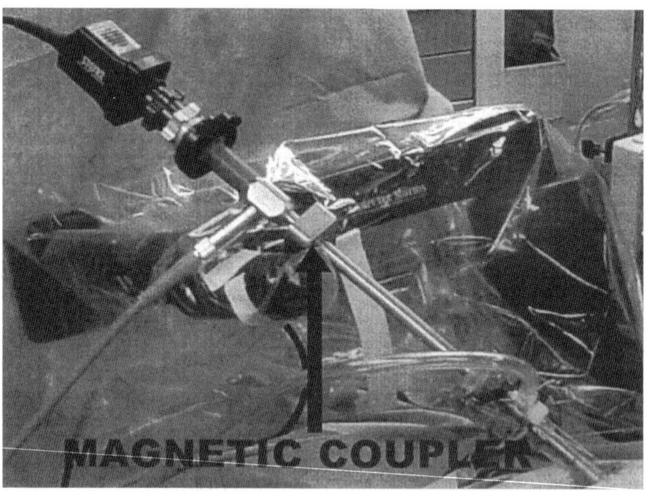

Figure 1 AESOP (Computer Motion Inc., Santa Barbara, CA) is a voice-controlled robot that holds the video telescope. The surgeon directs the movements of the telescope with simple voice commands. The telescope is linked to the robotic arm with a pressure-sensitive magnetic coupler. Should the movements of the telescope be impeded by anatomic structures, the telescope is disengaged from the robotic arm, thereby minimizing the risk of a penetrating injury.

tomies using a robotic surgical assistant [8]. The surgeon, sitting in a remote room and viewing the operation on a monitor, controlled the six degrees of freedom with a joystick. Gagner and colleagues reported additional experience with this prototype in 1995 [9]. They successfully accomplished eight laparoscopic cholecystectomies with cholangiography in humans between September 1, 1993, and October 10, 1994. The FDA approved AESOP for clinical use in 1994 and a wide clinical experience has subsequently been documented [10]. Initially, the surgeon controlled the AESOP either manually or remotely with a foot switch or hand controller [11,12]. In more recent generations, the surgeon controls AESOP with a proprietary voice-recognition system [13,14]. The surgeon directs movements of AESOP with simple commands, such as ''move up,'' ''move in,'' and ''move right.'' AESOP has proven successful in facilitating solo surgeon laparoscopic general surgery. Geis and colleagues, for example, used AESOP to perform 24 solo surgeon laparoscopic inguinal hernia repairs, cholecystectomies, and Nissen fundoplications [15]. As work hours for surgical residents become truncated and the cost of qualified surgical assistants increases, this may prove to be an important role of robotic assistants.

TELEROBOTIC SURGICAL SYSTEMS

The rapid evolution and miniaturization of computers has given rise to a new type of surgical robot. The robotic surgical assistants described above, such as AESOP, are controlled directly by the operating surgeon, who remains at the bedside [16]. Telerobotic surgical systems actually perform the operation and are controlled by a surgeon from a remote location. The surgeon sits at a computer console that displays a three-dimensional image of the operative field. Joysticks on the computer console translate the motions of the surgeon's hands into digital computer signals. The computer then transmits these digital directions to the remote robotic arms directly through fiberoptic cables or indirectly via telecasting systems. In the United States, the FDA demands that the surgeon remain in the same operating room. Nonetheless, the feasibility of having a remote surgeon perform a telerobotic operation was first demonstrated as early as 1991 [17]. More recently, Marescaux demonstrated that these systems could function with vast distances separating surgeon and patient by performing a laparoscopic cholecystectomy on a patient in Strasbourg, France, while sitting at a Zeus (Computer Motion Inc., Santa Barbara, CA) computer console in New York City [18–20]. The FDA has approved two telerobotic surgical systems for clinical use in the United States: the da Vinci (Intuitive Surgical Inc., Mountain View, CA) and the Zeus.

Da Vinci

Cadierre and colleagues reported the first successful clinical implementation of telerobotics in March 1997 by performing a laparoscopic cholecystectomy using a prototype of the Da Vinci robotic surgical system [21]. The FDA approved da Vinci for clinical use in all abdominal operations in June 2000. Intuitive Surgical Inc. designed da Vinci from scratch specifically to perform telerobotic surgery. Da Vinci consists of three parts: the surgeon's console, the robotic tower with three robotic arms, and an electronics tower (Fig. 2). The surgeon sits in an ergonomically comfortable position at the console. He or she views the surgical field through a binocular system that projects a true three-dimensional image, much like field binoculars. The surgeon inserts his or her hands into glove-like master devices that control the surgical instruments (Fig. 2 inset). All motions of the surgeon's hands are translated into identical motions of the robotic instruments. Buttons on the console allow the surgeon to select 1:1, 3:1, and 5:1 motion-scaling ratios. When a 5:1 ratio is selected, 5-in. motions of the surgeon's hands are reduced to 1-in. motions by the robotic instruments. The computer also filters

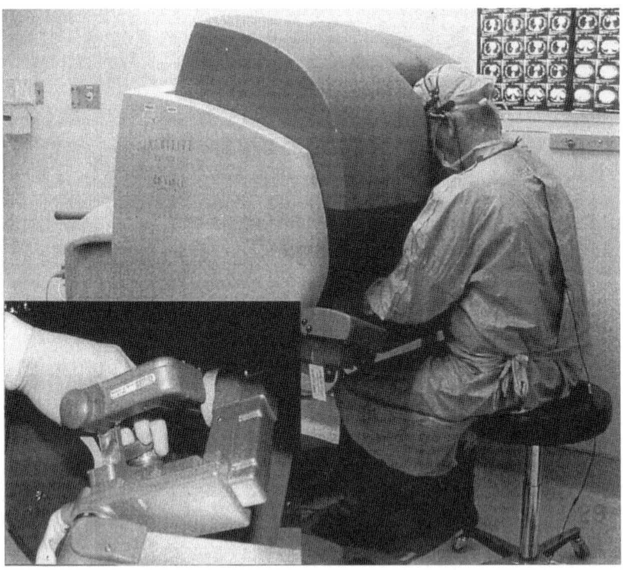

FIGURE 2 The da Vinci surgeon's computer console. In telerobotic surgery, the surgeon sits at a remote position away from the surgical table and patient. The surgeon views the virtual three-dimensional operating field through a binocular system in the console. This console intends to isolate the surgeon from his or her surrounding environment and to give the surgeon the perception of immersion within the operative field. INSET: The masters: the mechanical device that translates the motions of the surgeon's hands into motions of the remote robotic surgical instruments.

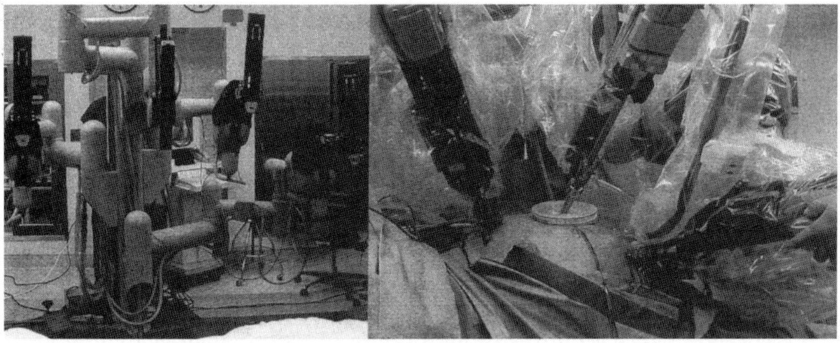

FIGURE 3 The left panel shows the da Vinci robotic tower supporting four robotic arms. The right panel shows the four robotic arms with sterile drapes being used to perform a telerobotic-assisted laparoscopic right hemicolectomy. The telescope is inserted through a 12-mm trocar placed within a hand-assisted surgery device (Lapdisk, Ethicon Endosurgery, Cincinnati, OH). At one time, the surgeon can control any two of the three robotic arms holding surgical instruments or move the telescope. The surgeon determines which robotic arms he or she is controlling by toggling a foot pedal.

out resting tremors in the surgeon's hands. The da Vinci masters provide some tensile feedback, but the tension on tissues generated by the robotic arms is best judged at this point by visual clues seen on the video image. The original robotic tower held three robotic arms: one to hold the video telescope and two for surgical instruments. A tower holding four robotic arms was recently approved by the FDA and reached the market in January 2003 (Fig. 3). The da Vinci robotic instruments move with seven degrees of freedom, producing motions very similar to those of the human hand. The electronics tower typically holds a video monitor, a carbon dioxide insufflator, and two video systems for the stereoscopic telescope.

Zeus

Zeus evolved from the clinically successful and reliable AESOP robotic camera holder during the late 1990s. In 1998, Margossian and colleagues sutured uterine horn anastomoses in six pigs using Zeus [22]. Over the last 5 years, several groups have assessed Zeus as a means for instructing medical students, surgical residents, and surgeons in techniques of advanced laparoscopic surgery. [23–25]. Unfortunately, Zeus received FDA clearance for abdominal operations only in October 2002; as a result, very few clinical studies using Zeus have been published. Zeus consists of a surgeon's computer console and three robotic arms. Zeus uses an open architecture that does not isolate the surgeon from the surrounding operating room. The surgeon sits in an ergonomically comfortable position (Fig. 4), viewing a three-dimensional projection of the operating field on the main monitor, which telecasts alternating video frames from the right and left video cameras. An active screen on the front of the monitor alternates between clockwise and counterclockwise polarizing filters synchronizing these filters with the right and left video frames, respectively. The surgeon wears sunglasses with a clockwise polarizing filter over the right eye and a counterclockwise filter over the left eye. This allows the right eye to see only the right video frames and the left eye the left video frames. The surgeon's brain reconstructs a three-dimensional video image from these two images that seems to project from the video monitor. A touch screen next to the surgeon's head controls programming functions such as motion scaling. Zeus also filters out resting tremors detected in the surgeon's hands. The surgeon wears a microphone through which he or she controls the robotic camera

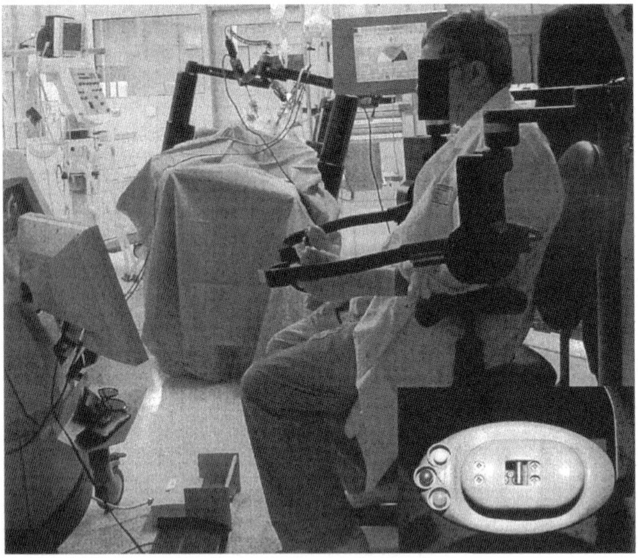

FIGURE 4 The Zeus surgeon's console, hand control, and three robotic arms. The surgeon sits in a comfortable chair, with instrument controllers in hand, viewing the three-dimensional operating field projected from the main monitor. A touch screen near the surgeon's head regulates functions such as motion scaling. The three Zeus robotic arms attach directly to the surgical table in the background. INSET: The Zeus hand controls, which translate the motions of the surgeon's hand into motions of the remote robotic surgical instrument. The buttons direct the video telescope to preset positions.

holder. Zeus's three robotic arms attach directly to the surgical table (Fig. 4). The camera holder is a voice-controlled AESOP. The two other robotic arms are AESOPs modified to hold surgical instruments. The Zeus robotic surgical instruments move with six degrees of freedom.

FUTURE DIRECTIONS IN ROBOTIC AND TELEROBOTIC SURGERY

The future direction of the utilization of robots can be speculated by analogy to other industries. While there has always been the fear of malfunction of a robot (a favorite scenario for science fiction stories and movies), a review of the safety of industrial robots favors just the opposite—they are reliable and fault-tolerant. Most robots have redundant systems or automatic shut-down, fail-safe mechanisms. According to ABB Robotics (Asea, Brown, Boveri, Ltd., Milwaukee, WI) [26], the largest producer of industrial robots, which has over 100,000 robots in the workplace, the average useful ''life expectancy'' for an industrial robotic system is more than 20 years (frequently working more than 12–18 hr/day continuously). The Occupational Safety and Health Administration (OSHA) has established numerous regulations [27,28] regarding safety in the workplace, including safe behavior in working near or cooperatively with robotic and automated systems. Injuries due to malfunction of robotics are virtually unheard of in the industrial sector; when accidents are investigated, human error or disobedience of rules or regulations is the principal causative factor. There have been no reports of any surgical robotic systems that have caused harm. In the case of anecdotal reports of a malfunction, as when a robot stopped working, no harm was done. Thus the prospect is bright for increasing the use of robotic systems, with anticipation that it may be possible to program them is such a way as to decrease or entirely avoid technical errors. Decision support systems, which run in real time and observe performance, can monitor the surgeon's performance during an operation and alert the surgeon or suggest options when his or her performance varies from actions during similar cases. This ''online, real-time'' assistance has the potential to reduce errors; in the same way a mentoring surgeon can make suggestions during a surgical procedure to help a resident avoid errors. In combination with surgical simulators, which will be used to train residents in the use of robotic surgical systems, improvement in patient safety through reduced errors can be accomplished. In addition, the opportunities to integrate the robot into all the operating room systems as well as the overall hospital information systems can broaden the value of the system.

COMPLICATIONS RELATED TO ROBOTIC CAMERA HOLDERS

A number of surgeons have published clinical experiences with AESOP [29–32]. No specific complications generated by the AESOP system have been reported.

At Hackensack University Medical Center, we have routinely used AESOP for laparoscopic cholecystectomies and laparoscopic inguinal hernia repairs since 1994 and for other advanced laparoscopic operations since 1997 [33,34]. Similarly, we are unaware of any injuries to our patients inflicted by AESOP. This is not surprising, since Computer Motion designed a number of features into the construction of AESOP to prevent the most likely problems.

Penetrating Injuries from the Telescope

The AESOP's robotic arm is extremely strong. AESOP could easily drive the tip of the telescope through vital structures such as the liver. To prevent this, Computer Motion designed a magnetic coupling device that separates at very low forces. A magnetic collar attaches the telescope to the robotic arm (Fig. 1). If the tip of the telescope pushes against a structure such as the liver, the resistance of the organ rapidly separates the magnetic collar from the robotic arm. We have found this mechanism to be reliable in preventing penetrating injuries.

Crush Injuries from the Robotic Arm

AESOP's robotic arm makes complex movements outside of the patient to move the tip of the telescope to the desired location. The robotic arm often makes large excursion arcs to accomplish this task. During these motions the arm could, theoretically, easily hit into the patient, causing bruising or crush injuries. In addition, the sweeping arcs of AESOP's arm could knock into and dislodge the endotracheal tube. In order to prevent these types of complications, the surgeon must manually set a ''lower limit'' for the motions of AESOP's arm. After setting this lower limit, we move the robotic arm across the patient to make sure that it does not hit the patient or endotracheal tube or prevent the respiratory movements of the chest. AESOP will not move below the lower-limit set point.

Voice-Recognition Errors

The surgeon controls the movements of AESOP through verbal commands. Random conversation in the operating room could therefore cause unexpected and dangerous robotic movements. In order to minimize this risk, Computer Motion developed a proprietary voice-recognition system that controls AESOP's motions. Each surgeon must record into a computer the set of AESOP commands, and the unique features of the surgeon's voice are burned onto a computer card. This card is required for any use of AESOP. AESOP's computer is extremely reliable in responding only to a particular surgeon's recorded voice. Naturally, no system is foolproof. We often encounter unexpected robotic movements. These can be immediately terminated through the voice command ''stop.'' Even if these random motions cause the telescope to hit an anatomical structure or the external arm to move toward the patient, the uncoupling system and the setting of a lower limit have always protected our patients.

COMPLICATIONS RELATED TO TELROBOTIC SURGERY

Da Vinci and Zeus evolved from different design concepts. The da Vinci telerobot was designed specifically to perform closed-chest internal mammary artery harvests and coronary artery bypass grafting. The use of da Vinci for abdominal operations changes the orientation of the robotic tower in relation to the patient and requires the use of the robotic surgical instruments for complex dissection. This leads to a variety of possible complications not generally encountered in cardiac surgery with the use of da Vinci. Zeus descended from AESOP. As a result, Zeus has inherited the safety features detailed above and avoids some of the robotic arm–generated problems discussed below. Other potential complications are shared by both systems.

Crush Injuries from the Robotic Arms

The da Vinci robotic arms can easy bruise the patient. When set up for thoracic operations, the patient is placed in a lateral position. The robotic tower is positioned at a perpendicular angle to the patient and the robotic arms project out away from the patient's chest. Only the cephalad robotic arm can hit the patient because the shoulder limits its excursion arcs. During abdominal operations, on the other hand, all three robotic arms sweep arcs over the patient's torso. All three arms can hit the patient, but this is most commonly seen with the two lateral arms, which hold the surgical instruments. Unlike AESOP, Zeus has no lower-limit set points for the excursion arcs of the robotic arms; the bedside assistant surgeon must monitor their motions. If collisions between the robotic arms and the patient are observed, the bedside assistant must manually reset the ''shoulders'' and ''elbows'' of the robotic arms. These problems are avoided with Zeus if the surgeon properly sets the lower limit on each of the three Zeus arms.

Wound Infections at the Camera Trocar Site

Da Vinci's central arm holds the video telescope and is locked to a 12-mm disposable trocar (Ethicon Endosurgery, Cincinnati, OH). If the locking device is set too close to the skin, the motions of the robotic arm will macerate the skin and subcutaneous fat surrounding the trocar site. We have found this to be a particular problem when the camera trocar site is near the umbilicus. During upper abdominal operations such as Nissen fundoplication, cholecystectomy, or gastric bypass, the telescope becomes nearly parallel to the abdominal wall even when a 30-degree telescope is being used. Under these circumstances, the locking device is pushed down into the periumbilical skin, crushing the tissue. This problem is accentuated in obese patients. In 2 of our first 10 da Vinci laparoscopic cholecystectomies, the periumbilical tissue was severely bruised and the supraumbilical trocar site developed wound infections shortly after surgery. We have found that we can avoid this problem by using a long 12-mm disposable trocar (Ethicon Endosurgery, Cincinnati, OH). The extra length of the trocar allows us to set the locking device several inches above the skin. Since we adopted this practice, we have not encountered any more trocar site infections.

Zeus holds the video telescope in exactly the same manner as AESOP. The magnetic coupling device is fixed to the telescope and not to the trocar. This displaces the coupling device several inches away from the patient's abdominal wall. We have not observed tissue maceration at the camera trocar site following AESOP-assisted operations and believe that this is an unlikely problem with Zeus procedures.

Penetrating Injuries

Both the telescope and robotic surgical instruments can impale vital structures. Zeus and da Vinci use different mechanisms to control the camera. Zeus uses the same voice-control mechanism detailed above for AESOP. Voice-recognition errors can lead to unexpected movements of the camera that could injure tissues. A magnetic coupler is used to link the video telescope and the two surgical instruments to the Zeus robotic arms (Fig. 5). These low-resistance magnetic couplers minimize this risk of penetrating injuries. With da Vinci, the surgeon manually maneuvers the camera with the hand-held master controls. These two systems make telescope-induced injuries unlikely with either telerobot. Penetrating injuries from the robotic surgical instruments, however, remain possible with either system. This is best avoided by limiting the motions of the instruments when they are out of direct videoscopic view.

Bedside assistant surgeons exchange the robotic surgical instruments during the course of telerobotic operations. Just as in laparoscopic operations, this can lead to penetrating injuries when the instruments are introduced into the abdomen through the trocars. Intuitive Surgical, Inc., recently added a feature to da Vinci to minimize this risk. Da Vinci's computer remembers the three-dimensional position of the previous instrument at the point when it was removed. Once the new instrument is attached to the robotic arm, da Vinci returns the instrument tip to exactly the same location. The use of an experienced assistant surgeon or surgical assistant also minimizes this risk.

Tissue Avulsion

Both da Vinci and Zeus robotic arms are extremely strong. Although some tensile feedback is provided by the master controls into which the surgeon inserts his or her hands, the surgeon can easily avulse tissues. One of the authors (GHB)

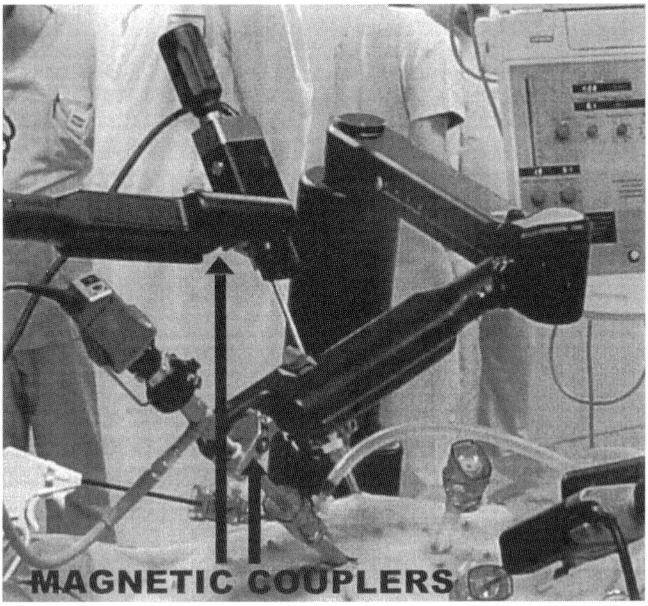

FIGURE 5 Zeus robotic arms. The video telescope and both robotic surgical instruments are attached to the robotic arms with low-resistance magnetic couplers. The couplers disengage when they encounter resistance to movement, as when hitting an anatomical structures. This minimizes the risk of penetrating injuries from the robotic surgical instruments.

observed a surgeon at another institution tear the gallbladder from its hepatic bed and snap the cystic duct during the first minute of his first telerobotic cholecystectomy. The surgeon must judge the tension placed on tissue by the robotic arms through visual clues. This is easily learned through experience.

Suture Shredding

Telerobots easily damage suture material, leading to insecure suture strength. This can cause an anastomotic leak, recurrence of a hiatal hernia, or separation of a fundoplication. The robotic needle holders and graspers can generate great crushing forces. The master devices do not transmit haptic feedback to the surgeon's hands. The surgeon cannot appreciate with what force the instrument is crushing the suture. Similarly, the surgeon must carefully judge the force exerted by the robotic arms while tying knots. Overzealous tightening may damage the suture material. Both excessive grasping and tightening can shred the suture, thereby reducing its tensile strength. During Nissen fundoplication, we attempt to minimize this risk by using a new suture for each stitch in the hiatal hernia repair and for constructing the fundoplication. In constructing a gastrojejunostomy for a gastric bypass with a continuous suture, the surgeon must take care to grasp the suture material very lightly. The bedside assistant surgeon can follow and maintain tension on the continuous suture, as in open or laparoscopic surgery.

Lost Cautery Tips

The original hook cautery used with da Vinci incorporated a disposable tip and reusable shaft (10 uses in the United States). On several occasions at Hackensack University Medical Center, this tip has caught on the grasping forceps of da Vinci's other hand. This was particularly easy with the Cadierre graspers because of their hollowed-out center. The great strength of the robotic arm easily pulled the tip out of the shaft. We used fluoroscopy to find the tips and to retrieve them. These events prolonged the operation but did not lead to any adverse patient events. Intuitive has released a newer version of the hook cautery in which the tip is permanently affixed to the shaft.

Laparoscopic Surgery Complications

Telerobotic operations are generally hybrid operations sharing robotic and laparoscopic technologies. As a result, operations performed with both da Vinci and Zeus are subject to all the complications associated with laparoscopic operations. The robotic instruments and telescopes for da Vinci and Zeus are inserted into the abdomen through standard laparoscopic trocars. We have experienced both significant hemorrhage and incisional hernias from trocar sites following telerobotic operations. We use the same precautions to prevent these complications following telerobotic operations that we use after standard laparoscopic operations. We decrease the intra-abdominal pressure and visually check the trocar sites for bleeding. We use a suture-passing device (Karl Storz Endoscopy, Los Angeles, CA) to close each of the 10- or 12-mm trocar sites with absorbable sutures.

Intra-abdominal hemorrhage can complicate any abdominal operation. National media recently focused attention on a death from hemorrhage following a telerobotic nephrectomy. The stapled closure of the renal pedicle bled in the early postoperative period. The pedicle was closed with a standard laparoscopic stapling device after the telerobotic portion of the operation was completed.

Laparoscopic and telerobotic operations often take longer than the equivalent open operations. Prolonged operation can lead to tissue necrosis from pressure in the dependent areas of the body. We have seen muscle necrosis in the buttocks following prolonged laparoscopic donor nephrectomies but fortunately have not seen this complication after telerobotic operations.

GRANTING CLINICAL PRIVILEGES FOR TELEROBOTIC OPERATIONS

At Hackensack University Medical Center, we have implemented a rigorous process for granting clinical privileges to perform telerobotic operations [35]. In general surgery, we require the surgeon to have clinical privileges to perform the equivalent laparoscopic operation before attempting the telerobotic operation. We grant telerobotic privileges as a technique of surgery similar to granting privileges for laser surgery. We do not grant privileges for each individual operation that might be performed telerobotically. We have based our process on the guidelines published by the Society of American Gastrointestinal Endoscopic Surgeons for granting privileges for advanced laparoscopic surgery [36,37].

We have set up a six-phase process. The surgeon must first pass an FDA-approved 2-day safety course on the use of the telerobot. This course includes didactic lectures, a dry laboratory, and live animated experience with the use of the telerobot. We encourage the surgeon to observe telerobotic operations at our hospital or at other centers. The surgeon then performs 10 operations on live animated or cadaveric models. The surgeon next acts as the bedside assistant surgeon for 5–10 operations. Once the surgeon commences his or her own clinical experience, he or she is proctored during the initial 5–10 telerobotic operations. After the surgeon is granted clinical privileges, the outcomes of the operations are monitored as part of our ongoing quality-assurance program. Using this system, we have achieved excellent clinical results. We believe that the best means to avoid complications during the learning-curve phase of the introduction of new operations into clinical practice is through a rigorous privileging process.

CURRENT STATUS OF ROBOTIC AND TELEROBOTIC SURGERY

Robotic camera holders and telerobotic surgical systems remain at different stages of evolution. Robotic camera holders are a routine and accepted part of our surgical suite at Hackensack University Medical Center. We have been routinely using AESOP for laparoscopic operations for nearly a decade. As the pool of surgical residents available to scrub on operations continues to dwindle and the cost of trained surgical assistants increases, AESOP and other similar robotic camera holders will become an increasingly common sight in operating rooms around the United States. Their ease of use, reliability and low cost of maintenance make them an attractive investment for busy surgical hospitals. In contrast, telerobots have not achieved the level of routine use.

The Da Vinci and Zeus robotic systems remain in a period of rapid evolution and exploration of clinical utility. Because telerobotic surgical systems are computer-based, they are likely to evolve at the same rate as computer chips, memory systems, and video graphics. The two currently available telerobotic systems have evolved with somewhat different philosophies. Da Vinci leads in dexterity, with its seven degrees of freedom for the motion of its surgical instruments and its true three-dimensional imaging system. The apparent reality of its virtual operative field is quite convincing and certainly facilitates accurate motions of the surgical instruments. Zeus leads in safety features and modularization. Having evolved from the safety conscious AESOP, Zeus contains the same lower-limit set points and pressure-sensitive magnetic couplers as AESOP. Zeus's three robotic arms attach directly to the surgical table, are relatively lightweight, and can be moved separately. Some surgeons prefer the telepresence virtual operative field of da Vinci while others prefer the open architecture of Zeus, which permits them to maintain direct visual contact with the surgical field and their patient. Hopefully, Computer Motion and Intuitive will learn from each other.

THE FUTURE

In regard to future directions for robotic and automated surgical systems, the first direction that needs to be addressed is integration. Other industries have integrated numerous robotic systems together, resulting in a cooperative environment of robots, called "robotic cells," that have replaced menial human labor (Fig. 6).

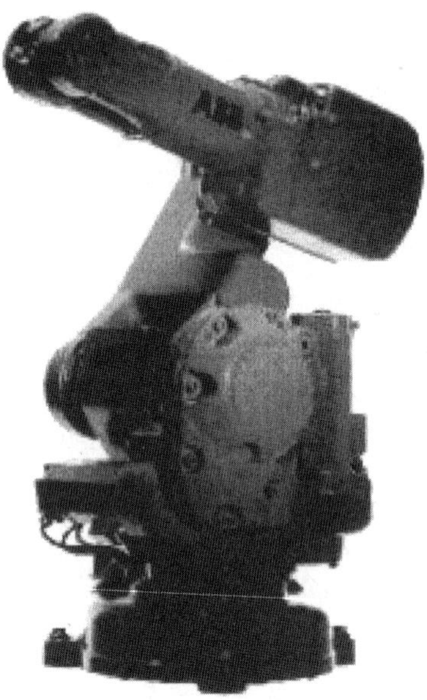

Figure 6 An industrial robot. Industrial robots are self-contained systems. They do not require assistants to change their active tools or supply materials. Industrial robots may serve as the model for future generations of surgical robots. (Courtesy ABB Robotics, Milwaukee, WI.)

Relevant to surgery is the integration of component robots into today's surgical robotic systems. In industry, there are no humans to hand different tools or instruments to the robot; rather, there is an automatic tool changer. In surgery, however, the scrub nurse changes instruments on the Zeus or da Vinci systems. Also in industry, there are no humans to hand ''parts'' to an industrial robot; there is an automatic inventory (or parts) dispenser. In surgery, however, there is a circulating nurse to hand mesh, suture, etc., to the robot. The handing of instruments and supplies is clearly a menial task, one that could certainly be replaced by an automated system. Thus, it can be anticipated that greater efficiency and safety can be gained by integrating a tool changer and inventory dispenser into the current surgical robotic systems. With no humans involved during the functioning of the robot, there is the prospect of significantly decreasing errors due to team interaction. An added benefit is that the nurses can be freed up to perform more important tasks, commensurate with their many years of educational training. The resulting reduction in personnel costs for the operating room could be substantial.

What will it take to achieve a higher integration of robotic systems? This currently exists with the Zeus system (Computer Motion, Inc., Santa Barbara, CA), which already has the integration of the Hermes (Computer Motion Inc., Santa Barbara, CA), voice-activated controller for the ancillary laparoscopic equipment and other operating room functions. In addition, Socrates (Computer Motion Inc., Santa Barbara, CA) is a video-conferencing system that is incorporated for mentoring and teletraining (Figs 7 and 8). In a similar fashion, OR-1 (Karl Storz Endoscopy, Los Angeles, CA) provides the same integrative functionality. Thus the infrastructure for total integration of systems is in place, and research is ongoing to integrate other components, as indicated above. With robotic systems evolving to having multiple arms that the primary surgeon can control (instead of requiring an assistant), there is high likelihood that within the next 5–10 years we will see systems integrated to a point where the surgeon can perform the entire procedure solo. Should tool changers and inventory dispensers be incorporated, perhaps the surgeon and one supervising nurse will be adequate for an entire surgical procedure.

There are additional advantages to the robotic systems once they are integrated. Today, nurses and physicians spend significant time in documentation—billing, coding, restocking the operating room, and reordering supplies. Not uncommonly there will be a miscommunication, resulting in incorrect billing or coding, or the operating room may not be restocked, etc. But the robot is an information system. Thus, for example, as the robotic system uses a new instrument from the tool changer or supply from the parts dispenser, the system can automatically bill the patient, send an order for the operating room to be restocked, and order a replacement from the inventory and supply office. All this is done autonomously, accurately, and instantaneously because the robot is integrated into the enterprisewide hospital information system. Some of the current major

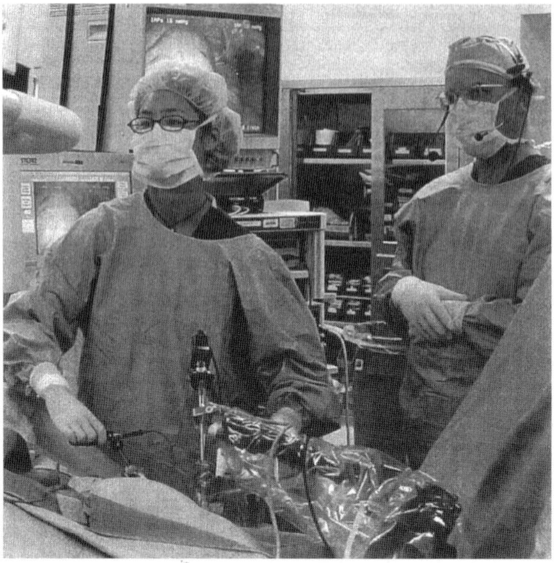

Figure 7 Preceptor supervising a novice laparoscopic surgeon. The preceptor controls the movements of AESOP through voice commands. This forces the novice surgeon to focus on the anatomical structures deemed important by the preceptor. This system permits the preceptor to safely direct the conduct of the operation.

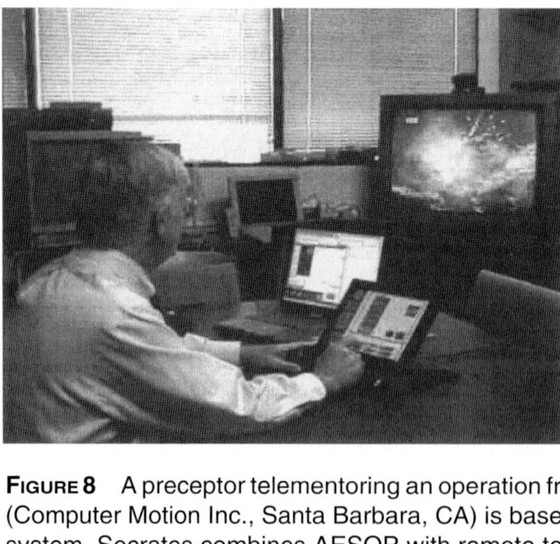

Figure 8 A preceptor telementoring an operation from a remote location. Socrates (Computer Motion Inc., Santa Barbara, CA) is based on this AESOP voice-control system. Socrates combines AESOP with remote telecasting systems and permits the preceptor to sit at a remote location and still direct the operation through voice commands that control the movement of the video telescope.

disadvantages of the robotic systems are that they are not integrated into the hospital system; thus they neither benefit from the other information systems nor enhance the efficiency of the entire hospital enterprise. Surgeons consider only the system's value as a mechanical device and ignoring its importance as an information system, thus not taking advantage of the robotic system's ability to enhance the entire spectrum of a surgical procedure (integration into all aspects of the operating room) and surgical practice (integration hospitalwide).

The above possibilities are based on the observation of standard practices in non–health care industries. While in concept such integration can be accomplished for operating rooms and hospitals, it must be stringently evaluated, especially for patient safety factors, before they are implemented. Yet the potential value of advanced robotic systems for efficiency, cost-effectiveness, and patient safety could be substantial.

REFERENCES

1. Paul H, Bargar WL, Mittestadt B, et al. Development of a surgical robot for cementless total hip arthroplasty. Clin Orthop 1992; 285:57–66.
2. Taylor RH, Joskowicz L, Williamson B, et al. Computer-integrated revision total hip replacement surgery: concept and preliminary results. Med Image Anal 1999; 3:301–319.
3. Jensen JF, Hill JW. Advanced telepresence surgery system development. Stud Health Technol Inform 1996; 29:107–117.
4. Moran ME. Stationary and automated laparoscopically assisted technologies. J Laparoendoscopic Surg 1993; 3:221–227.
5. Arezzo A, Ulmer F, Weiss O, Schurr MO, Hamad M, Buess GF. Experimental trial on solo surgery for minimally invasive therapy: Comparison of different systems in a phantom model. Surg Endosc 2000; 14:955–959.
6. Yavuz Y, Ystgaard B, Skogvoll E, Marvik R. A comparative study evaluating the performance of surgical robots AESOP and Endosista. Surg Laparosc Endosc Percut Tech 2000; 10:163–167.
7. Arezzo A, Testa T, Ulmer F, Schurr MO, Degregori M, Buess GF. Positioning systems for endoscopic solo surgery. Minerva Chir 2000; 55:635–641.
8. Gagner M, Bein E, Hurteau R, Pomp A. Robotic interactive laparoscopic cholecystectomy (letter). Lancet 1994; 343:596–597.
9. Begin E, Gagner M, Hurteau R, de Santis S, Pomp A. A robotic camera for laparoscopic surgery: Conception and experimental results. Surg Laparosc Endosc 1995; 5:6–11.
10. Ballantyne GH. Robotic surgery, telerobotic surgery, telepresence, and telementoring: Review of early clinical results. Surg Endosc 2002; 16:1389–1402.
11. Sackier JM, Wang Y. Robotically assisted laparoscopic surgery. From concept to development. Surg Endosc 1994; 8:63–66.
12. Jacobs LK, Shayani V, Sackier JM. Determination of the learning curve of the AESOP robot. Surg Endosc 1997; 11:54–55.

13. Johanet H. Voice-controlled robot: A new surgical aide? Thoughts of a user. Ann Chir 1998; 52:918–921.
14. Allaf ME, Jackman SV, Schulam PG, Cadeddu JA, Lee BR, Moore RG, Kavoussi LR. Laparoscopic visual field. Voice vs foot pedal interfaces for control of the AESOP robot. Surg Endosc 1998; 12:1415–1418.
15. Geis WP, Kim HC, Brennan EJ, McAfee PC, Wang Y. Robotic arm enhancement to accommodate improved efficiency and decreased resource utilization in complex minimally invasive surgery procedures. Stud Health Technol Inform 1996; 29: 471–481.
16. Satava RM, Jones SB. Preparing surgeons for the 21st Century. Surg Clin North Am 2000; 80:1353–1365.
17. Green PE, Piantanida TA, Hill JW, Simon IB, Satava RM. Telepresence: Dexterous procedures in a virtual operating field (abstr). Am Surg 1991; 57:192.
18. Marescaux J, Leroy J, Gagner M, Rubino F, Mutter D, Vix M, Butner SE, Smith MK. Transatlantic robot-assisted telesurgery. Nature 2001; 413:379–380.
19. Larkin M. Transatlantic, robot-assisted telesurgery deemed a success. Lancet 2001; 358:1074.
20. Marescaux J, Leroy J, Gagner M, Rubino F, Mutter D, Vix M, Butner SE, Smith MK. Transatlantic robot-assisted telesurgery. Nature 2001; 413:379–380.
21. Himpens J, Leman G, Cadiere GB. Telesurgical laparoscopic cholecystectomy (letter). Surg Endosc 1998; 12:1091.
22. Margossian H, Garcia-Ruiz A, Falcone T, Goldberg JM, Attaran M, Gagner M. Robotically assisted laparoscopic microsurgical uterine horn anastomosis. Fertil Steril 1998; 70:530–534.
23. Garcia-Ruiz A, Gagner M, Miller JH, Steiner CP, Hahn JF. Manual vs robotically assisted laparoscopic surgery in the performance of basic manipulation and suturing tasks. Arch Surg 1998; 133:957–961.
24. Nio D, Bemelman A, Kuenzler R, den Boer K, Gouma DJ, van Gulik TM. Efficiency of manual versus robotic (Zeus) assisted laparoscopic surgery in the performance of standardized task: A randomized trial (abstr). Surg Endosc 2001; 15:S-150.
25. Sweeney T, Rattner D. The Zeus system improves performance of complex laparoscopic skills irrespective of prior training (abstr). Surg Endosc 2001; 15:S-164.
26. http://www.abb.com/robots.
27. OSHA Technical Manual. Section 1: Safety Hazards, Chapter 4: Industrial Robots and Robot System Safety. http://www.osha-slc.gov/dts/osta/otm/otm_extended_toc.html.
28. The updated ANSI/RIA (American National Standards Institute/Robotics Industries Association) specificationS (June 21, 1999) for industrial Robots and Robot Systems—Safety Requirements. http://www.automatedconcepts.com/osha_req.htm.
29. Partin AW, Adams JB, Moore RG, Kavoussi LR. Complete robot-assisted laparoscopic urologic surgery: A preliminary report. J Am Coll Surg 1995; 181:552–557.
30. Mettler L, Ibrahim M, Jonat W. One year of experience working with the aid of a robotic assistant (the voice-controlled optic holder AESOP) in gynaecological endoscopic surgery. Hum Reprod 1998; 13:2748–2750.
31. Hubens G, Ysebaert D, Vaneerdewerg W, Chapelle T, Eyskens E. Laparoscopic adrenalectomy with the aid of the AESOP 2000 robot. Acta Chir Belg 1999; 99: 125–127.

32. Piazza L, Caragliano P, Scardilli M, Sgroi AV, Marino G, Giannone G. Laparoscopic robot-assisted adrenalectomy and left ovariectomy (case reports). Chir Ital 1999; 51: 456–466.
33. Trivedi A, Ballantyne GH. Laparoscopic hernia repair. In LeBlanc KA, ed. Laparoscopic Hernia Repair: An Operative Guide, Arnold Publishers, London, 0, 2003.
34. Ballantyne GH, Merola P, Weber A, Wasielewski A. Robotic solutions to the pitfalls of laparoscopic colectomy. Ospedali d'Italia Chirurgia 2001; 7:405–412.
35. Ballantyne GH, Kelley W. Granting clinical privileges for telerobotic surgery. Surg Laparosc, Endosc Percut Tech 2002; 12:17–25.
36. SAGES Guidelines. Guidelines for granting of privileges for laparoscopic (peritoneoscopic) general surgery. Surg Endosc 1993; 7:67–68.
37. SAGES Guidelines. Guidelines for granting of privileges for laparoscopic and/or thoracoscopic general surgery. Surg Endosc 1998; 12:379–380.

23

Small Intestine

Miguel Angel Carbajo Caballero, Juan Carlos Martín del Olmo, and Miguel Toledano Trincado
Medina del Campo Hospital, Valladolid, Spain

INTRODUCTION

To date, primary small intestinal laparoscopic surgery has been uncommon and the references in the literature are frequently limited to case reports regarding specific small bowel pathology. Few laparoscopic surgical texts or monographs adequately delineate specific small bowel pathology and the appropriate laparoscopic treatment modalities. These subjects are usually included in the discussion of the large intestine or within the chapters dedicated to emergent laparoscopic procedures. Consequently, there is little available information that has been derived from systematic studies regarding the complications from primary small bowel procedures.

There have multiple reports about the small bowel complications associated with the laparoscopic approach as it relates to trocar insertion, electrosurgical dissection, or of the use of all types of dissection or grasping instruments. It can be said, however, that the number and proportion of such complications seems to be low despite the rapid growth of laparoscopic procedures. The exact incidence of these complications is unknown because of the lack of dedicated studies. However, the analysis of such complications as well as their prevention, diagnosis, and treatment are of paramount importance. The immediate consequences can take the patient to a critical situation, making emergency intervention necessary.

Additionally, there is the real threat of the development of intra-abdominal sepsis and the possibility of a fatal outcome.

Although the true cost of small bowel complications is unknown, they are an important factor in morbidity and mortality associated with any type of laparoscopic procedure. Probably the specific characteristics of the small bowel—its topographic distribution, adhesive capacity, wide mobility, and easy volvulation or incarceration, as well as its weakness, in some circumstances—make surgeons reluctant to use the laparoscopic approach for small bowel pathology. On the other hand, it is necessary to appreciate the degree of difficulty in a complete exploration of the small intestine and understanding the findings and consequences derived from incorrect management, iatrogenic injury, or any postoperative complications.

Small bowel laparoscopic surgery, although delayed in relation to other procedures, has gained popularity in the therapeutic field of minimally invasive surgery because of the improvement of technology and the increased operative experience acquired over the last few years. Nevertheless, good laparoscopic training and an adequate knowledge of the technical resources continue to be necessary for a correct approach to the small intestine.

OBSTRUCTION

Postoperative small bowel obstruction, usually caused by visceral or parietal adhesions, has traditionally been treated by conventional open methods. The laparoscopic approach still generates much skepticism among many surgeons. Nevertheless, in our experience as well as in recent publications [1–3], laparoscopic adhesiolyis seems to be not only easier and safer but also associated with a lower incidence of intraoperative complications and a more comfortable postoperative outcome than open procedures. Additionally, the laparoscopic route diminishes the probability of new intra-abdominal adhesions because there is less manipulation of the small bowel as well as fewer resulting foreign-body reactions.

We have had the opportunity to observe a considerable number of patients with incisional hernias in whom chronic abdominal pain and repeated obstructive symptoms were frequently present. Following laparoscopic adhesiolysis and hernia repair, they have remained asymptomatic after more than 5 years [4]. In fact, obstructive problems are seldom seen after most laparoscopic procedures [5]. The more frequent and serious presentations of laparoscopic postoperative obstruction are due to small bowel herniation through an abdominal wall trocar port [5], fundoplication [6,7], postoperative small bowel volvulus [8], or the more serious mesenteric herniation and strangulation following a laparoscopic gastric bypass. There is an incidence of approximately 5% following the Roux-en-Y procedures [9], which presents as a blind-loop syndrome. These are emergency situations that require immediate intervention.

Identification of Complications

Acute obstruction of the small bowel after laparoscopic surgery usually presents as a clear clinical picture, making it relatively easy to make arrive at the correct diagnosis. Obviously the quick postoperative recovery that usually takes place in laparoscopic patients makes any problem more evident in that the usual postoperative course is significantly altered. Therefore any patient who experiences crampy abdominal pain, nausea, emesis, and the absence of intestinal transit should immediately raise suspicion of an intestinal complication or obstruction.

Usually a supine plain abdominal roentgenogram can achieve the diagnosis, although more complex studies could be necessary. Particularly evident is the small bowel incarceration through mesenteric defects created in the gastric bypass and Roux-en-Y procedures. The early appearance of a blind-loop syndrome, with a dilated gastric pouch (Fig. 1) and severe pain, presents the most characteristic symptoms. These are sometimes associated with nausea, emesis, and, more infrequently, diarrhea. Intervention must take place emergently. It is better to try a new laparoscopic procedure in those patients with an early diagnosis and without severe compromise of the incarcerated bowel. If the mechanical problem persists for more than 48 hr, it can trigger leakage of the gastric pouch, associated, peritonitis, and a fatal result.

The diagnosis of occlusive problems caused by the adhesions of previous surgery is more difficult. The routine therapeutic tools can be ineffective; sometimes only the presence of chronic abdominal pain or an abdominal wall hernia will determine the necessity of a laparoscopic exploration of the abdominal cavity. This procedure can be both diagnostic and therapeutic in most cases.

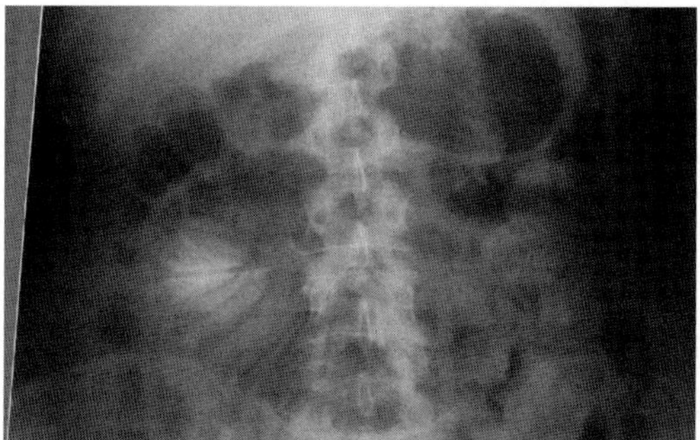

Figure 1 Dilated gastric pouch in blind-loop syndrome after gastric bypass.

Preoperative Evaluation and Prevention of Small bowel Complications

At the moment, there is no specific preoperative tool that allows us to evaluate the patient for the purpose of avoidance of a postoperative small bowel obstruction. However, some considerations should be kept in mind. In thin patients, intestinal occlusion secondary to herniation through a trocar orifice can occur relatively easily. If the trocar is introduced through the weakest areas of the abdominal wall and the patient produces an excessive amount of intra-abdominal pressure, the risk of trocar herniation increases proportionally to the size of stab wound.

In patients with an incisional hernia repair (especially if it has been repaired with mesh that was placed via an open laparotomy) or those with multiple prior abdominal surgeries, the development of a severe adhesive obstruction can be a significant problem. Another issue that should be identified during the evaluation of the patient is whether there has been any previous radiotherapy to the abdomen. In these patients, the possibility of radiation enteritis as the cause of an occlusive picture is significant. In those cases, laparoscopic surgery is extremely difficult due to the especially complex adhesiolysis that is necessitated by the severe fibrosis and inflammatory reaction that follows irradiation of the bowel (Fig. 2).

Intraoperative Measures to Prevent Obstructive Problems

The best prevention of small bowel incarceration and secondary obstruction is the elimination of any parietal or mesenteric defects that could be transformed into the site of a herniation. Therefore it is advisable that the larger trocar orifices and mesenteric or omental defects be closed. Another method of prevention is the avoidance of the passage of the small intestine through any mesenteric or omental defects unless necessary. In some cases this may require modification

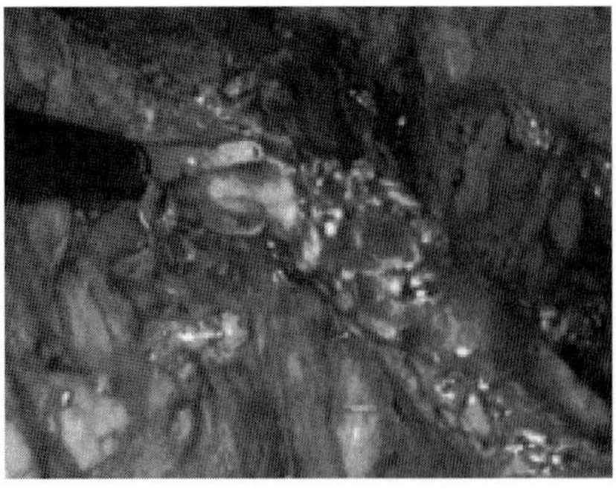

FIGURE 2 Severe adhesive process in the setting of radiation enteritis.

of the surgical strategy and the utilization of alternative intestinal routes, such as antecolic or antegastric procedures for gastrointestinal anastomosis. This technique has been employed by others and ourselves in the laparoscopic surgery for morbid obesity [10,11]. For the enteroenterostomy anastomosis, the correct position of the intestinal limbs is of paramount importance to prevent rotation and volvulus and a resulting obstruction. Proper placement and identification of each limb of the intestine will avoid this type of complication.

The laparoscopic handling of the small bowel must be with atraumatic grasping instruments that allow the manipulation and release of the soft adhesions (Fig. 3). It is important to avoid excessive traction and unnecessary tension on the bowel wall, which can produce serosal injuries that can be the source of future adhesions. This is especially important in the setting of a distended or edematous wall of the small intestine. While it is important to maintain hemostasis, electrosurgical diathermy is not advisable during the dissection of the adherent intestinal loops or in any acute inflammatory process. In these situations, the better option is the use of ultrasonic energy, as this disperses less energy and heat than electrocautery. However, caution is advised if this device is used near the small bowel wall, as this, too, can perforate the intestine if used incorrectly.

Meticulous lavage of the peritoneal cavity is prudent at the completion of the procedure. Some surgeons will finalize the procedure with the instillation of hyaluronic acid solution (Intergel, Ethicon, Somerville, NJ) into the abdominal cavity in an effort to prevent new adhesions [1,12].

The indiscriminate use of intra-abdominal drains that are in direct contact with intestinal loops is not advisable, especially in the inframesocolic space, where the risk of intestinal obstruction is greater than in the supramesocolic one. If determined to be necessary, the drains should be removed as soon as possible in order to prevent undesirable additional septic complications.

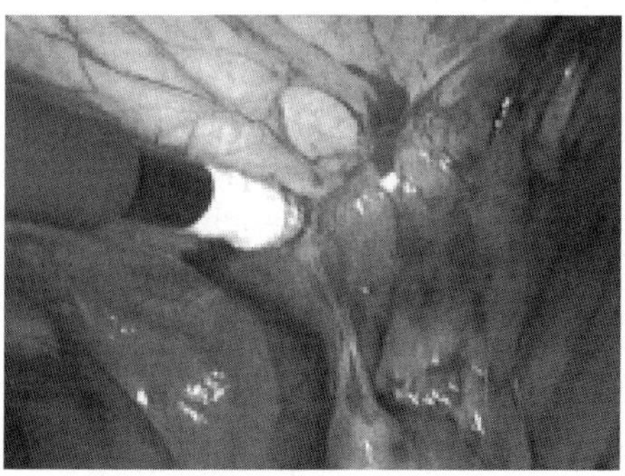

FIGURE 3 Release of adhesions with atraumatic dissection.

Postoperative Measures to Prevent Obstructive Small Bowel Problems

Unfortunately, there are no measures that let us prevent postoperative small bowel obstruction, especially following laparoscopic surgery. The minimally invasive procedure frequently does not require the use of nasogastric suction because the ability to institute early mobilization allows an earlier return to oral intake. Because the procedures result in a shortened hospital stay, any obstructive problem that may occur will do so in an outpatient situation. In this scenario, the patient may present with advanced obstruction and with an emergency situation.

Only in some procedures, such as those that involve a gastroenteric anastomosis, which require radiologic studies prior to the resumption of oral feeding, can the surgeon be alerted to the presence of an early intestinal obstruction. However, these findings are frequently nonspecific at that early postoperative period. It is evident that with a suspicious x-ray study or clinical data of small bowel obstruction, the standard medical treatment with nasogastric suction, electrolyte replacement, and sometimes total parenteral nutrition must be established. Nevertheless, in our experience, immediate postoperative laparoscopic exploration and a definitive solution of the problem is the best strategy.

Clinical Data and Workup in Suspected Small Bowel Obstruction

An understanding of the symptoms and physical findings in patients with postoperative small bowel obstruction is critical for making management decisions. The main feature of the acute obstructive picture is that of abdominal pain. The patient with an acute intestinal obstruction presents with intense crampy pain, sometimes referred to the back, and associated to nausea, emesis, opstipation, and abdominal distention. Initially, the patient can be stable, without fever, abnormal laboratory data, or cardio-respiratory compromise. Oliguria can be an early sign and is due to the third-spacing of fluids.

The typical radiological pattern of distended small bowel with air-fluid level interfaces always accompanies the clinical picture early in the clinical course. A computed tomography (CT) scan may be helpful in patients with indeterminate findings, and it can also identify the presence of intra-abdominal fluid collections. In advanced cases, the abdominal signs will be more evident and associated with general malaise, with respiratory and cardiovascular impairment, oliguria, fever, and leukocytosis. This represents a stage of severe metabolic compromise that mandates urgent surgical measures to prevent complications of the obstructive process, such as ischemic changes, intestinal perforation, peritonitis, and generalized sepsis.

With clinical suspicion or evidence of an acute postoperative obstruction, the patient should be treated with immediate digestive rest, nasogastric suction, correction of intravascular volume, and appropriate radiological studies. If clinical and radiological signs persist, early laparoscopic exploration is the best way of managing this problem. This approach will identify and solve the problem without excessive delay. Any delay can be associated with increased risk of complications. In the setting of a chronic obstructive picture, it may be judicious to begin with conservative medical treatment, combined with repeated abdominal radiological evaluations to access the evolution of the process. Such a strategy may make more aggressive and urgent measures unnecessary, thereby allowing the patient undergo a definitive elective operation.

Specific Management of Small Bowel Obstruction

There is a significant amount of published literature regarding the laparoscopic treatment of intermittent or chronic intestinal obstruction. Comparative studies have shown the effectiveness and advantages of the laparoscopic approach for this entity [3,13–17]. Based on our experience in the management of a long series of patients, we concur with these observations [4]. We have found that the procedure is associated with few conversions to laparotomy and with low morbidity, despite the fact that some of these cases are very complex.

In these patients, the first operative decision is determination of the most appropriate site of puncture of the abdomen to create the initial pneumoperitoneum. We prefer to place the Verress needle in the left subcostal space in the anterior axillary line because iatrogenic injury of any abdominal contents is thus less probable. The pneumoperitoneum must be established with a pressure of at least 14 mmHg. This maneuver makes it easier to identify any intestinal loops that may be adherent to abdominal wall (Fig. 4). The port site for the laparoscope is inserted in the same place used for the Verress needle. It is then necessary to make a careful exploration of the entire abdominal cavity to evaluate the degree of adhesions, the type of intestinal occlusion, and the free areas of the abdomen for the placement of additional trocars under direct vision.

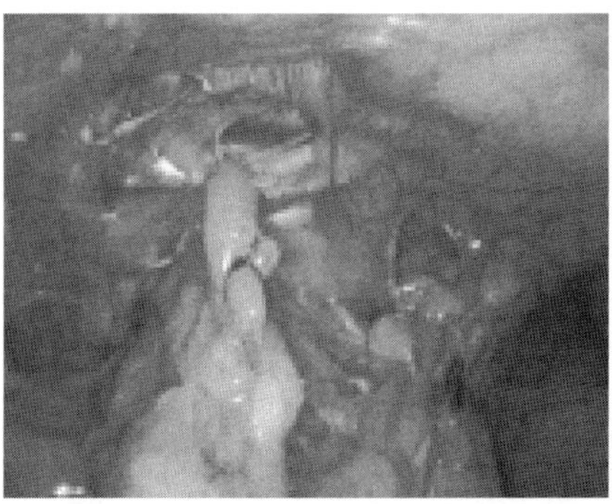

FIGURE 4 Firm small bowel adhesions to the abdominal wall.

Generally, two 5-mm trocars located on the left flank are sufficient to perform the parietal and visceral adhesiolysis and to handle the intestinal contents with comfort. When the main adhesive problem is situated in the left flank, we place the trocar on the right side. An ultrasonic scalpel can be used to lyse fatty and vascularized adhesions, but we avoid the use of any kind of surgical energy for visceral adhesions. This concept is very important for the prevention of unsuspected burns that can develop into either acute peritonitis or a late postoperative fistula. Sharp dissection with scissors and nontraumatic traction are the primary techniques to identify the dissection plane and release the incarcerated or twisted loops (Fig. 5). The avoidance of any traction on the small bowel wall is essential, because any type of laparoscopic clamp can lead to a visceral perforation. It is necessary to handle the abdominal contents delicately, with indirect traction, while looking for an adequate plane of dissection.

In difficult cases, it is better to avoid serosal tears by changing the dissection plane at the abdominal wall. In these situations, a peritoneal ''patch'' will remain on the intestinal surface, rather than an injury to the intestinal serosa (Fig. 6). Because we usually work with a dilated or inflamed small bowel wall, it is important to inspect the intestinal serosa prior to finishing the procedure. All denuded intestinal surfaces must be checked carefully and any seromuscular tears repaired.

Occasionally one will note that the serosal layers of the small intestinal wall are fused, which makes identification of the anatomical planes quite difficult. Excessive bleeding during dissection of these sites usually implies that we are not within the proper anatomic dissection plane. If the mesenteric border is firmly attached to the abdominal wall or to a scar, it is better avoid its mobilization, since the potential for vascular injury is very high, and this can lead to necrosis in the immediate postoperative period. In high midline processes, it is necessary to locate the transverse colon to prevent unintentional injury.

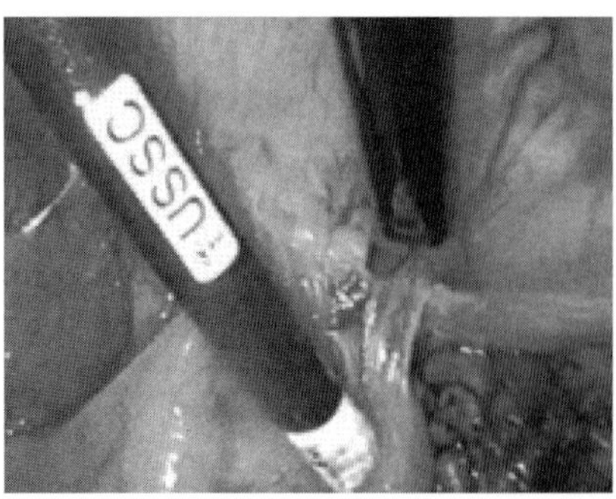

Figure 5 Sharp dissections by means of scissors and blunt dissection.

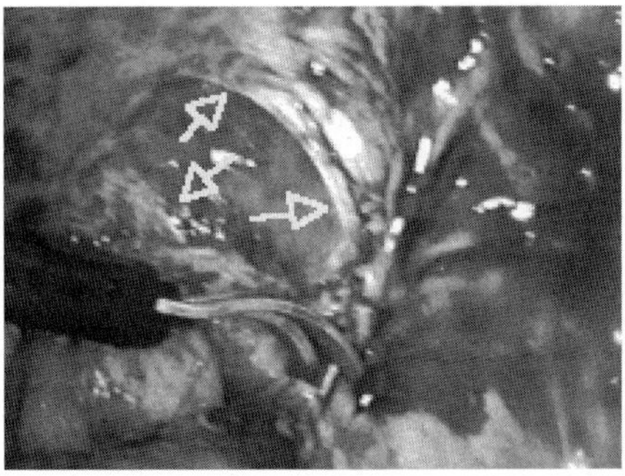

Figure 6 Peritoneal patch on the small bowel wall.

There are abdominal areas that present difficult access sites for a full evaluation and surgical dissection, such as inside the low pelvis, as well as the high midline, subxiphoid, and left subcostal regions. In these instances it may be necessary to add a supplementary trocar or change the laparoscopic access so that a complete and accurate visualization is had before beginning the dissection.

If, during adhesiolysis, a wide enterotomy is produced, the repair should be approached once the affected loop is completely released of its attachments and adhesions. Once it is mobilized, one can then evaluate the severity of the injury. If feasible, one may perform a laparoscopic enterorrhaphy. Only a severe enterotomy with vascular compromise necessitates a bowel resection. One may need to convert to the open procedure, but an alternative can be to enlarge one trocar port site (3–4 cm) and perform the repair at this incision once the small bowel has been exteriorized.

Laparoscopic management of the acute postoperative occlusion is less complex, since we are usually aware of the site of the obstruction. The exceptions are those cases involving early adhesions or severe volvulus. If the occlusive picture is very immediate, we can gain access through the same ports used for the primary procedure and look for the source of the problem based on the previous surgery. The recommendations regarding intestinal handling are the same as in the previous description and abundant lavage is equally necessary.

If one is faced with an intra-abdominal hernia or a transmesenteric or transmesocolic herniation with severe intestinal dilatation and an ischemic intestinal wall, conversion to open surgery is preferred to prevent the inadvertent perforation of the intestine with any clamp or maneuver. If there is a postbypass blind-loop problem, the remnant stomach must be drained by the placement of a gastrostomy tube for several days.

In general, small hernias at a trocar port or limited internal ones can be treated laparoscopically without difficulty, as can any adhesions showing no signs of necrosis. However, any anastomotic axial rotations, significant volvulus, or obstructive cases that include a segment of large intestine generally require conversion to open surgery and the usual postoperative resuscitative treatment.

RESECTION

Laparoscopic resective surgery of the small bowel is infrequently performed. The reasons are the low incidence of primary small bowel pathology and technical considerations, such as those previously mentioned (e.g., difficult laparoscopic handling and the need for laparoscopic suturing skills). Relatively simple techniques, such as resection of Meckel's diverticulum have been described for diverticular complications like diverticulitis or obstruction, but the incidence of all these combined is only 4% [17,18]. The presence of a carcinoid tumor in a diverticulum is very rare, requiring a later extended resection [18]. In our experience, the fortuitous finding of a Meckel's diverticulum during laparoscopic appendectomy or other surgical procedures does not present any problems for its laparoscopic resection. Primary small bowel malignances are rare conditions, and there are no data about their laparoscopic treatment except for rare case reports [19].

The chronic small bowel inflammatory pathology of terminal ileal disease or refractory Crohn's disease is more frequently seen. Randomized studies about the surgical treatment of ileocolic Crohn's disease have shown a decreased incidence of complications and shorter hospital stays in patients treated laparoscopically route compared to those treated with conventional open surgery [20]. Nevertheless, collective data on laparoscopic small bowel resection in inflammatory disease are scarce owing to the difficulties in evaluating the degree of small bowel involvement. The emergent laparoscopic management of various small bowel problems including perforations, parasites, or mesenteric ischemia, etc.—has not been validated or standardized at the present time.

Identification of Complications

The most serious complication after any intestinal resection is anastomotic dehiscence with or without the development of a postoperative fistula. The former problem can progress to an acute abdominal emergency that requires immediate surgery. Localization of a small bowel fistula can be more difficult. If the abdominal cavity has not been drained, the first evidence of this complication can be the development of a suppurative discharge from one of the trocar orifices or an intense inflammatory process at that site. If it is a consequence of a gastrojejunal anastomosis, it can easily be identified radiologically by (via an upper GI series and CT scan), as noted in several series on laparoscopic obesity surgery [21]. Unfortunately, we cannot evaluate other portions of the intestinal tract with the same studies as consistently and must be guided by indirect clinical, radiological, or other analytical data.

Luminal bleeding and anastomotic strictures are other potential complications after intestinal resection, especially when mechanical staples are used. This problem has been detected in large series of jejunojejunal anastomoses when a Roux-en-Y is performed [22]. Intestinal bleeding after stapler techniques can be especially important, because this can lead to a serious hypovolemic state requiring blood transfusion or reoperation. Food impaction at the site of an anastomotic stricture has been described but is a rare complication [23]. More frequent problems are anastomotic rotation or volvulation (see above). Anastomotic dehiscence caused by ischemia and necrosis can occur more frequently in patients with previous mesenteric ischemia. While this has been seen in open procedures, there are no reports of this complication in laparoscopic surgery.

Preoperative Evaluation and Preventive Measures of Complications

There are no specific preoperative measures for the prevention of postoperative complications after laparoscopic small bowel resection except for adequate surgical preparation: optima nutritional state, absence of immunosuppression, and absence of an acute inflammatory process or sepsis. Obviously, these cannot be prevented in emergency situations but must be evaluated carefully because the high incidence of fatal complications in these patients.

Intraoperative Measures to Prevent Resection Complications

A vigilant laparoscopic exploration of the gastrointestinal tract is necessary to adequately determine the need and length of intestinal resection, the degree of inflammation or fibrosis, and the vascular supply so that an adequate anastomosis can be performed. Once the necessity of resection is confirmed, it is very important to determine the length of the affected segment, since the laparoscopic handling of large segments of small bowel is difficult. Where there is doubt, the use of a minilaparotomy will assist the procedure and can solve this problem. In general, the use of the 2.5-mm endostapler provides great anastomotic and hemostatic security during small bowel resection (Fig. 7). Division of the mesentery can also be achieved with this type of stapler or with a specific laparoscopic vascular sealant (Ligasure-United States Surgical Corp/Tyco International, Norwalk, CT).

Extraction of the surgical specimen requires enlargement of some of the 12-mm ports. In those situations where the security of the anastomosis is uncertain, this incision can allow use of the open-assisted procedure to remove the excised tissues.

The execution of a laparoscopic jejunojejunal anastomosis requires experience and intracorporeal suturing skills. We advise that if there is any doubt about

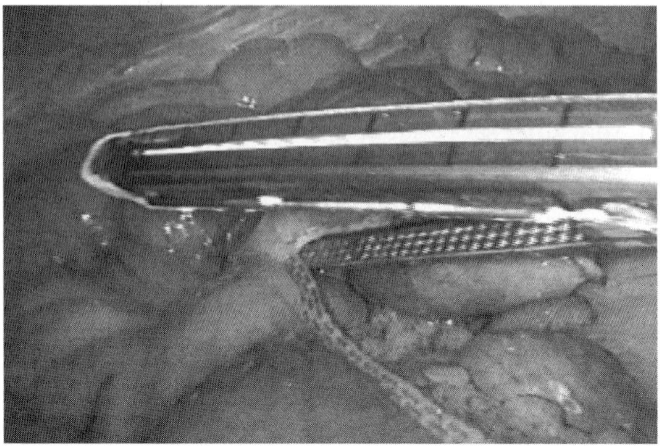

Figure 7 Small bowel transection with 2.5-mm endostapler.

the limb of the bowel, it should be marked. This will allow the surgeon to align the loops properly by avoiding any confusion of which limb is proximal and which distal, so that a blind-loop syndrome will not be created. Both limbs should be aligned in parallel, so that the endostapler can be placed gently and without tearing them (Fig. 8). As previously mentioned, it is important to use a 2.5-mm device to avoid undesirable hemorrhage at the anastomosis. One may inspect the anastomosis by lavage to identify any bleeding points at the staple line.

The anterior line of the anastomosis must be carefully sutured using absorbable material, with special attention to the corners. Mesenteric closure should

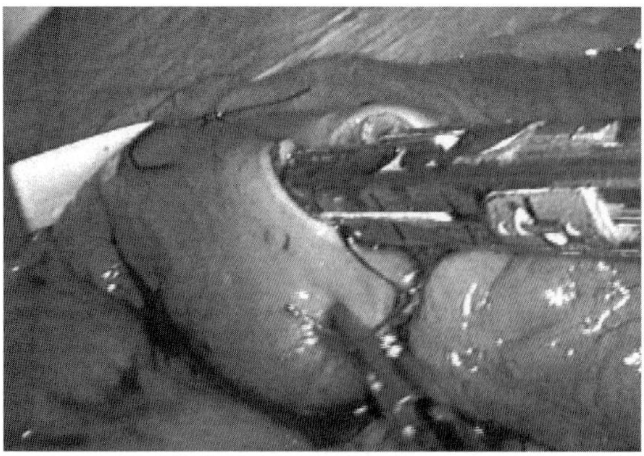

Figure 8 Jejunojejunal anastomosis with endostapler.

also not be forgotten. If we opt to carry out a laparoscopic hand-sewn anastomosis without endostaplers, the complications derived from those staplers are relatively rare [24]; however; the complexity is increased and specific training is necessary. In emergency situations or in unusual cases with a high-risk anastomosis, an enterostomy can be done rather than a risky anastomosis. This maneuver can save the patient's life. It is easy to close this by the laparoscopic approach secondarily [23].

Clinical Data and Workup in Small Bowel Resection Complications

Limited anastomotic leakage or a small postoperative fistula can become sequestered by intestinal and omental adhesions, thereby preventing the development of any clinical evidence initially. As noted earlier, an intense inflammatory process or suppuration at the site of one of the trocar ports can be the first clinical manifestation of this complication, although this can be accompanied by systemic symptoms such as fever, tachycardia, elevated white blood cell count, and sometimes diarrhea. With a foregut fistula, a left pleural effusion or atelectasis are frequent features. Increasing intestinal tenderness—but without rebound tenderness or general malaise—may be seen. Sometimes constipation and anorexia are not present early but may become apparent when the complete clinical picture is evident. These clinical signs indicate that the postoperative course is abnormal and call for radiological studies as well as the appropriate medical treatment. Obviously, the more aggressive course seen with a high-output fistula or anastomotic dehiscence requires an emergent operation.

Serious intestinal bleeding from a midgut anastomosis can become manifest by the development of melena. However, similar hemorrhage by a foregut anastomosis may not be associated with melena but present with syncope secondary to hypovolemia as the initial indication of that complication. Close observation of the vital signs in the first 24 hr postoperatively and laboratory data, when necessary, can be the keys to the diagnosis in the absence of external signs.

Specific Management of Complications

Treatment of the complications derived from laparoscopic resection of the small bowel depends not only on the severity of the complication but also on the primary pathology and its effects on the patient's general condition.

If we have an early fistula that has drained spontaneously or through an abdominal drain without generalized peritonitis, we initiate absolute digestive rest and the maintenance of good drainage of the fistula, which sometimes can be achieved with a simple nontraumatic probe. Antibiotic therapy, thromboembolic prophylaxis, and other medical measures are necessary, as well as total parenteral nutrition (TPN) in most cases. If the fistula coexists with a defined intra-abdominal collection confirmed on ultrasound or CT scan, percutaneous guided drainage alone can solve the problem. Laparoscopic exploration is not indicated initially and conservative treatment with close follow-up is adequate treatment if no other generalized complications arise.

If the fistula originates from a gastrojejunal anastomosis and the radiological diagnosis has been established early, the usual measures of digestive rest and conventional therapy can lead to the resolution of the fistula in few days. The most serious problem arises when the fistula has not been diagnosed and the patient resumes oral intake; the immediate consequences can be magnification of the output fistula's partial or total necrosis of the anastomosis, and massive subphrenic or intraabominal abscesses, followed by sepsis and shock. An emergency reintervention with adequate drainage of the collections, the anastomotic area, and the abdominal cavity is necessary in an attempt to save the patient's life. It is inadequate to attempt a reconstruction of the anastomosis.

In high-output fistulas, derived from colojejunal or jejunojejunal anastomosis with intra-abdominal involvement and a septic condition, it is necessary to try to save the patient's life by means of an intestinal resection and peritoneal lavage. The possibility of performing a new anastomosis or an alternative procedure (enterostomy or colostomy) must be based on factors such as peritoneal sepsis, small bowel wall, inflammation of the and the location of that anastomosis within the gastrointestinal tract.

Intraluminal continuous and uncontrolled bleeding necessitates prompt postoperative laparoscopic exploration to evaluate the anastomosis. Another option is to perform this inspection with the assistance of a minilaparotomy. Postoperative intraperitoneal bleeding is an infrequent event if the mesenteric division is carried out cleanly. As remarked above, volvulus or anastomotic rotations can take place and are usually due to technical errors during the anastomotic construction. Once the problem is recognized, initial medical management, including TPN, can be the implemented. If the problem persists, it is best to respond early with surgical intervention. We advise beginning with a laparoscopic exploration to evaluate and treat the problem. However, reconstruction of the anastomosis by minilaparotomy is recommended if it becomes necessary.

ENTEROSTOMY

Laparoscopic iatrogenic small bowel injuries of variable degrees are complications that have been reported in different series [25–30]. The injury is usually caused by the trocar or Verress needle. Nevertheless, all the authors agree on the relatively low incidence of this problem in spite of the great number of laparoscopic procedures performed. The real incidence is unknown because of the lack of a registry to record them. It is surprising that—despite the hundreds of thousands of trocars and needles that have been introduced into the abdominal cavity since the introduction of laparoscopic cholecystectomy—the percentage of injuries to the small bowel is so low [30,31]. The most important study performed to

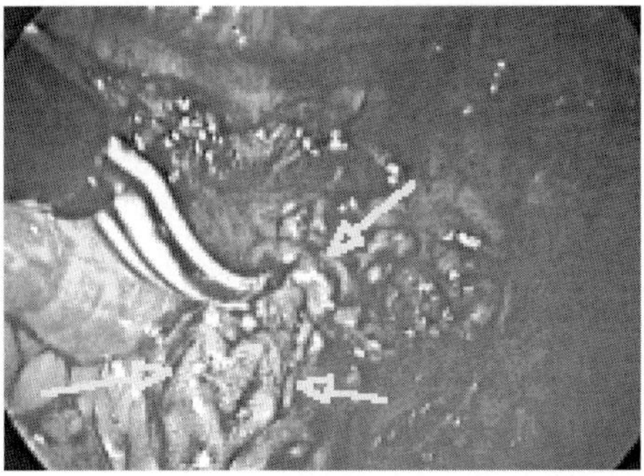

FIGURE 9 Small bowel injury in difficult adhesiolysis.

date, which analyzed over 14,243 laparoscopic procedures in Switzerland between 1995 and 1997, showed that 0.18% (22 cases) of injuries are produced by the insertion of either the trocar or the Veress needle. In these 22 cases, there were only six small bowel lesions [27].

More common are small bowel injuries produced in the course of a difficult adhesiolysis or with handling of the small bowel in patients with several previous open procedures (Fig. 9) [1,32,33]. Because there is no registry for such data, including thermal injury, we have no firm knowledge of the exact incidence of these complications [30,31]. In any case, inadvertent injuries of this kind can prove fatal if they go unrecognized. A higher mortality is associated with injuries affecting the duodenal segment [28,34].

Identification of Complications

The key to the identification of any complication is to acknowledge its existence and take whatever intraoperative steps are necessary to avoid its potential implications. If the intestinal lesion is unrecognized, the patient will experience an abnormal postoperative course rather than the usual recovery following laparoscopic surgery. If early peritoneal signs develop, they are associated with fever, tachycardia, opstipation, diarrhea, nausea, and emesis. Laboratory or radiological data are not always conclusive in establishing a diagnosis. If sufficient suspicion exists, an emergency laparoscopy is advisable. This can be both diagnostic and therapeutic and can save the patient's life.

If the intestinal injury is the result of vascular or thermal trauma or due to an ischemic process, the clinical signs of peritoneal inflammation become evident in the first 24–48 hr of the postoperative course. The injury can also become manifest by generalized sepsis. In such cases, immediate surgical exploration is necessary to avoid multiple organ system failure and septic shock.

During complex adhesiolysis, small serosal tears are commonplace and are usually not repaired. However, in the presence of an inflammatory component or a prosthetic biomaterial, a perforation can develop in the first few postoperative days or can later present as a cutaneous fistula or intestinal obstruction. If the immediate etiology is associated with a mesh product, a more complex surgical problem exists.

Preoperative Evaluation and Prevention Measures of Enterotomy Complications

The surgeon must understand that previous abdominal surgery (laparotomy rather than laparoscopic procedures), a history of intra-abdominal sepsis, inflammation, adhesions, or radiation injury will increase the risk of an iatrogenic enterotomy during the entry into the abdomen and during adhesiolysis. There are no rules for avoiding injuries in these cases, since open surgery too can result in these complications, sometimes with even greater frequency. One can never be free of this risk, even with the use of the Hasson entry for laparoscopy. Our advice is to carefully evaluate the type(s) of previous surgery and the existing incisions in choosing the point of the initial entry. Usually this will result in the creation of the pneumoperitoneum with a Veress needle in the left subcostal space, because this is the location that has the least likelihood of intestinal adhesions from prior surgeries. If this it not feasible, it is possible to start in the right subcostal area or at a site devoid of scars.

If we suspect a complex adhesive process—as is seen with large incisional hernias, prior hernia repairs with an intraperitional polypropylene mesh, chronic inflammatory bowel disease, or following abdominopelvic irradiation—we prepare the patient with preoperative intestinal cleansing for the purpose of diminishing contamination should an accidental enterotomy occur. For some incisional hernias it is helpful to evaluate the anterior abdominal wall with either CT or magnetic resonance imaging. Important information can be obtained which can identify the presence of intestinal herniation, the position of the large intestine, and the size and position of abdominal wall defects (Fig. 10). Antibiotic and thrombotic prophylaxis is essential when indicated.

Intraoperative Measures to Prevent Enterotomy Complications

Once the initial entry into the abdomen is performed, it is important to observe the progression and speed of the development of the pneumoperitoneum. Diffusion of the gas in a nonuniform manner or elevation of the required pressures during insufflation can indicate that the needle orifice is blocked by the omentum. However, this phenomenon can easily be caused by the penetration of the needle into an adhesive block, mesenteric fat, or a visceral organ. In these instances, it is advisable to change to a new insertion area. These sites should be inspected after the introduction of the laparoscope to assure that no injury has occurred.

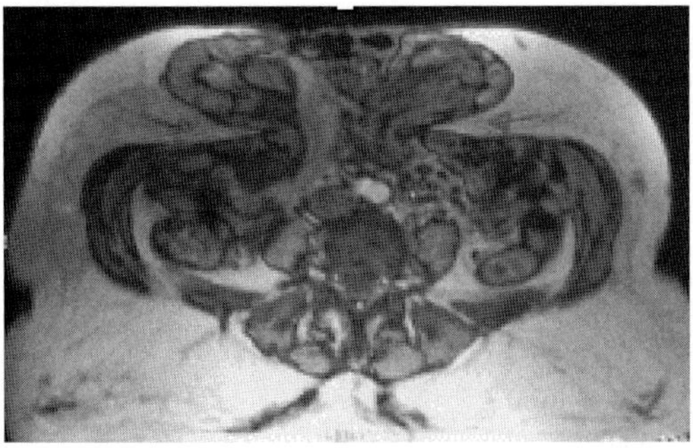

FIGURE 10 Preoperative MRI of incisional hernia.

If it is not possible to establish an adequate pneumoperitoneum, an option other than the Hasson trocar or direct-vision trocars is direct dissection at a site where adhesions are less likely. The camera is placed through a trocar to which the insufflator is connected. As the trocar is pushed forward through the peritoneal layer, the progressive increase of gas pressure will improve visual control of the abdominal cavity. Adhesions of previous surgery or other inflammatory processes must be carefully evaluated, as adhesiolysis may be required to allow the planned procedure to be completed as intended. The other trocars must be placed under direct vision, avoiding abrupt penetrations that can cause intra-abdominal injury. In the case of uncontrolled trocar placement, it is necessary to explore the port entry and the underlying intestine to detect any problem that may have been produced.

It is important to keep in mind that no laparoscopic device is not completely atraumatic. The surgeon must be careful to prevent iatrogenic injury during the use of these instruments. The use of smooth-tipped atraumatic graspers and the avoidance of unnecessary tissue traction will minimize this hazard. In general, if the pressure exercised by the grasper is excessive and associated with inadequate traction, a partial or complete tear of the intestinal serosal is possible (Fig. 11). A full-thickness injury is also possible. If it is necessary to lift the tissues significantly, we try to use countertraction with rubber material, such as might be used for an abdominal drain, without touching the intestinal wall with the forceps (Fig. 12).

During the procedure, it is important to carefully control any instrument connected to an energy source. If it is necessary to employ diathermy, we advise that the instrument be connected with a power source only when needed in order to avoid its accidental activation and unintended contact with any abdominal viscera. During diathermy utilization, it is also advisable to ensure that the entire length of the clamp or scissors does not cause capacitance coupling, which can result in a remote burn. Since the camera can be focused only at in the tip of the instrument, an undesirable burn of the abdominal contents can be caused by the

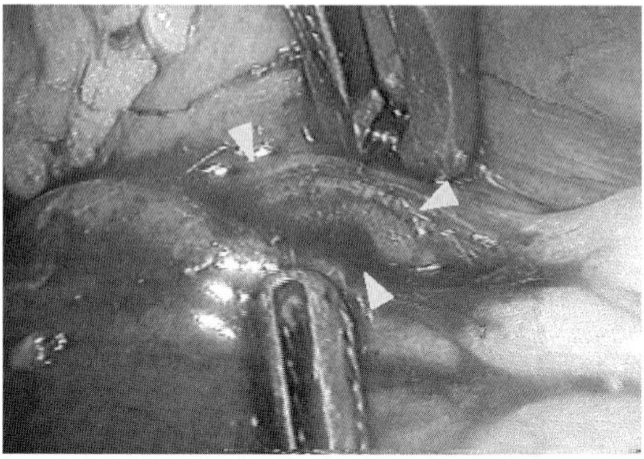

Figure 11 Serosal tear by excessive grasper traction.

metallic part of any instrument that may not be visualized by the camera. All insulated instruments should also be inspected preoperatively to ensure that the insulation is intact throughout the entire length of the instrument. Although the ultrasonic energy does not eliminate the risk of thermal injury, it does reduce this risk because no electrical grounding is necessary for this instrument.

During the use of an endostapler, it is necessary to control each entry of the device into the abdomen. The position of the intestine must be properly planned so that jaws of the instrument penetrate without traction, which could result in a perforation of the bowel wall at the tip of the jaws. Both portions of

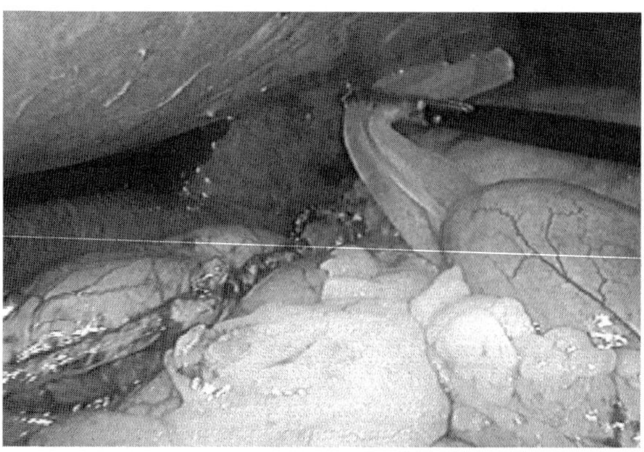

Figure 12 Atraumatic manipulation of the small bowel with a rubber drain.

the jaws must enter the intestine easily and gently so as to prevent an intestinal perforation, which would greatly complicate the completion of the anastomosis.

In performing small bowel surgery that includes parietal or visceral adhesiolysis, it is necessary to follow certain principles to prevent accidental injury in the presence of severe adhesions, obstruction, inflammation, or radiation enteritis. Fatty adhesions can be freed quickly and safely with an ultrasonic scalpel. In complicated cases, where the abdominal wall and the serosa of the intestine appear to the fused, it is easier to cause an accidental enterotomy. In such situations we recommend employing traction and countertraction with atraumatic graspers or a drain around the intestine and avoiding the use of electrosurgical energy for the lysis of the adhesions. Scissors are the best option to begin the surgical dissection (Fig. 13). The scissors must be used with the curve facing the abdominal wall. If necessary, it is better to excise a parietal peritoneal patch that remains on the bowel wall than to produce an enterotomy.

Minor bleeding during dissection is possible, but sudden and profuse bleeding demands an investigation for a possibly significant injury to the intestinal wall. If such an injury is confirmed, we recommend a complete evaluation before continuing the intestinal dissection, so that a small enterotomy is not transformed into a large intestinal opening. Repair of a small serosal tear, control of any bleeding, and a change of the dissection plane will avoid the the need to convert to an open procedure or prevent a difficult laparoscopic closure of the injury. If the small intestine is densely adherent to the abdominal wall, surgical dissection will be very difficult (Fig. 14). Particular attention must be paid to the vascularity of the small bowel, because severe fibrosis and lack of elasticity can eventuate in a vascular injury that will affect the viability of an intestinal loop. One must be certain that the vascular supply is sufficient to prevent ischemia and necrosis. Generally, viscerovisceral adhesions are simple to treat, but if they are firm or matted and there is no indication of stenosis, it is prudent not to attempt their

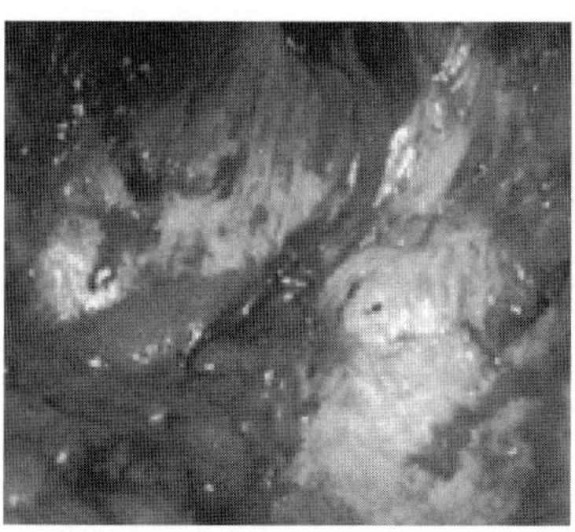

FIGURE 13 Ahesiolysis with Metzenbaum-type scissors.

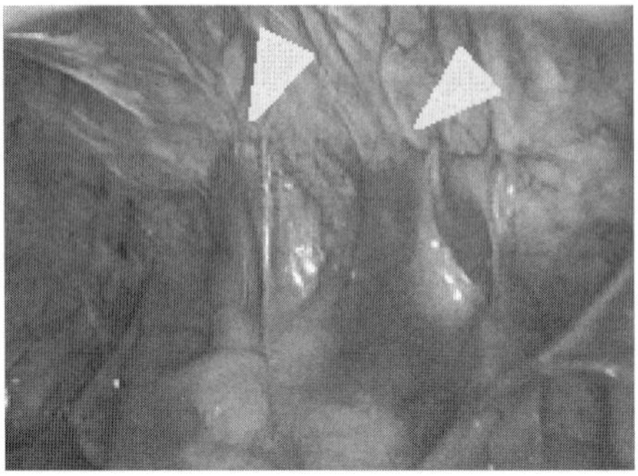

Figure 14 Small bowel completely fixed to the abdominal wall.

separation, since there may be no plane of dissection between the two walls (Fig. 15). This can easily result in an enterotomy.

Postoperative Measures to Prevent Enterotomy Complications

There are very few postoperative measures that can prevent these complications, since everything relative to the occurrence of an enterotomy as well as its identification and repair should occur during surgery. Serosal tears repaired during surgery may make it advisable to maintain postoperative digestive rest, based on the clinical course of the patient. Nasogastric decompression with intravenous therapy is usually effective in these cases. No type of prevention exists in the case of an inadvertent small bowel lesion, since the evolution of the patient's clinical picture will be that of an acute surgical abdomen.

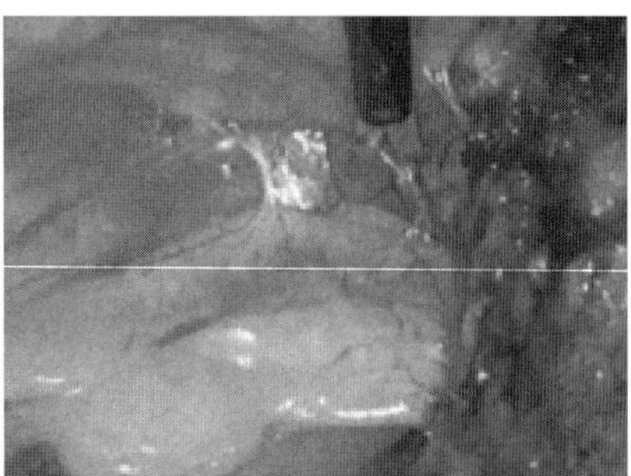

Figure 15 Soft adhesions between small bowel loops.

Clinical Data and Workup in Suspected Enterotomy Complications

There are two main clinical pictures of small bowel leakage resulting from an enterotomy. These depend upon the severity of the injury, the coexistence of an intestinal blockage, the presence or absence of an abdominal drain, the previous type(s) of surgery, and the individual factors of the patient. Less severe fistula formation appears as a small supurative process and follows leakage through an enterotomy repaired in suboptimal conditions or serosal tears that were not identified or incorrectly repaired. This usually becomes evident several days after surgery. These fistulas will frequently present by drainage through the nearest trocar site. They can become evident by the development of inflammation associated with cellulitis or by frank suppurative discharge. If a spontaneous opening does not develop, one should be created so as to allow for the needed drainage (Fig. 16).

The patient will present with fever, local and possibly abdominal pain, abdominal distention, opstipation, and general malaise. If this site becomes sealed by the peritoneal contents, the peritoneal symptoms could be hidden. In general, however, the patient remains stable. In these cases the initial treatment guidelines should include conservative measures comprising digestive rest, antibiotherapy, and TPN. Of course, radiological evaluation (plain radiographs and CT scanning) is mandatory to screen for the presence of significant intraperitoneal abscesses. In our experience with these measures, such fistulas will close in 1–2 weeks. If intestinal discharge persists despite these efforts, other etiologies such as volvulation, obstruction, or stenosis below the fistula level should be considered, because these factors can prevent spontaneous healing. One should also be aware that the use of an excessive TPN protocol can trigger bacterial translocation and potentially lead to sepsis and cardiovascular collapse. Should this occur, a surgical approach becomes necessary.

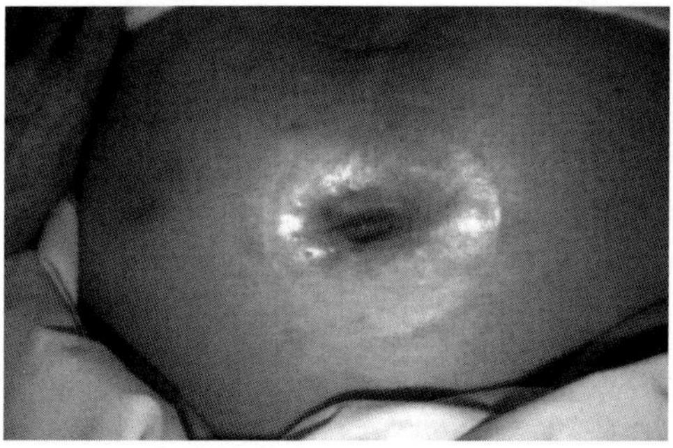

FIGURE 16 Enterocutaneous fistula after drainage of trocar scar abscess.

The other type of clinical presentation results from a large iatrogenic, unrecognized injury caused by a direct or indirect instrumental laceration, a thermal burn, or an ischemic insult. The consequences are usually immediate; however, a thermal or ischemic injury man present a few days later than a direct injury. At the onset of the loss of the integrity of the bowel lumen, the patient will present signs of peritoneal irritation, fever, opstipation, abdominal distention and possibly sepsis. Initial radiological evaluation may not be diagnostic. Nevertheless, the clinical picture must dictate the clinical decision-making process. If deemed necessary, a minimal procedure will be a second laparoscopic procedure for diagnostic purposes. Depending on the operative findings, a repair can be performed when feasible. The laparoscopic option has the benefit of a quicker recovery of the patient. However, when necessary, conversion to laparotomy may be the best approach to repair the enterotomy and adequately explore the entire abdomen effectively.

Specific Management of Enterotomy-Derived Complications

One of the biggest problems associated with any laparoscopic procedure is the morbidity and mortality due to inadvertent intraoperative or delayed enterotomy. It is therefore, extremely important to identify and treat such a complication intraoperatively. In this manner, a potentially serious complication can be resolved with a primary repair (Fig. 17)—laparoscopic repair beings preferred. If the surgeon does not have sufficient experience with laparoscopic suturing, an alternative is to perform the repair via a minilaparotomy, then closing that incision and continuing with the laparoscopic procedure. If the enterotomy occurs in the context of complex adhesiolyis, it may be impossible to complete the repair ade-

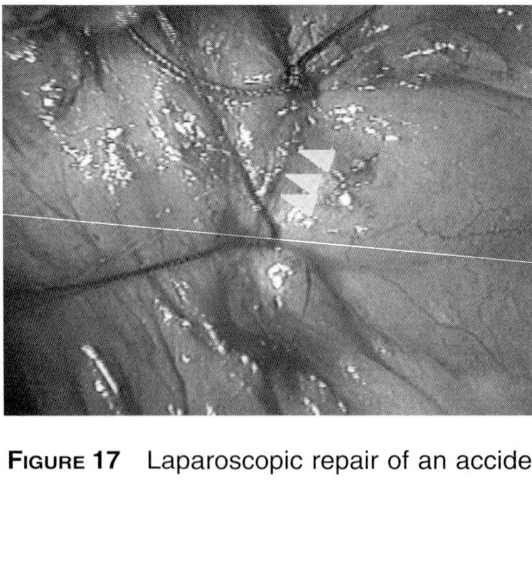

FIGURE 17 Laparoscopic repair of an accidental perforation.

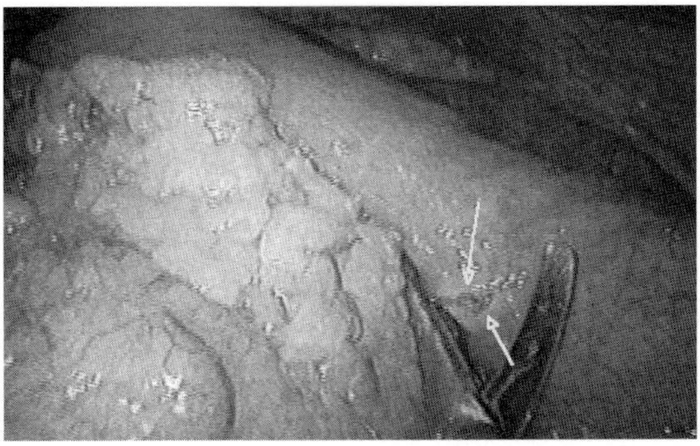

Figure 18 Thermal injury during difficult adhesiolysis.

quately if the involved intestinal is densely adherent to the abdominal wall. In these cases it is necessary to look for another surgical plane of dissection to avoid enlargement of the enterotomy. This is critically important if one is to suture the intestine with comfort and security. If the small bowel cannot be sufficiently released from the adhesions, the suture of the injured loop will be very difficult and can be jeopardized. Conversion to open surgery is then recommended.

If a thermal injury has occurred on the intestinal serosal layer, the resulting postoperative ischemia at that site can produce a delayed enterotomy. Because of this potential late complication, all injuries of this type require a serosal suture (Figs 18 and 19). The most devastating problem is the management of a delayed

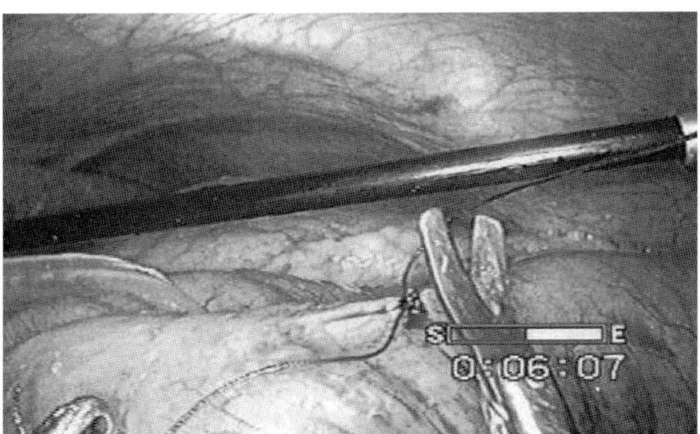

Figure 19 Laparoscopic repair of thermal injury.

or incorrectly treated enterotomy. An inadvertent lesion will probably not be suspected when the patient begins to have immediate problems, particularly if a postoperative acute abdomen is not very evident. This could result in a potentially fatal therapeutic delay. Immediate laparoscopic exploration based on clinical data can be decisive in therapeutic decision making at this juncture. Additionally, the surgeon can effect a repair of the injury or injuries before the need of an intestinal resection and/or the development of severe peritoneal contamination. A special circumstance is that involving ischemic injuries caused by thermal or vascular necrosis. In these cases, the enterotomy will not be immediate but can appear violently on the second or third postoperative day. Urgent exploration will be necessary to treat this.

CONCLUSION

In spite of the excitement surrounding the development of the laparoscopic approach to the digestive tract, primary small bowel laparoscopic surgery is seldom performed, with a paucity of published literature dealing with this issue. Usually, the small bowel plays a secondary role in the setting of laparoscopic surgery, and the complications with this organ in laparoscopic surgery usually result from other abdominal procedures. Although infrequent, these could become a serious surgical problems that can threaten the life of the patient. Judgment, good clinical decision making, and preventive measures like nontraumatic dissection and the avoidance of electrosurgical energy as much as possible are the best options. One must keep in mind that any abnormal postoperative course could be the first indication of a serious small bowel complication. Once the complication is confirmed, early surgical treatment will be the cornerstone of the management of the small bowel complications. If reintervention is considered necessary, the first option will be to perform a new laparoscopic procedure; but in severe and complicated cases, a formal laparotomy must be considered.

REFERENCES

1. Carbajo M, Martín del Olmo JC, Blanco JI, Martín F, Toledano M, de la Cuesta C. Therapeutic value of laparoscopic adhesiolysis. Surg Endosc 2001; 15(1):102.
2. Chosidow D, Johanet H, Montariol T, Kliet R, Manceau C, Marmuse E, Benhamou G. Laparoscopy for acute small-bowel obstruction secondary to adhesions. J Laparoendosc Adv Surg Tech 2000; 10(3):155–159.
3. Sato Y, Ido K, Kumagai M, Isoda N, Hozumi M, Nagamine N, Ono K, Shibusawa H, Togashi K, Sugano K. Laparoscopic adhesiolysis for recurrent small bowel obstruction long-term follow-up. Gastrointest Endosc 2001; 54(4):476–479.
4. Carbajo M, Martín del Olmo JC, Blanco JI, Toledano M, de la Cuesta C, Ferreras C, Vaquero C. Laparoscopic approach to incisional hernia. Surg Endosc. 2003; 17(1): 118–122.

5. Romagnolo C, Minelli L. Small-bowel occlusion after operative laparoscopy: Our experience and review of the literature. Endoscopy 2001; 33(1):88–90.
6. Malas MB, Katkhouda N. Internal hernia as a complication of laparoscopic Nissen funduplication. Surg Laparosc Endosc Percutan Tech 2002; 12(2):115–116.
7. Talhouk AS, Sorin A. Small bowel herniation around an anterior gastropexy for a gastric volvulus: A case report. JSLS 2000; 4(3):271–273.
8. Cuadra SA, Khalife ME, Char DJ, Wax MR, Halpern D. Intestinal obstruction from midgut volvulus after laparoscopic appendicectomy. Surg Endosc 2002; 16(1):215.
9. Filip JE, Mattar SG, Bowers SP, Smith CD. Internal hernia formation after laparoscopic Roux-en-Y gastric-bypass for morbid obesity. Am Surg 2002; 68(7):640–643.
10. Rutledge RL. The mini-gastric bypass: Experience with the first 1,274 cases. Obes Surg 2001; 11(6):276–280.
11. Champion JK. The route of the Roux in laparoscopic gastric bypass: Does it matter (abstr). Obes Surg 2001; 11(2):159.
12. Levard H, Boudt MJ, Msika S, Molkhou JM, Hay JM, Laborde Y, Fingerhut A. Laparoscopic treatment of acute small bowel obstruction: A multicentre study. Aust NZ J Surg 2001; 71(11):641–646.
13. Agresta F, Piazza A, Michelet I, Michelet I, Bendin N, Sartori CA. Small bowel obstruction. Laparoscopic approach. Surg Endosc 2000; 14(2):154–146.
14. Willemsen P, Appeltans B, Vanderveken M. Laparoscopic management of acute small bowel obstruction. Acta Chir Belg 1999; 99(6):289–291.
15. Suter M, Zermatten P, Halkic N, Martinet O, Bettschart V. Laparoscopic management of mechanical small bowel obstruction: Are there predictors of success or failure. Surg Endosc 2000; 14(5):478–483.
16. Fischer CP, Doherty D. Laparoscopic approach to small bowel obstruction. Semin Laparosc Surg 2002; 9(1):40–45.
17. Sarli L, Costi R. Laparoscopic resection of Meckel's diverticulum: Report of two cases. Surg Today 2001; 31(9):823–825.
18. Anderson DJ. Carcinoid tumor in Meckel's divertculum: Laparoscopic treatment and review of the literature. J Am Osteopath Assoc 2000; 100(7):432–434.
19. Tanimura S, Higashino M, Fukunaga Y. Laparoscopy-assisted resection for jejunal carcinoma. Surg Laparosc Endosc Percutan Tech 2001; 11(4):287–288.
20. Milsom JW, Hammerhofer KA, Bohm B, Marcello P, Elson P, Facio J. Prospective, randomized trial comparing laparoscopic vs. conventional surgery for refractory ileocolic Crohn's disease. Dis Colon Rectum 2001; 44(1):1–8; discussion 8–9.
21. Blachar A, Federle MP, Pealer KM, Ikramuddin S, Schauer PR. Gastrointestinal complications of laparoscopic Roux-en-Y gastric bypass surgery: Clinical and imaging findings. Radiology 2002; 223(3):625–632.
22. Nguyen NT, Neuhaus AM, Ho HS, Palmer LS, Furdui GG, Wolfe BM. A prospective evaluation of intracorporeal laparoscopic small bowel anastomosis during gastric bypass. Obes Surg 2001; 11(2):196–199.
23. Lauter DM. Laparoscopic enterocolostomy for palliation of malignant bowel obstruction. J Laparoendosc Adv Surg Tech 2000; 10(5):275–276.
24. Higa KD, Boone KB, Ho T. Complications of the laparoscopic Roux-en-Y gastric bypass: 1040 patients—What have we learned. Obes Surg 2000; 10(6):509–513.

25. Schafer M, Lauper M, Krahenbuhl L. Trocar and Veress needle injuries during laparoscopy. Surg Endosc 2001; 15(3):275–280.
26. Ostrzenski A. Laparoscopic intestinal injury: A review and case presentation. J Natl Med Assoc 2001; 93(11):440–443.
27. El-Banna M, Abdel-Atty M, El-Meteini M, Aly S. Management of laparoscopic-related bowel injuries. Surg Endosc 2000; 14(9):779–782.
28. Orlando R, Lirussi F. Delayed recognition of inadvertent gut injury during laparoscopy. Surg Endosc 2000; 14(12):1188.
29. Corson SL, Chandler JG, Way LW. Survey of laparoscopic entry injuries provoking ligation. J Am Assoc Gynecol Laparosc 2001; 8(3):341–347.
30. Bida B, Manger T. The iatrogenic small bowel perforation as a complication of laparoscopic cholecystectomy. Zentralbl Chir 2002; 127(6):554–558.
31. Dexter SP, Miller GV, Davides D, Martin IG, Sue Ling HM, Sagar P, Larvin M, McMahon MJ. Relaparoscopy for the detection and treatment of complications of laparoscopic cholecystectomy. Am J Surg 2000; 179(4):316–319.
32. Swank DJ, van Erp WFM, Repelaer van Driel OJ, Hop WCJ, Bomjer HJ, Jeekel J. Complications and feasibility of laparoscopic adhesiolysis in patients with abdominal pain. Surg Endosc 2002; 16:1468–1473.
33. Koehler RH, Voeller G. Recurrences in laparoscopic hernia repair: A personal series and review of the literature. JSLS 1999; 3(34):293–304.
34. Avrutis O, Meshoulam J, Yutkin O, Mikchalevski V, Haskel L, Adler M, Durst A. Brief clinical report: Duodenal laceration presenting as massive hematemesis and multiple intraabdominal abscesses after laparoscopic cholecystectomy. Surg Laparosc Percutan Tech 2001; 11(5):330–333.

24

Laparoscopic Gastric Surgery

Ricardo Vitor Cohen, José Carlos Pinheiro Filho, Carlos Aurélio Schiavon, and José Luis Lopes Correa
Hospital São Camilo, São Paulo, Brazil

The official history of laparoscopic gastric surgery dates from 1992, when Peter Goh of Singapore performed the first entirely laparoscopic Billroth II distal gastrectomy on a patient with a chronic gastric ulcer [1].

Since that time, laparoscopic gastric resections have not met with the same enthusiasm as other procedures, and laparoscopic gastrectomy for cancer has accounted for only a small fraction of minimally invasive interventions. Among the many reasons for its slow acceptance are the great skill required to perform advanced laparoscopic surgery and the fear that laparoscopy cannot accommodate basic oncological principles of open surgery. Other procedures were employed, such as gastric wedge resections and hand-assisted laparoscopic surgery (HALS), with reasonable experience in Japan, the United States, and Latin America (Brazil) [2,3].

This chapter describes the main complications related to different approaches in gastric surgery as well as their recognition and management.

COMPLICATIONS RELATED TO GASTRIC RESECTION

The techniques of minimal-access gastric resection and their complications may be categorized as follows:

The Interventional flexible endoscopic approach, suitable for superficial gastric neoplasms. Its complications are not addressed here.

Laparoendoluminal resection, combining peroral endoscopic resections and laparoscopy.

Bleeding is the major complication of this technique, besides problems of laparoscopic access and CO_2 insufflation discussed elsewhere in this book. Although bleeding is relatively frequent [4], transfusions are rarely required.

Other possible complications include unrecognized or delayed gastric perforation (excessive electrocoagulation with collateral damage) at the site of local submucosal excision. In full-thickness local resections, suture-line leakage is also possible. These complications must be approached surgically—if the patient's stability permits, preferably laparoscopically. Resection or closure of the defect followed by drainage is the common way of managing them.

LAPAROSCOPIC PARTIAL OR TOTAL GASTRECTOMY

Pneumothorax can occur if the pleural space is entered during mobilization of the mediastinal esophagus. CO_2 is then insufflated into the pleural space and tension pneumothorax may result. Placement of a chest tube corrects cardiopulmonary compromise but may impair peritoneal insufflation. If this happens, intermittent occlusion of the chest tube allows the operation to be completed.

Bleeding from a suture line may be due to staples, which are commonly employed to perform gastric resections and bariatric surgery. Expertise in handling them and choosing the correct cartridges for each organ's wall thickness is very important. Oozing from staple lines is common but almost never requires any surgical maneuver or transfusion and generally stops without intervention. Some advocate the use of staple-line reinforcement with biological or synthetic materials [5], but this has no clear advantage. If hand suture techniques are employed, the incidence of oozing and major bleeding is very low.

Anastomotic leakage results in a localized collection in the supracolic compartment, with fever and leukocytosis. Diagnosis may easily be made through meglumine diatrizoate (Gastrografin) studies (Fig. 1). Drainage, either percutaneously or with an open technique, is often followed by an external fistula. Clinical and nutritional support may be required to treat this.

Less common are ''acute'' leaks, which can lead to generalized peritonitis and thus require immediate re-exploration. If systemic conditions are favorable, reoperation may be conducted laparoscopically with a good outcome.

Mediastinitis, a severe complication, may occur following total gastrectomy and Roux-en-Y reconstruction, when the phrenoesophageal membrane is opened and there is continuation to the anterior mediastinum. Any incidental contamination or leak from the esophagojejunal anastomosis can lead to this critical condi-

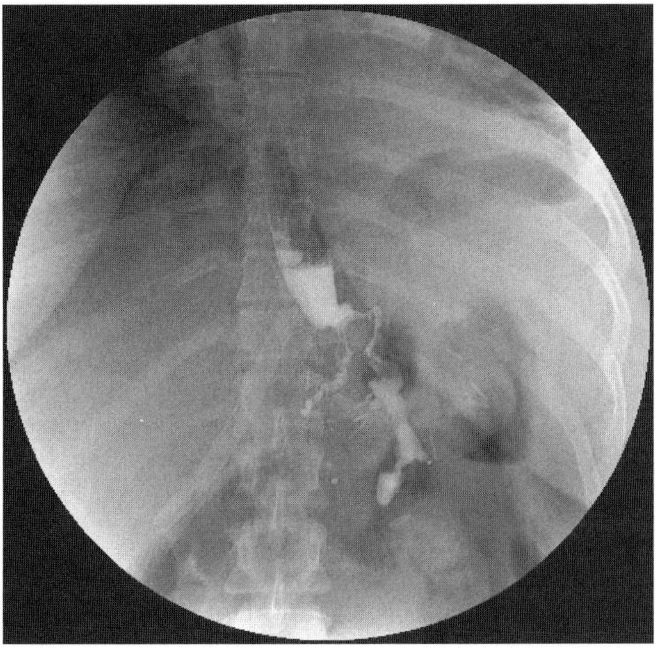

FIGURE 1 Meglumine Diatrizoate study showing an anastometic leak.

tion. Mediastinitis is a severe illness and many reoperations may be required to achieve good results and same the patient's life.

Pancreatic injury usually declares itself in the postoperative period with ileus, pain, and hyperamylasemia. It may be severe and necrotizing, making clinical measures very important. Surgery may be indicated, depending on several factors—such as systemic conditions, findings on computed tomography, and clinical evolution. Repair may be done either open or laparoscopically.

Splenic injury is usually due to a wound secondary to a stapler injury to the hilum or inferior pole when the gastric transection is being completed. If it is not recognized, bleeding may continue, requiring transfusion and reoperation.

Dudodenal stump fistula is a very rare occurrence after gastric resection for cancer because there is usually no inflammation surrounding the first duodenal segment. If not drained, as is normally done in those situations, peritonitis will develop and reoperation will be mandatory. If local conditions permit, closure of the duodenal defect should be performed during re-exploration and drains placed. Clinical measures with parenteral nutrition and clinical support will help to manage this problem.

Postgastrectomy syndromes, or poor functional results, are common after gastrectomy regardless of the type of reconstruction. Patients should be approached from several diagnostic perspectives. There are many pitfalls in the evaluation of these patients, whose complaints may be due to previous operation(s), to a pre-existing medical or surgical condition (previous treatment that was either ineffective or inappropriate), or to unrelated "new" problems [6].

Vomiting and Postprandial Discomfort

Loop syndromes, both afferent and efferent, are conditions that occur only after a Billroth II gastrectomy or gastroduodenostomy. The acute afferent loop syndrome is a symptom of an acute blowout of the duodenal stump. The most common cause of this complication is obstruction of the afferent loop, possibly due to kinking, a retroanastomotic hernia, or technical misadventure.

The chronic afferent loop syndrome is an important cause of postoperative vomiting. The typical complaint is postprandial vomiting of bilious material without any of the food recently eaten. Retroanastomotic hernias may cause this condition; surgery with reduction of the herniated loop alleviates the symptoms. If there is chronic and increased luminal hypertension of the duodenum secondary to compression/twisting of the afferent loop, the patient may show signs of hyperbilirrubinemia as well as clinical pancreatitis [7].

Efferent limb syndrome is due to incomplete obstruction of the loops of bowel draining the stomach. Adhesions, recurrent cancer, and/or carcinomatosis are the most common reasons for this complication. Jejunogastric intussusception is a rare cause of efferent block. Its diagnosis as well as its reduction may be made by endoscopy. Local loop conditions, such as edema in the jejunal segment, may prevent the success of this approach. Laparoscopic reoperation and correction may be required.

Dumping syndrome is among the most common causes of morbidity after gastric surgery; it is characterized by both gastrointestinal and vasomotor symptoms. Patients with severe dumping syndrome may limit their food intake to minimize symptoms. As a result, they lose weight and become malnourished. For patients unresponsive to medical therapy or unwilling to continue medical therapy, remedial surgery may be considered.

Many different remedial operations have been designed. They may be done laparoscopically and include narrowing of the gastrojejunal stoma, conversion of Billroth II anastomosis to Billroth I gastroduodenostomy, jejunal interpositions, conversion to Roux-en-Y gastrojejunostomy, and pyloric reconstruction [8].

COMPLICATIONS AFTER OTHER GASTRIC PROCEDURES

Gastrostomy

This procedure is generally indicated when a percutaneous approach cannot be performed.

Leakage

The gastrostomy can leak if the tube and the stomach are not close enough to the abdominal wall. The balloon of the gastrostomy tube should be inflated and pulled with gentle traction to approximate the anterior gastric wall to the abdominal wall. This is confirmed by direct visualization through the laparoscope. If a stapled tube is constructed, an incomplete staple line may result in leakage.

If visualization of the stomach to the abdominal wall is not satisfactory during the operation, one may inject dye through the tube while visualizing the abdominal wall. If any leak is seen, inadequate approximation between the stomach and abdominal wall is present and better fixation should be provided.

Gastric Perforation

This injury can be secondary to surgical manipulation or tension between the stomach and the abdominal wall leading to gastric laceration. Intraoperative recognition is important, so that the perforation can be sutured and another site that is tension-free selected. These steps usually resolve the problem.

Laparoscopic Vagotomy

Gastric perforation may occur from an electrocautery injury or by clipping the branch of the nerve of Latarjet on the serosa of the lesser curvature. This can usually be prevented by careful dissection and isolation of the nerve's branches as well as the avoidance of excessive electrocauterization. If a seromyotomy vagotomy is performed, the area should be oversewn with a continuous suture. Esophageal perforation may occur during hiatal dissection, particularly if manipulations are performed blindly.

During laparoscopic vagotomy, particular attention should be given to the presence of bleeding along the lesser curvature, avoiding excessive use of cautery. Misuse of electrocautery may lead to a delayed perforation. In that instance the patient may present with intra-abdominal sepsis 2–5 days after the operation. The perforation can be confirmed by a Gastrografin study. If no leak is identified and the patient is stable or improving, clinical observation may be adopted. If a leak is demonstrated and/or the clinical status worsens, surgical exploration, laparoscopic or not (depending on patient's systemic condition), is indicated. Oversewing of the area of perforation or even a gastric resection may be needed.

Other complications, such as delayed gastric emptying and diarrhea, can require surgical intervention if medical control is not possible.

Delayed gastric emptying is more frequent after selective or truncal vagotomy, mainly if any drainage procedure was performed (pyloromyotomy). After highly selective vagotomy, although rare, delayed gastric emptying may occur.

The surgical treatment consists of endoscopic pyloric dilatation. If this fails, pyloromyotomy or resection and gastrojejunostomy will be the option of choice [9].

For severe postvagotomy diarrhea that is unresponsive to medical therapy, remedial surgery may be considered. Two options having mixed results have been described. The first strategy may be the construction of a 10-cm antiperistaltic jejunal segment located 100 cm from the ligament of Treitz. The other possibility is the distal-onlay reversed ileal graft. Human experience with the latter procedure is extremely limited [10,11].

Laparoscopic Suture of Perforated Ulcer

Problems with this procedure include incorrect diagnosis (which can be avoided if the laparoscopist is scrupulously careful to visualize the site of perforation), recurrent ulcer, and inadvertent plication of a malignancy. These complications can be avoided by exercising good surgical judgment and converting to formal laparotomy if the diagnosis is unclear or suture of the perforation does not appear feasible [12]. Gastric outlet obstruction may result if the sutures are placed too deeply, or if the ulcer has produced significant pyloric stenosis.

Hand-Assisted Surgery: Its Role and Complications

Minimally invasive surgery offers the benefit of reduced hospital stay, less postoperative discomfort, and decreased wound complications. One drawback of a purely laparoscopic approach is the need to morcellate tissue for removal. If tumor resection is planned, morcellation makes it more difficult to assess the margin of resection. Another disadvantage to a purely laparoscopic approach is the loss of tactile feedback, making exploration more difficult.

The benefits of hand-assisted laparoscopic surgery (HALS) are numerous. Introduction of the hand may allow laparoscopic completion of a procedure that otherwise would be converted to a laparotomy.

HALS is also useful when intact specimens are required, as in cancer surgery. The HALS technique returns tactile feedback to the surgeon. The use of the hand allows rapid exploration of the abdomen, retraction, dissection, and swift and easy control of bleeding. The type of surgery planned guides the selection of the incision site.

There are no complications linked to HALS, such as the worst postoperative results in any of the procedures listed above. There are some complications related to the hand-assisted approach and devices employed to put the surgeon's hand inside the abdominal cavity. Some have described [13] more postoperative pain, due to the 7 to 9-cm incision, as well as more wound complications. Digital dissections may be carried out in a more ''aggressive'' fashion with the hand. As a result, incorrect placement of the hand can be disastrous, requiring conversion to open laparotomy. Regarding gastric surgery, including bariatric surgery, no paper has reported any advantage to the HALS technique. Regarding gastric resection for cancer, no improved outcomes have been demonstrated. Gastric procedures—unlike colorectal surgery, splenectomy with massively large spleens, and live-donor nephrectomy—can be safely accomplished by a purely laparoscopic approach.

Gastric Resection in Cancer: Particular Aspects

Port-site recurrence (PSR), or the metastasis of cancer cells to incisional sites of the abdominal wall, has been reported after curative laparoscopic operations for many gastrointestinal malignancies. This has probably been the single most important factor discouraging the widespread use of laparoscopy in the treatment of gastrointestinal cancers so far.

The implantation of malignant cells at incisional sites has long been known to occur after conventional surgery, but whether laparoscopy actually increases the risk of such implantation remains unclear [14].

There have been several reports concerning the potential causes of PSR. Local effects at port sites; transportation of tumor cells; mechanical factors; and immunological, systemic, and peritoneal and CO_2 aerolization are elements that were and currently are the focus of studies to determine the real effect of laparoscopy in the treatment of cancer. What has already been proven [15] is the importance of the surgeon's role in the oncological outcome. As in open operations, bad technique and lack of respect for basic principles are probably the chief factors contributing to poor results in laparoscopy generally and cancer in particular.

Regarding Ballesta-Lopez, Huscher, and Reyes et al. [16–18], there was no difference in lymph nodes harvested, blood loss, and free margins in comparing their series of laparoscopic gastric resections for cancer to other ''open'' series.

Much knowledge that has yet to be gained in the field of laparoscopy and gastric cancer. In today's perspective, however; if the operation is conducted by a skilled laparoscopic surgeon, patients will undergo operations that have the advantage of being less invasive which also producing satisfactory oncological results.

REFERENCES

1. Goh P, Tekant Y, Isaac J, Kum CK, Ngoi SS. The technique of laparoscopic Billroth II gastrectomy. Surg Laparosc Endosc 1992; 2:258–260.
2. Neufang T, Post S, Markus P, Becker H. Manually assisted laparoscopic surgery—Realistic evolution of the minimally invasive concept? Initial experience. Chirurgie 1996; 67:952–958.
3. Litwin D, Darzi A, Cohen RV. and the HALS Study Group. Hand-assisted laparoscopic colorectal surgery. Surg Endosc 2000; 14(10):877–995.

4. Cushier A. Gastric resections. In Cuschieri A , Buess G , Perissat J, eds. Operative Manual of Endoscopic Surgery. New York: Springer-Verlag, 1993.
5. Shikora S. The use of ''Peristrips'' during gastric partition. Proceedings of the 7th meeting of IFSO (International Federation of Societies for Surgery of Obesity). São Paulo. Brazil, September 2002:87–90.
6. Donahue P. Early postoperative and postgastrectomy syndromes. Gastroenterol Clin North Am 1994; 23(2):215–226.
7. Matsusue S, Kashihara S, Takeda H. Three cases of afferent loop obstruction: The role of ultrasonography in the diagnosis. Jpn J Surg 1988; 18:709–713.
8. Miranda R, Steffes B, O'Leary JP. Surgical treatment of postgastrectomy dumping syndrome. Am J Surg 1980; 139:40–47.
9. Legrand M, Dentroz B, Honore P, Jacquet N. Laparoscopic highly selective vagotomy. Surg Endosc 1992; 6:90–94.
10. Carvajal SH, Mulvihill SJ. Postgastrectomy syndromes: Dumping and diarrhea. Gastroenterol Clin North Am 1994; 23(2):261–279.
11. Henley FA. Experiences with jejunal interposition for correction of postgastrectomy syndrome. In Harkins HM , Nyhus LM, eds. Surgery of the Stomach and Duodenum. Boston: Little Brown, 1969, 777.
12. Mouret P, Francois Y, Vignal J, Barth X, Lombard-Plalet R. Laparoscopic treatment of perforated peptic ulcer. Br J Surg 1990; 77:1006–1010.
13. Watson DI, Game PA. Hand-assisted laparoscopic vertical banded gastroplasty. Surg Endosc 1997; 11:1218–1220.
14. Litwin DM, Willsher PC. Laparoscopy and gastric cancer: Perspectives and controversies. In Eubanks S , Cohen R , Younes R , Brody F, eds. Endosurgery for Cancer. Austin. TX: Landes Bioscience, 1999, 112.
15. Wittich PH, Bonjer HJ. Port-site recurrences in laparoscopic surgery. In Reymond MA , Bonjer HJ , Kockerling F, eds. Port-Site and Wound Recurrences in Cancer Surgery. New York: Springer-Verlag, 2000, 12–20.
16. Ballesta-Lopez C, Bastida-Vila X, Catarci M. Laparoscopic Billroth II subtotal gastrectomy with gastric stump suspension for gastric malignancies. Am J Surg 1996; 171:289–292.
17. Huscher GCS, Anastasi A, Crafa F, Recher A, Lirici MM. Laparoscopic gastric resections. Semin Laparosc Surg 2000; 7:26–54.
18. Reyes CD, Webe KJ, Gagner M, Divino CM. Laparoscopic vs open gastrectomy. Surg Endosc 2001; 15:928–931.

25

Splenectomy

John M. Whitaker
Minimally Invasive Surgery Institute, Baton Rouge, Louisiana, U.S.A.

INTRODUCTION

In 1991 and 1992 European, North American, and Japanese centers published the first reports of laparoscopic splenectomy [1–4]. It was the hope of these pioneers that patients would ultimately realize the similar benefits of shortened hospital stays, less pain, and improved cosmesis that were demonstrated with other laparoscopic procedures such as laparoscopic cholecystectomy and laparoscopic appendectomy. The early accounts of laparoscopic splenectomy consistently pointed out the technical difficulties encountered by surgeons using rudimentary laparoscopic instruments to dissect and manipulate such a vascular and fragile structure. Over time, technical advances—including the use of ultrasonic dissectors, endoscopic vascular stapling devices, and adoption by most surgeons of the lateral approach to laparoscopic splenectomy—have shortened operative times and decreased complications. Although there are no prospective, randomized trials comparing open and laparoscopic splenectomy, a number of retrospective and case studies provide evidence that laparoscopic splenectomy results in shorter hospital stays and fewer complications than open surgery [5–7]. I think it is safe to say that laparoscopic splenectomy is the procedure of choice for the removal of all but the most massively enlarged spleens [8]. Despite the advantages that laparoscopic splenectomy offers, the procedure presents technical challenges due to the vascular nature and frail texture of the spleen. The close proximity of the spleen to the pancreas, stomach, colon, and diaphragm—coupled

TABLE 1 Complications of Laparoscopic Splenectomy

Gastric perforation
Hemorrhagic
Hemoperitoneum
Abdominal wall hematoma
Subdiaphragmatic hematoma
Hemopneumothorax
Pancreatic injury
Residual splenic function
Missed accessory spleens
Splenosis
Overwhelming postsplenectomy infection (OPSI)
Diaphragmatic injury
Other
Portal and/or mesenteric vein thrombosis
Deep venous thrombosis
Pneumonia
Atelectasis
Bowel obstruction
Ileus
Subdiaphragmatic abscess
Wound infection

with the specific features of the hematological diseases for which the splenectomy is being done (thrombocytopenia and malignancy to name a few)—contributes to postoperative morbidity, which is largely technique-related [9]. It is with this in mind that this chapter attempts to address the measures one must take to minimize the intraoperative and postoperative complications of laparoscopic splenectomy and the means to manage them should they occur (Table 1).

INDICATIONS, CONTRAINDICATIONS, AND PATIENT SELECTION

The indications for laparoscopic splenectomy are essentially the same as those for open splenectomy. Laparoscopic splenectomy is generally done for benign and malignant hematological diseases as well as a number of nonhematological indications (cysts, abscesses, etc.). The indications for laparoscopic splenectomy are listed in Table 2. There are no specific disease processes that require or should not be done by a laparoscopic approach, but there are a few relative contraindications to consider (Table 3).

TABLE 2 Indications for Laparoscopic Splenectomy

Hematologic
Benign
Idiopathic thrombocytopenic purpura (ITP)
Autoimmune hemolytic anemia
Hereditary spherocytosis
Evans syndrome
Thrombotic thrombocytopenic purpura (TTP)
HIV-related ITP
HIV-related hypersplenism
HIV-related splenomegaly and possible malignancy
Malignant
Lymphoma, Hodgkin's and non-Hodgkin's
Leukemia, myeloid and lymphoid
Hairy cell leukemia
Myelofibrosis
Trauma
Other
Splenic cyst
Splenic abscess
Angioma
Hydatid cyst
Hematoma

TABLE 3 Relative Contraindications to Laparoscopic Splenectomy

Coagulopathy (including thrombocytopenia)
Adhesions
Trauma
Pregnancy
Massive splenomegaly
Portal hypertension
Inflammatory conditions (splenic abscess)
Obesity
Calcified splenic artery

Coagulopathy, particularly that associated with thrombocytopenia, is frequently the indication for splenectomy and can usually be corrected preoperatively with the aid of platelet transfusions, corticosteroids, gamma globulin, and the administration of clotting factors. In fact, laparoscopic splenectomy is now considered by most as the procedure of choice for idiopathic thrombocytopenic purpura (ITP) [10].

Other relative contraindications include scarring and adhesions from previous upper abdominal surgeries, trauma, pregnancy, splenomegaly, and portal hypertension. Most surgeons with advanced laparoscopic skills would agree that scarring and adhesions should not deter one from at least attempting laparoscopic splenectomy, yet they would also set limits on how long one should persevere in the face of dense adhesions before deciding to convert to an open procedure. The patient's general condition and comorbidities must also be considered as the duration of the operation lengthens. Laparoscopic splenectomy and partial splenectomy for external trauma has been described [11], but concerns exist relative to the ability to detect other intra-abdominal injuries and to the length of operative time. With improvements in preoperative evaluation [rapid computed tomography (CT) scans and ultrasound] as well as instrumentation that facilitates hemostasis, perhaps an endoscopic approach to external splenic trauma will become more commonplace. Procedures such as laparoscopic cholecystectomy during pregnancy have proven to be safe, but splenectomy is a longer and more technically challenging operation that requires unusual positioning, which may affect uterine blood flow and limit rapid control of massive bleeding should it occur. Fortunately splenectomy is rarely required during pregnancy, but a laparoscopic approach should be considered if the occasion arises, keeping in mind the aforementioned caveats.

It is clear that massively enlarged spleens present the greatest technical challenge to surgeons during laparoscopic splenectomy, and splenomegaly is cited in many series as the most common reason for conversion to open splenectomy [12–14]. Enlarged spleens make hilar control, splenic mobilization, and removal difficult; therefore splenomegaly should be considered a relative contraindication to the laparoscopic approach. There are, however, no established, uniform parameters to define splenomegaly. Splenic diameter as measured by ultrasound or CT is a reliable measure and is used by most to compare spleen sizes and define splenomegaly [11]. Spleen weight is a less reliable variable. In open splenectomy, spleens can be weighed after removal and compared, but in laparoscopic removal the specimens are almost always are fragmented, with a significant amount of blood lost to suction, thus decreasing spleen weight and resulting in an underestimation of spleen size. Others use less exact criteria, defining splenomegaly as a spleen extending to the midline or to the iliac crest on physical examination. Targarona, in a large series of laparoscopic splenectomies, concluded that laparoscopic splenectomy is technically feasible in cases with spleen weights as great as 3000 g [15], and Schlachta, in a series of 64 splenectomies, found the only limitation to be splenic size greater than 27 cm in polar diameter [11]. Hand-assisted laparoscopic splenectomy has been shown to be a safe and efficacious compromise for cases of extreme splenomegaly, with spleens up to 3500 g being removed by this method [14,15]. Splenomegaly is certainly not an absolute contraindication to a laparoscopic approach; as the surgeon gains experience, this should be only a minor deterrent.

Several other conditions warrant consideration prior to proceeding with laparoscopic splenectomy. These include inflammatory conditions such as splenic abscess as well as obesity and portal hypertension. These are not contraindications, but only surgeons with advanced laparoscopic skills should attempt laparoscopic surgery on such patients.

PERIOPERATIVE MANAGEMENT

Perioperative preparation of patients undergoing laparoscopic splenectomy depends on the indication for surgery and the overall medical condition of the patient. With careful planning, intraoperative and postoperative complications can be significantly reduced. Practically speaking, most patients are managed medically by their primary care physician or the hematology oncologist; but, for optimal care, the surgeon must be familiar with all aspects of the patient's therapy.

In an effort to reduce the incidence of postsplenectomy sepsis, at least 1 week before surgery the patient should receive polyvalent pnuemococcal, meningococcal, and *Haemophilus influenzae* type b vaccines. Postsplenectomy sepsis is discussed in more detail further on. Suffice it to say here that although the incidence of postsplenectomy sepsis is relatively low, the resulting morbidity and mortality warrant the routine use of perioperative vaccination. Transfusion of platelets is individualized according to the patient's preoperative platelet count. In patients with ITP and ''borderline'' platelet counts, administration of immunoglobulin G (400 mg/kg administered 3–5 days prior to surgery) results in platelet counts greater than 60,000 in 72% of cases [16]. In patients who cannot sustain a platelet count greater than 50,000, platelets should be ordered preoperatively and occasionally transfused when abnormal surgical bleeding or lack of coagulation is noted. Preoperative platelet transfusions in patients with severe thrombocytopenia and ITP should be avoided due to the rapid destruction of platelets by the spleen. Patients receiving therapeutic doses of corticosteroids preoperatively should receive stress doses prior to surgery. Prophylactic antibiotics are given immediately before surgery.

The issue of spleen size as a relative contraindication was discussed earlier, and the determination of whether splenomegaly exists can be important in the avoidance of the complications associated with splenomegaly. However, the routine use of CT or ultrasound to establish a more exact spleen size prior to laparoscopic splenectomy is not generally necessary, since—to most experienced surgeons—an enlarged spleen is not a deterrent to the laparoscopic approach. Probably the single best indicator of an enlarged spleen and a potentially difficult operation is the presence of a palpable spleen tip on physical examination. In the early days of laparoscopic splenectomy, preoperative angiographic embolization of the splenic artery was frequently utilized to decrease the risk of intraoperative bleeding. However, with the current levels of experience and technical refinement, most surgeons have come to realize that favorable outcomes can be obtained without embolization [16]. The embolization process itself is not without complication and may result in pain from splenic infarction, necrosis of surrounding tissue, contrast allergies, and arterial puncture site complications, to name a few. Though preoperative splenic artery embolization may be of value in selected situations, as when the surgeon is inexperienced or massive splenomegaly exists [16], it is generally agreed that embolization is unnecessary in most patients.

Certain perioperative technical factors have been shown to influence the incidence of postoperative complications. Several retrospective reviews consistently demonstrate the benefits of placing the patient in the full lateral position [12,15,17]. Targarona et al. demonstrated a reduction in the incidence of complications when they switched from the supine to the full lateral position [15]. The lateral position facilitates dissection of the splenic hilum, reduces operative time, and avoids manipulation of the spleen, thereby decreasing the likelihood of splenic tears and subsequent bleeding. Once the surgeon becomes familiar with the lateral position, exposure of the pancreatic tail is also superior to that achieved with the supine position, which lessens the risk of pancreatic complications (discussed later). Improvements in instrumentation, such as the use of ultrasonic dissectors and endoscopic vascular stapling devices, have facilitated dissection, allowed better hemostasis, and reduced the incidence of thermal injury. The use of these instruments obviates the need for hemostatic clips, which may become dislodged, and simplifies control of the short gastric vessels. The introduction of the endoscopic vascular stapler has simplified the control and division of the major splenic vessels, particularly when combined with the lateral position, which allows placement of the stapler without tension. The use of nonbladed trocars, particularly the 5-mm variety, has reduced the incidence of trocar-related hernias and bleeding, problems discussed in Chapter 3.

SURGICAL TECHNIQUE

Although the purpose of this chapter is to addresses the complications one might encounter during laparoscopic splenectomy, a brief discussion of the technical aspects of the procedure will provide a better understanding of how and why these problems occur. The procedure is done under a general endotracheal anesthesia. A nasogastric or orogastric tube is placed to deflate the stomach, and pneumatic compression stockings are applied. Appropriate patient positioning is of paramount importance to the successful completion of a laparoscopic splenectomy. The literature is replete with discussions comparing the supine with the right lateral decubitus position. From this it would seem safe to conclude that most surgeons see the most important innovation in the technique of laparoscopic splenectomy to be simply moving the patient from a supine to a lateral position on the operating table [18]. The patient is placed over a kidney rest, a right axillary roll is used, the left arm is stabilized, and the table is broken 20–30 degrees below level in both the caudad and cephalad directions. ''Breaking'' the table and elevating the kidney rest widen the space between the left costal margin and left iliac crest, providing more room between trocars and preventing ''fencing'' between instruments. The table is then placed in a reverse Trendelenburg position to facilitate gravity retraction of the viscera away from the left upper quadrant. The patient's position is further secured with either rolls or a beanbag. Video monitors are placed on each side of the table, at or above the patient's shoulder level.

Trocar selection and placement is important and may be influenced by spleen size and patient body habitus. We routinely use three 5-mm trocars and one 12-mm trocar. The 12-mm trocar is placed in the anterior axillary line near the left costal margin and is used for insertion of the endoscopic stapler and retrieval of the spleen. One 5-mm trocar is placed in the midline and a second in the midclavicular line, both near the left costal margin. The third 5-mm trocar is placed laterally in the midaxillary line. The operation begins with a thorough search of the abdominal cavity for accessory splenic tissue (see ''Residual Splenic Function,'' discussed later). This being completed, the splenic flexure of the colon is dissected away from the lower pole of the spleen and the splenophrenic and splenorenal attachments are freed enough to expose the posterior aspect of the splenic vessels. The lesser sac is entered along the medial border of the spleen. This allows the short gastric vessels, the main vascular pedicle, and the tail of the pancreas to be visualized. The short gastric vessels are divided by means of an ultrasonic dissector, hemoclips, or an endoscopic stapling device. We prefer using the ultrasonic dissector, as the endoscopic stapling device is usually not necessary on these small vessels and, as discussed below, the use of clips is not recommended, as they can become dislodged and may interfere with future applications of an endoscopic stapler.

After the short gastric vessels are divided, the splenic pedicle is carefully dissected on both the medial and lateral aspects (this is facilitated by the lateral position). In most patients the main vascular trunks branch 2 to 3 cm from the hilum; for that reason, we generally keep our dissection 2 cm from the spleen but are careful not to injure the tail of the pancreas. The hilar vessels are divided by several applications of the endoscopic stapling device. The spleen is now completely devascularized and is suspended by avascular splenophrenic attachments. These attachments are left in place to facilitate placement of the spleen into a sac for extraction. A puncture-resistant nylon bag is introduced through the 12-mm port site and opened within the abdominal cavity; the spleen is then placed in the bag. At this point the drawstring is closed, leaving only the superior pole attachments to be divided. The open end of the bag is brought outside the abdomen through the 12-mm trocar site. The spleen is then morcellated with ring forceps and digitally removed piecemeal. In situations requiring pathological evaluation of a relatively intact spleen (e.g., to document a hematological disease or tumor), the puncture wound will have to be enlarged to enable removal of the bag containing the intact spleen. In all cases care must be taken to avoid spillage of any spleen fragments into the abdominal cavity or the wound. A final assessment of hemostasis is now undertaken, and a drain can be placed if deemed necessary.

SPECIFIC COMPLICATIONS—AVOIDANCE, RECOGNITION AND MANAGEMENT

Gastric Perforation

A review of the literature relative to laparoscopic splenectomy indicates that gastric injury is an uncommon complication. However, the fact that the stomach is in close proximity to the spleen and receives a significant portion of its blood supply from the spleen via the short gastric vessels places it in harm's way during laparoscopic splenectomy. Injury to the stomach can occur as a result of direct trauma to the gastric wall or due to an ischemic phenomenon. Direct injury can be immediately apparent, as would occur with aggressive instrumentation, or its manifestation can be delayed, as might occur in the case of delayed necrosis and perforation as a result of an injury from an energy source. One of the initial maneuvers of laparoscopic splenectomy involves grasping the stomach and pulling it medially to place the short gastric vessels on tension. Overaggressive grasping can result in direct injury to the stomach in the form of partial- or full-thickness disruption of the stomach wall (Fig. 1). Dissection near the stomach, as during division of the short gastric vessels or separation of the stomach from the upper pole of the spleen, can also result in gastric injury. The management of such an injury will depend on the depth of injury. A superficial tear involving injury to the serosal surface or outer muscle layers can be left alone or closed using either Lembert sutures or an endoscopic stapling device. Obviously, full-thickness perforations will require closure. Problems arise when an intraoperative perforation is unrecognized or a perforation related to thermal injury and necrosis is delayed. A missed perforation will be apparent in the immediate postoperative period, which results in signs and symptoms of peritonitis soon after surgery. However, the signs of a perforation resulting from thermal injury and necrosis

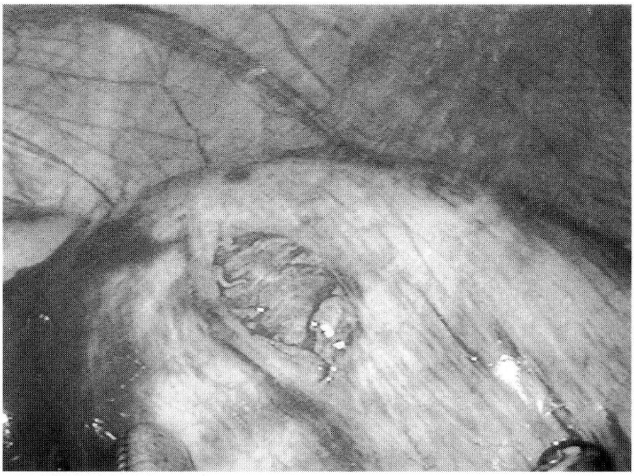

FIGURE 1 Overaggressive grasping of the stomach can result in direct injury to the stomach, as shown in this partial-thickness injury. A superficial injury such as this can be safely observed.

may not become manifest for several days into the postoperative period. Since hospital stays can be short following laparoscopic splenectomy, patients and their family members must be given careful instructions relative to the clinical signs of a delayed perforation. Should perforation be suspected, immediate reoperation and repair is indicated.

A rare but documented form of gastric injury following laparoscopic splenectomy is delayed perforation due to ischemic necrosis of the gastric wall. The stomach has a rich blood supply, but anatomical variations can cause a predisposition to ischemia and subsequent gastric perforation after ligation of the short gastric vessels. Martinez et al. of São Paulo, Brazil, reported a case of necrosis of the stomach with formation of a gastrocutaneous fistula following splenectomy [19]. They reviewed the literature relative to gastric necrosis and perforation and point out that this complication is associated with a mortality rate as high as 60%, stressing the importance of prompt diagnosis and immediate treatment of this unusual complication.

Gastric perforation during and after laparoscopic splenectomy can be prevented by following well-known principles of surgical technique and by using instrumentation that will reduce the likelihood of thermal injury. Gentle traction on the stomach and the use of atraumatic graspers will reduce the incidence of direct injury to the stomach. The upper pole of the spleen can be very close to the greater curvature of the stomach, and care must be taken not to injure the stomach during the process of dissecting it from the spleen. I recommend using sharp dissection only and avoiding the use of any energy source during this part of the dissection. Decompressing the stomach with either an orogastric or nasogastric tube will facilitate gastric manipulation and improve visibility. The use of the right lateral decubitus position allows the stomach to fall away from the spleen, decreasing the need for aggressive traction on the stomach and improving exposure of the short gastric vessels [12]. The advantage to the lateral position was first recognized during laparoscopic left adrenalectomy. During this procedure, it is necessary to mobilize the spleen medially; in doing so, it was noted that the surgeon gained superior exposure of the splenic hilum as well as better angles of approach for dissection compared with the anterior approach [18]. Electrocautery has long been a tool utilized in surgical dissection and hemostasis, but one of the disadvantages of this modality is the large heat field these instruments generate, which results in a greater risk of thermal injury (immediate and delayed) to surrounding structures. The incidence of thermal injury has been greatly reduced with the advent of instruments such as ultrasonic dissectors, using alternate energy sources. The overall temperature produced by the ultrasonic dissectors is well below the 250–400°C produced by electrosurgical instruments, and lateral thermal damage produced by ultrasonic energy is usually less than 1 mm, a fraction of that produced by electrosurgery. Today laparoscopic splenectomy can be performed safely and efficiently without electrosurgery by using ultrasound, thus reducing the incidence of thermal injury. Furthermore, ultrasonic surgery can replace surgical clips and scissors in many cases.

Pancreatic Complications

Pancreatic injury is a potentially lethal complication known to occur with open splenectomy, given the close proximity of the tail of the pancreas to the splenic hilum [20]. It logically follows that a similar occurrence can be expected with laparoscopic splenectomy, although no prospective analysis has been performed for either operative approach. Depending on the definition of pancreatic injury, this complication can occur in as many as 15% of cases of laparoscopic splenectomy [17]. The mechanism of pancreatic injury is related to direct trauma that occurs during the dissection of the pancreas away from the splenic hilum or during the process of dissection and transection of the hilar vessels. As pointed out above, technical advances—such as the use of stapling devices—have significantly reduced the incidence of complications associated with laparoscopic splenectomy. However, it has been suggested by Chand and others at the Cleveland Clinic that the incidence of pancreatic injury during laparoscopic splenectomy may, in fact, be increased by the use of these very same instruments [17]. Since the splenic hilar vessels do not need to be individually dissected before they are transected with an endoscopic stapling device, it is more likely that the tail of the pancreas will not be seen and thus damaged during the transection process.

In Chand's review, it was found that this was particularly the case in patients with splenomegaly. In the setting of splenomegaly, limited exposure to a broad hilum leads to less than ideal placement of multiple staples across the hilum, increasing the risk of an injury to the pancreatic tail. The use of an anterior approach may also result in increased difficulty in identifying the exact location of the pancreatic tail.

Pancreatic injury should be suspected in any patient with postoperative hyperamylasemia or complications referable to the pancreas. This would include patients with atypical postoperative pain that extends the length of hospital stay, peripancreatic fluid collections, pancreatic abscess, or amylase-rich drain fluid. Chand's definition of pancreatic injury may be too broad, because he included any patient who had an elevated postoperative serum amylase. In his review, half the patients with hyperamylasemia recovered without any further findings on laboratory or radiological workup, but the other half had a complicated postoperative course due to a pancreatic injury manifest by atypical postoperative pain, fever, and leukocytosis. Since most patients undergoing laparoscopic splenectomy will be discharged on the first or second postoperative day, it may be wise to obtain an amylase level routinely in the immediate postoperative period, so as to alert the surgeon of potential problems. If a pancreatic injury is suspected, a CT scan should be obtained to determine whether any intra-abdominal or peripancreatic fluid collections exist. Treatment will depend on the patient's clinical course. If the patient's abdominal pain resolves and the serum amylase returns to normal, no further intervention is indicated. If, however, the pain and hyperamylasemia persist and especially if there is an associated fever, the fluid collection should be aspirated and evaluated for evidence of infection. Should the fluid be infected or the pain and leukocytosis persist, a CT-guided drainage of the collection is indicated. The drain should be left in place until the fever and leukocytosis resolve and the volume of drainage falls below 50 mL in 24 hours.

Though the reported incidence of pancreatic complications associated with laparoscopic splenectomy is relatively low (0–6%) [21–23], patients who did develop significant complications required additional interventions. This outcome serves to underscore the importance of avoiding injury to the pancreas when possible. A thorough knowledge of the anatomy is important, with the presumption that the tail of the pancreas is intimately associated with the splenic hilum. Armed with this anatomical knowledge, the surgeon should identify the necessary landmarks and always apply the stapling device in close proximity to the hilum. It is also the opinion of most surgeons that placing the patient in the right lateral decubitus position allows the tail of the pancreas to be more easily identified and, if necessary, dissected off the splenic pedicle to avoid injury while ligating and dividing the vessels. If a pancreatic injury is suspected, a closed suction drain should be placed and exited through a trocar site. Chand recommends the routine check of serum amylase levels on postoperative day 1 to alert the surgeon to a possible pancreatic injury. If the patient's clinical course suggests pancreatitis or a pancreatic injury, further workup and longer in-hospital observation should be considered.

Hemorrhagic Complications

Nothing can be more intimidating than significant hemorrhage during an operation, particularly a laparoscopic procedure. The sometimes difficult nature of the operative dissection, the rich blood supply to the spleen, and the spleen's friable nature set the stage for rapid and potentially severe hemorrhage. In numerous reviews, hemorrhage has been cited as a common indication for conversion from a laparoscopic to an open approach. During the operative process, there are three major areas where hemorrhage is likely to occur. Trocar-related bleeding and abdominal wall hematomas are not discussed here, as these problems are addressed in the chapter devoted to complications common to all laparoscopic procedures (see Chapter 3). The first site of potentially problematic hemorrhage is the spleen itself. Early in the operative procedure, the spleen must be manipulated and its friability can lead to capsular tears and pesky bleeding. This is especially true in the presence of splenomegaly. Traction on structures attached to the spleen can also cause capsular disruption and bleeding. Various conditions—including splenic abscess, splenic infarction, splenic cysts, pancreatitis, and local irradiation—can lead to perisplenitis and hence local inflammation around the spleen. This, in turn, can cause the spleen to be enveloped by omentum and adhesions, making its manipulation more difficult and increasing the likelihood of bleeding.

Division of the short gastric vessels is the second area in which bleeding can complicate the process. The short gastrics can be divided by means of an ultrasonic dissector, hemoclips, suture ligatures, or an endoscopic stapling device. Most surgeons utilize an ultrasonic dissector for this purpose, since this device works as well as or better than the other modalities (Fig. 2). In particular, hemoclips have a tendency to become dislodged during the dissection process, and they can interfere with subsequent applications of an endovascular stapling device on the main splenic vessels. The stapler will not function properly if a clip is caught within its jaws, which risks significant bleeding from the splenic pedicle. Regardless of which device is utilized to control the short gastrics, traction must be applied to place these vessels on tension, so that they may be divided. Overzealous traction can result in disruption of the short gastric vessel and subsequent bleeding. Frequently, the proximal greater curvature of the stomach will directly abut the spleen. This makes the proximal short gastric vessels difficult to expose. Undue traction on the stomach to tent and isolate these vessels for division may result in bleeding.

The final major area in which there is a risk of significant bleeding is related to the splenic hilar vessels. Dissection of the splenic hilum may be relatively

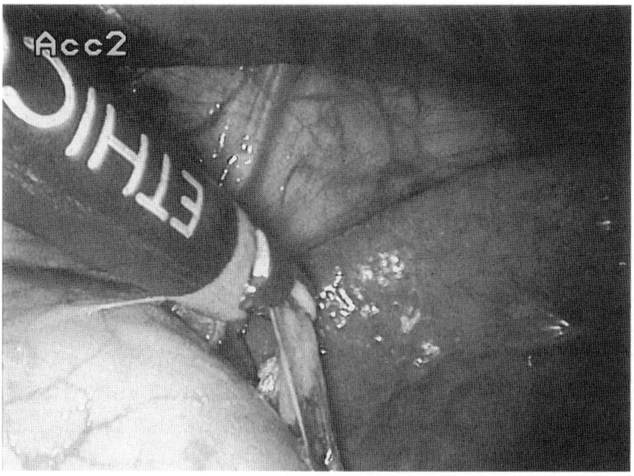

FIGURE 2 Short gastric vessels being divided with an ultrasonic dissector. Traction is placed on the vessels by retracting the stomach (to the left and below the ultrasonic dissector) medially. Care must be taken to avoid overzealous traction on the short gastric vessels, as this can result in disruption of the vessels and subsequent bleeding. Note also that the vessels are lifted away from the stomach and spleen to avoid thermal injury to these structures.

easy or treacherous depending on the size of the spleen, the patient's body habitus, the degree of coagulopathy, and the splenic artery anatomy. Unless one chooses to perform a splenic artery arteriogram on each patient, the anatomy of the splenic artery cannot be predicted. However, if, for example, a splenic artery has many terminal branches and the patient is obese, dissection of the hilum can be quite difficult and may lead to a hurried process in the face of troublesome hemorrhage. As mentioned earlier, use of clips in the hilar area is discouraged, as their presence may hamper the endovascular stapler. Minimization of hilar dissection will reduce the risk of hemorrhage (see later).

If bleeding occurs in any of the areas mentioned earlier, the key issue is for the surgeon to remain patient and not panic. With the patient in the lateral position, the surgeon can access the splenic pedicle from an anterior or posterior plane, allowing control of intraoperative bleeding by compressing the pedicle. A good suction apparatus is an absolute necessity even if this requires replacing a 5-mm with a 10-mm port so that a larger and more efficient suction apparatus can be used. Additionally, one should not hesitate to use additional trocars for retraction and exposure. These maneuvers will facilitate either a laparoscopic recovery of hemostasis or, if necessary, a controlled conversion to laparotomy. Bleeding from the spleen itself will usually stop spontaneously with the gentle pressure of a blunt instrument and/or the use of the omentum held against the area of bleeding. If this is unsuccessful, compression of the hilar vessels with an atraumatic clamp may be helpful. Absolute hemostasis here is ideal, but one must occasionally be satisfied with slowing the hemorrhage enough to allow transection of the hilar vessels, which, of course, will stop the bleeding from the spleen. The excessive use of topical hemostatic agents in an attempt to stop bleeding from the spleen itself is not logical, since the spleen will eventually be removed. A completely divided but uncontrolled short gastric vessel will bleed from both the gastric and splenic portions. Rolling the stomach anteriorly and grasping the vessel with an ultrasonic coagulation device or hemoclips can control the gastric portion of the vessels. Bleeding from the splenic side of a transected short gastric vessel can be more difficult. Adequate exposure of the bleeding site with suction, direct compression, and perhaps hilar compression may allow the surgeon to localize and control the bleeding site.

Hemorrhage encountered during dissection of the splenic hilum can be the most vigorous and difficult to control. The key to controlling this type of bleeding is the ability to obtain anterior and posterior exposure of the hilar vessels so that they can be compressed enough, with an atraumatic clamp, to slow or stop the bleeding, thereby allowing the surgeon to apply an endovascular stapling device accurately. It is critical to remember that the tail of the pancreas comes in direct contact with the spleen in as many 30% of cases, and this injury must be avoided.

It is obvious that the best way to manage intraoperative bleeding is to prevent its occurrence. Most bleeding can be avoided if the surgeon uses careful and gentle dissection techniques, maximizes exposure of vascular structures, and prepares the patient medically by correcting any existing coagulopathy (see ''Perioperative Management''), at the beginning of this chapter. As pointed out above, exposure of the short gastric and hilar vessels is best when the right lateral decubitus position is used. In this position, the vessels are essentially suspended and well exposed, so that the surgeon has access to both the anterior and posterior surfaces of the splenic pedicle, thus facilitating exposure prior to division and allowing compression to control bleeding. This position also allows the stomach to fall away from the spleen and reduces the need for traction on the short gastric vessels, diminishing the chance of tearing them and causing bleeding. Use of endovascular stapling devices has greatly reduced the risk of bleeding associated with the dissection and transection of the hilar vessels. A benefit of the endovascular stapling device is that it allows transection of the hilar vessels without individually dissecting each vessel. It is often this tedious dissection that results in bleeding around the hilum. If this dissection is not required, the bleeding may be avoided. There is one caveat, however; when the endovascular stapler is applied across the hilar pedicle, one must be careful not to partially include a vessel. If the stapler does not completely transect the vessel, significant bleeding will usually result when the instrument is fired. Therefore some dissection may be desirable to make sure that the vessels are completely within the jaws of the stapler prior to firing. A final technical issue that will reduce the chance of intraoperative bleeding bears repeating. The use of hemoclips near the splenic hilum should be avoided, as they may interfere with the operation of endovascular stapling devices. The clips can become lodged in the jaws of the stapler, causing it to misfire, with resultant bleeding.

A discussion of how to prevent intraoperative bleeding during laparoscopic splenectomy would not be complete without mentioning preoperative splenic artery embolization. This topic was touched on earlier with respect to splenomegaly, and there may be certain situations where one would want to consider this maneuver to reduce the chance of bleeding. An example would be the patient with portal hypertension, in whom the surgeon can expect to encounter dilated perisplenic veins and venous complexes that are friable and bleed easily. Preoperative splenic artery embolization may be helpful in such patients.

Residual Splenic Function—Missed Accessory Spleens and Splenosis

Locating and removing accessory spleens is often an important part of a laparoscopic splenectomy, particularly if the splenectomy is being done for hematological disease. In such cases, accessory splenic tissue is routinely removed, although it may be left in situ for other indications, such as trauma or splenic cysts, where the potential for residual splenic function is desirable. Several studies have questioned the ability to identify accessory splenic tissue during laparoscopic splenectomy, and early in the laparoscopic splenectomy experience it appeared that this issue might represent a major disadvantage of the laparoscopic approach. It was the contention of these critics that during such procedures it would be difficult to identify all accessory splenic tissue because all the areas where accessory spleens commonly occur could not be visualized. It would be logical to assume, particularly in hematological diseases such as ITP, that missing an accessory spleen would result in persistence or recurrence of the disease process. Since the majority of elective laparoscopic splenectomies are done for hematological disease and specifically for ITP, the issue of missed accessory spleens can be significant. The one early study that brings this issue to mind and is repeatedly quoted in the literature was published by Gigot et al. in 1998 [24]. By using denatured red blood cell scintigraphy, they were able to demonstrate a 50% incidence of missed accessory spleens after laparoscopic splenectomy; of patients with positive scans, one-third experienced recurrent disease. These scintigraphic studies were done 24 months after surgery and two-thirds of the patients with positive scans did not develop recurrent disease. Long-term follow-up evaluation is the only way to determine the effects of retained splenic tissue. While most recurrences are seen within the first 2 years of splenectomy, surgical failures have been reported up to 18 years later [25–27]. Accessory spleens often enlarge very slowly and have no effect on the platelet count for many years. These findings show that the significance of accessory splenic tissue is not fully defined.

In spite of Gigot's findings, it has been shown in multiple comparative studies that the frequency of accessory spleens is similar in open and laparoscopic surgery [28–32]. Accessory spleens are reportedly found in 4–27% of open splenectomies done specifically for ITP [25,26,33–35], and several larger laparoscopic studies have reported the localization of accessory splenic tissue in 11–21% of cases [32,36–38]. All in all, it is the general consensus that the ability to detect accessory splenic tissue via the laparoscopic approach is similar to that in previously published open splenectomy studies, and identification of accessory spleens should not be a deterrent to laparoscopic splenectomy.

How, then, can the surgeon avoid missing accessory spleens if finding them is desirable, and what can the surgeon do if he or she suspects missed accessory splenic tissue is responsible for persistent or recurrent disease following laparoscopic splenectomy? Several techniques have been used to detect accessory or residual splenic tissue, including preoperative technetium-99m or indium-111 scanning, CT, and laparoscopic ultrasonography. The routine use of preoperative scintigraphy is superfluous and not cost-effective, since these examinations are expensive and lack sensitivity and specificity. Endoscopic ultrasonography is becoming more commonplace, but it requires specially qualified operators and capital resources that not all hospitals can afford. Perhaps, therefore, the most indispensable tools that surgeons can arm themselves with are good standard laparoscopic instruments and a thorough knowledge of the most common sites for accessory spleens (hilum, retroperitoneum, greater omentum, and mesentery). Each operation should begin with a thorough search of the abdominal cavity for the presence of accessory splenic tissue. The stomach should be retracted medially to allow inspection of the gastrosplenic ligament (Fig. 3). The splenocolic ligament, greater omentum, and phrenosplenic ligament are carefully inspected next, followed by an examination of the small and large bowel mesenteries, pelvis, and adnexal tissues. The overall visualization obtained with laparoscopy is excellent; moreover, many feel that laparoscopic magnification actually may improve detection. Ironically, placing the patient in the right lateral decubitus position (a maneuver that almost all agree has greatly improved the technique of laparoscopic splenectomy) may make the exploration of the pelvis difficult and result in a missed accessory spleen. Accessory spleens have been found in the pelvis, but this is a rare occurrence and should not be a viewed as a reason to abort the use of the lateral approach. If an accessory spleen is found in the pelvis, the surgeon should be able to remove it laparoscopically. When recurrence or persistence of the hematological disease does occur and the presence of accessory splenic tissue is suspected as the cause, investigation with a radiolabeled red blood cell scan is indicated. Repeat laparoscopy, and resection is feasible.

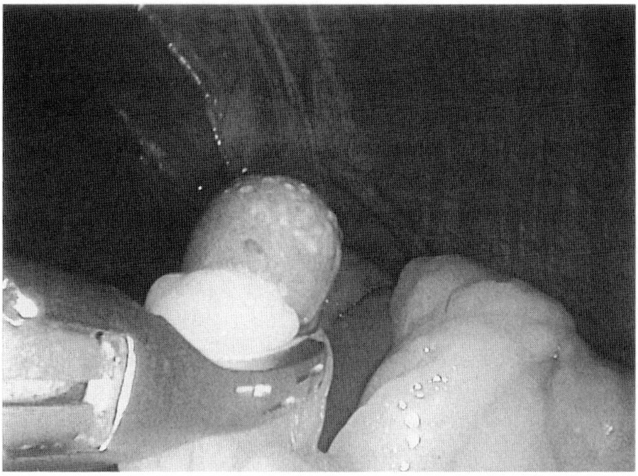

Figure 3 Detection of accessory spleens is important, particularly in the treatment of some hematological diseases. The surgeon should have a thorough knowledge of the most common sites for accessory spleens. This photograph demonstrates an accessory spleen in the gastrosplenic ligament, one of the more common areas in which to find accessory splenic tissue. This accessory spleen is about to be removed with the aid of an ultrasonic dissector.

A discussion of residual splenic function would not be complete without broaching the topic of splenosis. Splenosis is an autotransplantation of splenic tissue that usually occurs after splenic rupture and has been responsible for disease recurrence in cases of splenectomy done for ITP [39]. Its incidence in patients who have undergone splenectomy for trauma is as high as 76% [40–42], and it is estimated to occur in 15–20% of cases after open splenectomy for hematological disease [43]. During laparoscopic splenectomy, spillage of splenic tissue and subsequent implantation usually occurs after capsular tears resulting from manipulation of the spleen and during the process of morcellation and extraction. Data from an experimental rat model suggest that pneumoperitoneum may facilitate splenosis after laparoscopic splenectomy if the splenic capsule is ruptured or splenic tissue spills [44]. In addition to the diagnostic dilemma posed by splenosis, serious consequences have been described, including spontaneous rupture with massive bleeding into the abdominal cavity and gastrointestinal bleeding [45]. Kumar and Borzi reported a case of port-site splenosis in an 8-year-old child who underwent a laparoscopic splenectomy for congenital spherocytosis [46]. The child presented postoperatively with pain and a palpable nodule at a port site. The authors point out that port-site splenosis should be considered in the differential diagnosis of port-site pain after laparoscopic splenectomy.

Gentle dissection, minimal direct manipulation of the spleen, meticulous hemostasis, and the use of a durable bag in which to morcellate and extract the spleen are important factors in minimizing the risk of splenosis. Splenosis, therefore, should be considered in cases of unexplained postoperative pain, bleeding, or persistence/recurrence of hematological disease. Radionuclide scanning is a reliable, noninvasive preoperative study to help localize areas of splenosis when suspected; if splenosis is detected, removal of the splenic tissue should be approached laparoscopically.

Overwhelming Postsplenectomy Infection (OPSI)

OPSI can occur after either open or laparoscopic splenectomy, and there is no evidence to suggest that the laparoscopic approach to splenectomy alters the incidence of OPSI. However, since OPSI is among the more devastating sequelae of asplenia and is the most common fatal late complication of splenectomy [47], at least a brief discussion of it should be included in this chapter. It is highly likely that the incidence of infection following splenectomy is underreported, and the exact incidence of OPSI has been difficult to determine. However, one consistent observation is that the risk of OPSI is greater after splenectomy for malignancy or hematological disease than it is after splenectomy for trauma. The risk also appears to be greater in children below age 4 [48]. Infection may occur any time after splenectomy, but most cases are seen more than 2 years after splenectomy, while 42% occur more than 5 years later [49]. An episode of OPSI typically begins with a prodromal phase characterized by fever, chills, and nonspecific symptoms (sore throat, malaise, myalgias, nausea, vomiting, diarrhea); it progresses rapidly, with the development of hypotension, disseminated intravascular coagulation, respiratory coma, and death within hours of onset. Many cases have no identifiable focal site of infection. Despite aggressive therapy, the mortality rate is between 50 and 70% [50]. Those who survive often have long and complicated hospital courses with sequelae such as peripheral gangrene, requiring amputation; deafness from meningitis; bacterial endocarditis; and cardiac valvular damage.

Earlier in this chapter, the preoperative immunization recommended for patients undergoing elective splenectomy were discussed, but presplenectomy immunization is not possible in cases of splenic trauma. The immunization should be administered to these patients during the hospitalization in which the splenectomy occurred. High-risk patients without spleens should be considered for revaccination if more that 3–6 years have elapsed since their previous immunization. Rare cases of OPSI have been reported in vaccinated patients.

Miscellaneous Complications of Laparoscopic Splenectomy

A number of postoperative complications—not discussed here—are associated with many major abdominal procedures, including open and laparoscopic splenectomy. These include but are not limited to such problems as pneumonia, atelectasis, empyema, wound infections, subphrenic abscess and fluid collections, abdominal wall hematomas, ileus, bowel obstruction, pulmonary embolism, deep venous thrombosis, urinary complications, and cardiac complications. The issue that deserves mentioning relative to theses complications is that in many of the studies already cited in this chapter and in several others [10,32,51–53], the incidence of these complications was greater after open splenectomy, and they were usually more serious.

There are, however, a couple of complications associated with laparoscopic splenectomy that deserve particular mention. A rare but potentially dangerous complication that can occur during dissection of the spleen is diaphragmatic perforation. The phrenosplenic ligament can be very short, so that the spleen is in direct contact with the diaphragm. During dissection, especially with an energy source such as electrocautery, a perforation of the diaphragm can occur, and, as a consequence of the pneumoperitoneum, may enlarge. Acutely a pneumothorax will occur, with a resulting increase in peak airway pressures and paradoxical diaphragmatic motion. The patient will usually remain hemodynamically stable. Repair of the perforation is ideal, and placement of a chest tube or needle decompression of the pnuemothorax is mandatory. One can avoid this complication by using meticulous dissection techniques and good exposure. If the surgeon is unaware of a perforation but notices paradoxical diaphragmatic movement and/or anesthesia personnel report increases in peak airway pressures, he or she should look diligently for the perforation and repair it. Over the long term, a small cautery injury, mainly in the muscled part of the diaphragm, may enlarge and develop into a hernia. If this is the case, a laparoscopic repair should be attempted.

Another rare but potentially fatal complication of laparoscopic splenectomy is mesenteric and/or portal vein thrombosis. The exact incidence of portal vein thrombosis (PVT) associated with splenectomy (open or laparoscopic) is unclear; it appears to be influenced by the indication for splenectomy. In series that include splenectomies undertaken primarily for hematological diseases, the incidence of PVT ranges as high as 7–10% [54–56]. In those series where the indication for splenectomy included a large number of trauma patients, the incidence was lower (0.7–2%) [57–59]. In the December 2002 issue of the *American Journal of Surgery*, Winslow et al. reported an 8% incidence of PVT in a series of 101 splenectomies done primarily for hematological disease [54]. In this series, no significant difference in the incidence of PVT was noted between splenectomies done laparoscopically (5%) and those done open (9%); but when stratified by splenic weight, the rate of mesenteric and portal vein thrombosis increased as spleen size increased. In patients with splenic weights above 3000 g, the rate of PVT (50%) was significantly higher than that in those with spleens between 200 and 1000 g (6%). Patients with both a myeloproliferative disorder and a splenic weight greater than 3000 g had a 75% incidence of PVT. This particular subgroup appears to be at extraordinary risk for the development of this complication and would probably benefit from aggressive antithrombotic measures postoperatively (antiplatelet agents and heparin).

The exact etiology of portal and mesenteric vein thrombosis is not clear, but a number of related factors appear to lead to the development of the thrombosis after splenectomy, including the underlying disease process, presence of splenomegaly, postoperative thrombocytosis, and a hypercoaguable state. As mentioned above, the presence of splenomegaly and myeloproliferative disorders places a patient at significant increased risk for the development of PVT. Specifically, the association of splenomegaly with PVT may be due to the large splenic vein that serves as a low-flow cul-de-sac in which thrombosis occurs, subsequently propagating into the portal vein. The association between postsplenectomy thrombocytosis and PVT is unclear. Not all patients with postsplenectomy thrombocytosis develop PVT, and this complication has been described in patients with normal or even low platelet counts. In Winslow's study group, half of the patients had platelet counts in excess of 1 million upon presentation with PVT, suggesting that postoperative thrombocytosis may be an important risk factor. In screening for deficiencies of natural coagulation inhibitors (including protein C, protein S, antiphospholipid antibodies, and lupus anticoagulant), Denninger demonstrated that 72% of patients with portal or hepatic venous thrombosis (from any cause) had a previously undiagnosed systemic hypercoagulable state [60]. A systemic tendency toward thrombosis therefore may explain why a subset of patients experiences this complication after splenectomy.

The presenting symptoms of PVT after splenectomy are often vague, nonspecific, and insidious in onset, and it is the very vague nature of the presentation that often hinders a prompt diagnosis. A diagnosis of PVT should be considered in any patient who complains of vague or generalized abdominal pain, anorexia, or fever within the first 30 days after splenectomy. The most common physical findings are abdominal distention, mild to moderate diffuse tenderness, and heme-positive stools. Frank peritonitis is found in only one-fifth to one-third of presentations [61]. Initial laboratory studies are often of little value for securing the diagnosis of PVT, as they are frequently normal early on. If mesenteric or portal vein thrombosis is suspected, radiographic evaluation is the most accurate way of reaching the diagnosis. The diagnostic test of choice is an abdominal CT scan with intravenous contrast. This study not only generally confirms the diagnosis but also serves to exclude other intra-abdominal complications. Findings on CT include bowel wall thickening, abnormal gas collections either in the portal vein or bowel wall, ileus, or thrombus in the mesenteric or portal venous systems. Ultrasound, magnetic resonance imaging (MRI), and arteriography are also available but are limited by technician skill, cost, and invasiveness. Once the diagnosis is made, systemic anticoagulation should be started immediately. Recanalization can be anticipated in 90% of patients with acute portal or mesenteric vein thrombosis who are anticoagulated. The most difficult decision to make in the course of things is when to consider surgical intervention. This is an easy decision when peritonitis exists, but the goal is to identify those patients with intestinal gangrene and to intervene early on, when chances of recovery are better. Endoscopy has been shown to be beneficial in a limited number of cases [62,63], and laparoscopy should also be considered to help identify compromised bowel.

Ultimately, more effective measures are needed to prevent the development of PVT in high-risk patients, such as those with massive splenomegaly and myeloproliferative disorders. Administration of prophylactic subcutaneous heparin alone has been shown to be insufficient to prevent the development of PVT in this subgroup of patients [54,59]; therefore an aggressive approach to thrombotic prophylaxis should be considered, including the use of routine antiplatelet therapy with aspirin and administration of intravenous or low-molecular-weight heparin perioperatively followed by low-dose warfarin for the first several weeks after splenectomy.

REFERENCES

1. Delaitre B, Maignien B. Laparoscopic splenectomy: One case (letter). Presse Med 1991; 44:2263.
2. Delaitre B, Maignien B, Icard P. Laparoscopic splenectomy. Br J Surg 1992; 79: 1334.
3. Carroll BJ, Phillips EH, Semel CJ. Laparoscopic splenectomy. Surg Endosc 1992; 6:183–185.
4. Hashizume M, Sugimachi K, Ueno K. Laparoscopic splenectomy with an ultrasonic dissector (letter). N Engl J Med 1992; 327:438.
5. Diaz J, Eisenstat M, Chung R. A case-controlled study of laparoscopic splenectomy. Am J Surg 1997; 173:348–350.
6. Friedman RL, Hiatt JR, Korman JL, Facklis K, Cymerman J, Phillips EH. Laparoscopic or open splenectomy for hematologic disease: Which approach is superior. J Am Coll Surg 1997; 185:49–54.
7. Glasgow RE, Yee LF, Mulvihill SJ. Laparoscopic splenectomy: The emerging standard. Surg Endosc 1997; 11:108–112.
8. Terrosu G, Baccarani U, Bresadola M, Sistu A, Uzzau A, Bresadola F. The impact of splenic weight on laparoscopic splenectomy for splenomegaly. Surg Endosc 2002; 16:103–107.
9. Targarona E, Espert J, Bombuy E, Vidal O, Cerdan G, Artigas V, Trias M. Complications of laparoscopic splenectomy. Arch Surg 2000; 135:1137–1140.
10. Friedman RL, Fallas MJ, Carroll BJ, Hiatt JR, Phillips EH. Laparoscopic splenectomy for ITP: The gold standard. Surg Endosc 1996; 10:991–995.
11. Schlachta CM, Poulin EC, Mamazza J. Laparoscopic splenectomy for hematologic malignancies. Surg Endosc 1999; 13:865–868.
12. Torelli D, Cavaliere M, Casaccia M, Panaro F, Grondona P, Rossi E, Santini G, Truini M, Gobbi M, Bacigalupo A, Valente U. Laparoscopic splenectomy for hematologic diseases. Surg Endosc 2002; 16:965–971.

13. Targarona EM, Espert JJ, Cerdan G, Balague C, Piulachs J, Sugranes G, Artigas V, Trias M. Effect of spleen size on splenectomy outcome. Surg Endosc 1999; 13: 559–562.
14. Rosen M, Brody F, Walsh M, Ponsky J. Hand-assisted laparoscopic splenectomy vs conventional laparoscopic splenectomy in cases of splenomegaly. Arch Surg 2002; 137:1348–1352.
15. Targarona EM, Espert JJ, Balagué C, Piulachs J, Artigas V, Trias M. Splenomegaly should not be considered a contraindication for laparoscopic splenectomy. Ann Surg 1998; 228:35–39.
16. Flowers JL, Mastrangelo MJ. Laparoscopic splenectomy, anterior approach. In Zucker KA, ed. Surgical Laparoscopy. Philadelphia: Lippincott Williams & Wilkins, 2001, 609–624.
17. Chand B, Walsh RM, Ponsky J, Brody F. Pancreatic injuries following laparoscopic splenectomy. Surg Endosc 2001; 15:1273–1276.
18. Park AE. Lateral approach to laparoscopic splenectomy. In Zucker KA, ed. Surgical Laparoscopy. Philadelphia: Lippincott Williams & Wilkins, 2001, 625–634.
19. Martinez CA, Waisberg J, Palma RT, Bromberg SH, Castro MA, Santos PA. Gastric necrosis and perforation as a complication of splenectomy. Case report and related references. Arq Gastroenterol 2000; 37(4):227–230.
20. Baronofsky ID, Walton W, Noble JF. Occult injury to the pancreas following splenectomy. Surgery 1951; 29:852–865.
21. Gigot JF, De Ville de Goyet J, Van Beers BE, Reding R, Etienne J, Jadoul P, Michaux JL, Ferrent A, Cornu G, Otte JB, Pringot J, Kestens PJ. Laparoscopic splenectomy in adults and children: Experience with 31 patients. Ann Surg 1996; 119:384–389.
22. Katkhouda N, Hurwitz M, Rivera RT, Chandra M, Waldrep DJ, Gugenheim J, Mouiel J. Laparoscopic splenectomy: Outcome and efficacy in 103 consecutive patients. Ann Surg 1998; 228:568–578.
23. Tsiotos G, Schlinkert RT. Laparoscopic splenectomy for ITP. Arch Surg 1997; 132: 642–646.
24. Gigot JF, Jamar F, Ferrant A, van Beers BE, Lengele B, Pauwels S, Pringot J, Kestens PJ, Gianello P, Detry R. Inadequate detection of accessory spleens and splenosis with laparoscopic splenectomy: A shortcoming of the laparoscopic approach in hematologic diseases. Surg Endosc 1998; 12:101–106.
25. Akwari OE, Itan KMF, Coleman RE, Rosse WF. Splenectomy for primary and recurrent immune thrombocytopenia purpura (ITP). Ann Surg 1987; 206:529–541.
26. Cola B, Tonielli E, Sacco S. Surgical treatment of chronic idiopathic thrombocytopenic purpura: Results in 107 cases. Int Surg 1986; 71:195–198.
27. Johnson HA, Deterling RA. Massive splenomegaly. Surg Gynecol Obstet 1998; 168: 137.
28. Glasgow RE, Yee LF, Mulvihill JJ. Laparoscopic splenectomy: The emerging standard. Surg Endosc 1997; 11:108–112.
29. Delaitre B, Pitre J. Laparoscopic splenectomy versus open splenectomy: A comparative study. Hepato Gastroenterol 1997; 44:45–49.
30. Park A, Marcaccio M, Sternbach M. Laparoscopic splenectomy vs open splenectomy. Arch Surg 1999; 134:1263–1269.

31. Donini A, Baccarani N, Corno V. Laparoscopic versus open splenectomy in the management of hematologic disease. Surg Endosc 1999; 13:1220–1225.
32. Watson DI, Coventry BJ, Chin T. Laparoscopic versus open splenectomy for immune thrombocytopenic purpura. Surgery 1997; 121:18–22.
33. David PW, Williams DA, Shamberger RC. Immune thrombocytopenia: Surgical therapy and predictors of response. J Pediatr Surg 1991; 26:407–413.
34. Marassi A, Vignali A, Ziliani W, Biguzzi E, Bergamo C, Gianotti L, Carlo V. Splenectomy for idiopathic thrombocytopenic purpura: Comparison of laparoscopic and conventional surgery. Surg Endosc 1999; 13:17–20.
35. Winde G, Schmid KW, Lugering N, Fischer R, Brandt B, Berns T, Buunte H. Results and prognostic factors of splenectomy in ITP. J Am Coll Surg 1996; 183:874–879.
36. Harold KL, Schinklert RT, Mann DK, Reeder CB, Noel P, Fitch TR, Braich Camoriano JK. Long term results of laparoscopic splenectomy for immune thrombocytopenic purpura. Mayo Clin Proc 1999; 74:37–39.
37. Rege RV, Joehl RJ. A learning curve for laparoscopic splenectomy at an academic institution. J Surg Res 1999; 81:27–33.
38. Stanton CJ. Laparoscopic splenectomy for idiopathic thrombocytopenic purpura (ITP): A five-year experience. Surg Endosc 1999; 13:1083–1086.
39. Pace DE, Chiasson PM, Schlachta CM, Mamazza J, Poulin EC. Laparoscopic splenectomy of idiopathic thrombocytopenic purpura (ITP): Long term follow-up data. Surg Endosc 2003; 17:95–98.
40. Gunes I, Yilmazlar T, Sarchay A. Scintigraphic detection of splenosis superiority of tomographic selective spleen scintigraphy. Clin Radiol 1994; 12:115–117.
41. Nielson JL, Ellegrand J, Marqversen J. Detection of splenosis and ectopic spleens with ^{99m}Tc-labeled heat damaged autologous erythrocytes in 90 splenectomized patients. Scand J Haematol 1981; 27:51–56.
42. Normand JP, Rioux M, Dumont M. Ultrasonic features of abdominal ectopic splenic tissues. Can Assoc Radiol 1993; 44:179–184.
43. Spencer GR, Bird C, Prothero DL. Spleen scanning with ^{99m}Tc-labeled red blood cells after splenectomy. Br J Surg 1981; 68:412–414.
44. Espert J, Targarona E, Bombuy E, Setoain J, Visa J, Trias M. Evaluation of risk of splenosis during laparoscopic splenectomy in a rat model. World J Surg 2001; 25: 882–885.
45. Sikov WM, Schiffman F, Weaver M, Dyckman J, Schulman R, Torgan J. Splenosis presenting as occult gastrointestinal bleeding. Am J Hematol 2000; 65:56–61.
46. Kumar RJ, Borzi PA. Splenosis in a port site after laparoscopic splenectomy: A case report. Surg Endosc 2001; 15:413–414.
47. Horowitz J, Smith JL, Weber TK. Postoperative complications after splenectomy for hematologic malignancies. Ann Surg 1996; 223:290–296.
48. Styrt B. Infection associated with asplenia: Risks, mechanisms and prevention. Am J Med 1990; 88:5–33.
49. Cullingford GL, Watkins DN, Watts ADJ, Mallon DF. Severe late postsplenectomy infection. Br J Surg 1991; 78:716–721.
50. Beauchamp RD, Holzman MD, Fabian TC. Spleen. In Beauchamp RD, Evers BM, Mattox KL, eds. Sabiston Textbook of Surgery. Philadelphia: Saunders, 2001, 1144–1165.

51. Hashizume M, Omata M, Kishihara F. Laparoscopic splenectomy for idiopathic thrombocytopenic purpura: Comparison of laparoscopic surgery and conventional open surgery. Surg Laparosc Endosc 1996; 6:129–135.
52. Siromatsuya T, Horiuchi T. Laparoscopic splenectomy for treatment of patients with idiopathic thrombocytopenic purpura: Comparison with open splenectomy. Surg Endosc 1999; 13:563–566.
53. Cozano RR, Herrera MF, Vargas F, Lopez X. Laparoscopic versus open splenectomy for ITP. Am J Surg 1998; 176:366–369.
54. Winslow ER, Brunt ML, Drebin JA, Soper NJ, Klingensmith ME. Portal vein thrombosis after splenectomy. Am J Surg 2002:184.
55. Hassn AMF, Al-Fallouji MA, Ouf TI, Saad R. Portal vein thrombosis following splenectomy. Br J Surg 2000; 87:362–367.
56. Chaffanjon PCJ, Brichon PY, Ranchoup Y. Portal vein thrombosis following splenectomy for hematologic disease: Prospective study with Doppler color flow imaging. World J Surg 1998; 22:1082–1086.
57. Loring LA, Panicek DM, Karpeh MS. Portal system thrombosis after splenectomy for neoplasm or chronic hematologic disorders: Is routine surveillance imaging necessary. J Comput Assist Tomog 1998; 22:856–860.
58. Rattner DW, Ellman L, Warshaw AL. Portal vein thrombosis after elective splenectomy. An underappreciated, potentially lethal syndrome. Arch Surg 1993; 128: 565–570.
59. Van't Reit M, Burger JWA, van Muiswinkel JM. Diagnosis and treatment of portal vein thrombosis following splenectomy. Br J Surg 2000; 87:1229–1233.
60. Denninger MH, Chait Y, Casadevall N. Cause of portal or hepatic venous thrombosis in adults: The role of multiple concurrent factors. Hepatology 2000; 31:587–591.
61. Rhee RY, Gloviczki P, Mendonca CT. Mesenteric venous thrombosis: Still a lethal disease in the 1990s. J Vasc Surg 1994; 20:688.
62. Leiser A, Wysjenbeek A, Kadish U. Mesenteric venous infarction presenting as upper GI bleeding and diagnosed by upper GI endoscopy. Endoscopy 1985; 17:119.
63. Wade TP, Jewell WR, Andrus CH. Mesenteric venous thrombosis: Modern management and endoscopic diagnosis. Surg Endosc 1992; 6:283.

26

Vascular Surgery

Yves-Marie Dion

Université Laval, Centre Hospitalier Universitaire de Québec, Hôpital St-François d'Assise, and Québec Biomaterials Institute, Québec, Canada

Fabien Thaveau

Centre Hospitalier Universitaire de Québec, Hôpital St-François d'Assise, Québec, Canada

The surgical treatment of aortoiliac occlusive disease by aortofemoral or iliofemoral bypasses dates back to the early 1950s; since then, with the emergence of appropriate biomaterials for grafting in the 1960s and the improvement of anesthesiology, the frequency of this surgery gradually increased. The perioperative mortality rate is now of the order of 3.3%, with systemic morbidity varying around 8.3% [1]. Long-term patency rates are good. For claudication, the 5-year patency rate of aortobifemoral bypass (AFB) varies from 87.5–91%; at 10 years, from 81.6–86.8% of the bypasses are patent [1].

Following the excellent results of laparoscopic techniques in general surgery, we developed a laparoscopic treatment for aortoiliac disease. Our goal was to reduce mortality, morbidity, postoperative pain, and hospital stay while providing the same excellent patency rates attributed to standard bypass surgery. Along with the totally laparoscopic approach to the aortoiliac segment, laparoscopy-assisted techniques have been used. In this chapter, we describe our totally laparoscopic technique, the complications that may occur during laparoscopic treatment of the aortoiliac segment, and some of the instrumentation that helps to reduce or prevent these complications. We conclude by offering information on how to learn this new approach.

TECHNIQUE

General endotracheal anesthesia is induced and central venous and arterial lines are inserted. The patient is placed in the supine position with the left side elevated on pillows to provide adequate access to the left lateral abdominal wall (Fig. 1). The abdomen and groins are prepped and draped in the usual sterile fashion. During the procedure, the table is first mobilized to the left (right side up) to allow incision of the femoral regions when an aortobifemoral bypass is contem-

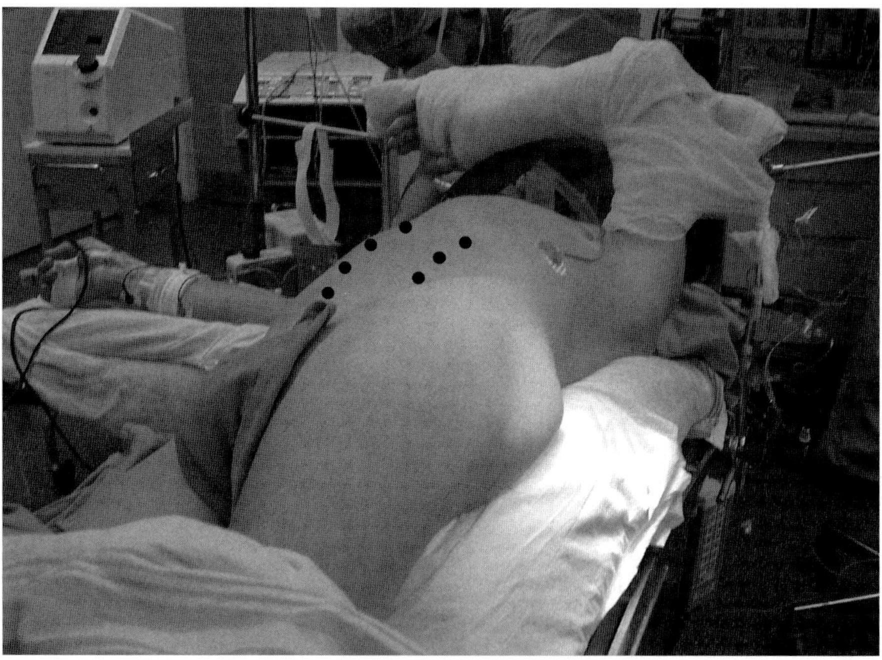

Figure 1 Patient being positioned on the table. Note that the table can be rotated to the left, when necessary, to allow femoral dissection. It can also be rotated to the right in cases where intraperitoneal organs would interfere with adequate visualization of the operative field. Black circles represent the sites of trocar insertion for a totally laparoscopic procedure done on the aortoiliac segment: four are located in the midline (one infraumbilical site, one umbilical, and two supraumbilical) and three laterally on a line slightly medial to the anterosuperior iliac spine.

plated. The right lateral decubitus position is then accentuated by elevating the left side of the table during the intra-abdominal procedure to facilitate movement of the intra-abdominal organs toward the left. This manuever as well as a 10-degree Trendelenburg position facilitates access to the left side of the abdomen and the aortic area for surgery.

CO_2 pneumoperitoneum is induced by means of a Veress needle through a small incision made at the umbilicus until the pressure reaches 15 mmHg. Then the Veress needle is replaced by a 10-mm trocar to allow insertion of a 30-degree laparoscope. The content of the peritoneal cavity is inspected and three other trocars are inserted in the midline: one 5-mm trocar is placed halfway between the symphysis pubis and the umbilicus and the two others are evenly distributed between the umbilicus and the xyphoid process.

A flap of parietal peritoneum (Fig 2A) used to be created and consisted of dissection alongside the left colon and sigmoid approximately 8 cm anterior to the Toldt line, beginning approximately 3 cm above the left internal inguinal ring and ending at the level of the spleen. We now dissect the Toldt line like in any hemicolectomy. The three lateral trocars are inserted on a line parallel and lateral to the rectus muscle and between the anterosuperior iliac spine and the lower costal margin (Fig. 1).

The incised peritoneal flap, the left colon, the sigmoid, and their mesentery are mobilized medially. The peritoneal flap is used for insertion of three sutures (2-0 nylon). This brings to the right the mobilized structures, which then cover the contents of the peritoneal cavity. This allows the further work to be unobstructed as it is performed through the retroperitoneum.

Once the apron is created and hides the abdominal content from view, one laparoscopic retractor is inserted in two midline trocars as described in a previous article [2]. Aortic dissection can begin proximally by visualizing the renal vein after incising the left Gerota's fascia. [3] Alternatively, the gonadal vessels and the left ureter can be visualized distally on the psoas muscle and then the left iliac artery, the aortic bifurcation, and the infrarenal aorta can be exposed.

When an aortobifemoral bypass is performed, a conventional bifurcated graft (Hemashield, Meadox Medicals, Oakland, NJ) is inserted in the retroperitoneal cavity through the left lower port and each limb tunneled using a specially designed laparoscopic clamp inserted from the femoral region (which had been incised before the abdominal part of the procedure commenced). The right limb of the prosthesis is first inserted and put into place. A small vascular clamp is placed on each of the limbs of the graft distally to prevent loss of CO_2. Systemic heparin is then administered.

An end-to-end or end-to-side aortic anastomosis is then performed for occlusive disease and an end-to-end anastomosis for aneurysmal disease using two running 3-0 polypropylene sutures starting posteriorly for the end-to-end and at the heel of the anastomosis for an end-to-side procedure.

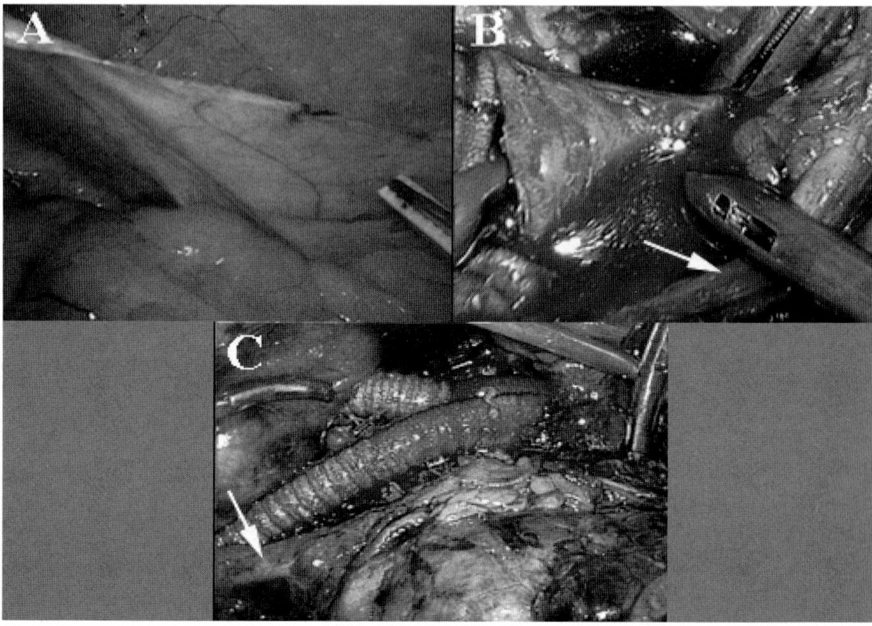

Figure 2 A. The left parietal peritoneum has been dissected using an ultrasonic device approximately 8 cm above the Toldt line. The left colon is seen in the left lower portion of the picture. Following peritoneal dissection, the left colon and sigmoid are mobilized medially to expose the retroperitoneum. B. Proximity of the ureter (arrow) to the anastomotic site. The technique has been modified so as to eliminate this proximity of the ureter to the working field. One can see a few milliliters of blood around the anastomotic site, which, when present, are eliminated by suction. C. The inferior pole of the kidney can be seen, as the aortic clamp has just been released. The gonadal vein (arrow) is visualized as a blue structure in the left lower corner of the picture. The ureter lies under the vein, and little dissection of it has been made in order to avoid potential ischemia. Note also how the ureter is protected from direct injury. A collagen sponge has been applied around the anastomotic site.

POTENTIAL DIFFICULTIES DURING LAPAROSCOPIC VASCULAR SURGERY

The following comments concern totally laparoscopic surgery performed for aortoiliac occlusive or aneurysmal disease using the previously described transabdominal retroperitoneal approach. Specific difficulties related to the transabdominal approach are mentioneal briefly, as well as those following the laparoscopy-assisted technique. At the time of writing, we have treated 86 patients laparoscopically with the technique described earlier in this chapter.

Instrumentation used to perform these techniques should be adequate to meet the needs of both the surgeon and the procedure itself. Specifically, a three-chip camera is recommended, and one should make every effort to record the entire procedure, so that it can be reviewed at a later time. The laparoscope should have a 30-degree viewing angle. The insufflator should provide at least 20 L of CO_2 per minute. Two television monitors should be available, one for the surgeon on one side of the table and one for his or her assistant on the other.

The assistant whose responsibilities will lie mostly in preserving exposure with the retractors during the phase of dissection, should be knowledgeable in vascular and laparoscopic surgery. Once adequate exposure is reached, a device fixed to the table holds the retractors. The assistant will have other responsibilities, such as using the suction device and holding the suture during performance of the anastomosis. The camera holder should be experienced in advanced laparoscopic surgery.

An important question is how long one should persist in the operation after the aorta is clamped before re-establishing blood flow to the limbs. There is a natural tendency to continue when success seems within reach. However, the surgeon should set a clamp time beyond which the procedure should be completed by open surgery. Although this is a rare occurrence for those surgeons familiar with the technique, as a rule the clamp time should not be allowed to exceed 2 hr before a decision is made to complete the procedure by either open or laparoscopy-assisted surgery.

Early in our experience, we attempted to reach the aortoiliac segment transabdominally by opening the retroperitoneum directly overlying the aorta. However, this proved difficult because there is no totally efficient way of retracting the small bowel or preventing the left colon from falling into the operative field. When that occurs, the operative field becomes obscure, rendering the procedure hazardous, since the bowel could be traumatized. Reperitonealization over the graft should not in itself be a major deterrent to this technique. However, when the transabdominal retroperitoneal approach is used, there is no need for reperitonealization, as the left colon is repositioned in the left side of the abdomen, covering the graft; with this approach, the bowel is kept away from the operative field.

Laparoscopy-assisted techniques can be used by surgeons who have not yet mastered suturing and feel more comfortable visualizing the aortic anastomosis directly after aortoiliac dissection has been performed. These assisted procedures have been claimed to facilitate patients' recovery [4–6]. They may be difficult to perform in obese patients due to subcutaneous fat, which reduces the operative view.

The surgeon beginning in this field should be open-minded, as was the case at the beginning of laparoscopic cholecystectomy in general surgery. When in doubt, make or enlarge the incision. The patient who would otherwise have received such an incision to begin with without the potential benefit of the laparoscopic approach will not misunderstand this operative change.

Potential complications of laparoscopic surgery for aortoiliac disease can be divided in two main categories: (1) complications related to access to the aortoiliac segment and (2) complications related to surgery of the infrarenal aorta and iliac arteries. The reader should know that most of these complications have tended to occur early in our experience as well as in that of others.

Potential Complications Related to Access to the Aortoiliac Segment

Prior to surgery, previous abdominal operations are carefully evaluated and all abdominal scars are inspected. As a rule, previous midline infraumbilical incisions are not a deterrant to using the Veress needle to create the pneumoperitoneum. For other, more extensive, or left-sided incisions, the aponeurosis should be opened and access to the abdominal cavity guaranteed before inserting the trocars. Prior left hemicolectomy, however, should be considered a contraindication to the transabdominal retroperitoneal approach at this time.

Once trocars have been inserted, care should be taken not to injure the small bowel when pushing it away from the operative field. In one of our first laparoscopy-assisted cases, done in 1993, we caused a small bowel laceration because the bowel was manipulated with an inadequate although atraumatic forceps. We then proceeded to a limited laparotomy, repaired the laceration, and completed the aortic bypass as planned.

After dissection of the parietal peritoneum, Gerota's fascia above and the gonadal vessels and ureter below become visible. Every effort should be made to keep the left kidney in situ by not dissecting behind and lateral to it. The plane should be kept anterior to the kidney, where the left renal vein will be dissected. If the kidney is mobilized, it will have a tendency to fall medially over the aorta because of the patient's position. The other reason to keep the kidney away from the aorta is to keep the ureter at a distance from this vessel. In an early description of our technique [2], the kidney was mobilized cephalad and automatically assumed a more medial location, which brought the ureter closer to the aorta. This could lead to two complications: direct trauma to the ureter due to its proximity to the aorta and possible ischemia due to traction and skeletonization (Fig. 2B).

Although we have severed the ureter, this complication has also been reported for conventional surgery and laparoscopic surgery [5]. Hence, meticulous dissection is recommended. We have encountered two cases of early transient hydronephrosis of the left ureter, which could be attributed to the second mechanism described above. [7]. Although these patients do not require intervention and can merely be watched during resolution of the hydronephrosis, we have modified this phase of the technique. We first identify the gonadal vein and manipulate the ureter, which can be seen beneath and lateral to these vessels (Fig. 2C), as minimally as possible.

At times, the small bowel may fall into the working space (Fig. 3A) and will have to be placed back in the peritoneal cavity (Fig. 3B). The causes for

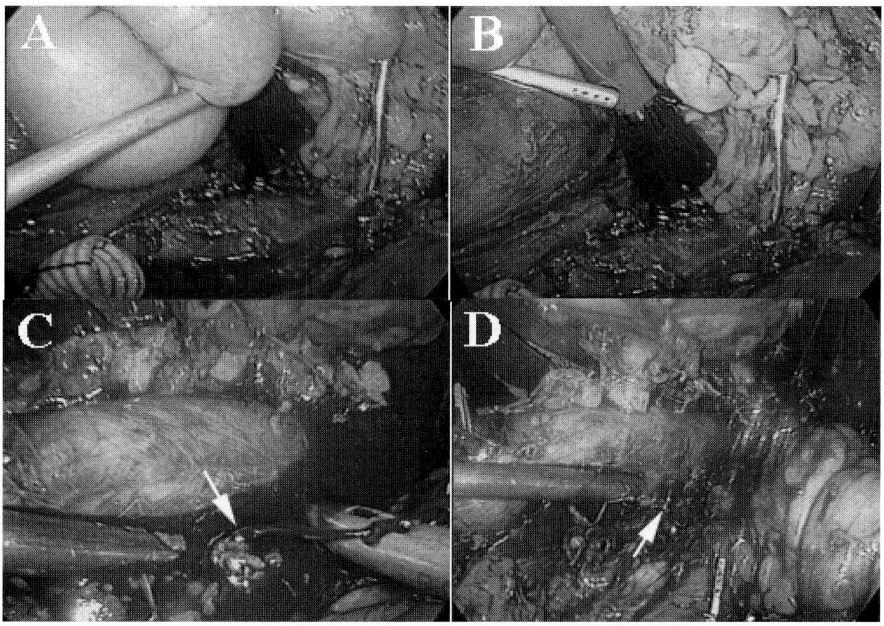

Figure 3 A. View of the retroperitoneal space and of the peritoneal "apron," over which the small bowel is seen dropping onto the operative field. In this case, The aortic clamp can be seen occluding the aorta. The body of the graft is visible in the lower left corner of the picture. At this point the small bowel becomes a major nuisance for the continuation of the procedure. B. The small bowel has been replaced in the intraperitoneal cavity using atraumatic DeBakey forceps. C. A branch of the gonadal vein has been severed, and the resultant bleeding site can be seen. Pressure with the instruments already present in the abdomen will stop the bleeding point until a hemostatic clip can be applied. This type of bleeding can be avoided by using the ultrasonic dissector. The aorta is seen in the middle of the picture. D. A clip has been applied to the bleeding vessel. Aortic dissection can now resume.

this problem may be inadequate positioning of the patient or movement to the left of the mobilized ''peritoneal apron'' due to badly positioned retractors or ineffective suture placement. Heavy suctioning or insufficient anesthesia are other causes.

Retroperitoneal bleeding is usually venous and due to trauma to the gonadal vein or a branch of this vein (Fig. 3C). These episodes of bleeding can be rapidly taken care of using hemoclips (Fig. 3D). Once one learns to follow the path of the gonadal vein and to work with an ultrasonic coagulating system in taking care of the collaterals, these minor complications should not occur.

Another although much less frequent source of bleeding may be the presence of a retroaortic left renal vein. Early in our experience, we were not doing CT scans to evaluate the possibility of great vein anomalies. When we traumatized such a vein (Fig. 4A), we were able to control the bleeding laparoscopically by first applying pressure with the instruments already present in the abdomen and carefully using the suction device. At this point, one has the choice of proceeding to a laparotomy for repair of the laceration or performing the venorrhaphy laparoscopically. We stopped the bleeding laparoscopically by applying hemoclips (Fig. 4B). Postoperatively, although asymptomatic, the patient developed left kidney edema, which later led to some kidney atrophy. Kidney edema is described in 2–3% of patients who undergo renal vein ligation, mostly in the course of aneurysm repair.

One potentially deadly complication is trocar-site bleeding, although it is of rare occurrence. Avoidance of this complication, which appears to be more common in the laterally placed trocars, can easily be ensured by looking at their sites at the end of the procedure (Fig. 4C). We speculate that heparinization during the procedure is a possibly incriminating factor. Using an endostitch will quickly resolve the matter (Fig. 4D). Confirmation of control of the bleeding site should be made laparoscopically.

Potential Complications Related to Surgery of the Infrarenal Aorta and Iliac Arteries

In dissecting the aorta, one must be careful not to traumatize the lumbar veins, which could lead to major bleeding (Fig. 5A). Although we have never encountered this complication, tamponade should first be performed, followed by clipping. In order to better visualize the bleeding site, a lumbar artery can be severed (Fig. 5B). We have clipped and incised the gonadal and lumbar veins at the level of the renal vein so as to allow visualization of the juxtarenal region (Fig. 5C).

In one case of laparoscopy-assisted aneurysm repair, a clip laparoscopically placed on a small tributary of the renal vein dislodged and caused immediate

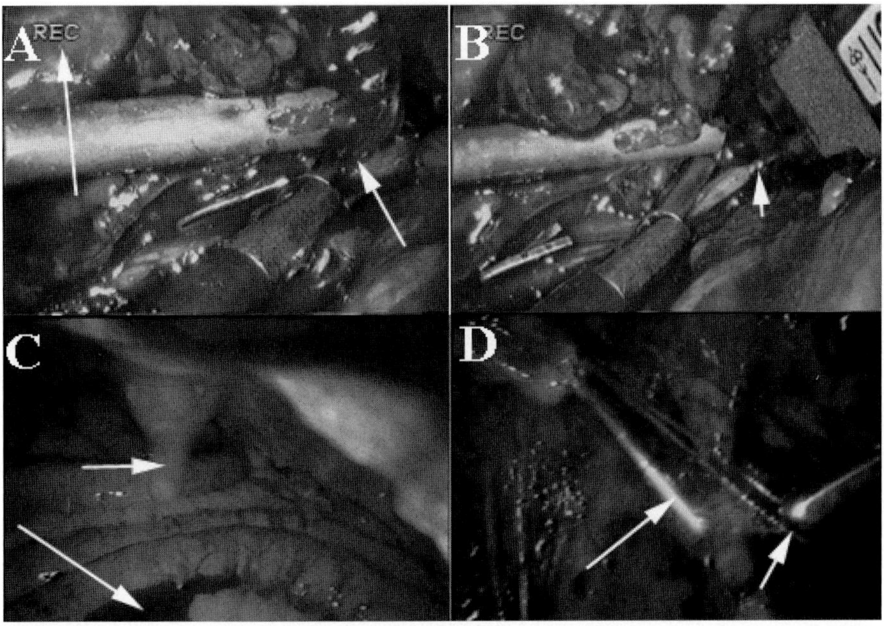

Figure 4 A. Trauma to a retroaortic left renal vein. A jet of blood can be seen originating from a traumatic venotomy (arrow). A forceps is about to close the wound. Since this case, we have operated without incident on two patients with a retroaortic renal vein. We recommend a CT scan for all patients to search for this anomaly preoperatively. B. Bleeding has been stopped with hemoclips (short arrow). A segment of aorta is visible in the extreme left upper corner of the picture. C. Blood dropping from the abdominal wall at a site of a lateral trocar (long arrow). If not recognized, such bleeding can be fatal. Note blood accumulating on the small bowel mesentery (short arrow). D. A 0-Vicryl stitch has been grasped with a forceps (short arrow) after having been brought through one side of the trocar wound by an Endostitch device (long arrow). The device will then be inserted through the other side of the wound, grasp the stitch, and bring it outside before tying.

postoperative bleeding, which needed operative control. We postulated that forceful wound retraction with sponges during the assisted part of the procedure caused release of the clip.

In one case, a tear in the renal vein caused by slippage of the aortic clamp necessitated a laparotomy. In this case, the mishap began when the aortic clamp had to be reapplied because of a lateral anastomotic leak. The clamp was not well applied and did not permit complete aortic control. However, as we knew

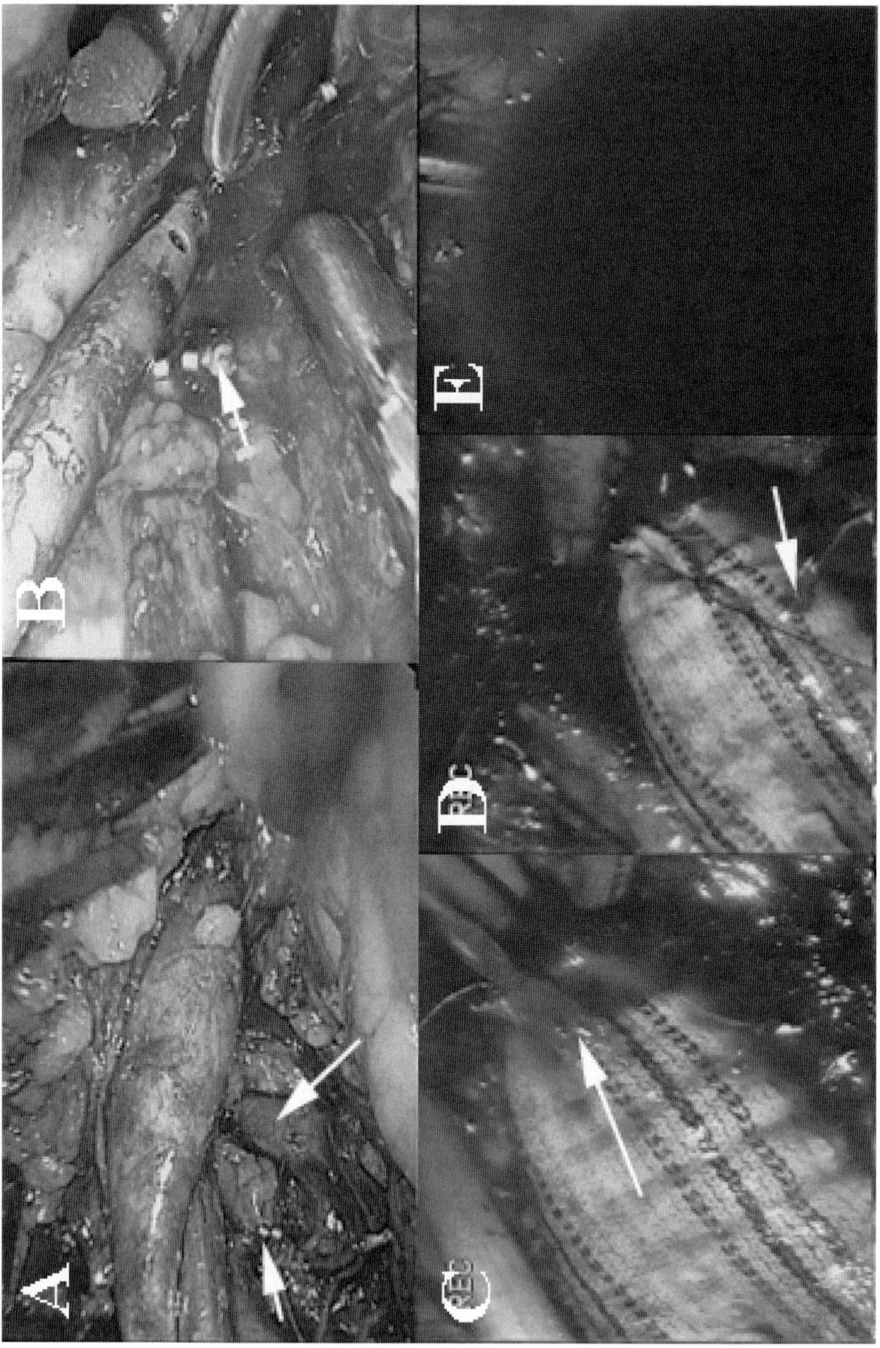
A
B
C
D
E

that only one suture would suffice to control the aortic leak, we elected to have the assistant press on the clamp. As we were finishing tying the knot on the aortic anastomosis and as a consequence of an involuntary twisting movement of the hand holding that clamp, the latter opened and slipped, causing a tear in the renal vein opposite the origin of the adrenal vein. At laparotomy, the aortic anastomosis was found to be adequate and the renal vein laceration was repaired. At present, such a mishap could not occur, since a protective mechanism impeding accidental opening of the clamp has been designed. Most of the dedicated vascular instrumentation is now available from Storz Endoscopy Tuttlingen, Germany.

Early in our experience, we were faced with an unusual situation. During insertion of the prosthesis into the abdomen through a trocar site, the body of the graft was injured by the atraumatic clamp (we are now using a laparoscopic DeBakey forceps). During unclamping, we noticed a hole in the anterior portion of the body of the graft (Fig. 5C). As we unclamped to evaluate the adequacy of the repair, we noticed a similar hole in the posterior aspect of the graft (Fig. 5D). Since this patient was young, we elected to replace his graft. This procedure was done through a laparotomy.

Lens soiling by spurting arterial blood can lead to a major complication (Fig. 5E). The camera holder should be told before surgery to withdraw the scope to the level of the trocar if blood spurting occurs. This will allow time to take appropriate actions to control the bleeding. If lens soiling occurs, the instruments present in the abdomen should be used to tamponade the bleeding site while the camera is rapidly cleaned.

FIGURE 5 A. The aorta has been lifted up with two forceps. Clips have been applied to a lumbar artery (short arrow), and a lumbar vein (long arrow) is visualized. B. When oozing occurs on the posterolateral aspect of the aorta, one pair of lumbar arteries can be severed (arrow) to allow better visualization of the bleeding site. C. At unclamping, a hole was discovered in the anterior portion of the body of the graft. Blood can be seen exuding from it (arrow). D. Upon a second unclamping to verify the adequacy of the repair, a second hole was noted posterior to the first. Blood can been seen coming from it (arrow). These wounds had been inflicted by the prosthesis during its insertion. It was therefore decided to replace the prosthesis. We now introduce the graft into the abdomen using laparoscopic DeBakey forceps. E. Blood soiling the lens of the laparoscope may be a dangerous event. In this case, one can still see the aortic cross clamp. One second later, the lens was totally soiled and vision of the working site was completely lost. In this situation, the bleeding site must be compressed with any instrument already present in the abdomen and the lens rapidly cleaned.

Another unexpected complication may occur during the arteriotomy. Uncontrollable but usually not heavy bleeding may be seen from the proximal stump. In that case a second aortic clamp should be inserted at the level of the aortotomy (Fig. 6A). As in open surgery, there are two possible courses of action. Either replace the first aortic clamp and see if bleeding is controlled, or bring down the first aortic clamp to take care of the bleeding lumbar artery (Fig. 6B). The second aortic clamp can then be removed.

During the performance of a totally laparoscopic anastomosis, the quality of the aortic stump must be inspected (Fig. 7A) and endarterectomy performed when necessary (Fig. 7B). The running suture should ideally be followed up with the assistant holding it and tightened with the nerve hook (Fig. 7C). Leaks can be rather easily taken care of in both end-to-end (Fig. 7D) and an end-to-side anastomoses (Fig. 7E).

In our experience, the most difficult anastomoses are those made into a calcified aorta. In one of these cases, although the CT scan led us to think we could clamp just infrarenally (Fig 8A and B), it proved totally impossible to do so at operation (Fig. 8C and D). We then had to perform a limited laparotomy, clamp suprarenally, and endarterectomize the juxtarenal aorta before performing the anastomosis.

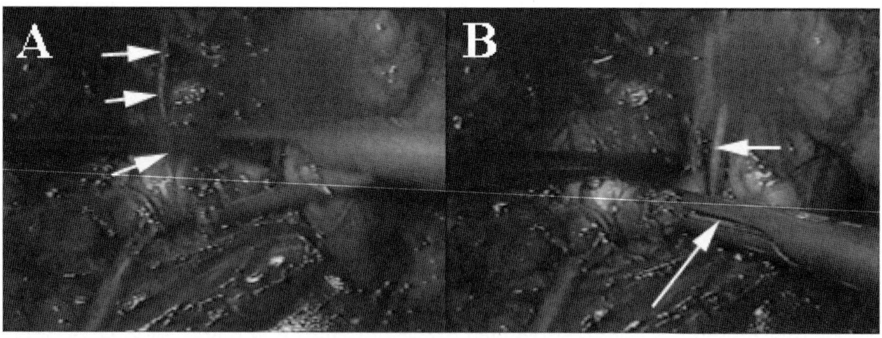

Figure 6 A. If bleeding occurs from the proximal stump after the aortotomy is made, as shown here, as blood is seen spurting (arrows) and a lumbar artery is not immediately apparent after lifting of the stump, the aorta must be clamped with another cross clamp placed below the first one. Note a drop of blood soiling the lens in the right upper corner of the picture and partially hiding view of the first aortic cross clamp. B. The first clamp is opened (short arrow) and brought down to occlude the bleeding lumbar artery, which is out of reach. The second aortic clamp (long arrow) is then removed and the anastomosis done.

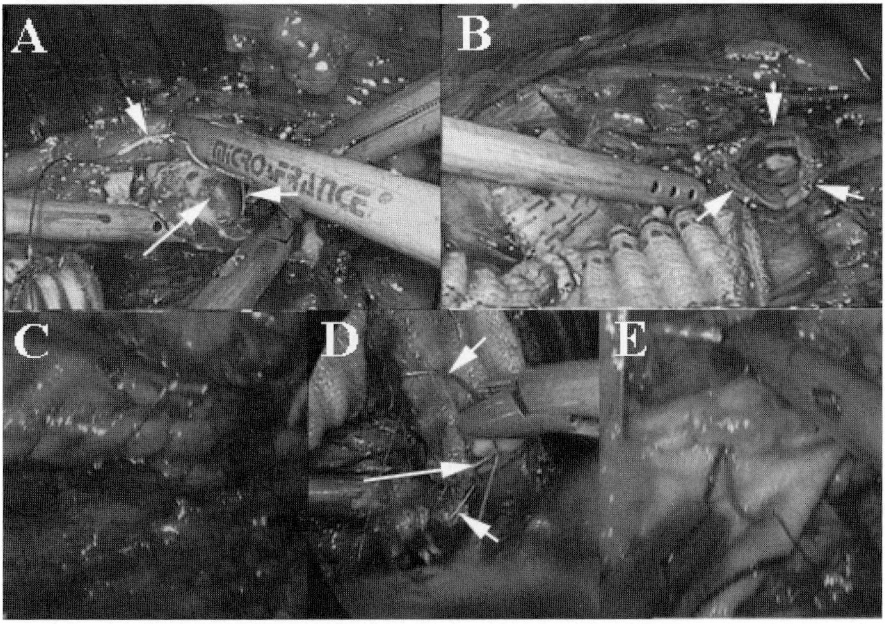

Figure 7 A. The needle (short arrows) of this 3-0 polypropylene suture cannot penetrate this calcified plaque (long arrow). B. The aortic stump is seen after endarterectomy (arrows). C. A nerve hook is used to tighten the anastomosis, end-to-side in this case. D. A posterior leak has been detected. The body of the graft is first elevated. Then a figure-of-eight is placed at the site of the leak, as shown here. The needle (short arrows) is seen after having penetrated both graft and aorta at the suture-line level (long arrow). E. The tip of the needle is being grasped after placement at the site of a leak in an end-to-side anastomosis.

In other cases, the laparoscopic GIA (USSC, Norwalk, CT) would not penetrate the calcified distal aorta to allow its occlusion. We then closed the distal aortic stump by suturing it laparoscopically.

INSTRUMENTS FOR LAPAROSCOPIC AORTOILIAC SURGERY

Instruments used for laparoscopy-assisted procedures are different from those employed for totally laparoscopic surgery. Since they are usually inserted through the main 8- to 12-cm incision or through small 2- to 3-mm skin incisions without trocars, instruments used in laparoscopy-assisted surgery can be bulkier than those

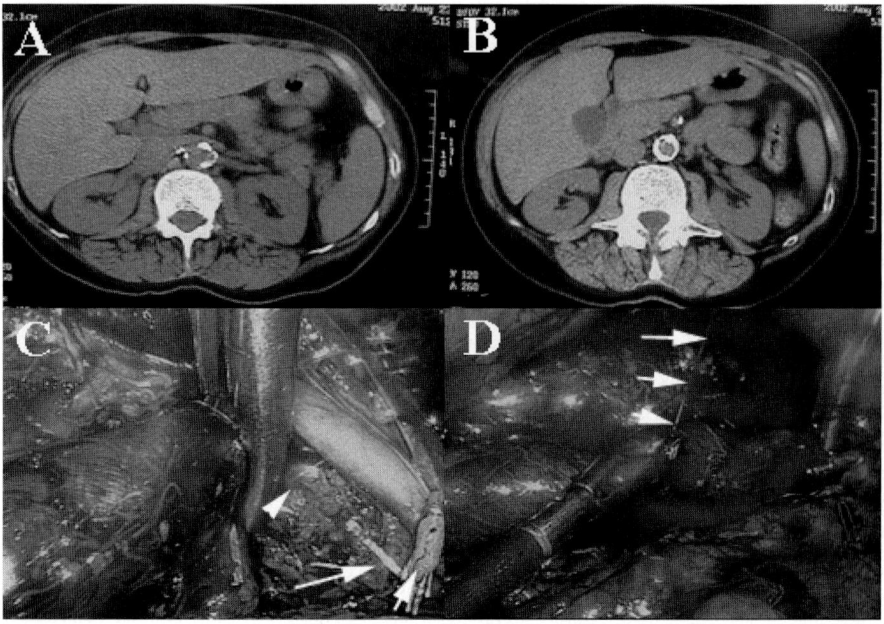

Figure 8 A. CT scan of a patient with aortoiliac occlusive disease. The left renal artery can be seen. Since there was no calcific ring covering the aortic circumference, it was felt that clamping could be performed at this level. B. Same patient. The infrarenal aortic wall is circumferentially calcified on its whole length, starting a few millimeters from the renal arteries. C. Infrarenal aortic clamping. The left renal artery is visualized (arrowhead). The left gonadal (short arrow) and lumbar (long arrow) veins in relation to the left renal vein have been clipped. D. Proximal clamping was found inadequate due to heavy calcifications. Blood can be seen spurting from the arteriotomy (arrows). The procedure was completed at open surgery by suprarenal clamping and endarterectomy of the infrarenal stump.

used for total laparoscopy. For instance, Satinsky aortic clamps can be of large size in assisted surgery. As a rule, when instruments are used for total laparoscopy, they must be inserted through trocars. In this section, some laparoscopic instruments used for totally laparoscopic procedures are shown.

Needle drivers (Fig. 9A) are the basis of advanced laparoscopic surgery. Ideally, their tips must be curved, so as to more easily allow for needle insertion into tissues, making knots, and grabbing tissue and other objects such as the vascular graft. The scissors should always be connected to a cautery device, and an ultrasonic apparatus should be available. Straight and curved DeBakey clamps (Fig. 9B) can be used to complete an endarterectomy done with a plaque elevator

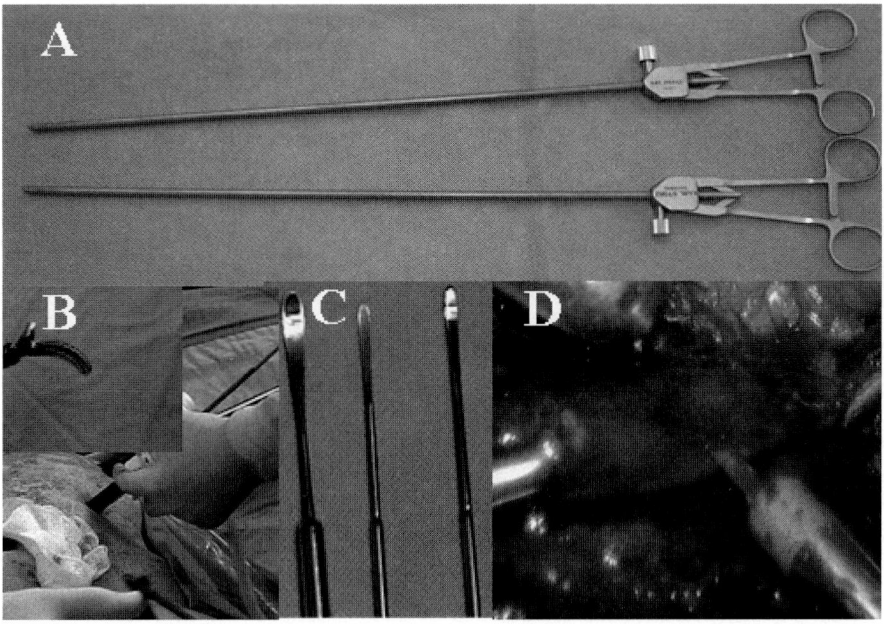

Figure 9 A. Specially designed curved needle drivers for anastomosis. B. Curved laparoscopic DeBakey forceps, which serve different purposes. Here they can be seen introducing a graft into the abdomen through the left lower trocar. C. Laparoscopic plaque elevators. D. In the middle of the picture, the arterial knife is penetrating the aortic wall in preparation for an end-to-side anastomosis.

(Fig. 9C). Fan-shaped retractors are useful to maintain exposure. An arterial knife is used for the arteriotomy (Fig. 9D). Potts scissors are available for end-to-side anastomosis (Fig. 10A). Vascular clamps are useful to cross-clamp large vessels such as the aorta and iliacs (Fig. 10B). Intracorporeal clamps can be left inside the abdomen and thus can be used in any number necessary without compromising any trocar site (Fig. 10C and D). They can then be retrieved at the appropriate moment. An instrument has also been designed for tunnellization during aortobifemoral bypass (Fig. 10B). Other instruments—such as the automatic clip applier, the linear stapling device (which interrupts the distal aortic stump during aortobifemoral bypass done with an end-to-end anastomosis), or the various grasping forceps made for general purposes—are also useful. Work is in progress to evaluate the possibility of stapling an aortic or iliac anastomosis. Anastomoses made by using a robotic system have also been reported [8].

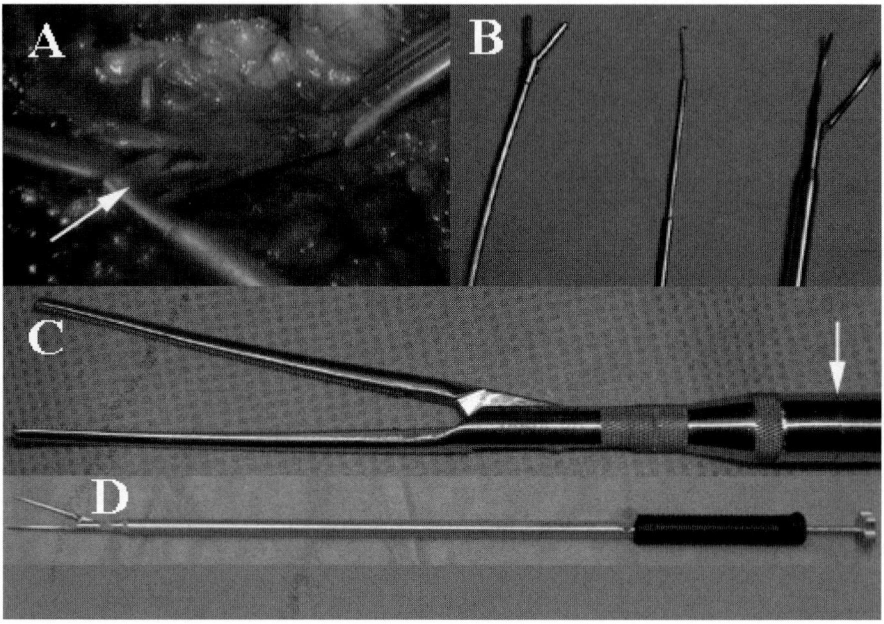

Figure 10 A. The lateral arteriotomy has begun. The Pott's scissors (arrow) are seen being reintroduced into the aorta to lengthen the arteriotomy cephalad. B. From left to right: tunneler, nerve hook, aortic clamp. C. Intracorporeal clamp. The clamp itself, which is the distal portion of the device, occludes the vessel. The site of insertion of the shaft is seen (arrow). D. Intracorporeal clamp. The clamp is not a bulldog. It has in its distal portion all the characteristics of a regular vascular cross clamp. When the shaft is removed, the clamp stays inside the abdomen without obstructing any trocar site.

LEARNING VASCULAR LAPAROSCOPY

The interest in the laparoscopic treatment of aortoiliac disease is increasing in many countries. Appropriate measures must be taken to ensure adequate teaching and learning. In that regard, the experience acquired during the introduction of laparoscopic cholecystectomy must be considered. Hands-on courses (Fig. 11) in this area offered in both America and Europe should be sought out and attended (www.vascularlaparoscopy.org). The surgeon should begin by observing actual procedures being performed. According to his or her prior level of expertise, the surgeon should then start using an assisted or a totally laparoscopic technique.

In summary, laparoscopic vascular surgery has the potential to benefit the vascular patient to a degree similar to that seen in general, gynecological, and

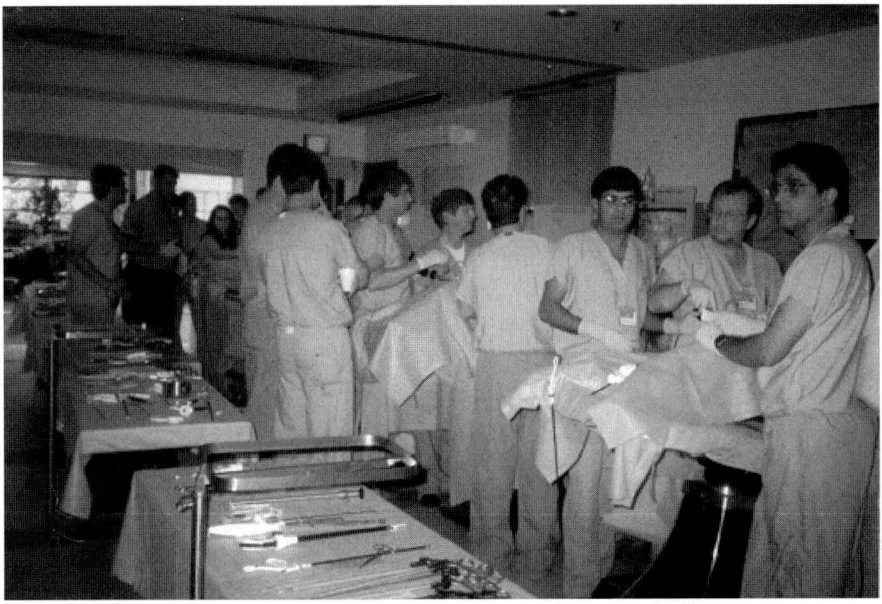

FIGURE 11 Day 3 of the hands-on course. Laparoscopic aortic procedures are being performed in the animal laboratory.

urological surgery, to name only a few specialties where it is used. It has to be carefully learned. We hope that the advice given in this chapter will be beneficial to anyone interested in this new treatment modality.

REFERENCES

1. De Vries SO, Hunink MGM. Results of aortic bifurcation grafts for aortoiliac occlusive desease: A meta-analysis. J Vasc Surg 1997; 26:558–569.
2. Dion YM, Gracia CR. A new technique for laparoscopic aortobifemoral graft in occlusive aortoiliac disease. J Vasc Surg 1997; 26:685–692.
3. Dion YM, Thaveau F, Fearn S. Technical note: current modifications to the totally laparoscopic ''apron technique.''. J Vasc Surg 2003; 38:403–406.
4. Kolvenbach R, Cheshire N, Pinter L, Da Silva L, Deling O, Kasper AS. Laparoscopy-assisted aneurysm resection as a minimal invasive alternative in patients unsuitable for endovascular surgery. J Vasc Surg 2001; 34(2):216–221.
5. Alimi YS, Hartung O, Valerio N, Juhan C. Laparoscopic aortoiliac surgery for aneurysm and occlusive disease: When should a minilaparotomy be performed?. J Vasc Surg 2001; 33(3):469–475.

6. Romanelli JR, Edoga JK, James KV, Resnikoff M. Laparoscopic surgery for infrarenal abdominal aortic aneurysms—The first 100 patients. Surg Endosc 2000; 14(suppl 1): S161.
7. Thaveau F, Dion YM, De Wailly GW, Dumont M, Laroche B. Early occurring transient hydronephrosis after laparoscopic aortobifemoral bypass grafting. J Vasc Surg 2003; 38:603–608.
8. Wisselink W, Cuesta MA, Gracia C, Rauwerda JA. Robot-assisted laparoscopic aortobifemoral bypass for aortoiliac occlusive disease: A report of two cases. J Vasc Surg 2002; 36:1079–1082.

Index